Acupuncture: Therapies and Clinical Case Studies

Acupuncture: Therapies and Clinical Case Studies

Editor: Patrick Lampard

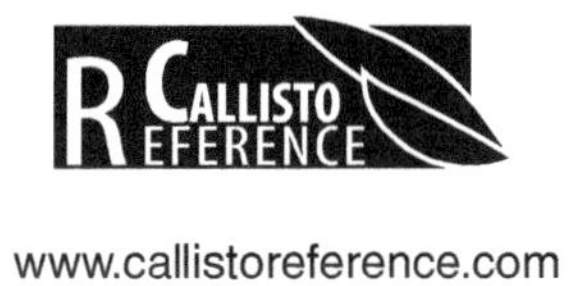

www.callistoreference.com

Callisto Reference,
118-35 Queens Blvd., Suite 400,
Forest Hills, NY 11375, USA

Visit us on the World Wide Web at:
www.callistoreference.com

ISBN: 978-1-63239-892-5 (Hardback)

The publisher's policy is to use permanent paper from mills that operate a sustainable forestry policy. Furthermore, the publisher ensures that the text paper and cover boards used have met acceptable environmental accreditation standards.

Printed in the United States of America.

Cataloging-in-Publication Data

Acupuncture : therapies and clinical case studies / edited by Patrick Lampard.
p. cm.
Includes bibliographical references and index.
ISBN 978-1-63239-892-5
1. Acupuncture. 2. Acupuncture--Case studies. 3. Alterative medicine. I. Lampard, Patrick.

RM184 .A28 2017
615.892--dc23

Table of Contents

Preface ... IX

Chapter 1 **Epidemiology, Quality and Reporting Characteristics of Systematic Reviews of Traditional Chinese Medicine Interventions Published in Chinese Journal** ... 1
Bin Ma, Jiwu Guo, Guoqing Qi, Haimin Li, Jiye Peng, Yulong Zhang, Yanqin Ding, Kehu Yang

Chapter 2 **Altered Hub Configurations within Default Mode Network following Acupuncture at ST36: A Multimodal Investigation Combining fMRI and MEG** ... 7
Youbo You, Lijun Bai, Ruwei Dai, Hao Cheng, Zhenyu Liu, Wenjuan Wei, Jie Tian

Chapter 3 **Effect of Acupuncture in Mild Cognitive Impairment and Alzheimer Disease: A Functional MRI Study** ... 19
Zhiqun Wang, Binbin Nie, Donghong Li, Zhilian Zhao, Ying Han, Haiqing Song, Jianyang Xu, Baoci Shan, Jie Lu, Kuncheng Li

Chapter 4 **Determining the Precise Cerebral Response to Acupuncture: An Improved fMRI Study** ... 32
Hua Liu, Jianyang Xu, Baoci Shan, Yongzhong Li, Lin Li, Jingquan Xue, Binbin Nie

Chapter 5 **Electroacupuncture for Moderate and Severe Benign Prostatic Hyperplasia: A Randomized Controlled Trial** ... 38
Yang Wang, Baoyan Liu, Jinna Yu, Jiani Wu, Jing Wang, Zhishun Liu

Chapter 6 **Risk of Bias Tool in Systematic Reviews/Meta-Analyses of Acupuncture in Chinese Journals** ... 44
Yali Liu, Shengping Yang, Junjie Dai, Yongteng Xu, Rui Zhang, Huaili Jiang, Xianxia Yan, Kehu Yang

Chapter 7 **Length of Acupuncture Training and Structural Plastic Brain Changes in Professional Acupuncturists** ... 50
Minghao Dong, Ling Zhao, Kai Yuan, Fang Zeng, Jinbo Sun, Jixin Liu, Dahua Yu, Karen M. von Deneen, Fanrong Liang, Wei Qin, Jie Tian

Chapter 8 **Acupuncture Induces Divergent Alterations of Functional Connectivity within Conventional Frequency Bands: Evidence from MEG Recordings** ... 58
Youbo You, Lijun Bai, Ruwei Dai, Chongguang Zhong, Ting Xue, Hu Wang, Zhenyu Liu, Wenjuan Wei, Jie Tian

Chapter 9 **Manipulation of and Sustained Effects on the Human Brain Induced by Different Modalities of Acupuncture: An fMRI Study**......68
Yin Jiang, Hong Wang, Zhenyu Liu, Yuru Dong, Yue Dong, Xiaohui Xiang, Lijun Bai, Jie Tian, Liuzhen Wu, Jisheng Han, Cailian Cui

Chapter 10 **Proteomic Response to Acupuncture Treatment in Spontaneously Hypertensive Rats**......78
Xinsheng Lai, Jiayou Wang, Neel R. Nabar, Sanqiang Pan, Chunzhi Tang, Yong Huang, Mufeng Hao, Zhonghua Yang, Chunmei Ma, Jin Zhang, Helen Chew, Zhenquan He, Junjun Yang, Baogui Su, Jian Zhang, Jun Liang, Kevin B. Sneed, Shu-Feng Zhou

Chapter 11 **Acupuncture Enhances the Synaptic Dopamine Availability to Improve Motor Function in a Mouse Model of Parkinson's Disease**......91
Seung-Nam Kim, Ah-Reum Doo, Ji-Yeun Park, Hyungjin Bae, Younbyoung Chae, Insop Shim, Hyangsook Lee, Woongjoon Moon, Hyejung Lee, Hi-Joon Park

Chapter 12 **Acupuncture Promotes Angiogenesis after Myocardial Ischemia through H3K9 Acetylation Regulation at VEGF Gene**......100
Shu-Ping Fu, Su-Yun He, Bin Xu, Chen-Jun Hu, Sheng-Feng Lu, Wei-Xing Shen, Yan Huang, Hao Hong, Qian Li, Ning Wang, Xuan-Liang Liu, Fanrong Liang, Bing-Mei Zhu

Chapter 13 **Impact of Including Korean Randomized Controlled Trials in Cochrane Reviews of Acupuncture**......111
Kun Hyung Kim, Jae Cheol Kong, Jun-Yong Choi, Tae-Young Choi, Byung-Cheul Shin, Steve McDonald, Myeong Soo Lee

Chapter 14 **A Systematic Review of Comparative Efficacy of Treatments and Controls for Depression**......121
Arif Khan, James Faucett, Pesach Lichtenberg, Irving Kirsch, Walter A. Brown

Chapter 15 **Electro-Acupuncture Stimulation Improves Spontaneous Locomotor Hyperactivity in MPTP Intoxicated Mice**......132
Haomin Wang, Xibin Liang, Xuan Wang, Dingzhen Luo, Jun Jia, Xiaomin Wang

Chapter 16 **Differences in Neural-Immune Gene Expression Response in Rat Spinal Dorsal Horn Correlates with Variations in Electroacupuncture Analgesia**......139
Ke Wang, Rong Zhang, Xiaohui Xiang, Fei He, Libo Lin, Xingjie Ping, Lei Yu, Jisheng Han, Guoping Zhao, Qinghua Zhang, Cailian Cui

Chapter 17 **CXCL10 Controls Inflammatory Pain via Opioid Peptide-Containing Macrophages in Electroacupuncture**......152
Ying Wang, Rebekka Gehringer, Shaaban A. Mousa, Dagmar Hackel, Alexander Brack, Heike L. Rittner

Chapter 18 **Laser Acupuncture Therapy in Patients with Treatment-Resistant Temporomandibular Disorders** 164
Wen-Long Hu, Chih-Hao Chang, Yu-Chiang Hung, Ying-Jung Tseng, I-Ling Hung, Sheng-Feng Hsu

Chapter 19 **Prolonged Repeated Acupuncture Stimulation Induces Habituation Effects in Pain-Related Brain Areas: An fMRI Study** 170
Chuanfu Li, Jun Yang, Kyungmo Park, Hongli Wu, Sheng Hu, Wei Zhang, Junjie Bu, Chunsheng Xu, Bensheng Qiu, Xiaochu Zhang

Chapter 20 **Practitioner Perspectives on Strategies to Promote Longer-Term Benefits of Acupuncture or Counselling for Depression** 180
Hugh MacPherson, Liz Newbronner, Ruth Chamberlain, Stewart J. Richmond, Harriet Lansdown, Sara Perren, Ann Hopton, Karen Spilsbury

Chapter 21 **Decreased Peripheral and Central Responses to Acupuncture Stimulation following Modification of Body Ownership** 187
Younbyoung Chae, In-Seon Lee, Won-Mo Jung, Dong-Seon Chang, Vitaly Napadow, Hyejung Lee, Hi-Joon Park, Christian Wallraven

Chapter 22 **Effects of Acupuncture at GV20 and ST36 on the Expression of Matrix Metalloproteinase 2, Aquaporin 4, and Aquaporin 9 in Rats Subjected to Cerebral Ischemia/Reperfusion Injury** 197
Hong Xu, Yamin Zhang, Hua Sun, Suhui Chen, Fuming Wang

Chapter 23 **Reporting Quality of Systematic Reviews/Meta-Analyses of Acupuncture** 207
Yali Liu, Rui Zhang, Jiao Huang, Xu Zhao, Danlu Liu, Wanting Sun, Yuefen Mai, Peng Zhang, Yajun Wang, Hua Cao, Ke hu Yang

Chapter 24 **Phantom Acupuncture: Dissociating Somatosensory and Cognitive/Affective Components of Acupuncture Stimulation with a Novel Form of Placebo Acupuncture** 214
Jeungchan Lee, Vitaly Napadow, Jieun Kim, Seunggi Lee, Woojin Choi, Ted J. Kaptchuk, Kyungmo Park

Permissions

List of Contributors

Index

Preface

In my initial years as a student, I used to run to the library at every possible instance to grab a book and learn something new. Books were my primary source of knowledge and I would not have come such a long way without all that I learnt from them. Thus, when I was approached to edit this book; I became understandably nostalgic. It was an absolute honor to be considered worthy of guiding the current generation as well as those to come. I put all my knowledge and hard work into making this book most beneficial for its readers.

Acupuncture is a medical procedure that primarily focuses on pain relief. The treatment involves undergoing a course of needles that are inserted to specific points. This therapy originated in traditional Chinese medicine. This book on acupuncture deals with the various therapies, ancient and modern, that have become popular among practitioners. Different remedies have different effects on the muscles according to the acuteness of the pain and the general condition of the patient have also been discussed. Case studies that reflect the varied ways in which acupuncture can be applied are elucidated in this book. Coherent flow of topics, student-friendly language and extensive use of examples make this book an invaluable source of knowledge.

I wish to thank my publisher for supporting me at every step. I would also like to thank all the authors who have contributed their researches in this book. I hope this book will be a valuable contribution to the progress of the field.

Editor

1

Epidemiology, Quality and Reporting Characteristics of Systematic Reviews of Traditional Chinese Medicine Interventions Published in Chinese Journals

Bin Ma[1], Jiwu Guo[1,2], Guoqing Qi[1], Haimin Li[1], Jiye Peng[3], Yulong Zhang[1,2], Yanqin Ding[1], Kehu Yang[1]*

1 Evidence-Based Medicine Center, Institute of Traditional Chinese and Western Medicine, School of Basic Medical Sciences, Lanzhou University, Lanzhou, Gansu, China, **2** Second School of Clinical Medicine of Lanzhou University, Lanzhou, Gansu, China, **3** The Library of Lanzhou University, Lanzhou, Gansu, China

Abstract

Background: Systematic reviews (SRs) of TCM have become increasingly popular in China and have been published in large numbers. This review provides the first examination of epidemiological characteristics of these SRs as well as compliance with the PRISMA and AMSTAR guidelines.

Objectives: To examine epidemiological and reporting characteristics as well as methodological quality of SRs of TCM published in Chinese journals.

Methods: Four Chinese databases were searched (CBM, CSJD, CJFD and Wanfang Database) for SRs of TCM, from inception through Dec 2009. Data were extracted into Excel spreadsheets. The PRISMA and AMSTAR checklists were used to assess reporting characteristics and methodological quality, respectively.

Results: A total of 369 SRs were identified, most (97.6%) of which used the terms systematic review or meta-analysis in the title. None of the reviews had been updated. Half (49.8%) were written by clinicians and nearly half (47.7%) were reported in specialty journals. The impact factors of 45.8% of the journals published in were zero. The most commonly treated conditions were diseases of the circulatory and digestive disease. Funding sources were not reported for any reviews. Most (68.8%) reported information about quality assessment, while less than half (43.6%) reported assessing for publication bias. Statistical mistakes appeared in one-third (29.3%) of reviews and most (91.9%) did not report on conflict of interest.

Conclusions: While many SRs of TCM interventions have been published in Chinese journals, the quality of these reviews is troubling. As a potential key source of information for clinicians and researchers, not only were many of these reviews incomplete, some contained mistakes or were misleading. Focusing on improving the quality of SRs of TCM, rather than continuing to publish them in great quantity, is urgently needed in order to increase the value of these studies.

Editor: Lisa Hartling, Alberta Research Centre for Health Evidence, University of Alberta, Canada

Funding: The authors have no support or funding to report.

Competing Interests: The authors have declared that no competing interests exist.

* E-mail: kehuyangebm2006@126.com

Introduction

The first systematic review addressing the effect of traditional Chinese medicine (TCM) that was published in a Chinese journal may be sourced back to Chen et al. in 1999 [1]. Since then, systematic reviews of TCM have become been increasingly published in China, and now with a large number. Given the implications of systematic reviews to policy making and clinical practice, achieving highest possible quality in design, conduct, analysis, and reporting is of paramount importance [2].

In the last decade, a few studies have examined the reporting of systematic reviews, and found that the quality of reporting was generally poor [3,4,5]. Three studies, using the Quality of Reporting of Meta-analyses (QUOROM) checklist, examined the quality of reporting of reviews of traditional Chinese medicine, and concluded with similar findings [6,7,8] Nevertheless, they were inherent with limitations, including the failure to report details about epidemiological characteristics of included reviews, and the failure to address methodological quality of those reviews.

In 2009, the newer standard of reporting systematic review, the Preferred Reporting Items for Systematic Reviews and Meta-Analyses (PRISMA) was released to replace the QUOROM for guiding the review reporting [9]. Earlier than that, an instrument, assisting the assessment of methodological quality of systematic reviews, Assessment of Multiple Systematic Reviews (AMSTAR) [10] was published in 2007. This instrument, developed on the biasis of the Oxman-Guyatt Overview Quality Assessment Questionnaire (OQAQ) [11] and Sack's Quality Assessment Checklist [12] is considered a validated tool in assessing the methodological quality of systematic reviews, and receives recognition from international agencies, including The Canadian Agency for Drugs and Technologies in Health (CADTH) [13].

Our study therefore aims to address the limitations of published studies, by assessing epidemiological and reporting characteristics, and methodological quality of systematic reviews of traditional Chinese medicine. We will particularly employ the new instruments for assessing the quality of reporting and methodological quality of those reviews.

Methods

Inclusion Criteria

We included all systematic reviews about TCM published in Chinese Journals. TCM interventions may have included herbal medicine, acupuncture/acupressure, moxibustion, Tuina massage, food therapy, and physical exercise such as tai chi and shadow boxing. TCM interventions may have been administered alone or in combination with conventional western medicine. We included publications described as systematic reviews or those that provided an overview of evidence from multiple studies and where authors described their methods in explicit detail.

Search Strategy(Text S1)

Four Chinese databases (Chinese Biomedicine Literature Database (CBM), Chinese Scientific Journal Full-text Database (CSJD), Chinese Journal Full-text Database (CJFD), and Wanfang Database) were searched from inception through Dec 2009. The search terms included "Systematic Review", "Meta-analysis", "Traditional Chinese Medicine" and "Chinese herbs" etc.

Screening

Two researchers independently screened the titles and abstracts of identified studies. One reviewer subsequently screened the full text articles of potentially included studies (Jiwu GUO) while a second reviewer independently screened a 20% random sample (Bin MA). Disagreement was resolved by discussion.

Data Collection and Analysis

Variables extracted included publication and reporting characteristics as well as items from the PRISMA and AMSTAR checklists. Reviews were classified according to their TCM focus as Herbal (e.g. bulk herbs, decoctions, pills) or Non-herbal (e.g. acupuncture, Tuina). Conditions studied were classified using the International Classification of Diseases (ICD-10). Data was collected using a standardized form and summarized using descriptive statistics (frequency, median, interquartile range (IQR)). Analyses were performed using Excel (version Microsoft Excel 2003; http://office.microsoft.com/zh-cn/) and SPSS (version 13.0; http://www.spss.com).

Results

Search

The searches identified 10,001 records. Screening excluded 9,621 reviews due to duplication, focus on non-TCM interventions, or for not being a SR. After examination of the full texts of 380 article, a further 11 reviews were excluded because they were quality assessments of systematic reviews and meta-analyses. A total of 369 publications were included (Figure 1, Text S2).

Epidemiological Characteristics (Table 1)

The 369 reviews were all written in Chinese and were published in 145 different Chinese Journals. Frequency of citation of each review ranged from 0 to 79; nearly half (46.1%) had not been cited and only 2.4% had been cited more than 15 times. Almost half (49.9%) of the reviews were written by clinicians. The reviews were classified as either Herbal interventions (84.3%) or Non-Herbal interventions. Non-herbal interventions included acupuncture (14.6%) and Tuina (1.1%). The most common conditions studied were diseases of the circulatory system (6.5%) and digestive system (5.7%).

Descriptive Characteristics (Table 2)

The reviews included a median of three authors (IQR: 2.0–5.0). Almost half the reviews (47.7%) were published in specialty journals although this differed significantly between reviews of herbal and non-herbal interventions (79.0% versus 21.0%,

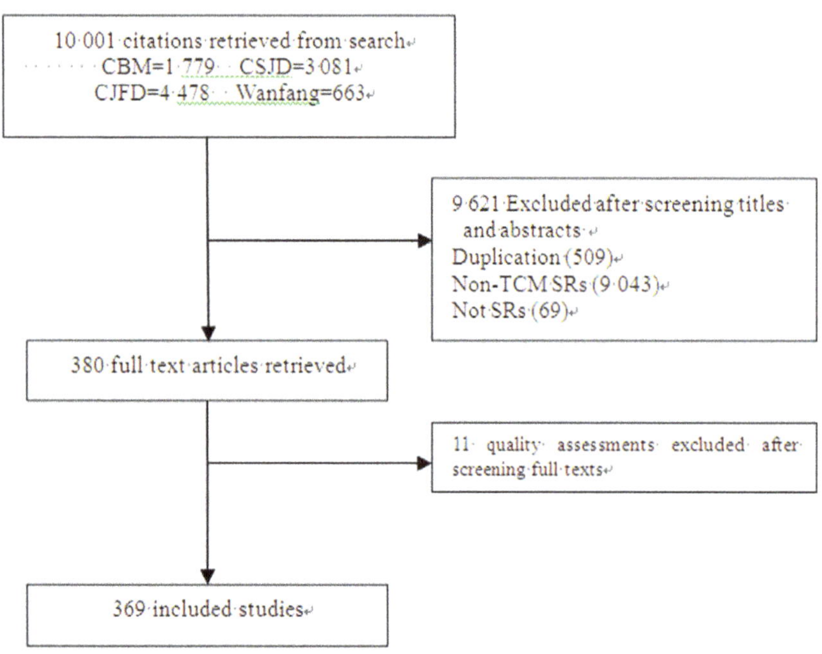

Figure 1. Flow chart of articles identified, included and excluded. SRs, Systematic Review.

Table 1. Epidemiology of Systematic Reviews.

Category	Characteristic	Number (%) of n = 369
Number of times cited	0	170 (46.1)
	1–5	137 (37.1)
	6–10	41 (11.1)
	11–15	12 (3.3)
	>15	9 (2.4)
Role of first author	Clinician	184 (49.9)
	Researcher	82 (22.2)
	Graduate student	54 (14.6)
	Other	49 (13.3)
Focus of reviews	Chinese Herbal Interventions[a]	314 (84.3)
	Non-Herbal Interventions[b]	55 (15.7)
Condition focused on in review (Common ICD-10[c])	Diseases of the circulatory system	24 (6.5)
	Diseases of the digestive system	21 (5.7)
	Diseases of the nervous system	18 (4.9)
	Diseases of the genitourinary system	17 (4.5)
	Diseases of the respiratory system	11 (3.0)
	Diseases of the blood and blood-forming organs and immune mechanism	14 (3.8)
	Diseases of the musculoskeletal system and connective tissue	9 (2.4)
	Mental and behavioural disorders	9 (2.4)
	Diseases of the skin and subcutaneous tissue	5 (1.4)
	Endocrine, nutritional and metabolic diseases	5 (1.4)
	Neoplasms	5 (1.4)
	Infectious and parasitic diseases	3 (0.8)
	Pregnancy, childbirth and the puerperium	2 (0.5)
	Diseases of the ear and mastoid process	1 (0.3)
	Diseases of the eye and adnexa	1 (0.3)
	Symptoms, signs and abnormal clinical and laboratory findings, not classified elsewhere	1 (0.3)

[a]Herbal interventions included bulk herbs, decoctions, pills;
[b]Non-herbal interventions included acupuncture and Tuina;
[c]Common ICD-10: International Classification of Diseases 10.

Table 2. Descriptive Characteristics of Included Systematic Reviews.

Category		All SRs n = 369	Herbal SRs[a] n = 314	Non-herbal SRs[b] n = 55
Number of authors, Median (IQR)		3 (2–5)	3.0 (2–4)	4 (3–5)
Journal type*	General, n (%)	193 (52)	175 (91)	18 (9)
	Specialty, n (%)	176 (48)	139 (79)	37 (21)
Indexed in CSCD[c] Yes n (%)*		120 (33)	91 (76)	29 (24)
Number of included studies Median (IQR)*		10 (7–17)	11 (7–19)	8 (6–13)
Number of participants in included studies	Median (IQR)	952 (562–1596)	1004 (583–1789)	890 (534–1273)
Meta-analysis	Yes (%)	343 (93)	292 (93)	51 (93)
Update of a previous review n (%)		0 (0)	0 (0)	0 (0)

[a]Herbal interventions included bulk herbs, decoctions, pills;
[b]Non-herbal interventions included acupuncture and Tuina;
[c]CSCD: Chinese Science Citation Database;
*indicates $p<0.05$.

respectively (p<0.05). Only one-third (32.5%) were published in journals cited by Chinese Science Citation Database (CSCD), which again varied significantly between herbal and non-herbal interventions (p<0.05). The reviews included a median of 10.0 studies each, involving 951.5 participants. Non-herbal SRs included significantly fewer studies (p<0.05) and participants compared to herbal SRs. Meta-analysis was conducted in almost all the reviews (93.0%) and did not differ significantly between groups. None of the reviews had been updated from a previous review.

PRISMA Checklist Assessment (Table 3)

Compliance with PRISMA checklist items ranged from 0–97.6%. Almost all reviews (97.6%) described themselves using the terms "systematic review" or "meta analysis". Most reviews were compliant with the following checklist items: included a clear rationale, described information sources, described method used for assessing risk of bias of individual studies, stated the principle of summary measures, described the results of individual studies, discussed limitations at study and outcome level, provided a general interpretation of results, and presented an available conclusion. More than half of reviews were compliant with the following checklist items: reported eligibility criteria, presented search strategy, stated the process for selecting studies, specified any assessment of risk of bias that may affect the cumulative evidence, described characteristics of included studies, or described risk of bias within studies. Less than half of reviews were compliant with the following checklist items: described data collection process, described synthesis of results, described additional analysis, described how the studies were selected, presented synthesis of results (although this varied across reviews category), presented results of any assessment of risk of bias across studies, or described sources of funding and other support. Few studies provided a description of objectives or purpose, lists of data items, or gave results of additional analysis. None of the studies provided a structured summary, protocol or registration information, or provided a summary of results in the discussion.

AMSTAR Checklist Assessment (Table 4)

Compliance with AMSTAR checklist items ranged from 0–70.2%. More than half of reviews were compliant with the following checklist items: reported that a comprehensive literature

Table 3. PRISMA Assessment of Reporting Characteristics.

Category	Item (Yes)	Overall, n = 369 n (%)	Herbs[a] n = 314 n (%)	Non-herbs[b] n = 55 n (%)
TITLE	1. Title	360 (97.6)	308 (98.1)	52 (94.6)
ABSTRACT	2. Structured summary	0 (0.0)	0 (0.0)	0 (0.0)
INTRODUCTION	3. Rationale	344 (93.2)	292 (93.0)	52 (94.6)
	4. Objectives	74 (20.1)	61 (19.4)	13 (23.6)
METHODS	5. Protocol and registration	0 (0.0)	0 (0.0)	0 (0.0)
	6. Eligibility criteria	214 (58.0)	185 (58.9)	29 (52.7)
	7. Information sources*	363 (72.1)	217 (69.1)	49 (89.1)
	8. Search*	208 (56.4)	165 (52.6)	43 (78.2)
	9. Study selection*	244 (66.1)	215 (68.5)	29 (52.7)
	10. Data collection process*	160 (43.4)	127 (40.5)	33 (60.0)
	11. Data items*	52 (14.1)	35 (11.2)	17 (30.9)
	12. Risk of bias in individual studies*	265 (71.8)	212 (67.5)	43 (78.2)
	13. Summary measures*	275 (74.5)	228 (72.6)	47 (85.5)
	14. Synthesis of results	143 (38.8)	126 (40.1)	17 (30.9)
	15. Risk of bias across studies	196 (53.1)	173 (55.1)	23 (41.8)
	16. Additional analyses	137 (37.1)	121 (38.5)	16 (29.1)
RESULTS	17. Study selection*	166 (45.0)	149 (47.5)	17 (30.9)
	18. Study characteristics	224 (60.7)	189 (60.2)	35 (63.6)
	19. Risk of bias within studies	227 (61.5)	187 (59.6)	40 (72.7)
	20. Results of individual studies	295 (80.0)	251 (79.9)	44 (80.0)
	21. Synthesis of results*	171 (46.3)	153 (48.7)	18 (32.7)
	22. Risk of bias across studies	151 (40.9)	133 (42.4)	18 (32.7)
	23. Additional analysis	78 (21.1)	71 (22.6)	7 (12.7)
DISCUSSION	24. Summary of evidence	0 (0.0)	0 (0.0)	0 (0.0)
	25. Limitations	346 (93.8)	296 (94.3)	50 (90.9)
	26. Conclusions	339 (91.9)	288 (91.7)	51 (92.7)
FUNDING	27. Funding	144 (39.0)	119 (37.9)	25 (45.5)

[a]Herbal interventions included bulk herbs, decoctions, pills;
[b]Non-herbal interventions included acupuncture and Tuina;
*indicates p<0.05.

Table 4. AMSTAR Assessment of Methodological Characteristics.

Category (Yes)	Overall, n=369 n (%)	Herbs, n=314 n (%)	Non- herbal interventions, n=55 n (%)
1. Was an 'a priori' design provided?	19 (5.2)	17 (5.4)	2 (3.6)
2. Was there duplicate study selection and data extraction? *	152 (41.2)	120 (38.2)	32 (58.2)
3. Was a comprehensive literature search performed? *	203 (55.0)	159 (50.6)	44 (80.0)
4. Was the status of publication (i.e. grey literature) used as an inclusion criterion?	10 (2.7)	9 (2.9)	1 (1.8)
5. Was a list of studies (included and excluded) provided?	13 (3.5)	10 (3.2)	3 (5.5)
6. Were the characteristics of the included studies provided?	221 (59.9)	182 (58.0)	39 (70.9)
7. Was the scientific quality of the included studies assessed and documented?	259 (70.2)	219 (69.8)	42 (76.4)
8. Was the scientific quality of the included studies used appropriately in formulating conclusions?	254 (68.8)	212 (67.5)	40 (72.7)
9. Were the methods used to combine the findings of studies appropriate? *	108 (29.3)	100 (31.9)	8 (14.6)
10. Was the likelihood of publication bias assessed? *	161 (43.6)	147 (46.8)	14 (25.5)
11. Was the conflict of interest stated?	30 (8.1)	27 (8.6)	3 (5.5)

a Herbal interventions included bulk herbs, decoctions, pills;
b Non-herbal interventions included acupuncture and Tuina;
*indicates $p<0.05$.

search was performed, provided the characteristics of included studies, assessed and documented the scientific quality of the included studies, or appropriately addressed the quality of included studies in formulating conclusions. Less than half of reviews were compliant with the following checklist items: reported that there were duplicated study selection and data extraction, used appropriate methods to combine the findings of studies (although this varied across reviews category), or assessed the likelihood of publication bias. Few studies provided an 'a priori' design, reported the status of publication used as an inclusion criterion, provided a list of studies, or stated if there was a conflict of interest or not. .

Discussion

Our study identified 369 systematic reviews of TCM interventions published since 1999, most of which evaluated herbal interventions. This study updates previous reviews of this topic [6,7,8] by including an additional 258 SRs. This review is also the first to examine compliance of Chinese SR authors with the PRISMA reporting guideline and AMSTAR tool for assessing methodological quality.

Our review examined some of the same variables described in Moher et al.'s investigation of SRs written in English and indexed in Medline [5]. In that study, the authors reported that the 300 SRs they included were published in 132 journals, including the Cochrane Library. In contrast to our review, only 8% of their included SRs were of complementary and alternative medicine (CAM) interventions. While most (91%) of their SRs were published in specialty journals, 45% of all 132 journals did not have an impact factor. Most (93%) of our SRs included a meta-analysis compared to 54% of the English studies and while 44% of our studies assessed for publication bias, only 23% of the English studies reporting doing so. Funding sources were reported in 39% of our studies compared to 59% of the English studies.

The range of diseases addressed in our reviews are similar with those in the three reviews [6,7,8] focusing on the Chinese literature. The three reviews, however, failed to report details about the epidemiological and study characteristics of systematic reviews, including number of times cited, journal type, number of studies included, number of participants, and whether it is an update of a published review. Moreover, one study [6] did not report the prevalence of reviews meeting each individual item of QUOROM. In addition we found that, despite the increasing use of the terms "systematic review" and "meta-analysis" in the title and subsequent manuscript sections, the quality of reporting remains poor.

While many deficits in reporting were evident in the Chinese SRs, we identified areas of particular concern. These included evidence that suggested that the SRs were not highly referenced by other researchers working in the same field. This may be due, in part, to the overall poor quality of this body of work, which may also be a reason that less than one third were indexed in the Chinese Science Citation Database (CSCD), which is similar to the Science Citation Index, in that indexed journals are considered of higher quality than non-indexed journals.

There is also evidence that even though SRs have become an increasingly popular source of up-to-date knowledge, they are under utilized by Chinese clinicians. Because although the Chinese Cochrane Center was established in 1997 by the Ministry of Health of the people's republic of China, recent studies reported that most clinicians and nurses had not heard of or did not understand the meaning of evidence-based medicine (EBM) [14,15]. In addition, not all medical schools have introduced EBM curricula in China.

Although it is well known that results from reviews are most useful when they are up-to-date [16], none of the reviews included in our SR reported being an update of a previous review. This may be due to lack of policies in China to encourage updates and reluctance of Chinese journals to publish updated reviews that are not substantially different from previous publications. The review by Moher et al. reported that 18% of the English SRs were updates, however, only those SRs published in the Cochrane Library had been updated [5], suggesting that this problem is not restricted to Chinese journals.

We have demonstrated that compliance with PRISMA reporting guidelines is low for many Chinese SRs. Items of particular concern included lack of appropriate abstracts or structured summaries and details of protocols or summaries of evidence. In order to improve the quality of reporting, we strongly recommend the use of reporting guidelines by authors. We also recommend that editors of medical journals recognize and promote use of reporting guidelines in their publications. Lastly, medical schools should introduce reporting guidelines into medical education as early as possible.

Reviews of numerous medical specialties, as well as comprehensive reviews, have concluded that the quality of SR and meta-analysis (MA) reporting is generally poor [6,7,17]. Examination of changes in reporting quality of MAs published in Medline, Embase and the Cochrane Database of Systematic Reviews, suggested that quality had improved after the release of the QUORUM reporting guidelines [18,19]. We anticipate that increased use of PRISMA by Chinese authors will be helpful in increasing the reporting quality of SRs published in Chinese journals.

Our study has also shown that the methodological quality of Chinese SRs of TCM is poor. Areas of particular concern include lack of report of an 'a priori' design, description of status of publication used as an inclusion criterion, as well as statement of conflict of interest, all factors which may be associated with biased results. In addition, statistical mistakes appeared in one-third (29.3%) of reviews. For instance, many reviews did not explore reasons for statistical heterogeneity but simply pooled results using a random effects model to account for heterogeneity. Where heterogeneity is substantial, an overall pooling of results may be inappropriate and may lead to the incorrect interpretation of results.

One explanation for limited compliance with methodological guidelines may be that AMSTAR has not been published or promoted in Chinese journals outside of a brief abstract published in the Chinese Journal of Evidence-based Medicine in September 2010 [20]. Broader promotion of methodological quality guidelines is a necessary step in enhancing dissemination and implementation of AMSTAR.

However, our study has limitations. First, the majority of articles failed to follow the PRISMA guideline. This is likely due to the fact that the PRISMA guideline had not yet been released at the time these studies were published. Second, our study included systematic reviews published only in Chinese journals, whereas Chinese investigators increasingly publish articles in international journals. Third, we have found differential results between systematic reviews addressing herbal versus non-herbal medicines. This is possibly because reviews addressing non-herbal medicines would have studies with fewer events, resulting in absence of statistical difference of comparisons. Last, in our search, we included the terms "systematic review" and "meta-analysis". Some potentially eligible systematic review (i.e., systematic reviews needs to be plural) may, however, not use these terms in their publications.

Our purpose was to provide readers with a broad overview of the reporting and methodological characteristics of SRs of TCM published in Chinese journals. Although many such SRs have been published, the quality of these reviews is troubling. As a potential key source of information for clinicians and researchers, not only were many of these reviews incomplete, some contained mistakes or were misleading. Focusing on improving the quality of SRs of TCM, rather than continuing to publish them in great quantity, is urgently needed in order to increase the value of these studies.

Supporting Information

Text S1 Four Chinese databases search strategy and hyperlink address.
(DOC)

Text S2 Three hundred and sixty-nine systematic review of traditional chinese medicine interventions published in Chinese journals
(DOC)

Acknowledgments

We thank Dr. Denise Adams (CARE Program, Department of Pediatrics, Faculty of Medicine, University of Alberta, Edmonton, Alberta, Canada.) and Prof. Xin Sun (Center for Health Research, Northwest, Portland, Oregon, United States) for providing assistance with editing the final manuscript. We thank the library of Lanzhou University for database access and acquiring full texts.

Author Contributions

Conceived and designed the experiments: BM KY J-WG G-QQ H-ML. Analyzed the data: J-WG BM J-YP Y-LZ Y-QD. Wrote the paper: BM J-WG. Extracted data from trials: J-WG BM. Final approval of manuscript: BM J-WG G-QQ H-ML J-YP Y-LZ Y-QD K-HY.

References

1. Chen ZH, Zhang JH (1999) Troditional Chinese herbs for precancerous lesion of esophagus: a meta analysis. TCM Res 12: 20–21.
2. Petticrew M (2000) Systematic reviews from astronomy to zoology: myths and misconceptions. BMJ 322: 98–101.
3. Jadad AR, McQuay HJ (1996) Meta-analyses to evaluate analgesic interventions: a systematic qualitative review of their methodology. J Clin Epidemiol 49: 235–2343.
4. Shea B, Moher D, Graham I, Pham B, Tugwell P (2002) A comparison of the quality of Cochrane reviews and systematic reviews published in paper-based journals. Eval Health Prof 25: 116–129.
5. Moher D, Tetzlaff J, Tricco AC, Sampson M, Altman DG (2007) Epidemiology and reporting characteristics of systematic reviews. PLoS Med 4: e78.
6. Li TQ, Liu XM, Zhang MM, Ma JX, Du L, et al. (2007) Assessment of Systematic Reviews and Meta-analyses on Traditional Chinese Medicine Published in Chinese Journals. Chin J Evid-based Med 7: 180–188.
7. Liu JP, Xia Y (2007) Quality appraisal of systematic reviews or meta-analysis on traditional Chinese medicine published in Chinese journals. Zhongguo Zhong Xi Yi Jie He Za Zhi 4: 306–311.
8. ZHZANGJuhua, SHANGHongcai, GAOXiumei, et al. (2007) Methodology and reporting quality of systematic review/meta-analysis of traditional Chinese medicine. J Altern Complement Med 13: 797–805.
9. Moher D, Liberati A, Tetzlaff J, Altman DG, PRISMA Group (2010) Preferred reporting items for systematic reviews and meta-analyses: the PRISMA statement. Int J Surg 8: 336–341.
10. Shea BJ, Grimshaw JM, Wells GA, Boers M, Andersson N, et al. (2007) Development of AMSTAR: a measurement tool to assess the methodological quality of systematic reviews. BMC Med Res Methodol 7: 10.
11. Oxman AD (1994) Checklists for review articles. BMJ 309: 648–651.
12. Sacks H, Berrier J, Reitman D, Berk A, Chalmers T (1987) Meta-analyses of randomized controlled trials. N Engl J Med 316: 450–455.
13. Bessa-Nogueira RV, Vasconcelos BC, Niederman R (2008) The methodological quality of systematic reviews comparing temporomandibular joint disorder surgical and non-surgical treatment. BMC Oral Health 8: 27.
14. Wang XP, Fan GH (2010) Investigation cognition about Evidence-based Medicine. Medical information 8: 2537–2539.
15. Liu K, Guo L, Zhang L (2010) Investigation into Nursing Staff's Cognition Status of Evidence- based Medicine. Journal of Liao ning Medical University 3: 259–262.
16. Moher D, Tsertsvadze A (2006) Systematic reviews: When is an update an update? Lancet 367: 881–883.
17. Moher D, Liberati A, Tetzlaff J, Altman DG, PRISMA Group (2009) Preferred reporting items for systematic reviews and meta-analyses: the PRISMA statement. BMJ 339: b2535.
18. Moher D, Cook DJ, Eastwood S, Olkin I, Rennie D, et al. (1999) Improving the quality of reports of meta-analyses of randomised controlled trials: the QUOROM statement. Quality of Reporting of Meta-analyses. Lancet 354: 1896–1900.
19. Delaney A, Bagshaw SM, Ferland A, Manns B, Laupland KB, et al. (2005) A systematic evaluation of the quality of meta-analyses in the critical care literature. Crit Care 9: R575–R582.
20. Xiong J, Du YH (2010) Assessing tool of methodology quality for systematic reviews and meta analysis: introduction of AMSTAR. Chin J Evid-based Med 9: 44–44.

2

Altered Hub Configurations within Default Mode Network following Acupuncture at ST36: A Multimodal Investigation Combining fMRI and MEG

Youbo You[1], Lijun Bai[1]*, Ruwei Dai[1], Hao Cheng[3], Zhenyu Liu[1], Wenjuan Wei[1], Jie Tian[1,2]*

1 Key Laboratory of Molecular Imaging and Functional Imaging, Institute of Automation, Chinese Academy of Sciences, Beijing, China, **2** Life Science Research Center, School of Electronic Engineering, Xidian University, Xi'an, Shaanxi, China, **3** Department of Anesthesiology, Beijing Ditan Hospital affiliated to Capital Medical University, Beijing, China

Abstract

Acupuncture, an externally somatosensory stimulation in the Traditional Chinese Medicine, has been proposed about its modulations on the brain's default mode network (DMN). However, it is still unknown on how the internal brain resting networks are modulated and what inferences can be made about the physiological processes underlying these changes. Combining high spatial resolution of functional magnetic resonance imaging (fMRI) with high temporal resolution of magnetoencephalography (MEG), in the current multimodal study, we sought to explore spatiotemporally whether or not band-specific DMN hub configurations would be induced by verum acupuncture, compared with sham control. Spatial independent component analysis was applied to fMRI data, followed by the discrete regional sources seeded into MEG data. Partial correlation analysis was further adopted to estimate the intrinsic functional connectivity and network hub configurations. One of the most striking findings is that the posterior cingulate cortex is not only validated as a robust DMN hub, but served as a hub only within the delta and gamma bands following the verum acupuncture, compared with its consistently being a DMN hub in sham control group. Our preliminary results may provide a new perspective to lend support for the specificity of neural mechanism underlying acupuncture.

Editor: Xi-Nian Zuo, Institute of Psychology, Chinese Academy of Sciences, China

Funding: This paper is supported by the National Basic Research Program of China (973 Program) under Grant 2011CB707700, the National Natural Science Foundation of China under Grant No. 81227901, 61231004, 30970771, 81000640, 81171314, 30970769, 81071217, the Fundamental Research Funds for the Central Universities (2011JBM226) and NIH (R01HD046526 & R01HD060595), the Beijing Nova program (grant number Z111101054511116), and Beijing Natural Science Foundation (grant number 4122082), the Fellowship for Young International Scientists of the Chinese Academy of Sciences under Grant No. 2010Y2GA03, the Chinese Academy of Sciences Visiting Professorship for Senior International Scientists under Grant No. 2012T1G0036, 2010T2G36, 2012T1G0039. The funders had no role in study design, data collection and analysis, decision to publish, or preparation of the manuscript.

Competing Interests: The authors have declared that no competing interests exist.

* E-mail: tian@ieee.org (JT); bailj4152615@gmail.com (LB)

Introduction

Acupuncture, an ancient healing modality in the Traditional Chinese Medicine, has the therapeutic effects in the treatment of a range of diverse disorders [1–2]. However, it has not gained a proper position so far in the modern biomedical disciplines. This is partly due to the fact that physiological mechanisms underlying acupuncture effects still remain elusive. Among all research interests, one of the most appealing is focused on the unresolved but fundamental issue in which the central representations of peripheral acupuncture stimulation with regard to its functional specificity. In other words, whether exerting acupuncture at certain acupoints can produce functionally specific effects in the brain compared to a sham or placebo control procedure. Although accumulating evidence emerges [3–7], the debate over such acupoint specificity continues [8–10]. In order to promote better acceptance of acupuncture as a viable clinical treatment, it is thus vital and necessary to explore the biological mechanisms of functional specificity underlying acupuncture.

It is remarkable to find that a large proportion of neuroimaging acupuncture researches have been carried out with the utilization of functional magnetic resonance imaging (fMRI). Indeed, its high spatial resolution (on the order of millimeters scale) has prominently paved the way to identify the induced activity of brain regions in the spatial dimension reliably [5]. However, the Blood Oxygen Level Dependent signal detected by fMRI only reflects the neuronal activity indirectly [11–12]. Due to the latency of the hemodynamic response, it is more or less handicapped in the temporal dimension, only examining correlations in the relatively slow neuronal oscillations [13]. Analysis conducted only within this low frequency domain in previous acupuncture researches thereby may be limited to unveil completely the underlying mechanism since most electrophysiological aspects of neural activities took place at a much faster time scale [14]. For instance, working memory is associated with neuron interactions in the theta band, while gamma synchronization is related to perception and consciousness [15–16]. Electrophysiological imaging technology such as magnetoencephalography (MEG), on the contrary, has the ability to bypass the hemodynamic response and measure the magnetic fields induced by synchronized current flows in neuronal assemblies [17]. It can provide a unique window into the neurophysiological processing on the milliseconds time scale [18] so as to capture the detailed temporal profile of neural

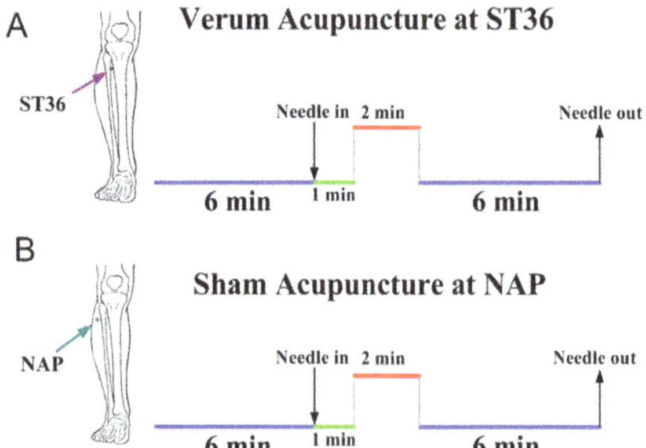

Figure 1. Experimental paradigm. Panel A indicated that acupuncture stimulation was performed at acupoint ST36 on the right leg (Zusanli, arrow pointing to dark pink dot). Panel B indicated that needling was performed at a nearby nonacupoint on the right leg (NAP, arrow pointing to dark cyan dot). The red line refers to needle administration, and the green line represents no acupuncture manipulation with needle inserted, the blue line indicates a 6-minute resting state or post-acupuncture resting state.

responses induced by acupuncture. However, its spatial resolving power does not match that of fMRI [19]. Since fMRI offers excellent spatial resolution with poor temporal resolution, while MEG provides excellent temporal resolution but poor spatial resolution, one feasible idea occurred that more exhaustive understanding of neural processes would be achieved by the combined employment of fMRI for localization and MEG for timing [20–22].

During the last decade, it has been gradually recognized that the brain is a complex network of dynamic systems with abundant functional interactions between local and remote regions [23–26]. One of the fast growing interests is related to the default mode network (DMN), which is identified as the distributed brain regions activated during rest but deactivated when specific goal-directed behavior is needed [27–28]. Accumulating evidence has typically demonstrated that several DMN regions play pivotal roles in connecting other regions and serve as network hubs with significant higher functional connectivity density [23,29]. In particular, recent investigations disclosed that the posterior cingulated cortex (PCC) constitutes one of the strongest DMN hubs in healthy subjects, with the highest degree of connectivity with other regions [29–32]. While substantial information has been gained about the prominent role of the hubs, the issues require more investigations on how these hubs interact with the rest of DMN regions and, more importantly, their alterations induced by acupuncture. The function of DMN has been considered to putatively engaged in self referential mental activity [33], stimulus-independent thoughts [34], and monitoring the environment among others [35] to maintain the body's homeostasis. In practice, the well-identified physical effects of acupuncture needling and its purported clinical efficacy also suggest that acupuncture acts in maintaining a homeostatic balance of the internal state within and across multiple brain networks [36]. Since the whole-brain hubs could be rearranged specifically following verum acupuncture compared with sham stimulation [37], furthermore, it has been increasingly elucidated that acupuncture could modulate spontaneous neural activities in wide resting brain networks, particularly within the DMN and its anticorrelated networks [5,38–40], therefore, further understanding of how such external intervention interacts with internal regulatory processes by regulating the DMN hubs may enlighten us to gain an appreciation of the physiological function and integrated mechanisms involved in acupuncture [5]. In recent electrophysiological studies, it is newly elucidated that functional connectivity between whole-brain regions would be modulated by acupuncture within specific frequency bands [41].

The current study attempted to spatiotemporally explore the specific DMN hub configurations following the verum acupuncture (Stomach Meridian 36, ST36), using sham acupuncture (non-

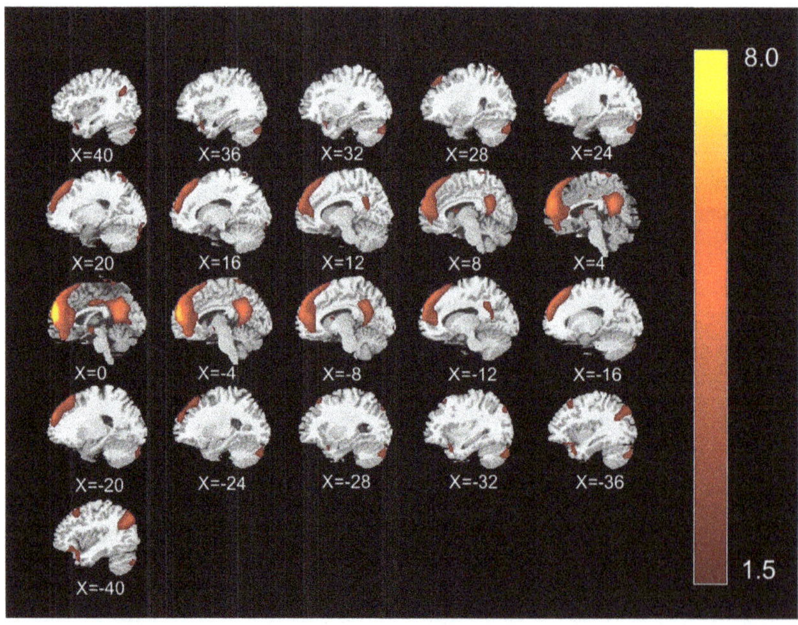

Figure 2. Spatial DMN components of group results extracted from fMRI data. Images are Z statistics overlaid on the average high-resolution scan transformed into standard (MNI 152) space. Red to yellow are Z values, ranging from 1.5 to 8.0.

Table 1. Talairach coordinates of the regional sources used to model the MEG data (P<0.05, FDR corrected).

Regions of Interest	Hem	Talairach			Z value	V voxels
		x	y	z		
MFG	L	−2	57	21	5.54	422
	R	2	57	8	4.94	341
SFG	L	−2	57	23	5.57	495
	R	4	58	25	3.19	742
ACC	L	−2	54	−1	3.71	77
	R	4	47	9	2.75	57
PCC	L	−2	−49	25	3.14	65
	R	2	−50	19	3.36	82
STG	L	−38	17	−19	2.21	56
	R	38	17	−19	2.27	33
AG	L	−49	−63	31	2.43	19
	R	51	−63	31	2.00	16
IPL	L	−46	−50	52	2.40	206
	R	50	−42	56	1.52	15
MTG	L	−49	−63	29	2.41	39
	R	53	−59	25	2.10	22

Abbreviations: Hem, hemisphere; L, left; R, right; MFG, medial frontal gyrus; SFG, superior frontal gyrus; ACC, anterior cingulate cortex; PCC, posterior cingulate cortex/precuneus; STG, superior temporal gyrus; AG, angular gyrus; IPL, inferior parietal lobule; MTG, middle temporal gyrus.

meridian point, NAP) as a control. Moreover, since previous investigations demonstrated the modulation on band-specific functional connectivity among the whole-brain network, it is proposed here that whether such regulations would specifically exist within conventional frequency bands, that is, delta (0.5–4 Hz), theta (4–8 Hz), alpha (8–13 Hz), beta (13–30 Hz) and gamma bands (30–48 Hz). To test this hypothesis, we attempted to employ fMRI for spatially identifying the DMN component and MEG for temporally evaluating the hub configurations so that more comprehensive knowledge would be dug out on the specific physiological mechanism underlying acupuncture.

Table 2. The DMN hub configurations during the resting state (REST), following sham acupuncture (NAP) and verum acupuncture (ST36) within the 5 frequency bands respectively.

Frequency band	Conditions		
	REST	NAP	ST36
Delta	PCC, IPL	PCC, MTG	PCC, SFG
Theta	PCC	PCC, STG	MFG, STG, SFG
Alpha	PCC, ACC,STG, SFG	PCC, ACC,STG, SFG, MFG	STG, SFG
Beta	PCC, ACC, SFG	PCC, ACC, SFG	ACC, SFG
Gamma	PCC	PCC, ACC	PCC, STG

Abbreviations as in Table 1.

Materials and Methods

Subjects

In order to reduce inter-subject difference, 28 right-handed healthy college students (14 males, 14 females, aged 24.5±1.8 years) from a homogeneous group were enrolled. All of them were acupuncture naïve. Participants were screened to exclude individuals with a history of major medical illness, head trauma, neuropsychiatric disorders or used any prescription medications within the last month. All subjects gave written, informed consent after the experimental procedures being fully explained. The Tiantan Hospital Subcommittee on Human Studies approved the methods and procedures, all of which was in accordance with the Declaration of Helsinki.

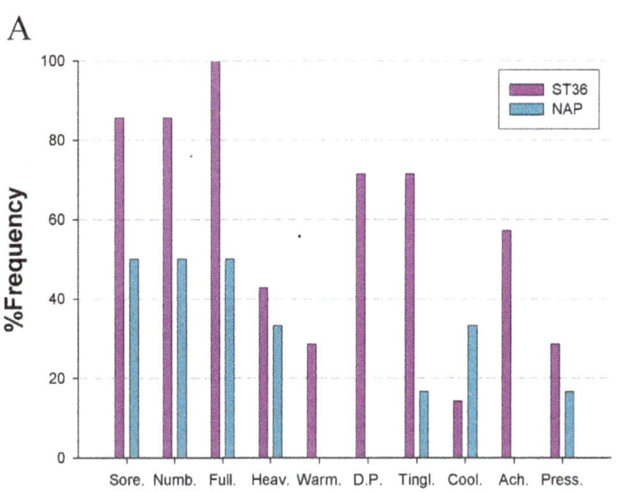

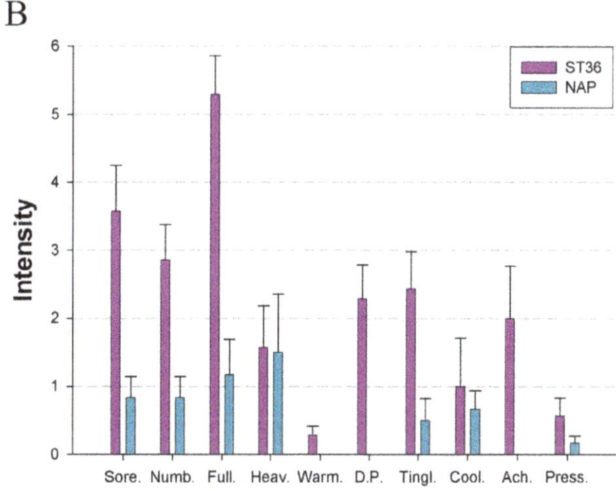

Figure 3. Averaged psychophysical response. A. The percentage of subjects that reported the given sensations. The frequency of aching was found greater following acupuncture at ST36. B. The intensity of sensations measured by average score (with standard error bars) on a scale from 0 denoting no sensation to 10 denoting an unbearable sensation. Sore, soreness; Numb, numbness; Full, fullness; Heav, heaviness; Warm, warmth; DP, dull pain; Tinl, tingling; Cool, coolness; Ach, aching; Press, pressure.

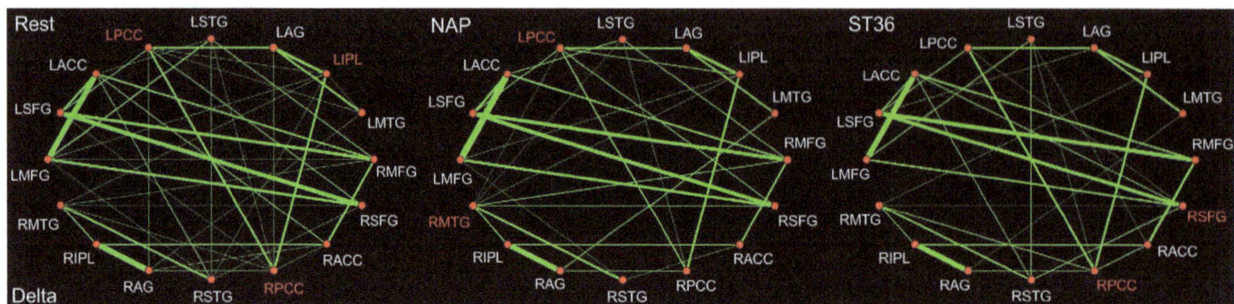

Figure 4. DMN hub configurations preceding acupuncture and following acupuncture at ST36 or NAP within the delta band (P<0.05, FDR corrected). The DMN hubs are indicated in red which are denoted as at least one standard deviation greater than the average degree of the network. The strength of the functional connectivity was expressed by the thickness of the green line. L, left; R, right; MFG, medial frontal gyrus; SFG, superior frontal gyrus; ACC, anterior cingulate cortex; PCC, posterior cingulate cortex/precuneus; STG, superior temporal gyrus; AG, angular gyrus; IPL, inferior parietal lobule; MTG, middle temporal gyrus.

Experimental paradigm

Twenty-eight participants were evenly divided into two groups, one for ST36 and the other for NAP, being matched by age and gender. All participants underwent firstly resting state functional MRI scanning for 6 min, followed by MEG data collection, during which the manual acupuncture was exerted at either ST36 or NAP. The whole MEG data collection lasts for 15 min, with the first 6 min for resting-state scanning and the other 9 min for acupuncture intervention. Both verum and sham manual acupuncture employed the single-block design paradigm, incorporating 2 min needle manipulation, preceded by 1 min rest epoch and followed by 6 min rest (without acupuncture manipulation) scanning. The experimental paradigm of MEG scanning can be found in Fig. 1. All participants were asked to remain relaxed without engaging in any mental tasks. To facilitate blinding, they were also instructed to keep their eyes closed to prevent from actually observing the procedures.

Verum acupuncture was performed at ST36 on the right leg (Zusanli, located four finger breadths below the lower margin of the patella and one finger breadth laterally from the anterior crest of the tibia) [42–43]. Verum acupuncture was delivered using a sterile disposable 38 gauge stainless steel acupuncture needle, 0.2 mm in diameter and 40 mm in length, which was inserted perpendicularly into the skin surface at a depth of 1.5–2.5 cm. Sham acupuncture was initially devised by an experienced and licensed acupuncturist (with 6 years of experience and had been trained to perform in the fMRI settings), with needling at non-meridian point (2–3 cm apart from ST36), with needle depth, stimulation intensity and manipulation procedure all identical to those used in verum acupuncture. A balanced "tonifying and reducing" technique was utilized as twirling the needle clockwise and counter-clockwise equally [44]. Stimulation consisted of rotating the needle clockwise and counterclockwise for 1 min at a rate of 60 times per min. The whole procedure was performed by the same acupuncturist on all participants.

According to Traditional Chinese Medicine, the sensation induced by twirling needles at the acupoints is asserted as "*De-qi*", which is essential to the efficacy of acupuncture [45]. As a concurrent psychophysical analysis, the MGH Acupuncture Sensation Scale (MASS) was utilized in the present study to quantify the subjective *De-qi* sensations [38,46]. The sensation rates ranged from 0 to 10 (0 = no sensation, 1–3 = mild, 4–6 = moderate, 7–8 = strong, 9 = severe and 10 = unbearable sensation). Spreading of any sensation was noted in a binary fashion and coded as follows: 1-spreading reported; 0-spreading not reported.

Table 3. The functional connectivity between the DMN key nodes and their alterations induced by acupuncture within the delta band (0.5–4 Hz).

Functional Connectivity	Delta				
	Rest	NAP	*P*-value	ST36	*P*-value
MFG-SFG	0.3643	0.4011	0.358	0.4299	0.723
SFG-ACC	0.2332	0.3016	0.231	0.1383	0.407
ACC-PCC	0.0546	0	–	0.0779	0.611
PCC-STG	0.0551	0.0710	0.841	0.0709	0.019
STG-AG	0	0	–	0	–
AG-IPL	0.6478	0.6209	0.635	0.6226	0.075
IPL-MTG	0.1289	0.1276	0.839	0.1199	0.699
MTG-MFG	0.0447	0.0817	0.125	0	–
MFG-ACC	0.6874	0.7952	0.575	0.6373	0.193
SFG-PCC	0.1176	0.0954	0.119	0.0953	0.623
ACC-STG	0.0823	0.0818	0.774	0.1167	0.053
PCC-AG	0.2077	0.2081	0.831	0.2145	0.752
STG-IPL	0.0504	0	–	0	–
AG-MTG	0.2146	0.2176	0.856	0.2438	0.648
IPL-MFG	0.0420	0.0632	0.742	0	–
MTG-SFG	0.0670	0.0806	0.248	0.0631	0.617
MFG-PCC	0	0	–	0	–
SFG-STG	0.0477	0	–	0.0975	0.161
ACC-AG	0.0516	0	–	0	–
PCC-IPL	0.2443	0.2363	0.684	0.2482	0.742
STG-MTG	0.2273	0.2622	0.396	0.2133	0.869
AG-MFG	0	0	–	0	–
IPL-SFG	0	0	–	0	–
MTG-ACC	0	0	–	0	–
MFG-STG	0.0755	0.0867	0.636	0.1219	0.195
SFG-AG	0	0	–	0.0475	–
ACC-IPL	0.1461	0.1228	0.395	0.1492	0.953
PCC-MTG	0.0685	0.0504	0.938	0.0843	0.872

The maximum of the 4 pairwise connections obtained between the two ROIs located in both hemispheres was defined as the connectivity between the two nodes (one sample *t*-test, $P<0.05$). Significant alterations induced by acupuncture at ST36 relative to NAP were based on the paired *t*-test ($P<0.05$) or with the emergence/suspension of functional connectivity following acupuncture compared with the resting state.

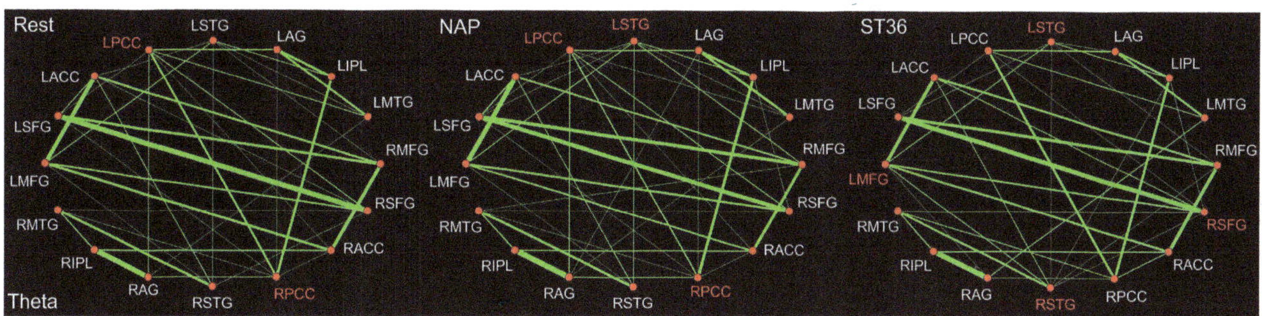

Figure 5. DMN hub configurations preceding acupuncture and following acupuncture at ST36 or NAP within the theta band ($P<0.05$, FDR corrected). The DMN hubs are indicated in red which are denoted as at least one standard deviation greater than the average degree of the network. The strength of the functional connectivity was expressed by the thickness of the green line. L, left; R, right; MFG, medial frontal gyrus; SFG, superior frontal gyrus; ACC, anterior cingulate cortex; PCC, posterior cingulate cortex/precuneus; STG, superior temporal gyrus; AG, angular gyrus; IPL, inferior parietal lobule; MTG, middle temporal gyrus.

fMRI and MEG data acquisition

All fMRI data were obtained with a 3.0 T MRI system (Allegra; Siemens, Erlangen, Germany). A custom-built head holder and foam padding were used to restricted head movements. The images were parallel to the AC-PC line and covered the whole brain. Thirty-two axial slices were obtained using a T2*-weighted single-shot, gradient-recalled echo planar imaging sequence (FOV = 240 mm×240 mm, matrix = 64×64, thickness = 5 mm, TR = 2000 ms, TE = 30 ms, flip angle = 75°). The total functional scanning was lasted for 6 minutes during the resting state. After the functional run, high-resolution structural information on each subject was also acquired using 3D MRI sequences with a voxel size of 1 mm^3 for anatomical localization (TR = 2700 ms, TE = 2.19 ms, matrix = 384×512, FOV = 256 mm×256 mm, flip angel = 7°, thickness = 1 mm).

The MEG data were recorded when participants comfortably seated inside an electromagnetically shielded room. The cortical responses were recorded with the whole head MEG system (CTF Systems Inc., Port Coquitlam, BC, Canada) consisting of 151 hardware first-order magnetic gradiometers. Two of the original 151 channels were not available due to technical problems during recording for all participants. The whole MEG scanning lasted 15 minutes, incorporating a 6 min resting state recording and followed by above-mentioned 9-min acupuncture procedure (Fig. 1). The head position was monitored during the measurement using head position indicator coils. MEG data were recorded at the sample rate of 600 Hz. The same acquisition settings were used for an empty-room recording without a subject in the MEG room to estimate the background noise [47]. During the recording, participants were instructed to close their eyes to reduce artifact signals due to eye movements, but remain awake as much as possible. The investigator and MEG technician checked the signal on-line and observed the participants using a video monitor. The head position relative to the MEG sensors was measured before and after each recording session by leading small alternating currents through three head position coils attached to the left and right pre-auricular points and the nasion on the subject's head. For all analyzed data sets, head displacements within a recording session were below 5 mm.

fMRI data analysis

The first five volumes of fMRI data were discarded to eliminate non-equilibrium effects of magnetization [48]. All images were subsequently pre-processed using the statistical parametric mapping (SPM5, http://www.fil.ion.ucl.ac.uk/spm/) [49]. Firstly, the image data underwent realignments for head motions using the least-squares minimization. None of subjects had head movements

Table 4. The functional connectivity between the DMN key nodes and their alterations induced by acupuncture within the theta band (4–8 Hz).

Functional Connectivity	Theta				
	Rest	NAP	*P*-value	ST36	*P*-value
MFG-SFG	0.3450	0.3848	0.405	0.3490	0.894
SFG-ACC	0.0922	0.1727	0.105	0.1204	0.142
ACC-PCC	0.0760	0.0691	0.055	0.0841	0.317
PCC-STG	0	0	–	0	–
STG-AG	0	0	–	0.0596	–
AG-IPL	0.6085	0.6289	0.064	0.2721	0.000
IPL-MTG	0.1433	0.1499	0.779	0.1399	0.833
MTG-MFG	0	0.0452	–	0	–
MFG-ACC	0.4756	0.5512	0.772	0.4608	0.132
SFG-PCC	0.0850	0.0883	0.314	0.0694	0.854
ACC-STG	0.0753	0.0841	0.714	0.0929	0.302
PCC-AG	0.2061	0.1669	0.208	0.1778	0.269
STG-IPL	0.0922	0.0818	0.545	0.0895	0.685
AG-MTG	0.2387	0.2929	0.057	0.2614	0.544
IPL-MFG	0	0	–	0	–
MTG-SFG	0.0553	0.0598	0.340	0.0679	0.533
MFG-PCC	0	0	–	0	–
SFG-STG	0.0472	0.0641	0.301	0.0614	0.463
ACC-AG	0.	0	–	0	–
PCC-IPL	0.2790	0.3263	0.091	0.5980	0.000
STG-MTG	0.2744	0.3002	0.628	0.2436	0.921
AG-MFG	0	0	–	0.0455	–
IPL-SFG	0	0.0410	–	0.0498	–
MTG-ACC	0	0	–	0	–
MFG-STG	0.0832	0.0817	0.818	0.0971	0.807
SFG-AG	0	0	–	0	–
ACC-IPL	0.1580	0.1509	0.981	0.1656	0.988
PCC-MTG	0.0773	0.0549	0.716	0.0904	0.998

The maximum of the 4 pairwise connections obtained from the two ROIs located in both hemispheres was defined as the connectivity between the two nodes (one sample *t*-test, $P<0.05$). Significant alterations induced by acupuncture at ST36 relative to NAP were based on the paired *t*-test ($P<0.05$) or with the emergence/suspension of functional connectivity following acupuncture compared with the resting state.

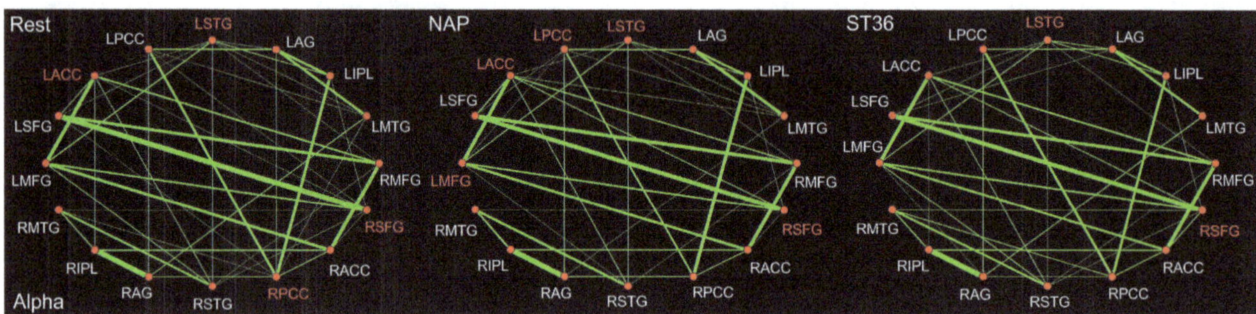

Figure 6. DMN hub configurations preceding acupuncture and following acupuncture at ST36 or NAP within the alpha band (P<0.05, FDR corrected). The DMN hubs are indicated in red which are denoted as at least one standard deviation greater than the average degree of the network. The strength of the functional connectivity was expressed by the thickness of the green line. L, left; R, right; MFG, medial frontal gyrus; SFG, superior frontal gyrus; ACC, anterior cingulate cortex; PCC, posterior cingulate cortex/precuneus; STG, superior temporal gyrus; AG, angular gyrus; IPL, inferior parietal lobule; MTG, middle temporal gyrus.

exceeding 1 mm on any axis or head rotation greater than one degree. A mean image created from the realigned volumes was coregistered with the subject's individual structural T1-weighted volume image. Secondly, the standard Montreal Neurological Institute (MNI) template provided by SPM5 was used in the spatial normalization. Then these data were resampled at 2 mm×2 mm×2 mm and filtered utilizing a finite-impulse response band-pass filter (0.01~0.08 Hz) in order to remove the effect of low-frequency drift and high-frequency noise [50–51]. Subsequently, the functional images were smoothed by a Gaussian kernel with a full width at half maximum of 6 mm (FWHM = 6 mm).

A data-driven method named independent component analysis (ICA), which is able to extract multiple functional connectivity networks [26,52], was performed on the preprocessed data of all subjects using the Group ICA of fMRI Toolbox (GIFT) [53–54]. To reduce the computational load of simply entering all subjects' data into an ICA analysis, two reduction steps were conducted, one on data from each subject and the other on an aggregate data set. In the first round of principal component analysis (PCA), the data for individual subject were dimension-reduced to 52 in the GIFT toolbox. After concatenation across subjects, the dimension was again reduced via the second round of PCA to 33 components estimated by the Minimum Description Length (MDL) criteria, followed by an independent component estimation using Infomax algorithm [54–55]. The mean ICs of all the subjects, the corresponding mean time courses and ICs for each subject were obtained from group ICA separation and back-reconstruction [53]. The maps of these ICs across all subjects were generated for a random effect analysis using a one-sample t-test. Thresholds were set at $P<0.05$ (correction with the FDR criterion). The intensity values in each spatial map were converted to Z scores to indicate the voxels that contributed most strongly to a particular IC. Voxels with absolute Z-values greater than 1.5 are considered active voxels of the IC [56]. The independent component was selected, which best matched the default mode network as previously reported [26,28]. Every template region was spherical with a radius of 5 mm (varying sphere size had no effect on component identification), and the average value of voxels within the template minus that of voxels outside the template was calculated for each component. Finally, the component with the greatest difference was determined to be the best-fit component and was designated as the DMN. The peak voxels of 8 core regions of interest (ROIs) were subsequently identified within the DMN component. These ROIs mainly include the bilateral medial frontal gyrus (MFG), superior frontal gyrus (SFG), anterior cingulate cortex (ACC), posterior cingulate cortex (PCC), superior temporal gyrus (STG), angular gyrus (AG), inferior parietal lobule (IPL) and middle temporal gyrus (MTG) [50,57–59]. See Fig. 2. Talairach coordinates of peak foci for each ROI are listed in the Table 1.

MEG data analysis

A third-order gradient noise reduction (computed with CTF software) was applied to the MEG signals on line. The raw data were then digitally filtered off-line with a band-pass of 0.5–48 Hz, followed by down-sampled at a rate of 300 Hz. Subsequently, the MEG data were band-passed into bands of interest: delta (0.5–4 Hz), theta (4–8 Hz), alpha (8–13 Hz), beta (13–30 Hz) and gamma band (30–48 Hz) [60–62]. To specifically highlight the temporal dynamics within and across different regions of the default mode network, discrete regional dipole source analysis [63] was applied in each frequency band to create a spatial filter to project into source space using the Brain Electrical Source Analysis (BESA, MEGIS Software GmbH, Germany) software package which implements a least squares algorithm to solve the overdetermined problem and estimate the activity contributed by each source to the scalp-recorded data [64–66]. This methodology overcomes some of the limitations associated with conducting analysis only in the sensor space and allows the spatiotemporal modeling of multiple simultaneous sources over defined intervals [67]. In our study, to represent brain activity within DMN preceding or following acupuncture, relevant fixed regional sources were seeded into a 3-layer spherical head model and source activity was estimated from each subject's continuous scalp data for further analysis [64,68]. Positioning of regional sources drew on the spatial localization of peak voxels in the DMN component obtained in fMRI. Talairach coordinates of these regional sources and proximate cortical structures are listed in Table 1.

Functional connectivity analysis and hub definition

Partial correlation analysis has been proven effective as a measure of the functional connectivity between a given pair of regions by attenuating the contribution of other sources of covariance [69–71]. Besides, partial correlations can be used to build undirected graphs, in which connections (edges) between nodes (vertices) depict their conditional dependence [69,72]. Given a set of N random variables, the partial correlation matrix is a symmetric matrix in which each off-diagonal element is the correlation coefficient between a pair of variables after partialling

Table 5. The functional connectivity between the DMN key nodes and their alterations induced by acupuncture within the alpha band (8–13 Hz).

Functional Connectivity	Alpha				
	Rest	NAP	*P*-value	ST36	*P*-value
MFG-SFG	0.3511	0.3768	0.564	0.3491	0.988
SFG-ACC	0.0997	0.1573	0.066	0.1103	0.078
ACC-PCC	0.0908	0.0778	0.034	0.1063	0.403
PCC-STG	0	0	–	0	–
STG-AG	0.0303	0	–	0.0800	0.148
AG-IPL	0.6003	0.6231	0.262	0.6070	0.768
IPL-MTG	0.1620	0.1753	0.362	0.1583	0.487
MTG-MFG	0	0	–	0	–
MFG-ACC	0.4672	0.3990	0.667	0.4492	0.116
SFG-PCC	0.0489	0.0460	0.912	0	–
ACC-STG	0.0925	0.0929	0.496	0.0908	0.684
PCC-AG	0.2084	0.1649	0.111	0.1593	0.157
STG-IPL	0.1000	0.0991	0.711	0.0984	0.689
AG-MTG	0.2778	0.3513	0.007	0.2971	0.731
IPL-MFG	0	0	–	0	–
MTG-SFG	0.0649	0.0544	0.482	0.0733	0.721
MFG-PCC	0	0.0451	–	0	–
SFG-STG	0.0388	0	–	0.0580	0.299
ACC-AG	0	0	–	0	–
PCC-IPL	0.3218	0.3922	0.197	0.3020	0.606
STG-MTG	0.2581	0.2926	0.501	0.2536	0.616
AG-MFG	0	0	–	0.0524	–
IPL-SFG	0.0604	0.0544	0.697	0.0622	0.696
MTG-ACC	0	0.0556	–	0	–
MFG-STG	0.1160	0.0957	0.155	0.1151	0.889
SFG-AG	0	0	–	0.0543	–
ACC-IPL	0.1708	0.1638	0.479	0.1697	0.749
PCC-MTG	0.0588	0.0508	0.633	0.0955	0.379

The maximum of the 4 pairwise connections obtained from the two ROIs located in both hemispheres was defined as the connectivity between the two nodes (one sample *t*-test, $P<0.05$). Significant alterations induced by acupuncture at ST36 relative to NAP were based on the paired *t*-test ($P<0.05$) or with the emergence/suspension of functional connectivity following acupuncture compared with the resting state.

out the contributions to the pairwise correlation of all other variables included in the dataset [71,73–75]. In our case, it was thus utilized within each frequency band to estimate the correlation coefficient between each pair of regions within DMN, factoring out the contribution to the pairwise correlations of the other 14 brain regions.

To estimate the partial correlation matrix within each frequency band for every participant, covariance matrix S was generated, using the 360s-long MEG data matrix Y on a subject-by-subject basis. Each component of S contains the sample covariance value between two brain regions (j, k) was $s_{j,k} = T^{-1} \sum_{t=1}^{T} (y_j(t)-\bar{y}_j)(y_k(t)-\bar{y}_k)$, where $\bar{y}_j$ denotes the average over time of the observations in a given region, T denotes the number of time points. Afterwards, the off-diagonal elements of the inverted matrix S^{-1} was rescaled to obtain the partial correlation matrix R: $r_{j,k} = -s^{-1}_{j,k} / \sqrt{s^{-1}_{j,j} s^{-1}_{k,k}}$ [71]. A Fisher's r-to-Z transformation was then applied on the partial correlation matrices in order to improve the normality of the partial correlation coefficients [76]. To test the null hypothesis that the partial correlation was zero between any pair of regions within DMN, we conducted multiple one-sample t-tests for the individually estimated partial correlations for each condition. False discovery rate (FDR) procedure was applied to restrict the expected proportion of type I errors to $q<0.05$ [77]. Subsequently, the partial correlation matrices obtained individually were averaged to obtain group mean inter-regional functional connectivity. Due to the lack of consensus as to the best method for defining network hubs, a pragmatic method was applied in which nodes were identified as network hubs if their degree values were at least one standard deviation greater than the average degree of the network [37,78]. Finally, significant alterations of functional connectivity induced by acupuncture for either ST36 or NAP group was evaluated for each band by means of a paired t-test with thresholded at $P<0.05$ in SPSS 17.0 software package for Windows.

Results

Psychophysical responses

The prevalence of subjective "*De-qi*" sensations was expressed as the percentage of individuals in the group who reported the given sensations (Fig. 3A). The intensity was expressed as the average score ± standard error (Fig. 3B). The occurrence frequency of all sensations except coolness was found to be greater for acupuncture at ST36 than NAP. The overall stimulus intensities (mean ± SE) were greater for ST36, exhibiting a stronger *De-qi* sensation in verum acupuncture ($P<0.05$, two sample t-test).

Band-specific DMN hub configurations

In the present study, the pairwise functional connectivity analysis between the 8 core brain regions within the default mode network were evaluated for each of the 5 conventional frequency bands (delta, theta, alpha, beta and gamma) preceding and following acupuncture, with the aim of exploring the band-specific alterations of DMN hub configurations induced by verum acupuncture at ST36, using a nearby non-acupoint (NAP, sham acupuncture) as a control. The summary of the DMN hub configurations within each frequency band was listed in the Table 2.

For the delta band (0.5–4 Hz), the PCC and IPL were identified as DMN hubs during the resting state (Fig. 4). Following acupuncture, either at ST36 or at NAP, it is of interest to find that little was modulated on the key role played by PCC in the DMN hub configurations. By contrast, the IPL no longer acted as a network hub within the DMN in either group during the post-stimuli acupuncture resting state. In addition, specific acupuncture-induced alterations on hub configuration were also exhibited. To be specific, the right MTG was identified as a hub following sham acupuncture, while the right SFG was spotted following verum acupuncture at ST36. Taken into account the acupuncture-induced alterations of functional connectivity, it can be found that the functional interactions were suspended between STG and IPL, ACC and AG following either sham or verum acupuncture. In the NAP group, the connectivity between ACC and PCC as well as SFG and STG was found to be interrupted. On the contrary, the

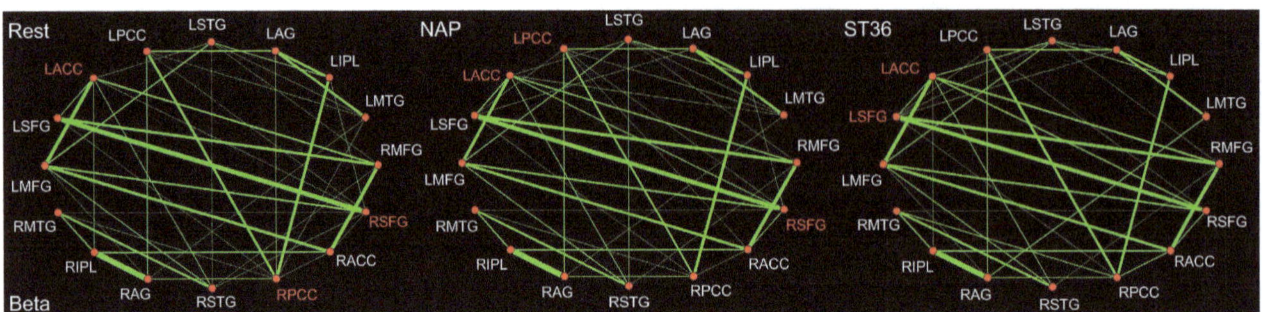

Figure 7. DMN hub configurations preceding acupuncture and following acupuncture at ST36 or NAP within the beta band (P<0.05, FDR corrected). The DMN hubs are indicated in red which are denoted as at least one standard deviation greater than the average degree of the network. The strength of the functional connectivity was expressed by the thickness of the green line. L, left; R, right; MFG, medial frontal gyrus; SFG, superior frontal gyrus; ACC, anterior cingulate cortex; PCC, posterior cingulate cortex/precuneus; STG, superior temporal gyrus; AG, angular gyrus; IPL, inferior parietal lobule; MTG, middle temporal gyrus.

Table 6. The functional connectivity between the DMN key nodes and their alterations induced by acupuncture within the beta band (13–30 Hz).

Functional Connectivity	Beta				
	Rest	NAP	*P*-value	ST36	*P*-value
MFG-SFG	0.3274	0.3446	0.725	0.3271	0.957
SFG-ACC	0.0915	0.1372	0.198	0.1281	0.221
ACC-PCC	0.0815	0.0717	0.023	0.0789	0.843
PCC-STG	0	0	–	0	–
STG-AG	0	0	–	0.0575	–
AG-IPL	0.6204	0.6424	0.256	0.6178	0.857
IPL-MTG	0.1534	0.1577	0.392	0.1481	0.631
MTG-MFG	0	0	–	0	–
MFG-ACC	0.4636	0.4153	0.107	0.4319	0.091
SFG-PCC	0.0642	0.0573	0.382	0.0529	0.443
ACC-STG	0.0914	0.0904	0.364	0.0897	0.598
PCC-AG	0.1979	0.1630	0.169	0.1771	0.392
STG-IPL	0.0969	0.0850	0.425	0.0878	0.441
AG-MTG	0.2357	0.3116	0.004	0.2517	0.750
IPL-MFG	0	0	–	0	–
MTG-SFG	0.0539	0.0491	0.793	0.0696	0.159
MFG-PCC	0	0	–	0	–
SFG-STG	0.0360	0	–	0.0458	0.694
ACC-AG	0	0	–	0	–
PCC-IPL	0.3118	0.3708	0.127	0.3059	0.610
STG-MTG	0.2575	0.2738	0.970	0.2535	0.667
AG-MFG	0.0429	0	–	0.0468	0.481
IPL-SFG	0.0446	0.0507	0.537	0	–
MTG-ACC	0	0.0514	–	0	–
MFG-STG	0.1121	0.0987	0.727	0.1020	0.642
SFG-AG	0	0.0458	–	0.0406	–
ACC-IPL	0.1566	0.1609	0.474	0.1405	0.595
PCC-MTG	0.0624	0.0533	0.776	0.0934	0.458

The maximum of the 4 pairwise connections obtained from the two ROIs located in both hemispheres was defined as the connectivity between the two nodes (one sample *t*-test, $P<0.05$). Significant alterations induced by acupuncture at ST36 relative to NAP were based on the paired *t*-test ($P<0.05$) or with the emergence/suspension of functional connectivity following acupuncture compared with the resting state.

relation between MTG and MFG together with IPL and MFG was disconnected following acupuncture at ST36. Meanwhile, there emerged the functional connectivity between the SFG and AG as well as increased interaction between PCC and STG in the ST36 group (Table 3).

Compared with the DMN hub configuration during the resting state in the delta band, it was recognized furthermore that the PCC constituted the only hub within the theta band (4–8 Hz). What's more, the most interesting difference lies in the fact that, following sham acupuncture at NAP, the bilateral PCC were still remained among the core hub regions, however, neither of them served as a hub following the verum intervention at ST36 (Fig. 5). Meanwhile, the STG was emerged to act as a network hub following either ST36 or NAP stimulation. In addition, it was remarkable that the SFG was specifically discerned as a DMN hub for the ST36 group. Following acupuncture at NAP, the connectivity between MTG and MFG was detected to be enhanced, while in the ST36 group, the relations between STG and AG, PCC and IPL, AG and MFG were found to be emerged, while the connectivity between AG and IPL was significantly decreased. Interestingly, the connection between IPL and SFG was detected to be strengthened following either acupuncture (Table 4).

Among the 5 frequency bands, it seems that there are the most hubs within the alpha band (8–13 Hz) during the resting state (Fig. 6), involving the ACC, STG, PCC as well as SFG. In line with the theta band, it is notable that the left STG served robustly as network hubs following either sham or verum acupuncture. Besides, it was also illustrated that the PCC acted as a hub specifically following the sham acupuncture. Moreover, what's different between the theta and alpha band is that the SFG not only emerged as a hub for the ST36 group, but also formed a network hub for the NAP group in the alpha band. In addition, it was noted that the ACC together with MFG formed the DMN hubs following acupuncture at NAP, none of which, on the contrary, was designated for the ST36 group. Moreover, the relations between ACC and PCC, STG and AG as well as SFG and STG were weakened, while the connections between AG and MTG, MFG and PCC, MTG and ACC were found to be strengthened following the sham stimulation. In the ST36 group, the connectivity between SFG and PCC was decreased while the relations between AG and MFG, SFG and AG were increased (Table 5).

To some extent similarity was found for the DMN hub configurations during the resting state between the beta band (13–30 Hz) and the alpha band (Fig. 7). First of all, the PCC was

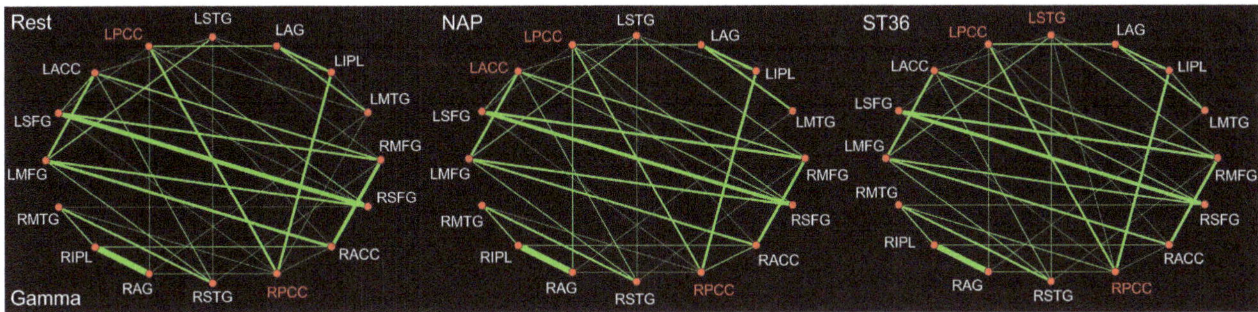

Figure 8. DMN hub configurations preceding acupuncture and following acupuncture at ST36 or NAP within the gamma band (P<0.05, FDR corrected). The DMN hubs are indicated in red which are denoted as at least one standard deviation greater than the average degree of the network. The strength of the functional connectivity was expressed by the thickness of the green line. L, left; R, right; MFG, medial frontal gyrus; SFG, superior frontal gyrus; ACC, anterior cingulate cortex; PCC, posterior cingulate cortex/precuneus; STG, superior temporal gyrus; AG, angular gyrus; IPL, inferior parietal lobule; MTG, middle temporal gyrus.

consistently identified as a hub. In addition, the ACC together with SFG was also designated for the beta band. Following either verum or sham acupuncture, it is noticeable that little was influenced on the role played by ACC and SFG for the DMN hub configurations. However, compared with the NAP group, the PCC did not serve as a network hub any more following acupuncture at ST36. There are also some shared alterations of the functional connectivity induced by acupuncture between the beta and alpha band. Following acupuncture at NAP, the connection between ACC and PCC, SFG and STG as well as AG and MFG were detected to be reduced, while the relations between AG and MTG, MTG and ACC, SFG and AG were enhanced. After stimulation at ST36, the connection between IPL and SFG was decreased, while the relations between STG and AG, SFG and AG were illustrated to be increased (Table 6).

In line with other frequency bands, the PCC was as well shown dominantly as the default mode network hub during the resting state within the gamma band (30–48 Hz). Following acupuncture, for either verum or sham stimulation, it is of interest to find that there was little acupuncture-induced modulation over the role played by PCC in the DMN hub configurations (Fig. 8). The PCC as well as the ACC was illustrated to be the network hubs following sham acupuncture. On the contrary, apart from the PCC, the STG was denoted specifically to work as a hub following acupuncture at ST36. Following acupuncture at either NAP or ST36, only a few significant alterations of functional connectivity were demonstrated within the gamma band. For the NAP group, the connection between MTG and SFG was decreased, while the connectivity between MTG and AG was significantly increased. For the ST36 group, significant increased connectivity was detected only between PCC and STG (Table 7).

Discussion

To the best of our knowledge, it is the first study to explore spatiotemporally the acupuncture effects on the DMN hub configurations within conventional frequency bands (delta, theta, alpha, beta and gamma) following stimulation at ST36, using a nearby non-acupoint (NAP) as a control, by combining fMRI and MEG analysis.Results exhibits differential alterations within the hub configurations of the DMN during the post-stimuli acupuncture resting state.

DMN hub configurations during the resting state

Among all DMN core regions, the PCC has been extensively denoted as the pivotal role in connecting other DMN brain regions for transmitting information under the mentioned cognitive processes, or optimizing the connectivity pattern to reduce cost of wiring and resources [23,29–30]. In the present study, by combining fMRI and MEG techniques, we not only confirmed the crucial function of the PCC in the DMN, but further extend previous knowledge about its hub configuration in the frequency domains. It is worthy to mention that the PCC constitutes the most attention-grabbing region as it is the only one which acted as a DMN hub consistently across the 5 conventional frequency bands (delta, theta, alpha, beta and gamma rhythm). Meanwhile, in line with previous fMRI studies, the IPL [79–80] and ACC, SFG [28] were validated as DMN hubs during the resting state. Moreover, with the advantage of MEG in providing amount of details in temporal dimension, it was further revealed that their crucial functions were exerted not across the 5 bands but within specific rhythms, especially with delta band for IPL and alpha, beta bands for both ACC and SFG.

Differential hub configurations following verum and sham acupuncture

Recently a number of noninvasive sham controls have been developed and tested [38,81–82]. While these hold promise in some respects, they also have limitations in what they can be used for, thus they should be used only when it is clear that their use matches the question for which sham treatment model is being selected [83]. Sham acupuncture is proved to a reasonable placebo control in many acupuncture fMRI setting, and can effectively reduce the subjects' bias toward the stimulation. In the current study, we also employed sham acupuncture as a control model. The comparison of the verum acupuncture, compared with the sham control, was expected to reveal the acupoint-specific response in the human brain and the observed differences between these two conditions may constitute a specific physiological effect.

As illustrated in aforementioned results (Fig. 4–8), the PCC constitute one of the most noteworthy DMN hubs with saliently differential alterations following either verum or sham acupuncture. Following sham acupuncture at NAP, the PCC remained to serve consistently as DMN hub across all 5 frequency bands. However, it is interesting to find out that the PCC was to a large extent regulated in specific bands by the verum acupuncture at ST36. Actually, it is only within delta and gamma bands that the PCC still acted as a DMN hub. As implicated typically in previous

Table 7. The functional connectivity between the DMN key nodes and their alterations induced by acupuncture within the gamma band (30–48 Hz).

Functional Connectivity	Gamma				
	Rest	NAP	*P*-value	ST36	*P*-value
MFG-SFG	0.2814	0.2980	0.669	0.2909	0.860
SFG-ACC	0.0775	0.1195	0.584	0.1283	0.092
ACC-PCC	0.0751	0.0760	0.191	0.0698	0.789
PCC-STG	0	0	–	0.0466	–
STG-AG	0	0	–	0	–
AG-IPL	0.6653	0.6769	0.303	0.6568	0.497
IPL-MTG	0.1366	0.1321	0.551	0.1397	0.796
MTG-MFG	0	0	–	0	–
MFG-ACC	0.3825	0.3614	0.495	0.3610	0.239
SFG-PCC	0.0842	0.0868	0.672	0.0718	0.583
ACC-STG	0.1050	0.1060	0.346	0.1039	0.592
PCC-AG	0.1843	0.1504	0.120	0.1756	0.578
STG-IPL	0.0594	0.0424	0.227	0.0517	0.066
AG-MTG	0.1843	0.2440	0.009	0.1883	0.828
IPL-MFG	0	0	–	0	–
MTG-SFG	0.0448	0	–	0.0561	0.125
MFG-PCC	0	0	–	0	–
SFG-STG	0	0	–	0	–
ACC-AG	0	0	–	0	–
PCC-IPL	0.2886	0.3226	0.127	0.2845	0.942
STG-MTG	0.2578	0.2568	0.166	0.2395	0.928
AG-MFG	0	0	–	0	–
IPL-SFG	0	0	–	0	–
MTG-ACC	0	0	–	0	–
MFG-STG	0.1073	0.0953	0.226	0.0930	0.611
SFG-AG	0	0	–	0	–
ACC-IPL	0.1130	0.1176	0.772	0.0976	0.491
PCC-MTG	0.0489	0.0533	0.772	0.0841	0.265

The maximum of the 4 pairwise connections obtained from the two ROIs located in both hemispheres was defined as the connectivity between the two nodes (one sample *t*-test, $P<0.05$). Significant alterations induced by acupuncture at ST36 relative to NAP were based on the paired *t*-test ($P<0.05$) or with the emergence/suspension of functional connectivity following acupuncture compared with the resting state.

neuroimaging studies, the PCC served as not only a DMN hub [28], but a core region for the whole brain network when engaging more brain regions within the whole brain network [23]. Recently, it is speculated that the brain regions are organized into interleaved networks to accomplish various functions or healing effects when a neural intervention is triggered [7]. Since DMN involves a mode of preparedness and alertness of possible changes in the internal milieu as well as external environment, the integrity of connectivity between the DMN and other brain networks may be central to the balance of brain functions [84]. Previous studies have shown alterations in the generalized activity and functional connectivity of the DMN in patients with various kinds of disorders [85–87]. Following stimulation at pain-control acupoints, it is demonstrated as well that there is increased DMN connectivity with pain related regions [40]. This suggests that specific brain networks may facilitate a correspondence between acupuncture stimulation and the central nervous system. Moreover, it has been proven, following acupuncture at vision-related acupoint, that the PCC performed intensive connections with other discrete core regions in vision networks [7]. Taken into account the ST36 is a commonly used acupoint for pain control in clinical practice, it is postulated that PCC would engage extensive interactions with the neural networks for both pain transmission and perception [88–89]. The connectivity was therefore believed to be enhanced between the PCC and those core regions within the pain matrix [90]. As a result, the role as a DMN hub played consistently by the PCC across the 5 frequency bands may be to some extent inhibited, supposed to be reallocated in order to balance the energy for the whole brain network to better exert the analgesia effect. In addition, it is for the first time revealed that the physiological regulations induced by acupuncture were dependent on the specific rhythms of neural activity. Compared with sham acupuncture, the acupuncture-induced modulation for PCC was mainly confined within the theta, alpha and beta bands.

Another striking finding is that, regarding to other core regions, to a certain extent shared DMN hub configuration patterns were observed following acupuncture at either ST36 or NAP. Given that acupuncture is a complex intervention that is intimately intertwined with placebo, patients, and practitioners. Therefore, it is logical that acupuncture may induce both specific and non-specific effects which contribute to its therapeutic effects [6]. That may support the clinical facts that acupuncture at sham points can also provide partial analgesia in chronic pain [91]. Moreover, in our present study, while the locations of these connectivity changes had overlap between verum and sham there were apparent differences as to the specific frequency bands between post-acupuncture modulation and post-sham modulation. Although STG were not among the DMN core regions during the resting state, it began to serve as a hub following both kinds of acupuncture. Nevertheless, it is implicated that sham intervention exerts such effect within only theta and alpha bands, while verum acupuncture produces additional influence for the gamma band. Likewise, the MFG demonstrates as well the acupuncture-evoked impacts on hub configurations within theta band following the verum intervention, in relative to the alpha band for the control group. In addition, the SFG constitutes as a DMN hub within the alpha and beta bands during the resting state. As illustrated in our results, the sham acupuncture seems to exert no effect on its hub configuration, remaining as a hub within the alpha and beta bands. Following verum intervention, however, the SFG served as a hub within not only these two bands, but additionally delta and theta rhythms.

In conclusion, the present study demonstrated differential alterations within 5 conventional frequency bands (delta, theta, alpha, beta and gamma) of DMN hub configurations following acupuncture at ST36 relative to NAP. With the complementary advantage of fMRI and MEG, we are able to explore spatiotemporally the specific biological mechanism underlying acupuncture, especially on the modulation of PCC as a DMN hub within the theta, alpha and beta bands. Overall, though it is a preliminary work, our results may provide additional evidence for the specificity of acupoint. We hope that this article serves as an introduction that will help to explore this fascinating topic in more depth and, as a consequence, shed more light on the specific neurophysiological mechanisms of acupuncture.

Acknowledgments

We would like to thank Fengbing Wang and Ying Jiang for valuable technical assistance in conducting this research.

Author Contributions

Conceived and designed the experiments: RD JT YY. Performed the experiments: YY LB HC. Analyzed the data: YY LB. Contributed reagents/materials/analysis tools: ZL WW. Wrote the paper: JT YY.

References

1. NCDP A (1998) NIH Consensus Conference. Acupuncture. JAMA 280: 1518–1524.
2. Witt CM, Manheimer E, Hammerschlag R, Ludtke R, Lao LX, et al. (2012) How Well Do Randomized Trials Inform Decision Making: Systematic Review Using Comparative Effectiveness Research Measures on Acupuncture for Back Pain. Plos One 7.
3. Bai L, Qin W, Tian J, Liu P, Li LL, et al. (2009) Time-varied characteristics of acupuncture effects in fMRI studies. Human brain mapping 30: 3445–3460.
4. Cho ZH, Chung S, Jones J, Park J, Park H, et al. (1998) New findings of the correlation between acupoints and corresponding brain cortices using functional MRI. Proceedings of the National Academy of Sciences 95: 2670–2673.
5. Bai L, Qin W, Tian J, Dong M, Pan X, et al. (2009) Acupuncture modulates spontaneous activities in the anticorrelated resting brain networks. Brain research 1279: 37–49.
6. Qin W, Tian J, Bai L, Pan X, Yang L, et al. (2008) FMRI connectivity analysis of acupuncture effects on an amygdala-associated brain network. Mol Pain 4: 1–17.
7. Qin W, Bai L, Dai J, Liu P, Dong M, et al. (2011) The temporal-spatial encoding of acupuncture effects in the brain. Mol Pain 11: 19.
8. Melchart D, Streng A, Hoppe A, Brinkhaus B, Witt C, et al. (2005) Acupuncture in patients with tension-type headache: randomised controlled trial. Bmj 331: 376–382.
9. Brinkhaus B, Witt CM, Jena S, Linde K, Streng A, et al. (2006) Acupuncture in patients with chronic low back pain: a randomized controlled trial. Archives of internal medicine 166: 450.
10. Linde K, Streng A, Jürgens S, Hoppe A, Brinkhaus B, et al. (2005) Acupuncture for patients with migraine. JAMA: the journal of the American Medical Association 293: 2118–2125.
11. Mandeville JB, Marota JJA, Ayata C, Zaharchuk G, Moskowitz MA, et al. (1999) Evidence of a cerebrovascular postarteriole windkessel with delayed compliance. Journal of Cerebral Blood Flow & Metabolism 19: 679–689.
12. Buxton RB, Wong EC, Frank LR (2005) Dynamics of blood flow and oxygenation changes during brain activation: the balloon model. Magnetic Resonance in Medicine 39: 855–864.
13. Rosen BR, Buckner RL, Dale AM (1998) Event-related functional MRI: past, present, and future. Proceedings of the National Academy of Sciences 95: 773–780.
14. Ghuman AS, McDaniel JR, Martin A (2011) A wavelet-based method for measuring the oscillatory dynamics of resting-state functional connectivity in MEG. Neuroimage.
15. Rodriguez E, George N, Lachaux JP, Martinerie J, Renault B, et al. (1999) Perception's shadow: long-distance synchronization of human brain activity. nature 397: 430–433.
16. Sarnthein J, Petsche H, Rappelsberger P, Shaw G, Von Stein A (1998) Synchronization between prefrontal and posterior association cortex during human working memory. Proceedings of the National Academy of Sciences 95: 7092–7096.
17. Cohen D (1972) Magnetoencephalography: detection of the brain's electrical activity with a superconducting magnetometer. Science (New York, NY) 175: 664.
18. Hämäläinen M, Hari R, Ilmoniemi RJ, Knuutila J, Lounasmaa OV (1993) Magnetoencephalography – theory, instrumentation, and applications to noninvasive studies of the working human brain. Reviews of modern Physics 65: 413.
19. Baillet S, Mosher JC, Leahy RM (2001) Electromagnetic brain mapping. Signal Processing Magazine, IEEE 18: 14–30.
20. Dale AM, Halgren E (2001) Spatiotemporal mapping of brain activity by integration of multiple imaging modalities. Current opinion in neurobiology 11: 202–208.
21. Dale AM, Sereno MI (1993) Improved localizadon of cortical activity by combining eeg and meg with mri cortical surface reconstruction: A linear approach. Journal of Cognitive Neuroscience 5: 162–176.
22. Liu AK, Belliveau JW, Dale AM (1998) Spatiotemporal imaging of human brain activity using functional MRI constrained magnetoencephalography data: Monte Carlo simulations. Proceedings of the National Academy of Sciences 95: 8945–8950.
23. Bullmore E, Sporns O (2009) Complex brain networks: graph theoretical analysis of structural and functional systems. Nature Reviews Neuroscience 10: 186–198.
24. Achard S, Bullmore E (2007) Efficiency and cost of economical brain functional networks. PLoS computational biology 3: e17.
25. Wang K, Liang M, Wang L, Tian L, Zhang X, et al. (2007) Altered functional connectivity in early Alzheimer's disease: A resting-state fMRI study. Human brain mapping 28: 967–978.
26. Damoiseaux J, Rombouts S, Barkhof F, Scheltens P, Stam C, et al. (2006) Consistent resting-state networks across healthy subjects. Proceedings of the National Academy of Sciences 103: 13848–13853.
27. Raichle ME, MacLeod AM, Snyder AZ, Powers WJ, Gusnard DA, et al. (2001) A default mode of brain function. Proceedings of the National Academy of Sciences 98: 676–682.
28. Buckner RL, Andrews-Hanna JR, Schacter DL (2008) The brain's default network. Annals of the New York Academy of Sciences 1124: 1–38.
29. Tomasi D, Volkow ND (2011) Functional connectivity hubs in the human brain. Neuroimage 57: 908–917.
30. de Pasquale F, Della Penna S, Snyder AZ, Marzetti L, Pizzella V, et al. (2012) A Cortical Core for Dynamic Integration of Functional Networks in the Resting Human Brain. Neuron 74: 753–764.
31. Hahn A, Wadsak W, Windischberger C, Baldinger P, Höflich AS, et al. (2012) Differential modulation of the default mode network via serotonin-1A receptors. Proceedings of the National Academy of Sciences 109: 2619–2624.
32. Miao X, Wu X, Li R, Chen K, Yao L (2011) Altered Connectivity Pattern of Hubs in Default-Mode Network with Alzheimer's Disease: An Granger Causality Modeling Approach. PloS one 6: e25546.
33. Wicker B, Ruby P, Royet JP, Fonlupt P (2003) A relation between rest and the self in the brain? Brain Research Reviews 43: 224–230.
34. Mason MF, Norton MI, Van Horn JD, Wegner DM, Grafton ST, et al. (2007) Wandering minds: the default network and stimulus-independent thought. science 315: 393–395.
35. Gilbert DT, Wilson TD (2007) Prospection: experiencing the future. science 317: 1351–1354.
36. Mayer DJ (2000) Acupuncture: an evidence-based review of the clinical literature. Annual review of medicine 51: 49–63.
37. Liu B, Chen J, Wang J, Liu X, Duan X, et al. (2012) Altered Small-World Efficiency of Brain Functional Networks in Acupuncture at ST36: A Functional MRI Study. PloS one 7: e39342.
38. Hui KKS, Liu J, Marina O, Napadow V, Haselgrove C, et al. (2005) The integrated response of the human cerebro-cerebellar and limbic systems to acupuncture stimulation at ST 36 as evidenced by fMRI. NeuroImage 27: 479–496.
39. Fang J, Jin Z, Wang Y, Li K, Kong J, et al. (2009) The salient characteristics of the central effects of acupuncture needling: Limbic-paralimbic-neocortical network modulation. Human brain mapping 30: 1196–1206.
40. Dhond RP, Yeh C, Park K, Kettner N, Napadow V (2008) Acupuncture modulates resting state connectivity in default and sensorimotor brain networks. Pain 136: 407–418.
41. You Y, Bai L, Dai R, Zhong C, Xue T, et al. (2012) Acupuncture Induces Divergent Alterations of Functional Connectivity within Conventional Frequency Bands: Evidence from MEG Recordings. PloS one 7: e49250.
42. Chen L, Tang J, White P, Sloninsky A, Wender R, et al. (1998) The effect of location of transcutaneous electrical nerve stimulation on postoperative opioid analgesic requirement: acupoint versus nonacupoint stimulation. Anesthesia & Analgesia 87: 1129–1134.
43. Han JS (2011) Acupuncture analgesia: areas of consensus and controversy. Pain 152: S41–48.
44. Hui KKS, Liu J, Makris N, Gollub RL, Chen AJW (2000) Acupuncture modulates the limbic system and subcortical gray structures of the human brain: evidence from fMRI studies in normal subjects. Human brain mapping 9: 13–25.
45. Xing C (1987) Chinese acupuncture and moxibustion. Beijing, China: Foreign Languages Press.
46. Kong J, Gollub R, Huang T, Polich G, Napadow V, et al. (2007) Acupuncture de qi, from qualitative history to quantitative measurement. The Journal of Alternative and Complementary Medicine 13: 1059–1070.
47. Montez T, Poil SS, Jones BF, Manshanden I, Verbunt J, et al. (2009) Altered temporal correlations in parietal alpha and prefrontal theta oscillations in early-stage Alzheimer disease. Proceedings of the National Academy of Sciences 106: 1614.
48. Castelli F, Glaser DE, Butterworth B (2006) Discrete and analogue quantity processing in the parietal lobe: A functional MRI study. Proceedings of the National Academy of Sciences of the United States of America 103: 4693–4698.
49. Friston KJ, Ashburner JT, Kiebel SJ, Nichols TE, Penny WD (2011) Statistical Parametric Mapping: The Analysis of Functional Brain Images: Academic Press.
50. Greicius MD, Krasnow B, Reiss AL, Menon V (2003) Functional connectivity in the resting brain: a network analysis of the default mode hypothesis. Proceedings of the National Academy of Sciences 100: 253.
51. Jiao Q, Lu G, Zhang Z, Zhong Y, Wang Z, et al. (2011) Granger causal influence predicts BOLD activity levels in the default mode network. Human brain mapping 32: 154–161.

52. Greicius MD, Srivastava G, Reiss AL, Menon V (2004) Default-mode network activity distinguishes Alzheimer's disease from healthy aging: evidence from functional MRI. Proceedings of the National Academy of Sciences of the United States of America 101: 4637–4642.
53. Calhoun V, Adali T, Pearlson G, Pekar J (2001) A method for making group inferences from functional MRI data using independent component analysis. Human brain mapping 14: 140–151.
54. Calhoun V, Adali T, Pearlson G, Pekar J (2001) Spatial and temporal independent component analysis of functional MRI data containing a pair of task-related waveforms. Human brain mapping 13: 43–53.
55. Hyvärinen A, Hurri J, Hoyer PO (2009) Independent component analysis. Natural Image Statistics: 151–175.
56. Liao W, Mantini D, Zhang Z, Pan Z, Ding J, et al. (2010) Evaluating the effective connectivity of resting state networks using conditional Granger causality. Biological cybernetics 102: 57–69.
57. Uddin LQ, Clare Kelly A, Biswal BB, Xavier Castellanos F, Milham MP (2009) Functional connectivity of default mode network components: correlation, anticorrelation, and causality. Human brain mapping 30: 625–637.
58. Gusnard DA, Akbudak E, Shulman GL, Raichle ME (2001) Medial prefrontal cortex and self-referential mental activity: relation to a default mode of brain function. Proceedings of the National Academy of Sciences 98: 4259.
59. Meindl T, Teipel S, Elmouden R, Mueller S, Koch W, et al. (2010) Test–retest reproducibility of the default-mode network in healthy individuals. Human brain mapping 31: 237–246.
60. Stoffers D, Bosboom J, Deijen J, Wolters E, Berendse H, et al. (2007) Slowing of oscillatory brain activity is a stable characteristic of Parkinson's disease without dementia. Brain 130: 1847–1860.
61. Douw L, Schoonheim M, Landi D, Van Der Meer M, Geurts J, et al. (2011) Cognition is related to resting-state small-world network topology: an magnetoencephalographic study. Neuroscience 175: 169–177.
62. Stam C, De Haan W, Daffertshofer A, Jones B, Manshanden I, et al. (2009) Graph theoretical analysis of magnetoencephalographic functional connectivity in Alzheimer's disease. Brain 132: 213–224.
63. Scherg M (1992) Functional imaging and localization of electromagnetic brain activity. Brain topography 5: 103–111.
64. Anderson KL, Ding M (2011) Attentional modulation of the somatosensory mu rhythm. Neuroscience.
65. Zhang Y, Ding M (2010) Detection of a weak somatosensory stimulus: Role of the prestimulus mu rhythm and its top–down modulation. Journal of Cognitive Neuroscience 22: 307–322.
66. Del Gratta C, Della Penna S, Ferretti A, Franciotti R, Pizzella V, et al. (2002) Topographic organization of the human primary and secondary somatosensory cortices: comparison of fMRI and MEG findings. Neuroimage 17: 1373–1383.
67. Keil A, Sabatinelli D, Ding M, Lang PJ, Ihssen N, et al. (2009) Re-entrant projections modulate visual cortex in affective perception: Evidence from Granger causality analysis. Human brain mapping 30: 532–540.
68. Nihashi T, Kakigi R, Kawakami O, Hoshiyama M, Itomi K, et al. (2001) Representation of the ear in human primary somatosensory cortex. Neuroimage 13: 295–304.
69. Whittaker J (1990) Graphical models in applied multivariate statistics: Wiley New York.
70. Hampson M, Peterson BS, Skudlarski P, Gatenby JC, Gore JC (2002) Detection of functional connectivity using temporal correlations in MR images. Human brain mapping 15: 247–262.
71. Salvador R, Suckling J, Coleman MR, Pickard JD, Menon D, et al. (2005) Neurophysiological architecture of functional magnetic resonance images of human brain. Cerebral Cortex 15: 1332–1342.
72. Stam CJ (2004) Functional connectivity patterns of human magnetoencephalographic recordings: a'small-world'network? Neuroscience letters 355: 25.
73. Marrelec G, Horwitz B, Kim J, Pélégrini-Issac M, Benali H, et al. (2007) Using partial correlation to enhance structural equation modeling of functional MRI data. Magnetic Resonance Imaging 25: 1181–1189.
74. Marrelec G, Krainik A, Duffau H, Pélégrini-Issac M, Lehéricy S, et al. (2006) Partial correlation for functional brain interactivity investigation in functional MRI. Neuroimage 32: 228–237.
75. Liu P, Zhang Y, Zhou G, Yuan K, Qin W, et al. (2009) Partial correlation investigation on the default mode network involved in acupuncture: an fMRI study. Neuroscience letters 462: 183–187.
76. He BJ, Snyder AZ, Zempel JM, Smyth MD, Raichle ME (2008) Electrophysiological correlates of the brain's intrinsic large-scale functional architecture. Proceedings of the National Academy of Sciences 105: 16039.
77. Benjamini Y, Yekutieli D (2001) The control of the false discovery rate in multiple testing under dependency. Annals of statistics: 1165–1188.
78. Gong G, He Y, Concha L, Lebel C, Gross DW, et al. (2009) Mapping anatomical connectivity patterns of human cerebral cortex using in vivo diffusion tensor imaging tractography. Cerebral Cortex 19: 524–536.
79. Buckner RL, Sepulcre J, Talukdar T, Krienen FM, Liu H, et al. (2009) Cortical hubs revealed by intrinsic functional connectivity: mapping, assessment of stability, and relation to Alzheimer's disease. The Journal of Neuroscience 29: 1860–1873.
80. Fransson P, Marrelec G (2008) The precuneus/posterior cingulate cortex plays a pivotal role in the default mode network: Evidence from a partial correlation network analysis. Neuroimage 42: 1178.
81. Sherman KJ, Hogeboom CJ, Cherkin DC, Deyo RA (2002) Description and validation of a noninvasive placebo acupuncture procedure. The Journal of Alternative & Complementary Medicine 8: 11–19.
82. Streitberger K, Kleinhenz J (1998) Introducing a placebo needle into acupuncture research. Lancet 352: 364–365.
83. Birch S (2003) Controlling for non-specific effects of acupuncture in clinical trials. Clinical acupuncture and oriental medicine 4: 59–70.
84. Hui KKS, Marina O, Claunch JD, Nixon EE, Fang J, et al. (2009) Acupuncture mobilizes the brain's default mode and its anti-correlated network in healthy subjects. Brain research 1287: 84–103.
85. Greicius MD, Menon V (2004) Default-mode activity during a passive sensory task: uncoupled from deactivation but impacting activation. Journal of Cognitive Neuroscience 16: 1484–1492.
86. Kennedy DP, Courchesne E (2008) The intrinsic functional organization of the brain is altered in autism. Neuroimage 39: 1877.
87. Lowe MJ, Phillips MD, Lurito JT, Mattson D, Dzemidzic M, et al. (2002) Multiple Sclerosis: Low-Frequency Temporal Blood Oxygen Level–Dependent Fluctuations Indicate Reduced Functional Connectivity – Initial Results1. Radiology 224: 184–192.
88. Bai L, Tian J, Zhong C, Xue T, You Y, et al. (2010) Acupuncture modulates temporal neural responses in wide brain networks: evidence from fMRI study. Mol Pain 6: 73.
89. Tracey I, Mantyh PW (2007) The cerebral signature for pain perception and its modulation. Neuron 55: 377–392.
90. Lewith GT, White PJ, Pariente J (2005) Investigating acupuncture using brain imaging techniques: the current state of play. Evidence-Based Complementary and Alternative Medicine 2: 315.
91. Richardson P, Vincent C (1986) Acupuncture for the treatment of pain: a review of evaluative research. Pain.

3

Effect of Acupuncture in Mild Cognitive Impairment and Alzheimer Disease: A Functional MRI Study

Zhiqun Wang[1], Binbin Nie[2], Donghong Li[3], Zhilian Zhao[1], Ying Han[4], Haiqing Song[4], Jianyang Xu[3], Baoci Shan[2], Jie Lu[1]*, Kuncheng Li[1,5]*

1 Department of Radiology, Xuanwu Hospital of Capital Medical University, Beijing, China, **2** Institute of High Energy Physics, Chinese Academy of Sciences, Beijing, China, **3** General Hospital of Chinese People's Armed Police Forces, Beijing China, **4** Department of Neurology, Xuanwu Hospital of Capital Medical University, Beijing, China, **5** Key Laboratory for Neurodegenerative Diseases, Ministry of Education, Beijing, China

Abstract

We aim to clarify the mechanisms of acupuncture in treating mild cognitive impairment (MCI) and Alzheimer disease (AD) by using functional magnetic resonance imaging (fMRI). Thirty-six right-handed subjects (8 MCI patients, 14 AD patients, and 14 healthy elders) participated in this study. Clinical and neuropsychological examinations were performed on all the subjects. MRI data acquisition was performed on a SIEMENS verio 3-Tesla scanner. The fMRI study used a single block experimental design. We first acquired the baseline resting state data in the initial 3 minutes; we then acquired the fMRI data during the procession of acupuncture stimulation on the acupoints of Tai chong and Hegu for the following 3 minutes. Last, we acquired fMRI data for another 10 minutes after the needle was withdrawn. The preprocessing and data analysis were performed using the statistical parametric mapping (SPM8) software. Then the two-sample t-tests were performed between each two groups of different states. We found that during the resting state, brain activities in AD and MCI patients were different from those of control subjects. During the acupuncture and the second resting state after acupuncture, when comparing to resting state, there are several regions showing increased or decreased activities in MCI, AD subjects compared to normal subjects. Most of the regions were involved in the temporal lobe and the frontal lobe, which were closely related to the memory and cognition. In conclusion, we investigated the effect of acupuncture in AD and MCI patients by combing fMRI and traditional acupuncture. Our fMRI study confirmed that acupuncture at Tai chong (Liv3) and He gu (LI4) can activate certain cognitive-related regions in AD and MCI patients.

Editor: Xi-Nian Zuo, Institute of Psychology, Chinese Academy of Sciences, China

Funding: This work was supported by the Project Sponsored by the Scientific Research Foundation for the Returned Overseas Chinese Scholars, the Natural Science Foundation of China (Grant No. 81000606, 61105118, 81141018) and Key Work of Special Project supported by the city government (Z101107052210002). The funders had no role in study design, data collection and analysis, decision to publish, or preparation of the manuscript.

Competing Interests: The authors have declared that no competing interests exist.

* E-mail: lujie@xwh.ccmu.edu.cn (JL); likuncheng@xwh.ccmu.edu.cn (KL)

Introduction

Alzheimer's disease (AD) is one of the most prevalent forms of dementia worldwide. The neuropathological changes of AD are characterized by amyloid-β plaques, neurofibrillary tangles and neuronal loss [1]. Mild cognitive impairment (MCI) is the most important at-risk state of AD. It has a high probability of degenerating into AD at a rate of 10–15% per year [2]. However, There are no effective therapy for AD and MCI. Acupuncture, a treatment of traditional Chinese medicine (TCM), remains promising as an investigational therapy to treat neurological diseases including chronic pain, drug addiction, stroke as well as dementia [3–5]. Despite its increasing usage of acupuncture, its underlying mechanisms are poorly understood.

Most recent findings hint that sensitive neuroimaging and network analysis played a special role for understanding the pathophysiological mechanism of MCI and AD. Several resting-state fMRI studies have investigated the neuronal integrity in the brain of the AD or MCI patients by different methods. By using regions of interest (ROI)-based functional connectivity approaches, the researchers found reduced functional integrity related to hippocampus [6–8], prefrontal regions [9] and posterior cingulate cortex (PCC) [10,11] in AD or MCI patients. Using independent component analysis (ICA), Greicius and colleagues [12] showed AD-related reduction of spontaneous brain activity within a default-mode network (DMN) including the PCC and medial prefrontal cortex (MPFC). Sorg et al. [13] found the DMN regions and executive attention network had markedly reduced brain activity in the MCI patients.

Neuroimaging, in particular functional magnetic resonance imaging (fMRI), is a versatile tool that has been applied to investigate the mechanisms of acupuncture. Accumulating neuroimaging studies in humans have shown that acupuncture can modulate a widely distributed brain network [14–23], for

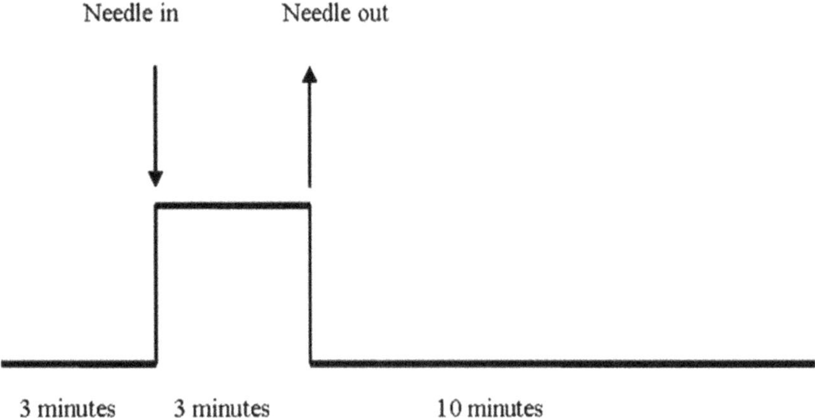

Figure 1. Experimental paradigm.

example, Feng et al. [14] sought to investigate the functional correlations throughout the entire brain following acupuncture at acupoint ST36, they found that increased correlations for acupuncture were primarily related with the limbic/paralimbic and subcortical regions, whereas decreased correlations were mainly related with the sensory and frontal cortex. Zhong et al. [15] investigated modulatory effects of acupuncture at GB40 (Qiuxu) and KI3 (Taixi) on resting-state networks and found that acupuncture at different acupoints could exert different modulatory effects. Zhang et al [23] found that stimulating PC6 (Neiguan) can change the amplitude of the intrinsic cortical activity of the brain. They concluded that stimulating PC6 may be a candidate method for improving cognitive impairment due to the consistent effect of acupuncture within PCC.

Based on the above knowledge, we can speculate that acupuncture may have a great effect on patients such as AD and MCI through modulating special brain network or brain regional activity. However, most of the acupuncture studies have been performed on healthy subjects, to the best of our knowledge; only two fMRI studies have been published on acupuncture effect in patients with AD and MCI [24–25].One previous study found that the temporal lobe, some regions of parietal lobe and cerebellum could be activated by acupuncture in AD patients [24]. Another recent fMRI study on MCI patients found the enhanced correlations in the memory-related brain regions following acupuncture [25]. In order to better understanding of the pathophysiology of AD and MCI, we sought to investigate the effect of acupuncture on the brain functional activity throughout the entire brain in AD and MCI patients compared to normal controls. We first identified regions showing abnormal brain activity in AD and MCI patients comparing to controls during the resting state. After that, we tested whether these regions could be modulated in AD and MCI patients in the procession of acupuncture. Finally, we explored whether there were any alterations or specific modulatory patterns after the acupuncture in AD and MCI patients by comparing the poststimulus resting state with the resting state.

Table 1. Characteristics of the AD, MCI patients and Normal controls.

Characteristics	**AD**	**MCI**	**NOR**	***P* value**
N (M/F)	14(4/10)	8(3/5)	14(6/8)	-
Age, years	66.92±8.91	66.37±10.96	66.07±5.78	0.96*
Education, years	10.07±3.38	10.62±3.54	11.00±4.52	0.82*
MMSE	15.92±4.32	25.37±1.30	28.00±1.41	<0.01*
AVLT(immediate)	11.35±3.95	14.13±3.52	26.86±5.24	<0.01*
AVLT(delayed)	2.64±1.59	4.37±1.59	11.07±2.76	<0.01*
AVLT(recognition)	3.35±1.55	7.38±3.11	12.71±2.09	<0.01*
CDR	1–2	0.5	0	-

MMSE, Mini-Mental State Examination; Plus-minus values are means ± S.D. AVLT, Auditory verbal learning test; immediate, immediate recall of learning verbal; delayed; delayed recall of learning verbal; recognition, recognition of learning verbal; CDR, clinical dementia rate.
*The *P* values were obtained by one-way analysis of variance tests.

Materials and Methods

Subjects

Thirty-six right-handed subjects participated in this study after giving written informed consent, including 14 patients with AD, 8 patients with MCI and 14 healthy controls. This study was approved by the Medical Research Ethics Committee of Xuanwu Hospital. The AD and MCI subjects were recruited from patients who had consulted the memory clinic at Xuanwu Hospital for memory complaints. The healthy elderly controls were recruited from the local community.

All AD patients underwent a complete physical and neurological examination, standard laboratory tests and an extensive battery of neuropsychological assessments. The diagnosis of AD fulfilled the Diagnostic and Statistical Manual of Mental Disorders 4th Edition criteria for dementia (American Psychiatric Association, 1994), and the National Institute of Neurological and Communicative Disorders and Stroke/Alzheimer Disease and Related Disorders Association

Table 2. Regions showing increased or decreased activities in MCI, AD subjects comparing to normal subjects in resting state.

Regions	BA	Cluster	Coordinates (MNI)			T-score
		Size	x	y	z	
MCI vs. NOR						
Lt. Middle Temporal Gyrus ↑	39	16	−57	−67	13	3.94
Rt. Inferior Frontal Gyrus ↑	44	127	60	5	16	5.46
Lt. Middle Frontal Gyrus ↑	6	8	−33	14	61	4.05
Lt. Middle Frontal Gyrus ↑	10	19	−39	59	7	3.78
Rt. Inferior Frontal Gyrus ↑	45	6	57	29	7	3.64
Lt. Inferior Frontal Gyrus ↑	46	7	−48	47	4	3.37
Lt. Superior Frontal Gyrus ↑	10	12	−18	62	25	3.30
Lt. Superior Frontal Gyrus ↑	6	16	−15	23	64	3.15
Lt. Lentiform Nucleus ↑	-	6	−15	2	−5	3.28
Rt. Cingulate Gyrus ↓	-	16	12	−4	28	−3.19
Lt. Fusiform Gyrus ↓	20	6	−30	−37	−23	−3.15
AD vs. NOR						
Lt. Temporal Lobe ↓	20	45	−42	−19	−17	−4.11
Lt. Middle Frontal Gyrus ↓	11	12	−36	50	−14	−3.19
AD vs. MCI						
Lt. Middle Temporal Lobe ↓	21	22	−48	−34	−2	−4.87
Lt. Middle Temporal Lobe ↓	21	8	−54	5	−23	−3.55
Lt. Inferior Parietal lobule ↓	40	54	−60	−49	43	−3.89
Lt. Middle Frontal Gyrus ↓	11	29	−30	35	−14	−3.54
Rt. Precentral gyrus ↓	6	8	63	−1	31	−3.34
Lt. Frontal Sub Gyral ↓	-	9	−12	20	−8	−3.24
Lt. Superior Frontal Gyrus ↓	8	6	−33	20	58	−3.08

(NINCDS-ADRDA) criteria for possible or probable AD (McKhann et al., 1984). The subjects were assessed with the Clinical Dementia Rating (CDR) score [26], CDR of 1 and 2 was assigned to the AD category.

Participants with MCI had memory impairment but did not meet the criteria for dementia. The criteria for identification and classification of subjects with MCI [27] was: a) impaired memory performance on a normalized objective verbal memory test; b) recent history of symptomatic worsening in memory; c) normal or near-normal performance on global cognitive tests (MMSE score>24), as well as on an activities of daily living scale; (d) global rating of 0.5 on the CDR Scale, with a score of at least 0.5 on the memory domain; e) absence of dementia.

Healthy controls met the following criteria: a) no neurological or psychiatric disorders such as stroke, depression and epilepsy; b) no neurological deficiencies such as visual or hearing loss; c) no abnormal findings such as infarction or focal lesion in conventional brain MR imaging; d) no cognitive complaints; e) MMSE score of 28 or higher; f) CDR score of 0.

Participants with contraindications for MRI such as pacemaker, cardiac defibrillator, implanted material with electric or magnetic system, vascular clips or mechanical heart valve, cochlear implant or claustrophobia were excluded. In addition, patients with a history of stroke, psychiatric diseases, drug abuse, severe hypertension, systematic diseases and intellectual disability were excluded.

Data acquisition

MRI data acquisition was performed on a SIEMENS verio 3-Tesla scanner (Siemens, Erlangen, Germany). The subjects were instructed to hold still, keep eyes closed and think nothing in particular. fMRI was acquired axially using an echo-planar imaging (EPI) [repetition time (TR)/echo time (TE)/flip angle (FA)/field of view (FOV) = 2000 ms/40 ms/90°/24 cm, image matrix = 64×64, slice number = 33, thickness = 3 mm, gap = 1 mm, bandwidth = 2232 Hz/pixel]. In addition, 3D T_1-weighted magnetization-prepared rapid gradient echo (MPRAGE) sagittal images were obtained (TR/TE/inversion time (TI)/FA = 1900 ms/2.2 ms/900 ms/9°, image matrix = 256×256, slice number = 176, thickness = 1 mm).

Our study used a single block experimental design. We first acquired the baseline resting state data in the initial 3 minutes; we then acquired the fMRI data during the procession of acupuncture stimulation for the following 3 minutes. A silver needle of 0.30 mm in diameter and 25 mm long was inserted and twirled at the four acupoints of the human body -Tai chong (Liv3) on the dorsum of the left and right foot; He gu

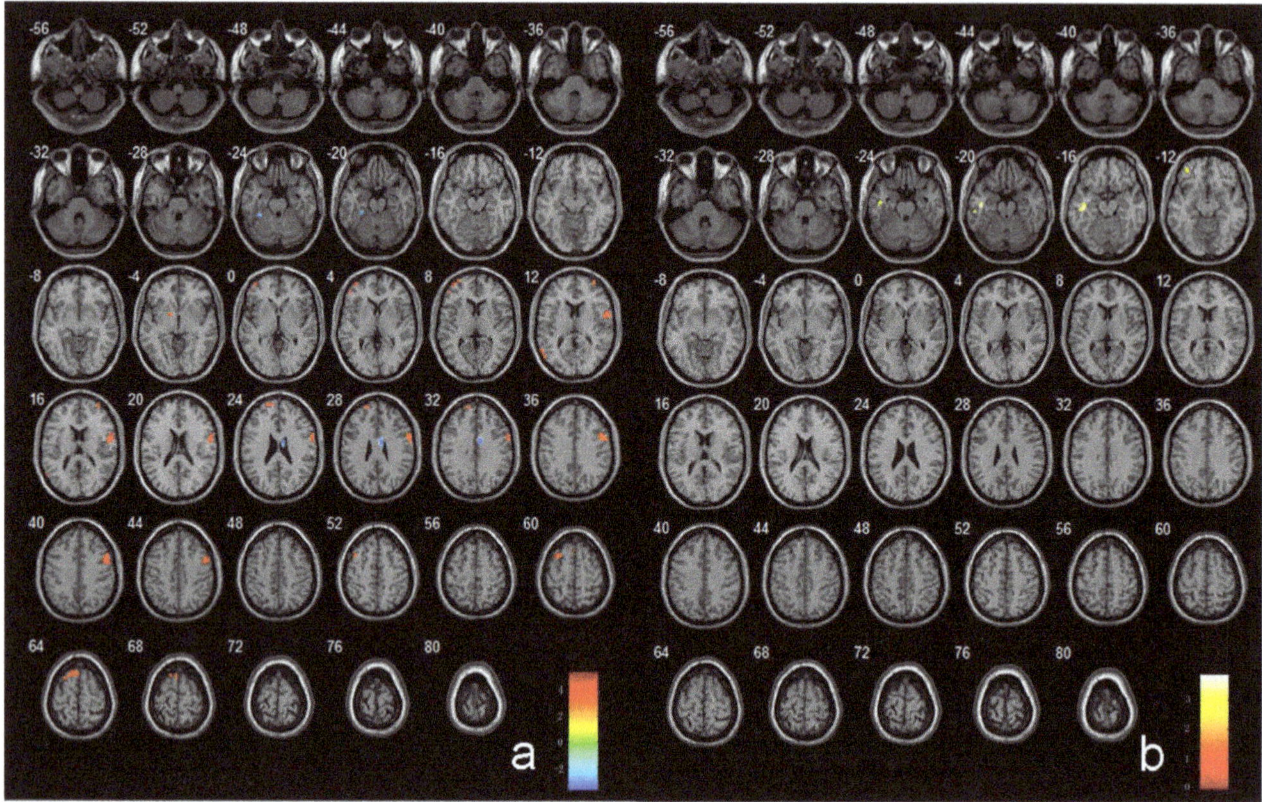

Figure 2. Regions showing abnormal activities in MCI subjects (a) and AD subjects (b) in resting state. Left in picture is left in the brain. The color scale represents t values.

(LI4) on the dorsum of the left and right hand. We acquired fMRI for another 10 minutes after the needle was withdrawn (Figure 1).

Data analysis

fMRI post-processing was performed by a single experienced observer, unaware to whom the scans belonged. The preprocessing and data analysis were performed using the statistical parametric mapping (SPM8) software (Wellcome Department of Imaging Science; http://www.fil.ion.ucl.ac.uk/spm). The functional datasets of all patients and healthy controls were preprocessed using the following main steps. 1) Slice timing: the differences of slice acquisition times of each individual were corrected using slice timing. 2) Realign: the temporal processed volumes of each subject were realigned to the first volume to remove the head motion, and a mean image was created over the 317 realigned volumes. All participants had less than 3 mm of translation in x, y, or z axis and 1° of rotation in each axis. 3) Spatial normalization: the realigned volumes were spatially standardized into the MNI (Montreal Neurological Institute) space by normalizing with the EPI template via their corresponding mean image. Then, all the normalized images were resliced by $3.0\times3.0\times3.0$ mm^3 voxels. 4) Smooth: the normalized functional series were smoothed with a Gaussian kernel of 8 mm full width at half-maximum (FWHM).

The first level, for each smoothed individual image, was fixed effects analysis based on the general linear model with a box-car response function as the reference waveform convolved with the canonical hemodynamic response function. There are three experimental conditions comprising resting state (baseline), acupuncture stimulation and the second resting state after withdraw of the acupuncture needle. The contrasts of cerebral areas activation during these three conditions were created. The subject-specific contrast images were then used to perform the second level analysis based on the random effects. The two-sample t-tests were performed (1) between AD and healthy controls of baseline; (2) between MCI and healthy controls of baseline; (3) between acupuncture stimulation and baseline of AD group; (4) between acupuncture stimulation and baseline of MCI group; (5) between the resting state after withdraw of the acupuncture needle and baseline of AD group; (6) between the resting state after withdraw of the acupuncture needle and baseline of MCI group. Brain regions with significant BOLD changes in patients of all the six statistical analysis demonstrated above were yielded based on a voxel-level height threshold of $p<0.001$ (uncorrected) and a cluster-extent threshold of 5 voxels.

Table 3. Regions showing increased or decreased activities in MCI subjects in the procession of acupuncture comparing to resting state.

Regions	BA	Cluster	Coordinates (MNI)			T-score
		Size	x	y	z	
MCI vs. NOR ↑						
Lt. Cerebellum Posterior lobe ↑	-	12	−27	−49	−50	4.77
Lt. Cerebellum Posterior lobe ↑	-	109	−36	−70	−41	4.45
Rt. Cerebellum Posterior lobe ↑	-	231	51	−64	−38	6.81
Rt. Cerebellum Posterior lobe ↑	-	11	36	−40	−44	3.78
Lt. Cerebellum Posterior lobe ↑	-	12	−9	−91	−26	4.03
Lt. Cerebellum Posterior lobe ↑	-	6	−3	−61	−17	3.46
Lt. Middle Temporal Gyrus ↑	38	24	−48	11	−41	4.35
Lt. Fusiform Gyrus ↑	19	92	−36	−76	−17	5.55
Lt. Inferior Temporal Gyrus ↑	20	5	−39	−13	−26	3.60
Rt. Parahippocampa Gyrus ↑	34	53	18	−10	−17	5.98
Rt. Middle Temporal Gyrus ↑	21	18	60	8	−20	4.47
Rt. Fusiform Gyrus ↑	19	20	36	−70	−17	4.78
Rt. Middle Temporal Gyrus ↑	21	7	63	−31	−14	3.41
Rt. Fusiform Gyrus ↑	19	10	21	−55	−8	3.36
Rt. Middle Temporal Gyrus ↑	21	43	66	−16	−5	4.39
Rt and Lt. Frontal Lobe ↑	10	9324	21	44	−2	7.35
Lt. Occipital Lobe ↑	17	25	−12	−106	4	4.21
Rt. Occipital Lobe ↑	19	54	45	−85	4	5.24
Rt. Occipital Lobe ↑	19	212	27	−97	22	6.09
Lt. Inferior Parietal Lobule ↑	40	12	−51	−40	25	3.85
Rt. Inferior Parietal Lobule ↑	40	10	54	−28	25	3.48
Rt. Postcentral Gyrus ↑	1	13	54	−28	43	3.85
Rt. Inferior Parietal Lobule ↑	40	26	51	−43	55	4.83
MCI vs. NOR ↓						
Rt. Cerebellum Posterior lobe ↓	-	5	33	−76	−50	−3.91
Lt. Cerebellum Posterior lobe ↓	-	20	−3	−70	−50	−4.53
Lt. Cerebellum Anterior lobe ↓	-	5	−36	−40	−41	−3.69
Rt. Cerebellum Anterior lobe ↓	-	31	42	−43	−32	−5.19
Rt. Cerebellum Posterior lobe ↓	-	10	24	−73	−17	−4.11
Rt. Temporal lobe ↓	42	7	66	−7	10	−4.56
Lt. Superior Frontal Gyrus ↓	6	60	−24	−10	73	−5.28
Rt. Middle Frontal Gyrus	6	7	27	5	70	−4.01
Rt. Superior Frontal Gyrus ↓	6	16	21	−10	70	−3.64
Lt. Precentral Gyrus ↓	6	5	−42	−10	61	−4.06
Lt. Paracentral Lobule ↓	6	52	−3	−28	52	−5.20
Rt. Postcentral Gyrus ↓	3	222	42	−28	61	−6.06
Lt. Superior Parietal Lobe ↓	5	66	−30	−55	67	−5.15
Lt. Paracentral Lobule ↓	3	18	−15	−28	76	−4.20
Rt. Lingual Gyrus ↓	18	8	6	−79	−11	−3.88
Rt. Limbic Lobe ↓	-	19	24	−10	−35	−4.16

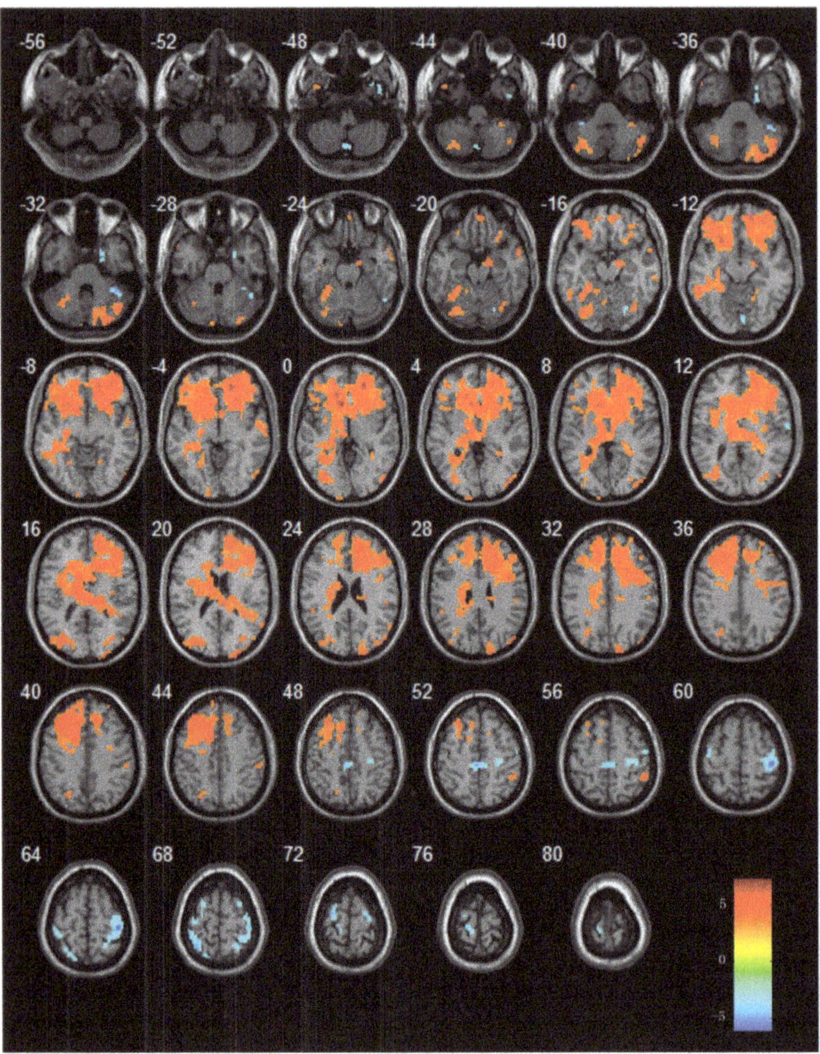

Figure 3. Regions showing increased or decreased activities in MCI subjects in the procession of acupuncture comparing to resting state. Left in picture is left in the brain. The color scale represents t values.

Results

Demography and neuropsychological test

Demographic characteristics and neuropsychological scores were shown in Table 1. There were no significant differences among the three groups in gender, age, and years of education, but the neuropsychological test such as Mini-Mental State Examination (MMSE) and Auditory verbal learning test (AVLT) scores were significantly different ($P<0.01$) among the three groups.

Regions showing increased or decreased activities in MCI, AD subjects comparing to normal subjects in resting state

When compared to normal subjects, increased activities in MCI patients were found in regions of the temporal lobe [left middle temporal gyrus(MTG)], frontal lobe [left superior frontal gyrus(SFG), left middle frontal gyrus (MFG) and bilateral inferior frontal gyrus(IFG)] and left lentiform nucleus; while decreased activities in MCI patients were found in regions of right cingulate gyrus and left fusiform gyrus(FG). In AD patients, left temporal lobe and left MFG showed decreased activities from that of normal subjects. The details of these regions see table 2 and Figure (2a, 2b).

Regions showing increased or decreased activities in MCI and AD subjects in the procession of acupuncture comparing to resting state

When compared to resting state, MCI patients showed increased activities in regions of bilateral cerebellum posterior lobe (CPL), temporal lobe [bilateral MTG, bilateral FG, right parahippocampus (PHG), left inferior temporal gyrus(ITG)], frontal lobe, parietal lobe[bilateral inferior parietal lobule (IPL) and right postcentral gyrus(PoCG)] and occipital lobe. Additionally, MCI patients showed decreased activities in regions of bilateral CPL, temporal lobe, frontal lobe [(bilateral SFG, right MFG, left precentral gyrus (PrCG)], parietal lobe [(right PoCG, left paracentral lobule (PCL), left superior parietal lobule (SPL)],

Table 4. Regions showing increased or decreased activities in AD subjects in the procession of acupuncture comparing to resting state.

Regions	BA	Cluster Size	Coordinates (MNI) x	y	z	T-score
AD vs. NOR ↑						
Rt. Cerebellum Posterior lobe ↑	-	7	51	−67	−32	4.14
Lt. Medial Frontal Gyrus ↑	11	18	0	53	−20	4.46
Lt. Inferior Frontal Gyrus ↑	47	31	−12	11	−14	4.78
Rt. Middle Frontal Gyrus ↑	47/11	61	27	38	−5	4.89
Rt. Superior Frontal Gyrus ↑	10	12	45	−85	1	3.74
Lt. Inferior Frontal Gyrus ↑	45	26	−57	29	7	4.31
Rt. Inferior Parietal lobule ↑	40	36	42	−58	58	4.37
Rt. Middle Occipital Gyrus ↑	19	12	21	62	−2	3.83
Rt. Middle Occipital Gyrus ↑	19	20	33	−91	25	4.44
AD vs. NOR ↓						
Lt. Cerebellum Posterior lobe ↓	-	8	−39	−79	−41	−4.69
Lt. Cerebellum Posterior Lobe ↓	-	11	−48	−67	−38	−3.59
Rt. Cerebellum Anterior Lobe ↓	-	66	30	−49	−35	−4.10
Rt. Middle Temporal Gyrus ↓	21	10	57	2	−29	−3.74
Rt. Superior Temporal Gyrus ↓	22	5	42	−58	13	−3.44
Rt. Middle Frontal Gyrus ↓	6	60	42	−1	46	−4.07
Lt. Medial Frontal Gyrus ↓	6	23	0	−10	55	−3.93
Lt. Brainstem ↓	-	5	−6	−25	−11	−3.40

right lingual gyrus and limbic regions. The details of these regions see table 3 and Figure 3

In AD patients, the regions of right CPL, bilateral frontal lobe, right inferior parietal lobule (IPL), right middle occipital lobe (MOG) showed increased activities from that of resting state. Additionally, In AD patients, the regions of right superior temporal gyrus (STG), right MTG, bilateral MFG and left brain stem showed decreased activities from that of resting state. The details of these regions see table 4 and Figure 4.

Regions showing increased or decreased activities in MCI and AD subjects in the second resting state after acupuncture comparing to resting state

In MCI patients, the regions of bilateral CPL, temporal lobe (bilateral FG, right MTG and right PHG), frontal lobe, right lentiform nucleus, left extra nuclear and right thalamus showed increased activity in the second resting state after acupuncture comparing to resting state. Additionally, decreased activity were showed in the regions of bilateral CPL, temporal lobe (bilateral MTG, left STG, right ITG and right FG), frontal lobe (left SFG, left IFG, bilateral PrCG, right MFG), parietal lobe (bilateral PoCG, left IPL, bilateral SPL, right angular) and occipital lobe [left superior occipital lobe(SOG), left cuneus]. The details of these regions see table 5 and Figure 5.

In AD patients, the regions of right CPL, temporal lobe (left ITG, right MTG), frontal lobe (bilateral SFG, left IFG, right MFG and bilateral PrCG), occipital lobe(right MOG), parietal lobe(bilateral SMG, right SPL) showed increased activity in the second resting state after acupuncture comparing to resting state. Additionally, decreased activity were showed in the regions of left CPL, bilateral PHG, right MFG, left lingual gyrus, right cingulate gyrus, left lentiform nucleus and right midbrain. The details of these regions see table 6 and Figure 6.

Discussion

Our study used fMRI to study the regional brain activities in MCI patients, AD patients and control subject under three conditions including resting state, acupuncture and resting state after acupuncture. All subjects underwent acupuncture at four acupoints of Tai chong (Liv3) and He gu (LI4) in left and right side. We found that during the resting state, brain activities in AD and MCI patients were different from those of control subjects. During the acupuncture, AD and MCI patients showed activation in regions consistent with impaired brain function. We also found that for the resting state after acupuncture, there are several regions showing increased or decreased activities in MCI, AD subjects comparing to normal subjects. Most of regions were involved in the temporal lobe and the frontal lobe, which were closely related to the memory and cognition.

Resting state brain activities in AD and MCI patients

Our study investigated the resting state activities in AD and MCI patients. Comparing to controls, the frontal lobe (SFG, MFG and IFG), the temporal lobe (MTG) and the lentiform nucleus showed increased activities in MCI patients. The frontal and temporal regions were considered as important components of

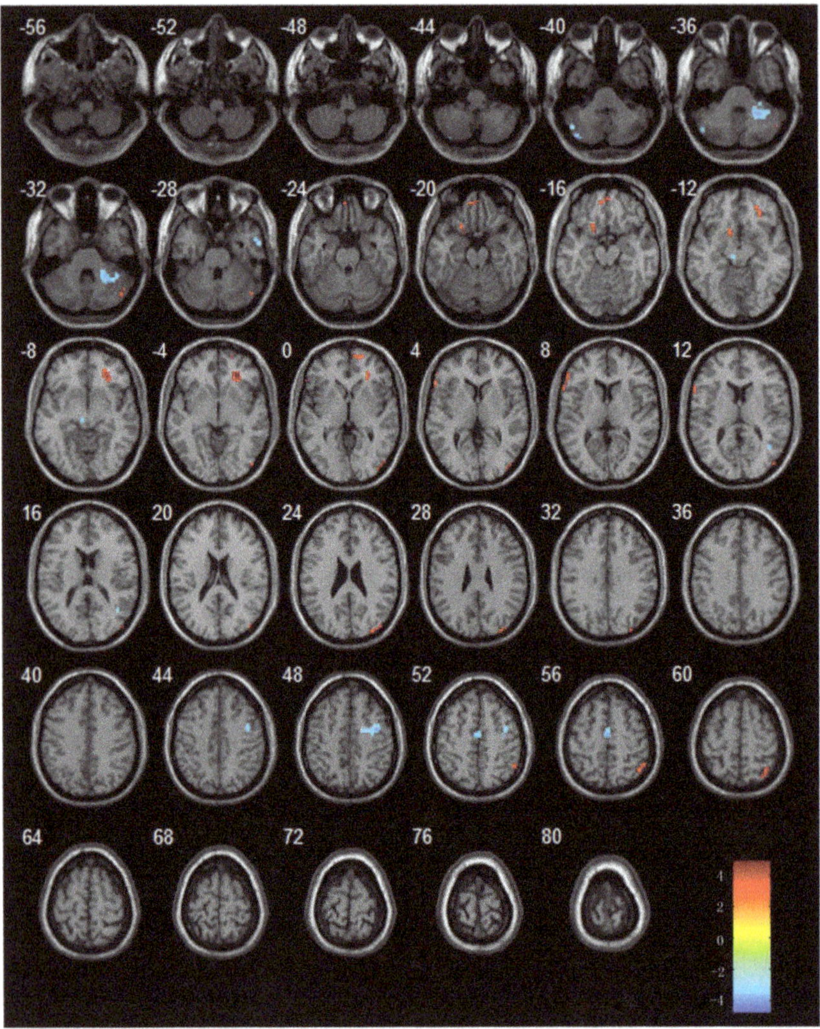

Figure 4. Regions showing increased or decreased activities in AD subjects in the procession of acupuncture comparing to resting state. Left in picture is left in the brain. The color scale represents t values.

human default-mode networks [28–30] and have been shown to exhibit AD- and MCI-related structural and functional abnormalities. These increases in frontal and temporal lobe could be interpreted as compensatory reallocation or recruitment of cognitive resource. This result is compatible to previous studies which showed increased temporal activation in MCI and at-risk subjects relative to healthy controls [31–34]. In addition, some regions such as cingulate gyrus and fusiform gyrus showed decreased activities in MCI patients comparing to controls, these changes represented the functional disruption of the above regions in the MCI patients.

Interestingly, AD patients showed different patterns of resting state activities from MCI patients. The temporal lobe and left MFG showed decreased activity in AD patients, which appeared to reflect a continuous breakdown of spontaneous brain activity during disease progression, consistent with previous studies [6,7,10,12, and 35]. Hence, the increased frontal lobe and temporal activation has been postulated as compensatory mechanisms in MCI patients. On the other hand, the temporal lobe and left MFG exhibited decreased activities with the progression of the disease in AD patients.

Brain activities in AD and MCI patients in the procession of acupuncture

In the current study, in order to demonstrate the value of acupuncture, we only focused on the regions which showed different activity in AD and MCI comparing to normal controls in the resting state. In MCI patients, we mainly explored changes of the left SFG, the left MFG and bilateral IFG, left MTG, the left lentiform nucleus as well as the right cingulate gyrus and left FG. In AD patients, we only focused on the left temporal lobe and left MFG.

During acupuncture, a lot of regions including the temporal lobe, the frontal lobe, the occipital lobe and the CPL showed increased activities in MCI patients comparing to the resting state. Most of these regions were related to the cognitive impairment. We noticed that the FG and cingulate gyrus were activated. On the other hand, several regions showed decreased activities in MCI patients, among these regions, we noticed that

Table 5. Regions showing increased or decreased activities in MCI after acupuncture comparing to resting state.

Regions	BA	Cluster Size	Coordinates (MNI) x	y	z	T-score
MCI vs. NOR ↑						
Lt. Cerebellum Posterior Lobe ↑	-	33	−36	−67	−41	4.57
Rt.Cerebellum Posterior Lobe ↑		17	51	−64	−35	4.51
Rt. Fusiform Gyrus ↑	19	31	36	−70	−20	5.49
Rt. Parahippocampa Gyrus ↑	28	32	21	−13	−17	5.34
Rt. Middle temporal Gyrus ↑	21	28	57	8	−23	4.65
Rt. Middle temporal Gyrus ↑	21	33	63	−31	−17	4.09
Lt. Fusiform ↑	19	7	−33	−73	−17	3.65
Rt. Frontal Lobe ↑	9,8,32	1128	12	23	16	5.54
Lt. Medial Frontal gyrus ↑	9	169	−18	29	34	3.95
Lt. Frontal lobe Sub-Gyral ↑	-	27	−27	−43	28	3.76
Lt. Superior Frontal Gyrus ↑	8	5	−9	26	49	3.37
Rt. Lentiform Nucleus ↑	-	17	30	−19	1	4.03
Lt. Extra-Nuclear ↑	-	165	−18	20	10	4.46
Rt. Thalamus ↑	-	89	6	−22	7	4.26
Rt. Right Cerebrum sub lobar ↑	-	15	0	8	13	3.38
MCI vs. NOR ↓						
Rt.Cerebellum Posterior Lobe ↓	-	7	33	−76	−50	−4.16
Lt. Cerebellum Posterior Lobe ↓		24	−3	−70	−47	−5.06
Lt. Cerebellum Anterior Lobe ↓		108	−42	−52	−29	−6.67
Lt. Cerebellum Posterior Lobe ↓		6	−18	−85	−35	−4.06
Rt.Cerebellum Posterior Lobe ↓		59	0	−70	−26	−4.69
Lt. Middle Temporal Gyrus ↓	39	39	−57	−70	7	−5.17
Rt. Fusiform Gyrus ↓	6	26	24	−73	−14	−4.32
Rt. Middle Temporal Gyrus ↓	21	73	54	−46	4	−4.20
Lt. Superior Temporal Gyrus ↓	22	9	−57	−10	7	−3.86
Rt. Inferior Temporal Gyrus ↓	37	8	63	−58	−8	−3.54
Lt. Superior Frontal Gyrus ↓	8	14	−15	59	−8	−5.61
Lt. Frontal lobe ↓	9	10	−6	−1	−14	−4.39
Lt. Superior Frontal Gyrus ↓	18	6	18	−100	−11	−3.69
Lt. Inferior Frontal Gyrus ↓	44	32	−54	8	28	−4.13
Rt. Precental Gyrus ↓	4	11	66	−13	31	−3.99
Rt. Precental Gyrus ↓	6	124	39	−25	61	−4.54
Rt. Middle Frontal Gyrus ↓	6	17	30	2	67	−4.04
Lt. Precentral Gyrus ↓	6	6	−42	−7	61	−3.72
Lt. Precentral Gyrus ↓	6	13	−36	−19	67	−4.41
Lt. Superior Frontal Gyrus ↓	6	30	−30	−7	70	−4.03
Rt. Postcentral Gyrus ↓	43	22	66	−10	13	−4.30
Lt. Postcentral Gyrus ↓	40	257	−54	−19	34	−4.93
Lt. Inferior parietal lobule ↓	7	17	−36	−76	49	−4.11
Rt. Angular ↓	7	9	36	−70	55	−3.83
Rt. Superior parietal lobule ↓	7	19	30	−55	52	−3.87
Lt. Superior parietal lobule ↓	7	276	−39	−40	61	−5.73
Rt. Postcentral Gyrus ↓	7	189	24	−55	70	−6.66
Lt. Occipital superior lobe ↓	7	6	−15	−85	46	−3.62
Lt. Cuneus ↓	19	22	−27	−94	28	−5.82

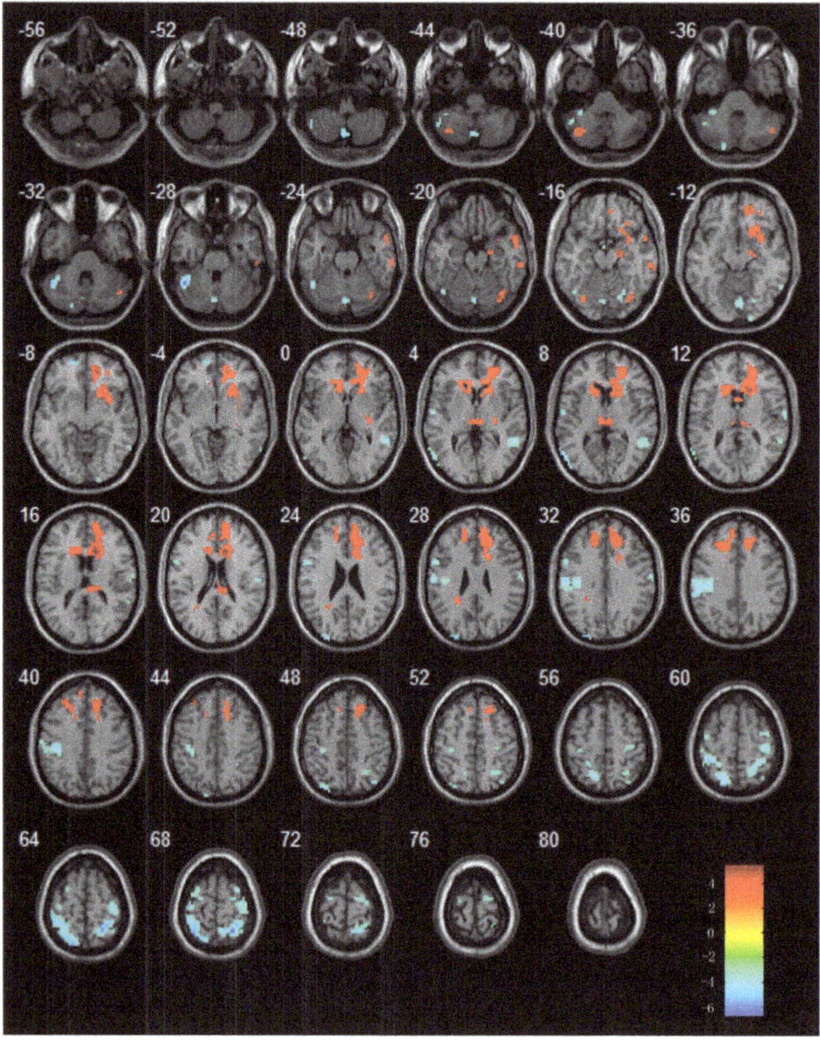

Figure 5. Regions showing increased or decreased activities in MCI subjects after acupuncture comparing to resting state. Left in picture is left in the brain. The color scale represents t values.

left SFG and right IFG showed decreased activities in MCI patients. To our knowledge, there were only a few previous studies using fMRI technique to explore the acupuncture effect on MCI patients. In our study we firstly found that acupuncture can modulate the brain activity in MCI patients bilaterally. That is to say, it can activate the regions which showed decreased activity in the resting state in MCI patients. It can also deactivate the regions which showed increased activity in the resting state in MCI patients.

During acupuncture, several regions showed increased or decreased activities in AD patients comparing to the resting state. However, the regions of left temporal lobe and left MFG were not be involved. We speculated that these regions probably can't be activated by the current acupoints. Future study is needed to elucidate its mechanism.

Brain activities in AD and MCI patients in the second resting state after acupuncture

In order to examine the post-effect of the acupuncture, we also studied brain activities in AD and MCI patients in the resting state after acupuncture. A lot of regions including the temporal lobe, the frontal lobe, the limbic regions and the CPL showed increased activities in MCI patients comparing to the resting state. Most of regions were involved in the temporal lobe and the frontal lobe, which were closely related to the memory and cognition, Except for these above regions, thalamus were also activated in the procession of acupuncture in MCI patients. Zhang et al. showed that thalamus is a vital region that integrates neural activity from widespread neocortical inputs and outputs, and modulate and facilitate communication in all areas of the cerebral cortex [36]. One of our

Table 6. Regions showing increased or decreased activities in AD subjects after acupuncture comparing to resting state.

Regions	BA	Cluster Size	Coordinates (MNI) x	y	z	T-score
AD vs. NOR ↑						
Rt. Cerebellum Posterior lobe ↑	-	29	48	−67	−29	4.48
Lt. Inferior Temporal Gyrus ↑	20	7	−60	−22	−26	4.43
Rt. Middle Temporal Gyrus ↑	21	10	−66	−43	−5	3.50
Lt. Inferior Frontal Gyrus ↑	47	7	−12	14	−14	3.49
Rt. Superior Frontal Gyrus ↑	10	32	21	62	1	5.08
Rt. Middle Frontal Gyrus ↑	47	45	30	35	−2	4.47
Lt. Superior Frontal Gyrus ↑	8	52	−15	29	46	4.27
Rt. Superior Frontal Gyrus ↑	6	11	3	32	61	3.42
Lt. Precentral Gyrus ↑	6	11	−9	−22	67	3.34
Rt. Precentral Gyrus ↑	6	30	21	−22	70	3.72
Lt. Medial Frontal Gyrus ↑	6	7	−3	−16	76	3.65
Rt. Middle Occipital Gyrus ↑	19	49	48	−82	−2	4.71
Lt. Middle Occipital Gyrus ↑	19/18	1365	−42	−79	13	4.81
Lt. Supramarginal Gyrus ↑	40	5	−54	−43	31	3.29
Rt. Supramarginal Gyrus ↑	40	23	48	−52	34	3.50
Rt. Superior Parietal lobule	7	23	39	−61	61	4.46
AD vs. NOR ↓						
Lt. Cerebellum Posterior Lobe ↓	-	7	−21	−61	−23	−3.64
Rt. Parahippocampa Gyrus ↓	35	12	21	−10	−14	−3.88
Lt. Parahippocampa Gyrus ↓	35-	5	−33	−28	−26	−3.68
Lt. Parahippocampa Gyrus ↓	35	100	−15	−25	−14	−4.10
Rt.Middle Friontal Gyrus ↓	6	23	42	−1	46	−3.58
Lt. Lingual Gyrus ↓	18	41	−3	−61	1	−3.95
Rt.Cingulate Gyrus ↓	-	11	12	−4	37	−3.40
Rt.Cingulate Gyrus ↓	-	15	6	−1	49	−3.57
Lt. Lentiform Nucleus ↓	-	36	−15	−4	7	−3.95
Rt. Brainstem ↓	-	5	6	−19	−14	−3.35

recent studies showed that disruption between the thalamus and posterior cingulate cortex (PCC) in MCI suggested the cognitive decline [37]. We noticed that the FG was activated, which showed decreased activity in the resting state. On the other hand, several regions showed decreased activity in MCI patients comparing to the resting state. Among these regions, we noticed left MTG and left IFG presented decreased activity, which showed increased activity in the resting state. This was similar with the brain activities in MCI patients in the procession of acupuncture.

After acupuncture, several regions showed increased or decreased activities in AD patients comparing to the resting state.

The activated regions include the frontal lobe, the occipital lobe, the parietal lobe and the temporal lobe. We noticed the region of left temporal lobe (ITG) was involved, which showed decreased activity in resting state. In addition, we also noticed the region of left temporal lobe (PHG) showed decreased activity after acupuncture. We speculated that the temporal lobe, as is subjected to be impaired in AD patients, was activated to compensate for the cognitive impairment.

Conclusions

In conclusion, we investigated the effect of acupuncture in AD and MCI patients by combing fMRI and traditional acupuncture. Our fMRI study confirmed that acupuncture at Tai chong (Liv3) and He gu (LI4) can activate certain cognitive-related regions in AD and MCI patients.

Author Contributions

Conceived and designed the experiments: JL KL. Performed the experiments: ZW DL ZZ. Analyzed the data: BN BS. Contributed reagents/materials/analysis tools: BN YH HS. Wrote the paper: ZW BN JL. Provided assistance in acupucture: JX.

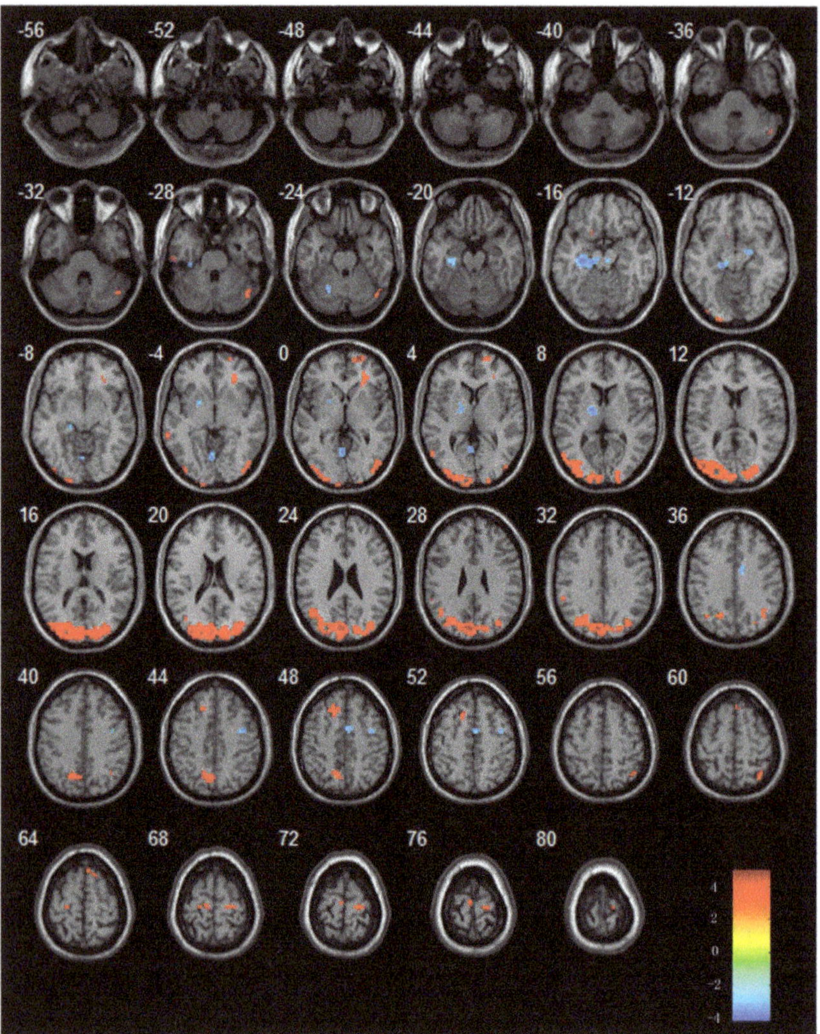

Figure 6. Regions showing increased or decreased activities in AD subjects after acupuncture comparing to resting state. Left in picture is left in the brain. The color scale represents t values.

References

1. Braak H, Braak E (1991) Neuropathological stageing of Alzheimer-related changes. Acta Neuropathol 82:239–259.
2. Petersen RC, Doody R, Kurz A, Mohs RC, Morris JC, et al. (2001) Current concepts in mild cognitive impairment. Arch Neurol 58:1985–1992.
3. Lu L, Liu Y, Zhu W, Shi J, Liu Y, et al. (2009) Traditional medicine in the treatment of drug addiction. Am J Drug Alcohol Abuse. 35(1):1–11.
4. Li G, Yang ES (2011) An fMRI study of acupuncture-induced brain activation of aphasia stroke patients. Complement Ther Med. 19 Suppl 1:S49–59.
5. Zhong XY, Su XX, Liu J, Zhu GQ (2009) Clinical effects of acupuncture combined with nimodipine for treatment of vascular dementia in 30 cases. J Tradit Chin Med. 29:174–6.
6. Allen G, Barnard H, McColl R, Hester AL, Fields JA, et al. (2007) Reduced hippocampal functional connectivity in Alzheimer disease. Arch Neurol 64:1482–1487.
7. Wang L, Zang Y, He Y, Liang M, Zhang X, et al. (2006) Changes in hippocampal connectivity in the early stages of Alzheimer's disease: evidence from resting state fMRI. Neuroimage 31:496–504.
8. Wang Z, Liang P, Jia X, Qi Z, Yu L, et al. (2011) Baseline and longitudinal patterns of hippocampal connectivity in mild cognitive impairment: evidence from resting state fMRI. Journal of the Neurological Sciences. 309:79–85.
9. Wang K, Liang M, Wang L, Tian L, Zhang X, et al. (2007) Altered functional connectivity in early Alzheimer's disease: a resting-state fMRI study. Hum Brain Mapp 28:967–978.
10. Zhang HY, Wang SJ, Xing J, Liu B, Ma ZL, et al. (2009) Detection of PCC functional connectivity characteristics in resting-state fMRI in mild Alzheimer's disease. Behav Brain Res 197:103–108.
11. Wang Z, Liang P, Jia X, Jin G, Song H, et al. (2012) The baseline and longitudinal changes of PCC connectivity in mild cognitive impairment: a combined structure and resting-state fMRI study. PLoS ONE 7: e36838.
12. Greicius MD, Srivastava G, Reiss AL, Menon V (2004) Default-mode network activity distinguishes Alzheimer's disease from healthy aging: evidence from functional MRI. Proc Natl Acad Sci U S A 101: 4637–4642.
13. Sorg C, Riedl V, Muhlau M, Calhoun VD, Eichele T, et al. (2007) Selective changes of resting-state networks in individuals at risk for Alzheimer's disease. Proc Natl Acad Sci U S A 104:18760–18765.
14. Feng Y, Bai L, Ren Y, Wang H, Liu Z, et al. (2011) Investigation of the large-scale functional brain networks modulated by acupuncture. Magn Reson Imaging. 29:958–65.
15. Zhong C, Bai L, Dai R, Xue T, Wang H, et al. (2012) Modulatory effects of acupuncture on resting-state networks: a functional MRI study combining independent component analysis and multivariate Granger causality analysis. J Magn Reson Imaging. 35:572–81.
16. Bai L, Qin W, Tian J, Dong M, Pan X, et al. (2009) Acupuncture modulates spontaneous activities in the anticorrelated resting brain networks. Brain Res. 1279:37–49.
17. Bai LJ, Qin W, Tian J, Dai JP, Yang WH (2009) Detection of dynamic brain networks modulated by acupuncture using a graph theory model. Prog Nat Sci 19:827–35.

18. Dhond RP, Yeh C, Park K, Kettner N, Napadow V (2008) Acupuncture modulates resting state connectivity in default and sensorimotor brain networks. Pain 136:407–18.
19. Yan B, Li K, Xu J, Wang W, Li K, et al. (2005) Acupoint-specific fMRI patterns in human brain. Neurosci Lett. 383(3):236–40.
20. Bai L, Tian J, Zhong C, Xue T, You Y, et al. (2010) Acupuncture modulates temporal neural responses in wide brain networks: evidence from fMRI study. Mol Pain 6: 73.
21. Hui KK, Liu J, Makris N, Gollub RL, Chen AJ, et al. (2000) Acupuncture modulates the limbic system and subcortical gray structures of the human brain: evidence from fMRI studies in normal subjects. Hum Brain Mapp. 9:13–25.
22. Wu MT, Hsieh JC, Xiong J, Yang CF, Pan HB, et al. (1999) Central nervous pathway for acupuncture stimulation: localization of processing with functional MR imaging of the brain a preliminary experience, Radiology. 212(1):133–41.
23. Zhang G, Yin H, Zhou YL, Han HY, Wu YH, et al. (2012) Capturing Amplitude Changes of Low-Frequency Fluctuations in Functional Magnetic Resonance Imaging Signal: A Pilot Acupuncture Study on NeiGuan (PC6). J Altern Complement Med. 18:387–93.
24. Zhou Y, Jin J (2008) Effect of acupuncture given at the HT 7, ST 36, ST 40 and KI 3 acupoints on various parts of the brains of Alzheimer's disease patients. Acupunct Electrother Res. 33:9–17.
25. Feng Y, Bai L, Ren Y, Chen S, Wang H, et al. (2012) FMRI connectivity analysis of acupuncture effects on the whole brain network in mild cognitive impairment patients. Magn Reson Imaging. 30:672–82.
26. Morris JC (1993) The Clinical Dementia Rating (CDR): current version and scoring rules. Neurology 43: 2412–4.
27. Petersen RC, Smith GE, Waring SC, Ivnik RJ, Tangalos EG, et al. (1999) Mild cognitive impairment: clinical characterization and outcome. Arch Neurol 56: 303–8.
28. Buckner RL, Andrews-Hanna JR, Schacter DL (2008) The brain's default network: anatomy, function, and relevance to disease. Ann N Y Acad Sci 1124: 1–38.
29. Raichle ME, MacLeod AM, Snyder AZ, Powers WJ, Gusnard DA, et al. (2001) A default mode of brain function. Proc Natl Acad Sci U S A 98: 676–82.
30. Greicius MD, Krasnow B, Reiss AL, Menon V (2003) Functional connectivity in the resting brain: a network analysis of the default mode hypothesis. Proc Natl Acad Sci U S A 100: 253–8.
31. Bookheimer SY, Strojwas MH, Cohen MS, Saunders AM, Pericak-Vance MA, et al. (2000) Patterns of brain activation in people at risk for Alzheimer's disease. N Engl J Med 343: 450–6.
32. Dickerson BC, Salat DH, Bates JF, Atiya M, Killiany RJ, et al. (2004) Medial temporal lobe function and structure in mild cognitive impairment. Ann Neurol 56: 27–35.
33. Dickerson BC, Sperling RA (2008) Functional abnormalities of the medial temporal lobe memory system in mild cognitive impairment and Alzheimer's disease: insights from functional MRI studies. Neuropsychologia 46: 1624–35.
34. Hamalainen A, Pihlajamaki M, Tanila H, Hanninen T, Niskanen E, et al. (2007) Increased fMRI responses during encoding in mild cognitive impairment. Neurobiol Aging 28: 1889–903.
35. He Y, Wang L, Zang Y, Tian L, Zhang X, et al. (2007) Regional coherence changes in the early stages of Alzheimer's disease: a combined structural and resting-state functional MRI study. Neuroimage 35:488–500.
36. Zhang D, Snyder AZ, Fox MD, Sansbury MW, Shimony JS, et al. (2008) Intrinsic functional relations between human cerebral cortex and thalamus. J Neurophysiol 100:1740–1748.
37. Wang Z, Jia X, Liang P, Qi Z, Yang Y, et al. (2012) Changes in thalamus connectivity in mild cognitive impairment: Evidence from resting state fMRI. Eur J Radiol., 81:277–285.

4

Determining the Precise Cerebral Response to Acupuncture: An Improved fMRI Study

Hua Liu[1,2,3*], Jianyang Xu[4], Baoci Shan[1,3], Yongzhong Li[5], Lin Li[1,3], Jingquan Xue[1,3], Binbin Nie[1,3]

1 Institute of High Energy Physics, Chinese Academy of Sciences (CAS), Beijing, China, 2 Graduate University of Chinese Academy of Sciences, Beijing, China, 3 Key Laboratory of Nuclear Analysis Techniques (LNAT), CAS, Beijing, China, 4 General Hospital of Armed Police Forces, Beijing, China, 5 Xuanwu Hospital, Capital Medical University, Beijing, China

Abstract

Background: In acupuncture brain imaging trials, there are many non-acupuncture factors confounding the neuronal mapping. The modality of the placebo, subjects' psychological attitude to acupuncture and their physical state are the three most confounding factors.

Objective: To obtain more precise and accurate cerebral fMRI mapping of acupuncture.

Design and Setting: A 2×2 randomized, controlled, participant-blinded cross-over factorial acupuncture trial was conducted at Xuanwu Hospital in Beijing, China.

Participants: Forty-one college students with myopia were recruited to participate in our study and were allocated randomly to four groups, Group A, Group B, Group C and Group D.

Interventions: Group A received real acupuncture (RA) and treatment instruction (TI); Group B received RA and non-treatment instruction (NI); Group C received sham acupuncture (SA) and TI; Group D received SA and NI.

Results: Stimulation at LR3 activated some areas of the visual cortex, and the cerebral response to non-acupuncture factors was complex and occurred in multiple areas.

Conclusions: The results provide more evidence regarding the credibility of acupuncture therapy and suggest that more precise experimental designs are needed to eliminate sources of bias in acupuncture controlled trials and to obtain sound results.

Editor: Wang Zhan, University of Maryland, United States of America

Funding: The authors have no support or funding to report.

Competing Interests: The authors have declared that no competing interests exist.

* E-mail: liuhua@ihep.ac.cn

These authors contributed equally to this work.

Introduction

Many studies have been performed using functional magnetic resonance imaging (fMRI) to investigate the cerebral matrix related to acupuncture therapy. [1,2,3,4,5] A rather variable pattern in blood oxygenation-level dependent (BOLD) signal changes were obtained in those studies, even at specific acupoints. These variable patterns are indicative of non-acupuncture factors that confound the results.

The creditability of the placebo is an important factor in acupuncture trials. [6] The most commonly used control modality is 'sham acupuncture', of which the depth of insertion and stimulation is the same as the RA, but the insertion points differ. During the procedure, sham acupuncture is matched as closely as possible with the real acupuncture. However, studies have pointed out that sham acupuncture appears to have an analgesic effect similar to that of real acupuncture. [7] Evidence from clinical trials suggests that sham acupuncture has little effect on nausea and is primarily a placebo. [6,8].

Patients participate in some studies, whereas healthy volunteers are involved in others. LI4 (Hegu) is one of the most common acupoints to be investigated in analgesic studies. The consistency of the experimental results is, however, not ideal. [2,9,10] For a specific acupoint, the physical status of a subject should be taken into greater consideration.

Psychological factors, especially an individual's expectations, can alter their physical condition and have treatment effects. [11] The same situation exists in acupuncture trials. [12] In acupuncture imaging trials, neither positive nor negative psychological tendencies should be eliminated.

In this fMRI study, we employed a 2×2 single-blind randomized cross-over factorial design to filter the cerebral responses from those non-acupuncture factors mentioned above and to obtain a more precise estimation of neuronal responses to acupuncture at LR3 (Taichong).

Table 1. Comparisons of behavioral results.

		RA		SA	
		Group A	Group B	Group C	Group D
Credibility scores comparison		QB QA		QB QA	
P value (χ^2)	Group A	–	–	0.42 0.56	–
Needling sensation scores	Mean (SD)	14.25 (7.44)	12.46 (7.02)	4.23 (5.01)	3.77 (3.58)
comparison	95% CI	8.96–18.35	6.45–16.91	2.57–7.38	2.09–6.88
	Mean (SD)	13.75 (7.23)		3.97 (4.35)	
	95% CI	6.45–18.35		2.57–7.38	

Scores of credibility and belief comparison between Group A and Group C, and needle sensation for all four interventions.
RA: real acupuncture; SA: sham acupuncture; QB: questions before treatment (How confident are you that this treatment can alleviate your complaint?); QA: questions after treatment (How confident would you be in recommending this treatment to a friend who suffered from the same complaint?).

Participants and Methods

1. Subjects

The study was approved by the Ethics Committee of the Chinese Academy of Sciences (Beijing, China). We obtained written informed consent from all participants involved in the study.

Forty-one college students with myopia (male/female = 21/20, age 25.7±3.7 years, all right-handed) were recruited to participate in our study. No subjects had a history of neurological or psychiatric illness and all were acupuncture naive. Subjects were free of any transient medical problems and did not take any medications the day prior to the study.

2. Experimental Groups and Acupuncture

All the subjects were divided into four groups randomly.

Subjects in Group A (n = 11) underwent real acupuncture (RA), and were told they would receive acupuncture treatment which would surely benefit their myopia before MRI scan (treatment instruction).

Subjects in Group B (n = 11) received RA stimulation, but were told they were participating in an experiment to estimate a medical machine's sensitivity of detecting tactile signals (non-treatment instruction).

Subjects in Group C (n = 10) received stimulation at the sham acupoint (SA) and treatment instruction.

Subjects in Group D (n = 9) received stimulation at the SA and non-treatment instruction.

Each subject underwent only one of the four interventions, and each participant received the individual instructions only before the MRI scan. Each subject participated in the trial individually to avoid inter-participant interaction.

The acupuncture point left LR3 (Taichong) is located in the muscle bulk between the 1st and 2nd phalangeals on the dorsum of the left foot. One sham acupuncture point was chosen approximately 10 mm anterior to the classical site.

For Group A and Group C, before scanning, participants were asked two questions regarding credibility rating. [13] Each question was measured on a 0–6 Likert scale with 6 being the most credible.

All subjects completed a needle sensation questionnaire (NSQ) after scanning. We adopted an NSQ scale system to evaluate the needling sensation during acupuncture, with scores ranging from 0 (minimum) to 75 (maximum). [14].

After entering the scanning room, all subjects underwent resting scanning for 186 seconds (62 scans) first. A sterile, single-use silver needle (25 mm in length ×0.30 mm in diameter) was then inserted into the real acupoint or the sham acupoint, and the needle was twirled manually clockwise and counterclockwise at 1 Hz with even reinforcing and reducing manipulation for 180 seconds (60 scans). The needle was subsequently extracted while fMRI scanning continued for a total of 402 scans for every subject. The depth of needle insertion was approximately 10 mm, and all the acupuncture manipulations were performed by the same acupuncturist (Dr. Jianyang Xu, the General Hospital of the Armed Police Forces).

3. fMRI Procedure and Data Analysis

The experiments were performed with a 1.5-T whole body MRI scanner (Siemens, Sonata, Germany), with a standard head coil. Images spanned the entire head and were parallel to the anterior commissure-posterior commissure line. Functional images were obtained using a BOLD T2*-weighted gradient-echo EPI sequence with an in-plane resolution of 3.59 mm (TR = 3000 ms, TE = 50 ms, flip angle 90°, field of view = 230 mm×230 mm, matrix = 64×64 mm, 6-mm slice thickness and 1.2-mm slice gap).

The data were analyzed with statistical parametric mapping (SPM2) software (Welcome Department of Imaging Neuroscience, London, UK). The first two scans were discarded, so every subject had a final total of 400 volumes. After realignment, the images were normalized to the Montreal Neurological Institute (MNI) space and then smoothed spatially using a 9 mm×9 mm×9 mm Gaussian kernel. The estimated data were analyzed at two levels. The first level, for each individual subject, was a fixed-effect analysis based on the general linear model with a box-car response function as the reference waveform convolved with the Poisson hemodynamic response function. The cerebral areas activated during acupuncture relative to the baseline were obtained. The second level was performed using random-effect analysis based on a one-way analysis of variance model with fixed effect results to obtain intergroup comparisons. The results were reported using Talairach space coordinates.

Results

1. Behavioral Results

Credibility. Credibility ratings were compared using a χ^2 test (Table 1). There were no statistical differences between scores for Group A and Group C.

Table 2. Spatial coordinates and levels of significance of the activations.

Contrasts	Anatomical structure	Side	Talairach space coordinates			Statistical significance
			x	y	z	Z
RA−SA>0	VII	R	4	−83	32	2.91
	Visual-parietal area	R	35	−54	23	2.49
EG−NE>0	MFG	L	−2	35	48	4.06
	OFC	R	44	19	−13	2.85
		L	−42	25	−15	3.27
	DLPFC	R	42	38	26	2.96
		L	−24	61	8	3.07
	SII	R	67	−7	13	2.85
		L	−61	−23	12	2.73
	Temporal pole	L	−24	4	−30	2.84
	VII	R	36	−93	0	3.16
	Cerebellum	R	4	−71	−13	2.62
		L	−18	−85	−19	2.71
	Uncus	L	−24	4	−30	2.7
Group A−Group C>0	VII	R	6	−80	32	3.04
	Cerebellum	R	18	−30	−15	4.04
		L	−34	−45	−40	2.64
Group B−Group D>0	VII	L	−14	−59	18	2.79
	OFC	R	26	38	−19	3.72
Group A−Group B>0	MFG	L	−1	33	35	3.09
	DLPFC	R	40	36	28	2.47
		L	−26	59	10	3.59
	OFC	R	46	19	−13	2.94
	SI/MI	L	−6	−39	65	2.55
		R	4	16	43	3.21
	SII	R	50	−52	50	2.79
		R	28	−65	60	3.42
	Temporal pole	L	−44	20	−23	2.88
	VI	R	20	−82	−11	3.57
	VII	R	28	−64	3	2.94
	Uncus	L	−24	2	−32	2.78
	Cerebellum	R	12	−59	−9	2.86
		L	−20	−85	−19	2.61
Group C−Group D>0	MFG	L	−4	37	50	3.36

$p<0.001$ uncorrected and $k=10$ continuous voxels.
VII: secondary visual cortex; MFG: medial frontal gyrus; OFC: orbital frontal cortex; DLPFC: dorsum lateral prefrontal cortex; SI/MI: first sensory-motor cortex; SII: secondary sensory cortex.

Needle sensation. The mean scores for needle sensation are shown in Table 1. There are no statistical differences between Group A and Group B or between Group C and Group D. RA did elicit significantly different sensations from SA.

2. fMRI Results

SPM maps of the random effect analysis threshold were at $p<0.001$ uncorrected and $k=10$ continuous voxels. Subjects receiving real acupuncture made up the RA group, and those receiving the sham acupuncture made up the SA group. Subjects receiving treatment instruction made up the EG group, and those not receiving treatment instruction made up the NE group. The comparison of spatial coordinates of area activations are listed in Table 2.

RA vs. SA. Activations occurred in the upper division of the right occipital cuneus, the secondary visual cortex (VII) (Fig. 1a).

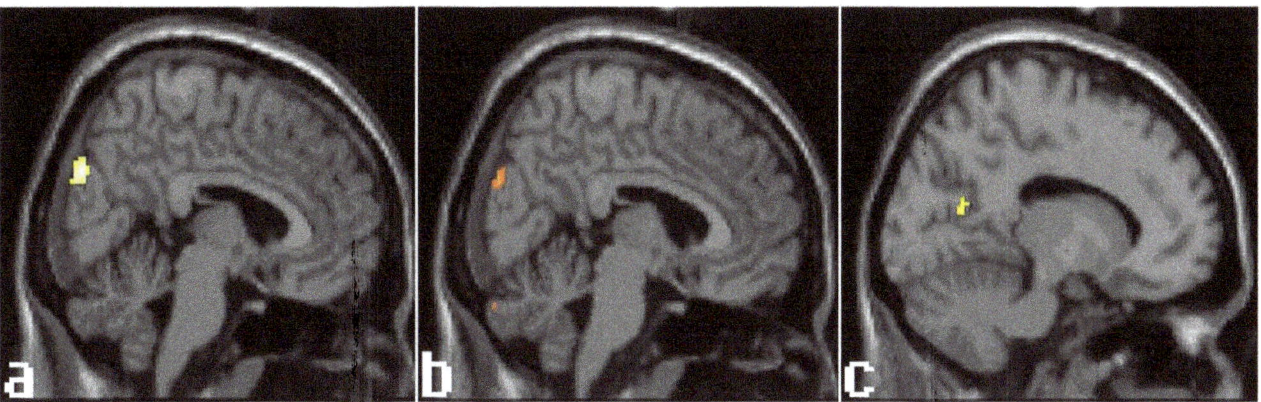

Figure 1. Activation of visual-related cortex by acupuncture. a: Activation in RA vs. SA. b: Activation in Group A vs. Group C. c: Activation in Group B vs. Group D. In both RA vs. SA and Group A vs. Group C, the activation occurred in the same right superior part of VII. The activation in Group B vs. Group D is in the interior part of the left VII. SPM maps the threshold at $p<0.001$, uncorrected for multiple comparison. See Table 2 for details. RA: real acupuncture (Group A with Group B). SA: sham acupuncture (Group C with Group D).

EG vs. NE. Areas in the left medial frontal gyrus (MFG) (Fig. 2 a1), bilateral dorsum lateral prefrontal cortex (DLPFC) (Fig. 2 a3), bilateral orbital frontal cortex (OFC) (Fig. 2 a2) and bilateral posterior lobe of the cerebellum were activated.

Group A vs. Group C. The right superior division of the cuneus, part of VII (Fig. 1b), the right culmen of the cerebellar anterior lobe and the left cerebellar tonsil were activated.

Group B vs. Group D. The left interior division of VII (Fig. 1c) and the right OFC were activated.

Group A vs. Group B. The left medial frontal cortex (Fig. 2 b1), right OFC (Fig. 2 b2), SII, the visual-temporal area, the inferior division of VII, the anterior lobe of the cerebellum, and the bilateral DLPFC (Fig. 2 b3) were activated.

Group C vs. Group D. Areas in the left MFG (Fig. 2 c1) were activated.

Discussion

The behavioral effect of acupuncture stimulation at the real acupoint is different from the effect at the sham acupoint. Furthermore, subjects receiving the treatment instruction exhibited sound expectancy due to the psychological effect of our instruction.

1. The Specific Effect of Acupuncture at LR3

According to Chinese traditional medicine, LR3 is a fundamental acupoint, and acupuncture at this point is used to treat many disorders including eye diseases. Some studies have found that acupuncture at LR3 decreases intraocular pressure. [15,16] Those studies suggested that acupuncture at visual-related acupoints could modulate optical physiology. In this study, the superior part of the secondary visual cortex (VII) was activated in two contrasting conditions (RA vs. SA and Group A vs. Group C), and the interior part of VII was activated in the other contrasting condition (Group B vs. Group D). VII plays an important role in the integration of visual information and visual physiology. [17] How stimulation at certain point(s) modulates certain organs is the secret of acupuncture. In many trials examining the anesthesia effect of acupuncture, some pain-related regions are mentioned. [2,18] Acupuncture may modulate central neural activity through a crossed spino-thalamo-cortico-limibic pathway or a direct uncrossed spino-thalmo-limibic pathway. [12,19,20] Acupuncture at LR3, an acupoint on the foot, may control eye-related cortex via those pathways; however, those studies did not give direct proof.

2. The Effect of Non-acupuncture

In this study, we adopted a "sham acupoint" as a placebo rather than other placebo modalities, such as minimal acupuncture, mock transcutaneous nerve stimulation (TENS) and Streitberger needle (SN). [21] TENS and SN can give subjects the impression of being pierced by an acupuncture, which are credible as placebos for psychological effects, but have no actually straight physiological effects. It means that the physical proprioception to needle stimulation is absent. We considered the "sham acupoint" as a placebo was credible and primarily acted as a placebo in this non-painful study.

The choice of subjects with myopia was based on the following consideration. Myopia is one relatively simple pathological condition and other systemic states are normal, so the complex response originating from irrelevant systems could be avoided. The output of cerebral mapping to acupuncture may be reflected in a normal physiological state. Moreover, to such a specific disorder, the psychological instruction could be implanted definitely and specifically.

Among the confounding factors in acupuncture studies, the most variable item is the psychological condition of subjects toward acupuncture therapy. Expectancy and belief have been proven to modulate the neuronal substrates of pain treated by acupuncture. [12] In this study, we introduced a distinct expectancy factor, not for its therapeutic efficacy for myopia but for its confounding effect in neuronal imaging of acupuncture stimulation. In all three contrasting conditions aimed to elicit cerebral responses to expectancy, the ipsilateral MFG, contralateral OFC, contralateral secondary sensory cortex (SII) and contralateral cerebellum were activated. The contralateral DLPFC, temporal pole and hippocampi uncus were activated in EG vs. NE and Group A vs. Group B. Many studies have validated the medial frontal gyrus- and DLPFC-related expectancy, emotion and cognitive control. [11,22,23] The temporal pole and hippocampi uncus are classical areas related to emotion. The activation of MFG is pronounced, so we proposed that the activity of the medial gyrus is involved in the modulation of acupuncture expectation. The function of the cerebellum has been confirmed to be not just limited to motor control but to play an important role in cognition and emotion including expectation. [23,24] Given the

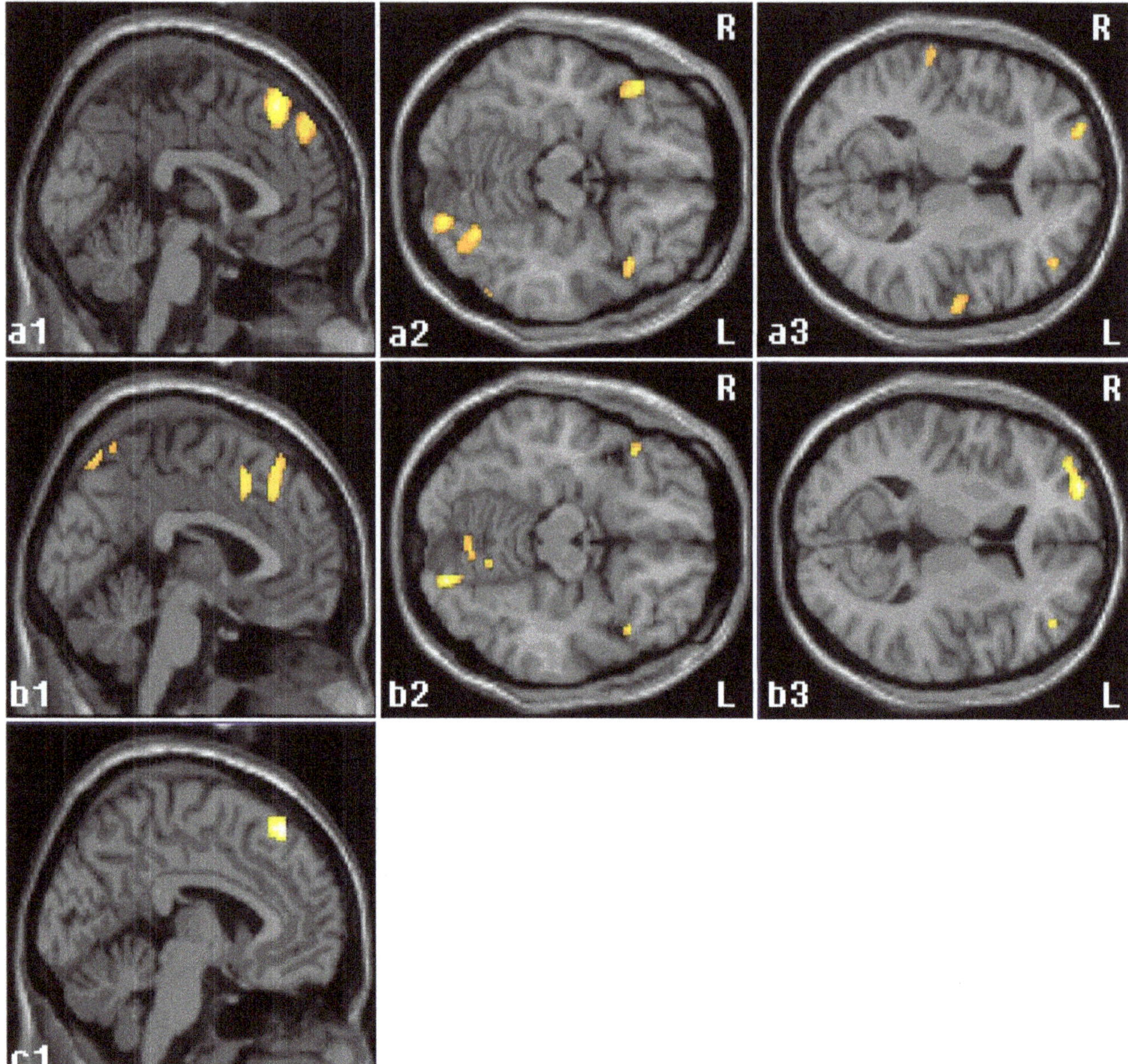

Figure 2. Activations related to the effect of expectancy interventions. a: Activations in EG vs. NE. b: Activations in Group A vs. Group B. c: Activations in Group C vs. Group D. In those three interventions, the left medial cortex, bilateral OFC and right posterior lobe of the cerebellum were activated (a1, a2, b1, b2, c1). In both EG vs. NE and Group A vs. Group B, bilateral DLPFC were activated (a3, b3). SPM maps the threshold at $p<0.001$ uncorrected. See Table 2 for details. EG: expectancy group (Group A with Group C). NE: no-expectancy group (Group B with Group D).

complicated function of the cerebellum and our experimental design, we argued that the activation of the cerebellum in this study was related to expectancy.

Conclusions

After filtering out confounding non-acupuncture factors, stimulation at LR3 was shown to activate some areas of the visual cortex. Such a result provided more evidence regarding the credibility of acupuncture therapy. On the other hand, cerebral responses to some non-acupuncture factors were complex and occurred in multiple areas, which may overlap with the neuronal responses to acupuncture. More precise experimental designs are needed to eliminate sources of bias in acupuncture controlled trials and to obtain sound results.

Author Contributions

Conceived and designed the experiments: HL. Performed the experiments: J. Xu LL. Analyzed the data: BS BN. Contributed reagents/materials/analysis tools: J. Xue YL. Wrote the paper: HL.

References

1. Fang B, Hayes JC (1999) Functional MRI explores mysteries of acupuncture. Diagn Imaging (San Franc) 21: 19–21.
2. Hui KK, Liu J, Makris N, Gollub RL, Chen AJ, et al. (2000) Acupuncture modulates the limbic system and subcortical gray structures of the human brain: evidence from fMRI studies in normal subjects. Hum Brain Mapp 9: 13–25.
3. Wu MT, Sheen JM, Chuang KH, Yang P, Chin SL, et al. (2002) Neuronal specificity of acupuncture response: a fMRI study with electroacupuncture. Neuroimage 16: 1028–1037.
4. Yan B, Li K, Xu J, Wang W, Li K, et al. (2005) Acupoint-specific fMRI patterns in human brain. Neurosci Lett 383: 236–240.
5. Yoo SS, Teh EK, Blinder RA, Jolesz FA (2004) Modulation of cerebellar activities by acupuncture stimulation: evidence from fMRI study. Neuroimage 22: 932–940.
6. Vincent C, Lewith G (1995) Placebo controls for acupuncture studies. J R Soc Med 88: 199–202.
7. Lewith GT, Machin D (1983) On the evaluation of the clinical effects of acupuncture. Pain 16: 111–127.
8. Dundee JW, McMillan CM (1992) P6 acupressure and postoperative vomiting. Br J Anaesth 68: 225–226.
9. Kong J, Ma L, Gollub RL, Wei J, Yang X, et al. (2002) A pilot study of functional magnetic resonance imaging of the brain during manual and electroacupuncture stimulation of acupuncture point (LI-4 Hegu) in normal subjects reveals differential brain activation between methods. J Altern Complement Med 8: 411–419.
10. Wu MT, Hsieh JC, Xiong J, Yang CF, Pan HB, et al. (1999) Central nervous pathway for acupuncture stimulation: localization of processing with functional MR imaging of the brain–preliminary experience. Radiology 212: 133–141.
11. Wager TD, Rilling JK, Smith EE, Sokolik A, Casey KL, et al. (2004) Placebo-induced changes in FMRI in the anticipation and experience of pain. Science 303: 1162–1167.
12. Pariente J, White P, Frackowiak RS, Lewith G (2005) Expectancy and belief modulate the neuronal substrates of pain treated by acupuncture. Neuroimage 25: 1161–1167.
13. Vincent CA, Richardson PH (1986) The evaluation of therapeutic acupuncture: concepts and methods. Pain 24: 1–13.
14. Park H, Park J, Lee H, Lee H (2002) Does Deqi (needle sensation) exist? Am J Chin Med 30: 45–50.
15. Kim MS, Seo KM, Nam TC (2005) Effect of acupuncture on intraocular pressure in normal dogs. J Vet Med Sci 67: 1281–1282.
16. Uhrig S, Hummelsberger J, Brinkhaus B (2003) Standardized acupuncture therapy in patients with ocular hypertension or glaucoma–results of a prospective observation study. Forsch Komplementarmed Klass Naturheilkd 10: 256–261.
17. Ghose GM, Yang T, Maunsell JH (2002) Physiological correlates of perceptual learning in monkey V1 and V2. J Neurophysiol 87: 1867–1888.
18. Zhang WT, Jin Z, Huang J, Zhang L, Zeng YW, et al. (2003) Modulation of cold pain in human brain by electric acupoint stimulation: evidence from fMRI. Neuroreport 14: 1591–1596.
19. Price DD (2000) Psychological and neural mechanisms of the affective dimension of pain. Science 288: 1769–1772.
20. Craig AD (2003) Interoception: the sense of the physiological condition of the body. Curr Opin Neurobiol 13: 500–505.
21. Streitberger K, Kleinhenz J (1998) Introducing a placebo needle into acupuncture research. Lancet 352: 364–365.
22. Ridderinkhof KR, van den Wildenberg WP, Segalowitz SJ, Carter CS (2004) Neurocognitive mechanisms of cognitive control: the role of prefrontal cortex in action selection, response inhibition, performance monitoring, and reward-based learning. Brain Cogn 56: 129–140.
23. Ueda K, Okamoto Y, Okada G, Yamashita H, Hori T, et al. (2003) Brain activity during expectancy of emotional stimuli: an fMRI study. Neuroreport 14: 51–55.
24. Schmahmann JD, Pandya DN (1997) The cerebrocerebellar system. Int Rev Neurobiol 41: 31–60.

5

Electroacupuncture for Moderate and Severe Benign Prostatic Hyperplasia: A Randomized Controlled Trial

Yang Wang[1], Baoyan Liu[2], Jinna Yu[1], Jiani Wu[1], Jing Wang[1], Zhishun Liu[1]*

1 Guang'anmen Hospital, China Academy of Chinese Medical Sciences, Beijing, China, 2 China Academy of Chinese Medical Sciences, Beijing, China

Abstract

Purpose: To evaluate the effects of electroacupuncture (EA) on the International Prostate Symptom Score (IPSS), postvoid residual urine (PVR), and maximum urinary flow rate (Qmax), and explore the difference between EA at acupoints and non-acupoints in patients with moderate to severe benign prostate hyperplasia (BPH).

Subjects and Methods: Men with BPH and IPSS ≥8 were enrolled. Participants were randomly allocated to receive EA at acupoint (treatment group, n = 50) and EA at non-acupoint (control group, n = 50). The primary outcome measure includes the change of IPSS at the 6th week and the secondary outcome measures include changes of PVR and Qmax at the 6th week and change of IPSS at the 18th week.

Results: 100/192 patients were included. At the 6th week, treatment group patients had a 4.51 ($p<0.001$) and 4.12 ($p<0.001$) points greater decline in IPSS than the control group in the intention to treat (ITT) and per-protocol (PP) populations. At the 18th week, a 3.2 points ($p = 0.001$) greater decline was found in IPSS for the treatment. No significant differences were found between the two groups in Qmax at the 6th week ($p = 0.819$). No significant difference was observed in PVR ($P = 0.35$).

Conclusion: Acupoint EA at BL 33 had better effects on IPSS, but no difference on PVR and Qmax as compared with non-acupoint EA. The results indicate that EA is effective in improving patient's quality of life and acupoint may have better therapeutic effects than non-acupoints in acupuncture treatments of BPH.

Trial Registration: ClinicalTrials.gov NCT01218243.

Editor: Praveen Thumbikat, Northwestern University, United States of America

Funding: This study is supported by a grant from the "Twelfth Five-Year Plan" of National Science and Technology Support Program (Project Number: 2012BAI24B01) and Guang'anmen Hospital (2009S208). No other potential conflict of interest related to this trial. The funders had no role in study design, data collection and analysis, decision to publish, or preparation of the manuscript.

Competing Interests: The authors have declared that no competing interests exist.

* E-mail: liuzhishun@yahoo.com.cn

Introduction

Benign prostate hyperplasia (BPH) is an enlargement of the prostate gland due to progressive hyperplasia of the stromal and glandular cells of the prostate. The prevalence of BPH is as high as 40% in men in their fifties and 90% in men in their eighties [1]. BPH is one of the most common causes of lower urinary tract symptoms (LUTS) which include frequent urination, urgent urination, nocturia, urinary stream hesitancy, straining to void, and dribbling [1]. Although the pathophysiology of BPH is characterized by non-neoplastic histological changes, urine storage and voiding problems increase patients' risk of urinary tract infection and chronic kidney diseases and adversely affect patients' quality of life [2,3]. Current treatment options for BPH include watchful waiting, lifestyle modifications, alpha blockers, 5 alpha-reductase inhibitors, phytochemicals, and BPH-related surgery [4]. Although most of the aforementioned therapies have various degrees of documented effectiveness in the management of BPH, the use of these interventions are limited to specific patient populations or have certain side effects that interfere with patient's quality of life [5].

Acupuncture is a traditional Chinese medicine treatment which has been commonly used in the management of LUTS in China for thousands of years. The effects of acupuncture on LUTS were well documented in Chinese medicine textbooks and are well-supported by modern research studies [6]. Ricci et al [7] found that electroacupuncture (EA) had better effects in decreasing number of voiding times of urinary urgency that persisted after transurethral resection of the prostate. Kubista et al [8] found that EA could significantly increase the closing pressure in women with stress incontinence as compared with placebo, and Philp et al [9] found that acupuncture increased the bladder capacity in patients with bladder instability. Besides effects on urinary storage problems, acupuncture was also found effective in the prevention of recurrent lower urinary tract infections in adult women [10,11], in improving the quality of life in patients with chronic prostatis [12], in primary monosymptomatic nocturnal enuresis [13].

BPH is clinically characterized by various LUTS which may include or be similar to urinary urgency, stress incontinence,

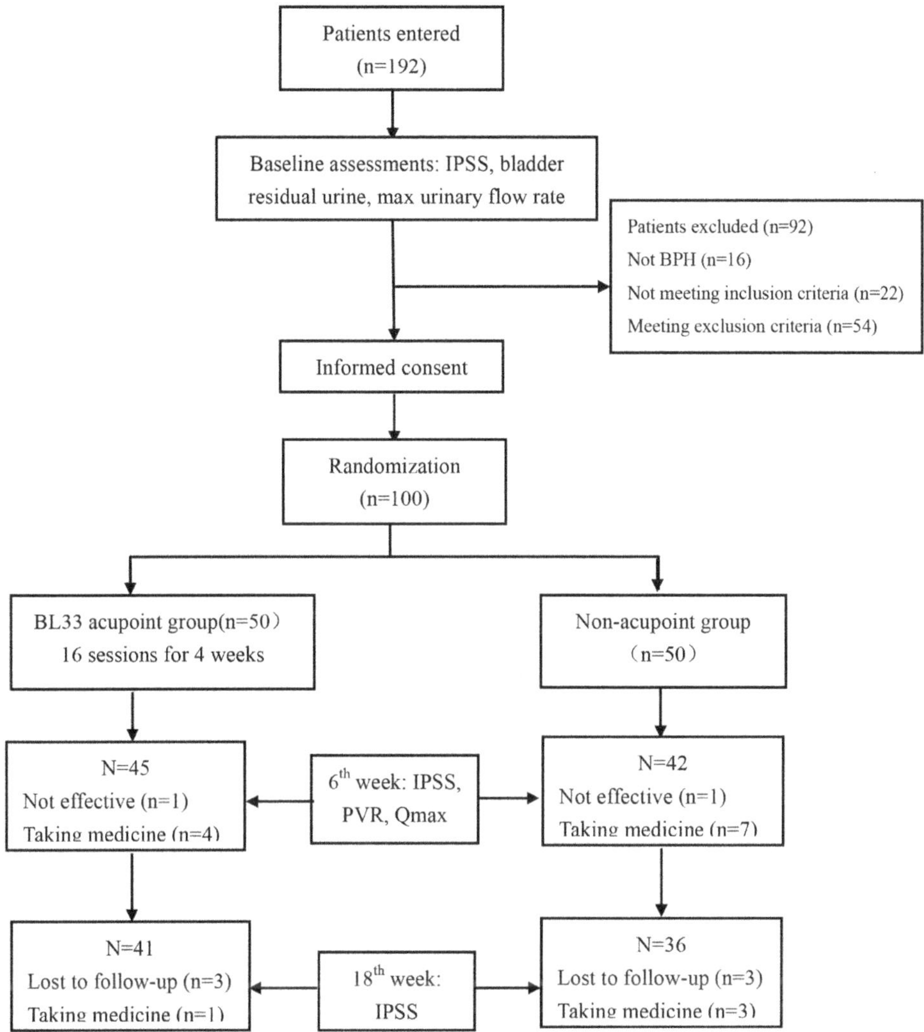

Figure 1. The flowchart of study participation.

bladder instability, and UTIs; therefore, we hypothesize that acupuncture may be effective in the management of BPH.

This hypothesis is supported by our previous studies in which we found that acupuncture at BL33 had better effects than terazosin in improving International Prostate Symptom Score (IPSS), post-void residual urine (PVR), and maximum urinary flow rate (Qmax) on patients diagnosed with mild to moderate BPH [14,15]. In addition, we also compared the therapeutic effectiveness of EA at bilateral acupoints of BL33 with EA at non-acupoints (2 cun [around 6.7 cm] lateral to BL33s) in a randomized controlled pilot study; the results demonstrated acupoint EA was more effective than non-acupoint EA in reducing IPSS [16]. However, terazosin is not necessarily the standardized treatment option for patients with BPH and the pilot study related to effects of acupoint on the EA treatment of BPH has a relative small sample size with efficacy measurements of IPSS only [14–16].

Theories of traditional Chinese medicine and results from modern studies indicate that acupoints of the fourteen meridians have specific functional regulatory effect on zang-fu organs [17–19]; however, studies in western countries found that dry needling, an acupuncture procedure at trigger points (including non-acupoints that do not belong to the meridian system), were effective in the management of various diseases [20–21]. Both dry needling and traditional acupuncture treat diseases via inserting stainless needles into the human body. However, differences between acupuncture at acupoints and acupuncture at non-acupoints have not been fully investigated. In the present study, we aimed to evaluate the effects of EA on IPSS, PVR, and Qmax, and explore the difference between EA at acupoints and non-acupoints in patients with moderate to severe BPH.

Methods

The protocol for this trial and supporting CONSORT checklist are available as supporting information; see Checklist S1 and Protocol S1.

Study Design

This was a randomized control trial which was performed at the Acupuncture Department of Guang An Men Hospital, China Academy of Chinese Medical Sciences. The study protocol was registered with ClinicalTrials. gov (Identifier: NCT01218243) and was previously published [22]. In the original study protocol, patients with IPSS score higher than 20 (including 20) were

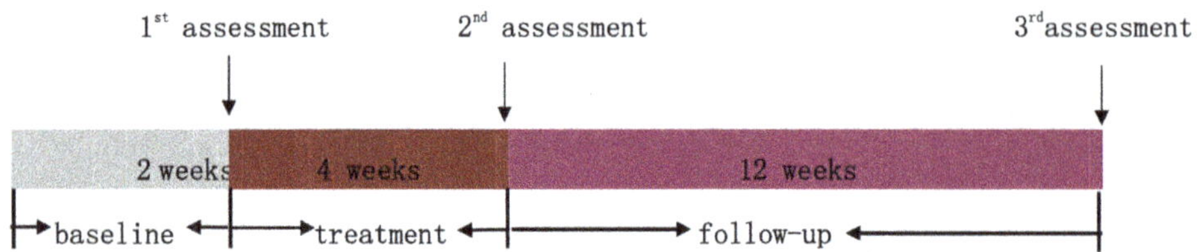

Figure 2. Time frame of each period. Figure 2 shows the time frame of baseline period, treatment period and follow-up period.

proposed to be excluded; however, we changed the inclusion criteria to patients with IPSS≥8 during the actual study, as most patients who visited the acupuncture department and were willing to participate in the study had moderate to severe BPH. The study design complies with the Consolidated Standards of Reporting Trials (CONSORT) and was approved by the hospital ethics committee. Participants were recruited through advertisements on local newspapers and posters and signed informed consent before study participation.

Sequentially numbered, opaque, sealed envelopes were distributed to patients by an investigator who was not involved in acupuncture procedures and data analyses. Based on odd or even numbers assigned in the envelope, participants were randomly allocated to receive EA at acupoint (treatment group, n = 50) and EA at non-acupoint(control group, n = 50).

Based on the results of our pilot study, the reduction of IPSS of the EA at acupointgroup was seven [16]. Therefore, in conjunction with methods and results of the studies by Chapple et al [23] and Yu et al [24], 50 patients will be needed for each group (1:1 allocation) in the present study to detect a seven point reduction in IPSS with a two-tailed significance level of 5% and a power of 90% while allowing for a 20% dropout rate. Sample size was calculated with a standard deviation (SD) of 2.30 as per reports in the epidemiology monograph by Wang [25].

Participants

For inclusion, the following criteria were fulfilled: 1) 50–70 years old; 2) mild to moderate BPH evaluated by I-PSS; 3) patients having urinary dysfunction more than 3 months; 4) patients with stable life signs; 5) not on any α1 receptor blocker, 5α-reductase inhibitor or traditional Chinese medicine for over 1 week; 6) volunteer to join this research and give informed consent prior to receiving treatment. For safety reasons, patients were instructed of possible emergency conditions and were told to seek appropriate medical help if happens.

The exclusion criteria included 1) urinary dysfunction caused by gonorrhea or urinary tract infection; 2) oliguria and anuria caused by urinary calculi, prostate cancer, bladder tumor and acute/chronic renal failure; 3) urinary dysfunction caused by neurogenic bladder, bladder neck fibrosis and urethral stricture; 4) failure of invasive therapy for prostatic obstruction; 5) injured local organs, muscle and nerve caused by pelvic operation or trauma; 6) upper urinary obstruction and hydrocoele combined with damaged renal function due to BPH diagnosed by B-ultrasound; 7) Patients unable to commit to treatment because of commuting problems to the hospital.

Table 1. Demographic Information and Baseline Characteristics.

	Acupoint group (n = 50)	Non-point group (n = 50)	P-value (two-tailed)
Age	64.80±7.05	65.94±6.74	0.411
Course of disease	76.08±57.59	73.66±57.72	0.834
IPSS	20.10±6.52	18.76±6.06	0.289
Qmax	13.04±6.73	15.93±7.33	0.051
PVR (ml)	20 (0,128)	16 (0,128)	0.260

Table 2. Descriptive Statistics of ITT Population.

		Acupoint group (n = 50)	Non-point group (n = 50)
IPSS	baseline	20.10±6.52	18.76±6.06
	6th week	12.84±5.87	16.42±6.80
	Change in IPSS	7.26±5.12	2.34±4.85
	18th week	14.62±5.76	16.96±6.47
	Change in IPSS	5.48±5.16	1.8±5.06
PVR (ml)	Baseline	20 (0,128)	16 (0,128)
	6th week	20 (0,300)	15(0,180)
	Change in PVR	0 (−172,84)	0 (−120,80)
Qmax,	Baseline	13.04±6.73	15.93±7.33
	6th week	12.63±6.11	15.00±6.50
	Change in Qmax	0.36±4.51	0.98±4.05

Initial diagnosis and assessment were made by an urologist who was not involved in the study. Patients on LUTS medications were requested to stop medications one week before baseline assessment. The baseline assessments included IPSS, PVR and Qmax.

Acupuncture protocol

Huatuo brand needles (size 0.30 mm×100 mm, manufactured by Suzhou Medical Appliance, Suzhou, Jiangsu Province, China) together with GB6805-2 Electro-Acu Stimulators (HuayiMedical Supply &Equipment Co., Ltd, Shanghai, China) were used. In traditional Chinese medicine, acupuncture at Baliao points (BL31-34) are commonly used as treatment options for LUTS, lumbodynia, and reproductive disorders [6]; our previous study confirmed the effects of acupuncture at BL33 on LUTS [14–16]. In the present study, BL33s were used in the acupoint treatment group; whereas the two points which are 2 cun (around 6.7 cm) lateral to BL33s were used in the non-acupoint control group. Localization of BL33 which corresponds with the third sacral foramen was reported previously [26]. In order to accuratelylocalize bilateral BL33, a line is drawn between the two posterior superior iliac spines (PSIS) which cross over at point A of the spinal column. Then, each PSIS and point A are connected to construct two separate lines. Finally, two different equilateral triangles are drawn inferiorly and the apexes B and C of these two equilateral triangles are the two BL33 acupoints. The acupuncturists inserted acupuncture needles at BL33obliquely at an angle of about 45° for about 6 cm–8 cm until the patient felt heaviness and numbness locally or even with radiation sensation to the genitalia. Acupuncture procedures were performed bilaterally at two BL33 acupoints and electrodes of the electric stimulator were attached to the handle of the needle bilaterally. Disperse-dense wave, 20 Hz electric current was used in the present study. The intensity of electric current was increased to the patients' maximum tolerance and then slightly reduced to a bearable level. Acupuncture treatment protocol and electric stimulator parameters were the same for non-acupoint acupuncture procedures in the control group, except for the genitalial radiating sensation upon acupuncture.

Patients received a total of 16 sessions of acupuncture treatment which include five sessions in the 1st and 2nd week, acupuncture once a day; three sessions in the 3rd and 4th week, acupuncture every other day. Acupuncture procedures were implemented by an acupuncturist with more than 10 years' clinical experience. Data management and analysis were performed by researchers who were blinded to the acupuncture procedures.

Outcome Assessment

All patients were evaluated during the first week for baseline values which include IPSS, PVR, and Qmax. The primary outcome involves the change of IPSS at the 6th week; secondary outcomes include the changes of PVR, Qmax at the 6th week and change of IPSS at the 18th week. Safety evaluation includes hematoma, fainting, severe pain, and local infection during and after acupuncture. In addition, emergency conditions which require catheterization were also recorded if any.

Statistical analysis

The statistical analysis was performed by a statistician blinded to treatment allocation in the Clinical Evaluation Center of China Academy of Chinese Medical Sciences. SPSS statistical package program (ver.16.0) was used and a significance level was set at $\alpha<0.05$. Data analysis of baseline characteristics was based on the intention-to-treat (ITT) population which included all participants who were randomized. Primary and secondary outcomes were mainly based on the data of the ITT population; however, primary outcome was also analyzed based on per-protocol (PP) population as an extra supportive analysis. Quantitative data of IPSS and Qmax were expressed with mean±SD; PVR was expresses as Range (Median) as the data was not normally distributed. For primary and secondary outcome measures, analysis of covariance was used to investigate the differences between acupoint acupuncture and non-acupoint acupuncture on IPSS and Qmax. Changes of the IPSS and Qmax after treatment were the dependent variable, the group was the fixed factor and the baseline data were the covariate. The Mann Whitney U test was used for the analysis of PVR.

Table 3. Descriptive statistics of PP population.

		Acupoint group (n = 45)	Non-point group (n = 42)
IPSS	Baseline	19.84±6.46	18.83±6.00
	6th week	12.60±5.85	16.05±6.83
	Change in IPSS	7.24±5.23	2.79±5.17

Results

From September, 2010 to May, 2012, a total of 192 patients with LUTS visited the Acupuncture Department at Guang'anmen Hospital in Beijing. 92 patients were excluded from the present study for the following reasons: 16 did not have BPH; 22 did not meet the inclusion criteria; 54 met the exclusion criteria. 100 of them were included and equally randomized to receive acupoint acupuncture and non-acupoint acupuncture treatments (Figure 1). Figure 2 details the time frames of recruitment, treatment and follow-up periods.

Demographic characteristics and baseline information of the 100 participants are shown in Table 1. 25 patients in the acupoint acupuncture group and 23 in the non-acupoint control group were diagnosed as severe BPH (IPSS≥20). No statistically significant differences were found between the two groups in age, gender, and baseline values. The mean age of all participants was 65.37±6.89 years old.

IPSS

Analyses of IPSS at the 6th week were based on both of ITT population and PP population (See Table 2 and Table 3). At the 6th week, the ITT analysis indicated that IPSS reduced from 20.10±6.52 at baseline to 12.84±5.87 for the acupoint treatment group, and from 18.76±6.06 at baseline to 16.42±6.80 for non-point control group. With the PP analysis, IPSS of the two groups reduced to 12.60±5.85 and 16.05±6.83 respectively. At the 6th week, acupoint group patients had a 4.51 ($p<0.001$) and 4.12 ($p<0.001$) points greater decline than the non-acupoint control group in the ITT and PP populations respectively (Table 4). At the 18th week, a 3.2 points ($p = 0.001$) greater decline was found for the acupoint treatment group as compared with the non-acupoint control group.

Qmax and PVR

No significant differences were found between the two groups in Qmax at the 6th week ($p = 0.819$, Table 4). PVR data followed a non-normal distribution and no significant difference was found ($P = 0.35$).

Adverse Events

No serious adverse events happened in eithergroups. Two cases of mild hematoma were reported in the non-acupoint control group during study. The patients were told to apply ice and compression within 24 hours and heat compression after 24 hours to the acupuncture treatment areas. Hematoma disappeared in about two weeks.

Discussion

The results of this trial showed that greater decrease in IPSS in the BL33 group than in the non-acupoint group, but no significant difference was found in Qmax and PVR. The change of IPSS indicates that EA at acupoints significantly improved the quality of life in patients diagnosed with BPH. The IPSS change matched the results of our previous studies and added further credence in the use of acupuncture for patients with BPH [14–16]. The IPSS was decreased by 7.26 (from20.10 to 12.84, $P = 0.000$) and 2.34 (from 18.76 to 16.42, $P = 0.001$) in BL33 acupoint EA group and

Table 4. ANCOVA estimation of outcomes.

		Treatment effect estimate (Mean difference)	Standard error	P-value
IPSS (ITT)	6th week	4.51	0.93	0.000
	18th week	3.20	0.93	0.001
IPSS (PP)	6th week	4.12	1.03	0.000
Qmax(ITT)	6th week	0.18	0.80	0.819

ANCOVA: Analysis of Covariance.

the non-point EA group respectively. Compared to the non-point control group, the acupoint group was associated with a 4.51-point greater decline in IPSS at the 6th week ($P<0.01$). The difference of IPSS decrease indicates that EA at acupoints had significantly better effects than EA at non-acupoint on the quality of life in patients diagnosed with BPH. As EA procedures at both acupoint and non-acupoint share the same electric stimulation parameters and same EA protocol, the specificity of needling site at BL33 acupoint may be accountable for the difference in IPSS in the present study. This echoed the results of our pilot study stating that acupoints have better effects than non-acupoints [16]. The results of the present study also increases the credibility of results of other related studies indicating that the acupoint of the meridian system seem to have specific functional regulatory effects compared to non-acupoints [17–19].

In a similar trial comparing EA with sham EA (shallow needle insertion of 2 mm) for BPH, greater increase of Qmax was found in the EA group than the sham EA group; whereas IPSS was similar in both groups [27]. With a close analysis, acupoints use, manipulation methods, parameters of EA and number, frequency and duration of treatment sessions could all cause the differences between the two studies. Nonetheless, both studies demonstrated that standard EA at acupoint had better effects than EA with shallow needle insertion of 2 mm or EA at non-acupoints on at least certain clinical parameter(s). In addition, IPSS improve in the present study is also supported by results from the study by Johnstone et al [28] in which some difference in IPSS ($p = 0.063$) was found between acupuncture and blank control. As only 20 out of 30 patients were treated with acupuncture in the study by Johnstone et al [28], the p value is likely to drop to lower than 0.05 if the sample size is increased. Consequently, we should believe the specificity of acupoints in acupuncture treatment even though the mechanism of acupuncture at acupoints has not been fully elucidated.

Studies demonstrate that sacral neuromodulation could improve symptoms of overactive bladder [29–30]. As BL33 is actually the third sacral nerve which travels through the 3rd sacral foramen, we should believe that EA at BL33 is actually one type of sacral neuromodulation. Sacral acupuncture was found to be effective in improving symptoms of acetic acid-induced bladder irritation in rats through inhibition of capsaicin-sensitive C-fiber activation [31]. Therefore, EA for BPH may be related to acupuncture sacral neuromododulation.

Although the exact mechanism of EA treatment for BPH has yet to be clarified, researchers believe that the effects of acupuncture are less likely to be related to histological changes of the prostate, as no difference was found in PSA levels, between sham and vera EA and between acupuncture and blank control [27,28]. As results of acupuncture fMRI studies showed a significant connection between brain activities and acupuncture procedures, and the human brain is closely involved in the sensation and control of the lower urinary system [32–34], we should also believe that brain modulation by acupuncture may also play a role in the effects of EA on BPH. This was confirmed by in-vivo animal study in which Chung et al [35] found that expression of c-Fos expression in the pontine micturition center (PMC), ventrolateral periaqueductal gray (vlPAG), and medial preoptic nucleus (MPA) was increased in stress urinary incontinence, and acupuncture significantly decreased c-Fos expression in these areas. Nonetheless, further studies are needed to explore the mechanism of acupuncture on BPH.

Limitations

As blinding is difficult in acupuncture studies, real randomized placebo controlled trials seem impossible. Although non-acupoint EA procedures were used as control in the present study, they are still acupuncture procedures; thus we could not rule out the confounding factor of needling and placebo effects in the present study. Patients in the present study were only treated for 4 weeks and followed up till the 18th week, long term effects and optimal treatment regimens of EA for BPH remain to be established. In addition, this RCT was performed in only one hospital rather than multi-centers; therefore, the results of the present study may not well-characterize the general response of patients with BPH in the world. To further test the therapeutic effects of EA on BPH, further large scale, multi-center, international cooperative studies are warranted.

Conclusion

In the present study, acupoint EA at BL 33 had better effects on IPSS, but no difference on PVR and Qmax as compared with non-acupoint EA. The results indicate that EA is effective in improving patient's quality of life and acupoint may have better therapeutic effects than non-acupoints in acupuncture treatments of BPH.

Supporting Information

Checklist S1 CONSORT Checklist.
(PDF)

Protocol S1 Trial Protocol.
(PDF)

Author Contributions

Conceived and designed the trial: ZL. Contributed materials: BL. Performed the trial: JY J. Wu. Analyzed the data: J. Wang. Wrote the paper: YW.

References

1. Nickel JC (2006) The overlapping lower urinary tract symptoms of benign prostatic hyperplasia and prostatitis. CurrOpinUrol 16: 5–10.
2. Hong SK, Lee ST, Jeong SJ, Byun SS, Hong YK, et al (2010) Chronic kidney disease among men with lower urinary tract symptoms due to benign prostatic hyperplasia. BJU Int 105(10): 1424–8.
3. Bruskewitz RC (2003) Quality of Life and Sexual Function in Patients with Benign Prostatic Hyperplasia. Rev Urol 5: 72–80.
4. Tanguay S, Awde M, Brock G, Casey R, Kozak J, et al (2009) Diagnosis and management of benign prostatic hyperplasia in primary care. Can UrolAssoc J 3(3 Suppl 2): S92–S100.
5. American Urology Association (2012) Guideline on the Management of Benign Prostatic Hyperplasia. http://www.auanet.org/content/guidelines-and-quality-care/clinical-guidelines/main-reports/bph-management/chap_1_GuidelineManagementof(BPH). pdf (accessed 1/31/2013).
6. Wang QC (2003) Acupuncture therapeutics. Beijing: China Traditional Chinese Medicine Publishing.
7. Ricci L, Minardi D, Romoli M, Galosi AB, Muzzonigro G (2004) Acupuncture reflexotherapy in the treatment of sensory urgency that persists after transurethral resection of the prostate: a preliminary report. NeurourolUrodyn 23(1): 58–62.
8. Kubista E, Altmann P, Kucera H, Rudelstorfer B (1976) Electro-acupuncture's influence on the closure mechanism of the female urethra in incontinence. Am J Chin Med (Gard City N Y) 4(2): 177–81.
9. Philp T, Shah PJ, Worth PH (1988) Acupuncture in the treatment of bladder instability. Br J Urol 61(6): 490–3.
10. Aune A, Alraek T, LiHua H, Baerheim A (1998) Acupuncture in the prophylaxis of recurrent lower urinary tract infection in adult women. Scand J Prim Health Care 16(1): 37–9.
11. Alraek T, Soedal LI, Fagerheim SU, Digranes A, Baerheim A (2002) Acupuncture treatment in the prevention of uncomplicated recurrent lower urinary tract infections in adult women. Am J Public Health 92(10): 1609–11.
12. Capodice JL, Jin Z, Bemis DL, Samadi D, Stone BA, et al (2007) A pilot study on acupuncture for lower urinary tract symptoms related to chronic prostatitis/ chronic pelvic pain. Chin Med 6;2: 1.
13. Karaman MI, Koca O, Küçük EV, Öztürk M, Güneş M (2010) Laser acupuncture therapy for primary monosymptomatic nocturnal enuresis. J Urol 185(5): 1852–6.
14. Yang T, Zhang XQ, Feng YW, Xu HR, Liu ZS, et al (2008) Efficacy of Electroacupuncture in Treating 93 Patients with Benign Prostatic Hyperplasia. Chinese Journal of Integrated Traditional and Western Medicine 28(11): 998–1000.
15. Yang T, Liu ZS, Zhang XQ, Feng YW, Xu HR, et al (2008) Evaluation on therapeutic effects of electroacupuncture for benign prostatic hyperplasia: A prospective randomized controlled study. Chinese Journal of Rehabilitation Medicine 23(11): 1028–1031.
16. Ding Y, Yu J, Liu Z (2011) A pilot trial of point speciality using electroacupuncture at Zhongliao point for benign prostatic hyperplasia. Journal of Clinical Acupuncture and Moxibustion 27(7): 1–4.
17. Shuran J, Zhongsuan H (1987) Specific effect of acupuncture at ST36 for visceral pain. Acupuncture Reaearch 1: 73–76.
18. Cheng K, Han Y (2004) Study on the Specificity of Effects of Acupuncture of Different Acupoints in Reducing Gentamycin Induced Ototoxicity in Guinea-pigs. Acupuncture Reaearch 29(3): 204–208.
19. Xu B, Yu XC, Chen CY, Wang LL, Liu JL, et al (2010) Relationship Between Efficacy of Electroacupuncture and Electroacupuncture Stimulation of Different Acupoints and Different Tissue Layers of Acupoint Area in Hypotension plus Bradycardia Rats. Acupuncture Reaearch 35(6): 422–428.
20. Dıraçoğlu D, Vural M, Karan A, Aksoy C (2012) Effectiveness of dry needling for the treatment of temporomandibularmyofascial pain: a double-blind, randomized, placebo controlled study. J Back MusculoskeletRehabil 25(4): 285–90.
21. Kalichman L, VulfsonsS (2010) Dry needling in the management of musculoskeletal pain. J Am Board Fam Med 23(5): 640–6.
22. Wang Y, Liu ZS, Yu JN, Ding TL, Liu X (2011) Efficacy of electroacupuncture at Zhongliao point (BL33) for mild and moderate benign prostatci hyperplasia: study protocol for a randomized controlled trial. Trials 12: 211.
23. Chapple RC, Montorsi F, Teuvo LJT, Wirth M, Koldewijn E, et al (2011) Silodosin therapy for lower urinary tract symptoms in men with Suspected Benign Prostatic Hyperplasia: Results of an International, Randomized, Double-Blind, Placebo- and Active-Controlled Clinical Trial Performed in Europe. European Urology 59: 342–352.
24. Yu HJ, Lin AT, Yang SS, Tsui KH, Wu HC, et al (2011) Non-inferiority of silodosin to tamsulosin in treating patients with lower urinary tract symptoms (LUTS) associated with benign prostatic hyperplasia (BPH). BJU INTERNATIONAL 108(11): 1843–1848.
25. Wang J (2001) Clinical Epidemiology-design, measurement and evaluation. Shanghai: Shanghai Science and Technology Press: 41–142.
26. Liu ZS, Zhou KH, Wang Y, Pan YX(2011)Electroacupuncture improves voiding function in patients with neurogenic urinary retention secondary to caudaequina injury: results from a prospective observational study. Acupunct Med 29(3): 188–192.
27. Yu JS, Shen KH, Chen WC, Her JS, Hsieh CL (2011) Effects of Electroacupuncture on Benign Prostate Hyperplasia Patients with Lower Urinary Tract Symptoms: A Single-Blinded, Randomized Controlled Trial. Evidence-Based Complementary and Alternative Medicine 20: 303198.
28. Johnstone PA, Bloom TL, Niemtzow RC, Crain D, Riffenburgh RH, et al (2003) A prospective, randomized pilot trial of acupuncture of the kidney-bladder distinct meridian for lower urinary tract symptoms. J Urol 169(3): 1037–9.
29. Wendy WL, Michael BC (2005) How does Nerve Stimulation Neuromodulation Works. UrolClin N Am 32: 11–18.
30. Vignes JR, De Seze M, Dobremez E (2005) Sacralneuromodulaiton in lower urinary tract dysfunction. Adv Tech Stand Neurosurg 30: 177–224.
31. Hino K, Honjo H, Nakao M, Kitakoji H (2010) The Effects of Sacral Acupuncture on Acetic Acid-induced Bladder Irritation in Conscious Rats. Urology 75: 730–734.
32. Fang J, Jin Z, Wang Y, Li K, Kong J, et al (2009). The salient characteristics of the central effects of acupuncture needling: limbic-paralimbic-neocortical network modulation. Hum Brain Mapp 30(4): 1196–206.
33. Fang J, Wang X, Liu H, Wang Y, Zhou K, et al (2012) The Limbic-Prefrontal Network Modulated by Electroacupuncture at CV4 and CV12. Evid Based Complement Alternat Med 2012: 515893.
34. Napadow V, Lee J, Kim J, Cina S, Maeda Y, et al (2012). Brain correlates of phasic autonomic response to acupuncture stimulation: An event-related fMRI study. Hum Brain Mapp 000: 00–00.
35. Chung IM, Kim YS, Sung YH, Kim SE, Ko IG, et al (2008) Effects of acupuncture on abdominal leak point pressure and c-Fos expression in the brain of rats with stress urinary incontinence. NeurosciLett 439(1): 18–23.

6

Risk of Bias Tool in Systematic Reviews/Meta-Analyses of Acupuncture in Chinese Journals

Yali Liu[1,2], Shengping Yang[1,3], Junjie Dai[1,3], Yongteng Xu[1,3], Rui Zhang[1,3], Huaili Jiang[1,3], Xianxia Yan[1,3], Kehu Yang[1,2]*

1 Evidence-Based Medicine Center, School of Basic Medical Sciences, Lanzhou University, Lanzhou, China, **2** Institute of Integrated Traditional Chinese and Western Medicine, Lanzhou University, Lanzhou, China, **3** The First Clinical Medical College of Lanzhou University, Lanzhou, China

Abstract

Background: Use of a risk of bias (ROB) tool has been encouraged and advocated to reviewers writing systematic reviews (SRs) and meta-analyses (MAs). Selective outcome reporting and other sources of bias are included in the Cochrane ROB tool. It is important to know how this specific tool for assessing ROB has been applied since its release. Our objectives were to evaluate whether and to what extent the new Cochrane ROB tool has been used in Chinese journal papers of acupuncture.

Methods: We searched CBM, TCM database, CJFD, CSJD, and the Wanfang Database from inception to March 2011. Two reviewers independently selected SRs that primarily focused on acupuncture and moxibustion, from which the data was extracted and analyzed.

Results: A total of 836 SRs were identified from the search, of which, 105 were included and four are awaiting assessment. Thirty-six of the 105 SRs were published before release of the Cochrane ROB tool (up to 2009). Most used the Cochrane Handbook 4.2 or Jadad's scale for risk or quality assessment. From 2009 to March 2011 69 SRs were identified. While "risk of bias" was reported for approximately two-thirds of SRs, only two SRs mentioned use of a "risk of bias tool" in their assessment. Only 5.8% (4/69) of reviews reported information on all six domains which are involved in the ROB tool. A risk of bias graph/summary figure was provided in 2.9% (2/69) of reviews. Most SRs gave information about sequence generation, allocation concealment, blindness, and incomplete outcome data, however, few reviews (5.8%; 4/69) described selective reporting or other potential sources of bias.

Conclusions: The Cochrane "risk of bias" tool has not been used in all SRs/MAs of acupuncture published in Chinese Journals after 2008. When the ROB tool was used, reporting of relevant information was often incomplete.

Editor: Neil R. Smalheiser, University of Illinois-Chicago, United States of America

Funding: The authors have no support or funding to report.

Competing Interests: The authors have declared that no competing interests exist.

* E-mail: kehuyangebm2006@126.com

Introduction

Assessment of internal validity, risk of bias, or methodological quality of studies included in systematic reviews (SRs) and meta-analyses (MAs) is a very important step in identifying limitations of individual studies. Randomized controlled trials (RCTs) are often included as the study type for SRs of interventions.

Since the 1980s, numerous tools involving scales and checklists have been developed for assessing the methodological quality of clinical trials [1], including the Cochrane Collaboration's "risk of bias" (ROB) tool which was published in 2008 [2]. It shows that "the ROB tool is composed of two parts, 'description' and 'judgment'. For parallel group trials, it addresses six specific domains: sequence generation, allocation concealment, blinding, incomplete outcome data, selective outcome reporting, and other sources of bias. In these six domains, the judgments of 'Yes', 'No', or 'Unclear' indicates 'low risk of bias', 'high risk of bias', and 'uncertain risk of bias', respectively" [2]. As an essential guide to writing a Cochrane SRs, use of the ROB tool has been encouraged and advocated [2]. Moreover, authors are encouraged to use the latest version, which is currently Handbook 5.1.0 [updated March 2011].

The ROB tool continues to be recommended and disseminated by the Cochrane Collaboration and its sub-centers in different countries. In determining the effect of the ROB tool, it is very important to know how effectively it has been applied. Accordingly, we evaluate whether and to what extent the Cochrane ROB tool has been used in SRs of acupuncture published in Chinese journals.

Methods

The protocol of this study was written in Chinese which has not published.

Inclusion Criteria

SRs or MAs of acupuncture/acupressure and moxibustion published on Chinese journals. We included studies that described their methods and results in detail.

Exclusion Criteria

SRs and MAs primarily focused on the other traditional Chinese medicine (TCM) (herbal medicine, massage, etc) rather than acupuncture.

Search Strategy (Text S1)

Five databases (Chinese Biomedicine Literature Database (CBM), Traditional Chinese Medicine database (TCM database), Chinese Journal Full-text Database (CJFD), Chinese Scientific Journal Full-text Database (CSJD), and Wanfang Database) were systematically searched from inception to March 2011. The main search terms were as follows: "systematic review", "meta-analysis", "acupuncture", "needling", "ear acupuncture", " electroacupuncture", "electro-acupuncture", "acupuncture points", "acupressure", "moxibustion", and "acupoint".

Screening

Two reviewers (Yongteng XU and Huaili JIANG) independently screened the title and abstract of each record. Full texts of potentially included articles were further assessed. Disagreements were resolved by discussion.

Data Extraction and Analysis

Data about general characteristics and "risk of bias" were independently extracted by two reviewers (Junjie DAI and Rui ZHANG). Discrepancies were resolved through discussion or settled by the third principal investigator (Yali LIU). Since the ROB tool was first published in February 2008 (Cochrane handbook 5.0.0) [3], we assessed the use of the ROB tool only in those reviews published since 2009.

Data was extracted into a standardized form by trained extractors. The forms was composed of two parts: (1) General information: publication, type of included studies, funding etc, and (2) Information related to risk of bias: name and version of assessment tool, risk of bias graph/summary; randomization sequence, allocation concealment, blinding, incomplete outcome data, selective reporting, and other potential sources of bias etc. Each domain was assessed as 'yes' (described in papers), or "no" (not described in papers).

Data was summarized using descriptive statistics (frequency, percentage). Analysis was carried out with Excel (version Microsoft Excel 2007; http://office.microsoft.com/zh-cn/) and SPSS software (version 13.0; http://www.spss.com).

Results

Search

Our search identified 837 SRs and MAs, of which 675 abstracts did not meet inclusion criteria. One hundred and sixty-two reviews were chosen for full text analysis and assessed for inclusion. Full texts were obtained for 158 reviews; 105 met inclusion criteria and four are awaiting assessment, as full text was not available (Figure 1, Text S2). All SRs and MAs were written by Chinese authors.

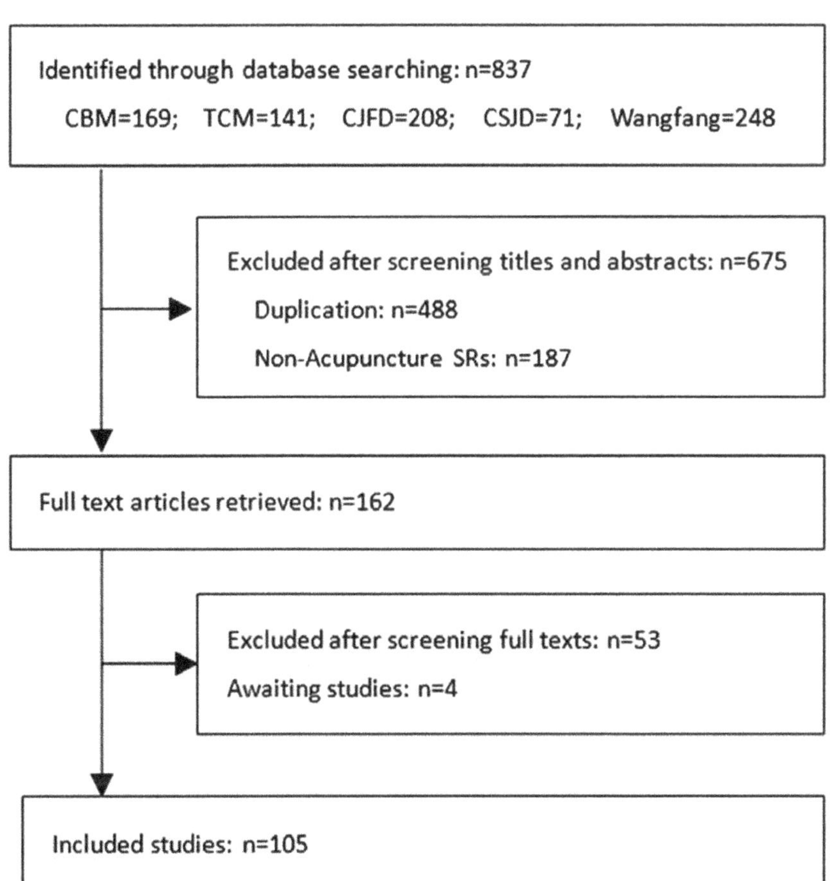

Figure 1. Flow chart of articles identified, included and excluded.

General Characteristics (Table 1)

The first systematic review and meta-analysis were published in 2002 and 2003, respectively. Since 2007, the number of SRs and MAs published annually has increased.

Of the 105 included reviews, 74 and 22 included "systematic review" and "meta-analysis" in their titles, respectively. However, there were nine reviews that included "evidence-based medicine analysis", "the curative effect comparison appraises", and other phrases in their titles, which were later identified as "systematic reviews" or "meta-analyses." All reviews concerned diseases defined from a western medicine perspective. In total, 15 different types of diseases were involved, with the majority [24.8% (26/105)] focused on treatment of diseases of the nervous system. Diagnostic criteria were reported in 55.2% (58/105) of the reviews. Of these 58 reviews, 41 reported their diagnostic criteria based solely on "Western disease" and two reviews reported their diagnostic criteria based solely on "TCM syndrome." The remaining 15 reviews included both "western disease" and "TCM syndrome" diagnostic criteria. Funding was supplied by at least one funding body for 56.2% (59/105) of reviews. Of these, 98.3% [58/59] were supported by funding from China and only one was funded by an international foundation (The China Medical Board, CMB). Most, 94.9% (56/59), failed to provide declarations of interest, while the remaining three reviews reported that there were no conflicts of interests.

While most [91.4% (96/105)] SRs and MAs restricted study design to RCTs, some included controlled clinical trials (CCTs) [36.2% (38/105)] and quasi-RCTs [13.3% (14/105)]. The number of trials included in the reviews ranged from three to 203, with a median of 12.7. And the number of included RCTs ranged from 0 to 67, with a median of 7.

Risk of bias tool (Table 2, 3)

Thirty-six SRs were published during the seven years from 2002 through 2008, and another 69 since 2009. Of the first 36 SRs, one-third [33.3% (12/36)] used the Jadad scale [4] and one-third [33.3% (12/36)] applied the Cochrane Handbook. Among the latter 12 reviews, seven used the Cochrane Handbook 4, and another five reviews used the Cochrane handbook but failed to report the exact version used. Most reviews assessed sequence generation, allocation concealment, blinding, loss of follow-up and intention-to-treat (ITT) analysis.

Of the 69 SRs published since 2009, 73.91% (51/69) applied the Cochrane Handbook as an assessment tool. Of these, 18.84% (13/69) used the Cochrane Handbook 5 and, 36.23% (25/69) used the Cochrane Handbook 4, and a further thirteen reviews used the Cochrane handbook but failed to report the version used. The Jadad scales were used by 57.97% (40/69) and of these, 25 used both the Cochrane Handbook and the Jadad scale. One review did not use any quality or ROB assessment for included studies. Methodological quality and ROB have been used interchangeably in the SRs and MAs. Most reviews used "quality assessment" rather than "risk of bias assessment" in their methods or results. Only two reviews specified a "risk of bias tool" as their assessment tool.

Few [5.8% (4/69)] reviews reported on all six domains of the Cochrane ROB tool. Most SRs gave information about baseline similarity; however, only four reviews described other potential sources of bias and selective reporting bias. A "risk of bias graph/summary" figure was provided in 2.9% (2/69) of the reviews.

Information about blinding was reported in 68 reviews, but 61 of these failed to report who was blinded in the trials. Most reviews reported loss of follow-up or ITT analysis, but failed to mention incomplete outcome data. None of the reviews reported verbatim quotes in their papers.

Discussion

An increasing number of SRs and MAs of acupuncture have been published, especially since 2007. In this study, we identified 105 SRs and MAs of acupuncture interventions in Chinese journals. In addition, there were 36 Cochrane SRs in the Cochrane Database of Systematic Reviews (CDSR) and 154 SRs and MAs have been published in international journals that

Table 1. Characteristics of included studies.

Category	Characteristic	Number (%) of n = 105
Title	Systematic review	74 (70.5)
	Meta analyse	22 (20.9)
	Others	9 (8.6)
Diagnostic criteria	Western medicine (diseases)	41 (39.0)
	Traditional medicine	2 (1.9)
	Using both disease and syndrome	15 (14.3)
	No diagnostic criteria reported	47 (44.8)
funding source	The number of reviews with funding source(s)	59 (56.2)
	Chinese foundation	58 (98.3*)
	International foundation	1 (1.7*)
	No declarations of interest	56 (94.9*)
	The number of funding sources	Median:1 (range: 0–5)
Trial types included	RCTs	96
	CCT	38
	quasi-RCTs	14

*n = 59.

Table 2. The use of numerous tools in studies.

Assessment tools	2000–2008 y (n = 36)	2009–2011.3 y (n = 69)
Cochrane Handbook version 4	7	25
Cochrane Handbook version 5	-	13
Cochrane Handbook (version not reported)	5	13
Jadad scale	12 (11+1*)	40 (15+25*)
Juni	3	1
PED pro	1	0
No mention assessment tool	7	2 (1+1#)
Others	2	0

*The number of reviews that applied both the Jadad scale and another.
#No use any assessment tool.

primarily focus on acupuncture. To our knowledge, this paper is the first to investigate the use of the Cochrane Collaboration's ROB tool in the acupuncture field. Although the study was not a classical systematic review, we tried to report it according to PRISMA Checklist [14] (Text S3).

We identified other studies that focused on use of the ROB tool. While most of these studies evaluated the ROB of RCTs and/or their influence in specific fields, such as dentistry [5], pediatrics [6], and persistent asthma treatment [7], other studies have assessed the internal validity of RCTs, inter-rater agreement [8,9], and concurrent validity [8,9]. Some reviews have contrasted the ROB tool with other tools, such as the Jadad scale [7,8], the Schulz approach [7,8], and the Effective Public Health Practice Project Quality Assessment Tool (EPHPP) [9]. Hartling et al. demonstrated low correlation and varied inter-rater agreements between the ROB tool assessments and the Jadad scale [7,8].

Other reviews of SRs and MAs published in Chinese journals have identified problems with methodological or reporting quality, however, these studies failed to pay attention to use of the ROB tool in their reviews [10–12].

The QUOROM statement [13] and the updated version of the PRISMA statement [14] encourage use of the terms systematic review or meta-analysis in titles of such studies, in order to maximize search success. Among the reviews we identified, most included these terms in their titles, however, nine SRs or MAs failed to use these terms in their titles in Chinese. In addition, most reviews did not declare whether a conflict of interest existed or not, which is a potential threat to validity.

Although acupuncture belongs to the domain of TCM, most SRs and MAs focus on "western disease" rather than "TCM syndrome" as their diagnostic criteria. Consequently, TCM practitioners may find it difficult to understand and apply evidence from such publications in their clinical practice because TCM places more emphasis on syndromes rather than on western disease classifications. Therefore, some researchers propose using both western disease and TCM syndrome in their diagnostic criteria in studies of TCM. This is an interesting issue worthy of serious discussion but it is beyond the scope of this paper.

Many instruments exist for assessing the "quality" of RCTs. While 25 scales and nine checklists were published prior to 1994

Table 3. Reporting of the six domains in the ROB tool in SRs and MAs after 2009.

ROB tool's domains	Systematic reviews (n = 50)	Meta-analyses (n = 13)	Others titles (n = 6)	Subtotal (n = 69)
Sequence generation	48	13	6	67
Allocation concealment	42	9	5	56
Blindness	49	13	6	68
Blinding participants	1	1	0	2
Blinding healthcare providers	0	1	0	1
Blinding outcome assessors	2	0	0	2
Blinding data analysts	2	0	0	2
Incomplete outcome data	7	1	0	8
Loss of follow-up	43	7	6	56
Intention-to-treat (ITT) analysis	14	4	1	19
Selective outcome reporting.	4	0	0	4
Other potential sources of bias	4	0	0	4
Using ROB graph/summary	2	0	0	2
Reported verbatim quotes	0	0	0	0

[15,16], more instruments focusing on methodological quality [2,4,17–20] or both methodological quality and reporting quality [21–24] have since been proposed. Despite the abundance of such instruments, assessment tools specifically for evaluating acupuncture RCTs are rare [23]. In addition, some items of these instruments are not directly related to internal validity. For example, whether a power calculation was done or not relates to the precision of the results rather than internal validity [2]. In our study, we concentrated on tools that focused on internal validity.

We found that the Cochrane Handbook and the Jadad scale were often chosen by Chinese reviewers. Although, the Jadad scale has been popular for many years, using the Cochrane Collaboration ROB tool instead of the Jadad scale should be recommended when performing SRs and MAs. There are several core reasons for this recommendation: 1) the Jadad scale is based on reporting quality rather than actual RCT conduct [4]; 2) while the Jadad scale focuses on randomization, double blinding, withdrawals or dropouts, we believe these criteria are insufficient to assess the internal validity of RCTs; 3) the Jadad scale tends to overestimate treatment effects because it ignores allocation concealment [25] and selective outcome reporting [26,27], which are very important to overall assessment of ROB; and 4) the term "double blind" is incomplete and lacks specificity for assessing "blinding" because it is not clear who is blinded [28].

We found that most Chinese SRs and MAs were written according to the Cochrane Collaboration's Handbook. The Cochrane Handbook is frequently updated, the most recent being version 5.1.0, published in March 2011 [2]. Although many scales and tools are available for assessing methodological quality of RCTs, the new version of the Cochrane handbook recommends that a specific ROB tool be used assess the risk of bias in each included study. It is not uncommon that authors of SRs and MAs use the terms "methodological quality" and "risk of bias" interchangeably. The term "bias" indicates a systematic error or deviation from the truth in a study's results or inferences [2]. Assessing ROB is to directly assess the extent that the results of included studies should be *believed* [2]. But not all parts of quality assessment have direct implications for ROB. Therefore, ROB is recommended for assessing "bias" instead of methodological quality, because "bias" may be different from "quality". For example, blinding is difficult or impossible for some interventions, such as surgery or Chinese herbal medicine. In these cases, the risk from lack of blinding may affect the trial's validity, however, it may be inappropriate to score these studies as "low quality" [2].

The Cochrane ROB tool was recommended in Cochrane handbook version 5.0.1, although 'selective reporting' and 'other potential sources of bias' were mentioned in Handbook 4.2.6. Few of the reviews we identified [18.8% (13/69)] reported that they used Cochrane Handbook 5 and only three of these also used all 6 domains. One review reported use of Cochrane Handbook 4.2.6 and also described the selective outcome reporting bias and the other potential sources of bias. Most SRs and MAs reported information about sequence generation, allocation concealment, blindness, and incomplete outcome data, however, major reviews ignored selective outcome reporting and other potential sources of bias. These studies that lack analysis of selective outcome reporting and other sources of bias have performed incomplete ROB assessment. Although baseline imbalance was described, many SRs and MAs failed to analyze the influence of other sources of bias. None of the SRs and MAs in our study analyzed early stoppage, conflict of interest, or other factors that are other potential threats to validity. Some of the SRs and MAs that reported using Cochrane Handbook 5 in their methods, actually used version 4 in their results. It is easy to mislead a reader because most clinicians may not know the differences between Cochrane Handbook 4 and Handbook 5.

With regards to blinding, we noticed that most reviews failed to describe the blinding process in detail. In a clinical trial, different types of personnel can be blinded, such as participants, healthcare providers, outcome assessors, and data analysts. If we do not know which types of personnel were blinded, it is difficult to accurately judge which bias (performance bias or measurement bias) may have occurred. In addition, use of the term "double blind" is ambiguous and authors often fail to state exactly who was blinded [28]. Some people assume "double blind" means that patients and clinicians were blinded, however, some authors reported "double blind", when patients and outcome assessors were blinded. Furthermore, for subjective outcomes, blinding outcome assessors is more important than blinding clinicians in order to avoid measurement bias.

While most reviews provided details of loss to follow-up (attrition/drop-out) and ITT analyses, few mentioned the term "incomplete outcome data". We recommend that future reviews include information about incomplete outcome data, not only the amount and distribution of drop-outs across study groups but also the reasons for outcomes being absent. This would help reviewers assess the risk of attrition bias.

The "risk of bias summary" figure was provided in few reviews. Reasons for this may be that reviewers are not be aware of this requirement or that journals may require specific layout specifications that authors are unable to comply with.

In order to improve assessment of risk of bias, we recommend that the most recent version of the Cochrane ROB tool be used by SR and MA authors. Reviewers should continue to update their knowledge according to the latest Cochrane Collaboration Handbook versions and other developing methodology and to clearly state which version of the tool or handbook was used in their reviews.

There are several limitations in the study. We included SRs and MAs that primarily focused on acupuncture. Those reviews involving acupuncture as a secondary intervention were excluded. We only selected SRs and MAs published in Chinese journals and therefore our results are only applicable to those journals. In addition, we did not analyze internal validity and inter-rater agreements between the ROB tool assessments and the Jadad scale or other assessment tools.

In conclusion, the Cochrane Handbook and the Jadad scale were the risk of bias or quality assessment instruments most commonly used by Chinese authors of systematic reviews and meta-analyses of acupuncture. In reviews published after 2008 in Chinese journals, Cochrane ROB tools were not always used. In cases where a Cochrane ROB tool was used, reporting was sometimes incomplete.

Supporting Information

Text S1 Five Chinese databases search strategy.
(DOC)

Text S2 One hundred and five SRs/MAs of acupuncture published in Chinese journals.
(DOC)

Text S3 PRISMA Checklist.
(DOC)

Acknowledgments

We thank Dr. Denise Adams (CARE Program, Department of Pediatrics, Faculty of Medicine and Dentistry, University of Alberta, Edmonton,

Alberta, Canada.) and Dr. Rongbin Wang (Zhejiang University) for providing assistance with editing the final manuscript.

Author Contributions

Conceived and designed the experiments: YLL KHY SPY. Performed the experiments: JJD RZ HLJ YTX. Analyzed the data: YLL SPY XXY. Wrote the paper: YLL KHY SPY.

References

1. Yang SP, Yan XX, Liu JQ, Yang KH, Yuan JQ, et al. (2010) Analysis of Quality Standards Assessing Randomized Controlled Trials. The Journal of Evidence-Based Medicine 10: 369–373.
2. Higgins JPT, Green S, eds (2008) Cochrane Handbook for Systematic Reviews of Interventions Version 5.1.0 [updated March 2011]. The Cochrane Collaboration, 2011. Available: http://www.cochrane-handbook.org.
3. Higgins JPT, Green S (2008) Cochrane Handbook for Systematic Reviews of Interventions Version 5.0.0 [updated February 2008]. The Cochrane Collaboration, 2011. Available: http://www.cochrane-handbook.org.
4. Jadad AR, Moore RA, Carroll D, Jenkinson C, Reynolds DJ, et al. (1996) Assessing the quality of reports of randomized clinical trials: Is blinding necessary?. Control Clin Trials 17: 1–12.
5. Ferreira CA, Loureiro CA, Saconato H, Atallah AN (2011) Assessing the risk of bias in randomized controlled trials in the field of dentistry indexed in the Lilacs (Literatura Latino-Americana e do Caribe em Ciências da Saúde) database. Sao Paulo Med J 129: 85–93.
6. Crocetti MT, Amin DD, Scherer R (2010) Assessment of risk of bias among pediatric randomized controlled trials. Pediatrics 126: 298–305.
7. Hartling L, Bond K, Vandermeer B, Seida J, Dryden DM, et al. (2011) Applying the risk of bias tool in a systematic review of combination long-acting beta-agonists and inhaled corticosteroids for persistent asthma. PLoS One 6: e17242.
8. Hartling L, Ospina M, Liang Y, Dryden DM, Hooton N, et al. (2009) Risk of bias versus quality assessment of randomised controlled trials: cross sectional study. BMJ 339: b4012.
9. Armijo-Olivo S, Stiles CR, Hagen NA, Biondo PD, Cummings GG, et al. (2010) Assessment of study quality for systematic reviews: a comparison of the Cochrane Collaboration Risk of Bias Tool and the Effective Public Health Practice Project Quality Assessment Tool: methodological research. J Eval Clin Pract;Available: http://www.ncbi.nlm.nih.gov/pubmed/20698919.
10. Li TQ, Liu XM, Zhang MM, Ma JX, Du L, et al. (2007) Assessment of Systematic Reviews and Meta-analyses on Traditional Chinese Medicine Published in Chinese Journals. Chin J Evid-based Med 7: 180–188.
11. Liu JP, Xia Y (2007) Quality appraisal of systematic reviews or meta-analysis on traditional Chinese medicine published in Chinese journals. Chinese Journal of Integrated Traditional and Western Medicine 4: 306–311.
12. Zhang JH, Shang HC, Gao XM, Zhang BL, Xiang YZ (2007) Methodology and reporting quality of systematic review/meta-analysis of traditional Chinese medicine. J Altern Complement Med 13: 797–805.
13. Moher D, Cook DJ, Eastwood S, Olkin I, Rennie D, et al. (1999) Improving the quality of reports of meta-analyses of randomised controlled trials: the QUOROM statement. Quality of Reporting of Meta-analyses. Lancet 354: 1896–1900.
14. Moher D, Liberati A, Tetzlaff J, Altman DG, The PRISMA Group (2009) Preferred Reporting Items for Systematic Reviews and Meta-Analyses: The PRISMA Statement. PLoS Med 6(6): e1000097.
15. Moher D, Jadad AR, Nichol G, Penman M, Tugwell P, et al. (1995) Assessing the quality of randomized controlled trials: An annotated bibliography of scales and checklists. Controlled Clinical Trials 16: 62–73.
16. Moher D, Jadad AR, Tugwell P (1996) Assessing the quality of randomized controlled trials: Current issues and future directions. International Journal of Technology Assessment in Health Care 12: 195–208.
17. Detsky AS, Naylor CD, O'Rourke K, McGeer AJ, L'Abbé KA (1992) Incorporating variations in the quality of individual randomized trials into meta-analysis. J Clin Epidemiol 45: 255–265.
18. Verhagen AP, de Vet HC, de Bie RA, Kessels AG, Boers M, et al. (1998) The Delphi list: a criteria list for quality assessment of randomized clinical trials for conducting systematic reviews developed by Delphi consensus. J Clin Epidemiol 51: 1235–1241.
19. Jüni P, Altman DG, Egger M (2001) Systematic reviews in health care: Assessing the quality of controlled clinical trials. BMJ 323: 42–46.
20. Scottish Intercollegiate Guidelines Network (2011) Methodology Checklist 2: Randomised Controlled Trials. Scottish Intercollegiate Guidelines Network. Available: http://www.sign.ac.uk/guidelines/fulltext/50/compchecklist.html. Accessed 2011 Nov 12.
21. Chalmers TC, Smith H, Jr., Blackburn B, Silverman B, Schroeder B, et al. (1981) A method for assessing the quality of a randomized control trial. Control Clin Trials 2: 31–49.
22. Evans M, Pollock AV (1985) A score system for evaluating random control clinical trials of prophylaxis of abdominal surgical wound infection. Br J Surg 72: 256–260.
23. Ter Riet G, Kleijnen J, Knipschild P (1990) Acupuncture and chronic pain: a criteria-based meta-analysis. J Clin Epidemiol 43: 1191–1199.
24. Dennison DK (1997) Components of a randomized clinical trial. J Periodontal Res 32(5): 430–438.
25. Moher D, Pham B, Jones A, Cook DJ, Jadad AR, et al. (1998) Does quality of reports of randomised trials affect estimates of intervention efficacy reported in meta-analyses? Lancet 352: 609–613.
26. Chan A, Hróbjartsson A, Haahr MT, Gøtzsche PC, Altman DG (2004) Empirical evidence for selective reporting of outcomes in randomized trials: comparison of protocols to published articles. JAMA 291: 2457–65.
27. Chan AW, Altman DG (2005) Identifying outcome reporting bias in randomised trials on PubMed: review of publications and survey of authors. BMJ 330: 753–756.
28. Schulz KF, Chalmers, Altman DG (2002) The landscape and lexicon of blinding in randomized trials. Annals of Internal Medicine 136: 254–259.

7

Length of Acupuncture Training and Structural Plastic Brain Changes in Professional Acupuncturists

Minghao Dong[1], Ling Zhao[2], Kai Yuan[1], Fang Zeng[2], Jinbo Sun[1], Jixin Liu[1], Dahua Yu[1,3], Karen M. von Deneen[1], Fanrong Liang[2], Wei Qin[1*], Jie Tian[1,4*]

1 School of Life Sciences and Technology, Xidian University, Xi'an, Shaanxi, China, **2** The 3rd Teaching Hospital, Chengdu University of Traditional Chinese Medicine, Chengdu, Sichuan, China, **3** Information Processing Laboratory, School of Information Engineering, Inner Mongolia University of Science and Technology, Baotou, Inner Mongolia, China, **4** Institute of Automation, Chinese Academy of Sciences, Beijing, China

Abstract

Background: The research on brain plasticity has fascinated researchers for decades. Use/training serves as an instrumental factor to influence brain neuroplasticity. Parallel to acquisition of behavioral expertise, extensive use/training is concomitant with substantial changes of cortical structure. Acupuncturists, serving as a model par excellence to study tactile-motor and emotional regulation plasticity, receive intensive training in national medical schools following standardized training protocol. Moreover, their behavioral expertise is corroborated during long-term clinical practice. Although our previous study reported functional plastic brain changes in the acupuncturists, whether or not structural plastic changes occurred in acupuncturists is yet elusive.

Methodology/Principal Findings: Cohorts of acupuncturists (N = 22) and non-acupuncturists (N = 22) were recruited. Behavioral tests were delivered to assess the acupuncturists' behavioral expertise. The results confirmed acupuncturists' tactile-motor skills and emotion regulation proficiency compared to non-acupuncturists. Using the voxel-based morphometry technique, we revealed larger grey matter volumes in acupuncturists in the hand representation of the contralateral primary somatosensory cortex (SI), the right lobule V/VI and the bilateral ventral anterior cingulate cortex/ventral medial prefrontal cortex. Grey matter volumes of the SI and Lobule V/VI positively correlated with the duration of acupuncture practice.

Conclusions: To our best knowledge, this study provides first evidence for the anatomical alterations in acupuncturists, which would possibly be the neural correlates underlying acupuncturists' exceptional skills. On one hand, we suggest our findings may have ramifications for tactile-motor rehabilitation. On the other hand, our results in emotion regulation domain may serve as a target for our future studies, from which we can understand how modulations of aversive emotions elicited by empathic pain develop in the context of expertise. Future longitudinal study is necessary to establish the presence and direction of a causal link between practice/use and brain anatomy.

Editor: Manabu Sakakibara, Tokai University, Japan

Funding: This paper is supported by the Project for the National Key Basic Research and Development Program (973) under Grant Nos. 2011CB707702, 2012CB518501, the National Natural Science Foundation of China under Grant Nos. 30930112, 30970774, 81000640, 81000641, 81101036, 81030027, 81101108, 31150110171, 30901900, 81271644, 31200837, the Fundamental Research Funds for the Central Universities. The funders had no role in study design, data collection and analysis, decision to publish, or preparation of the manuscript.

Competing Interests: The authors have declared that no competing interests exist.

* E-mail: wqin@xidian.edu.cn (WQ); tian@ieee.org (JT)

Introduction

"Plasticity is an intrinsic property of the human brain and gives an evolution's invention to enable the nervous system to escape restrictions of its own genome" [1]. Use is a pivotal factor initiating plastic reorganizations of cortical maps [2]. Indeed, imaging studies have provided compelling evidence that training/enhanced use of a body part or cognitive functions cause structural plastic changes in human central nervous system in the model of dancers [3], sports experts [4] and meditators [5]. These findings consolidated the concept of use-dependent plasticity in humans, according to which changes in cortical maps are dependent on the amount of use that an individual allocates to conform to the requirements of environmental constraints [2].

Acupuncturists forms a model par excellence for understanding tactile-motor plasticity, as well as plastic changes in the emotion regulation domain, which was demonstrated in a previous study [6]. Specifically, acupuncture process that relies mainly on the acupuncturists' tactile feedback to manipulating fingers to generate motor plans, which is to be implemented as fine finger movement (Figure 1). Also, acupuncture genuinely is an invasive procedure inflicting painful treatment to achieve therapeutic effects [7], such as inserting needles into the skull, into the bottom of feet or into the area around canthus, etc. Although this process seems unitary or even automatic for professional acupuncturists, it can be decomposed into several interacting components in sensorimotor and cognitive domains: 1) exceptional tactile discrimination ability which enable the acupuncture practitioners to distinguish subtle dynamic changes of manipulation sensation transmitted through fine needles because a patient's concurrent physical status and synchronous bodily response to each round of needling manipulation is constantly changing; 2) the ability of making precise adjustment and promptly generating precise motor plans/commands [8]; 3) fine/dexterous motor skills of manipulating fingers; 4) emotion regulation proficiency which is indispensable since acupuncture would induce empathic pain in acupuncturists and massive exposure to such situation would naturally induce negative emotions or personal distress in acupuncturists, which would eventually impair their professionalism [6].

Basically, acupuncturists, a major part of physicians in China, receive intensive training in national medical schools following standardized training protocols [7] and their behavioral expertise are corroborated during long-term clinical practice. It has been shown that, after extensive training/use, behavioral expertise is paralleled by a profound reorganization in brain architecture, characterized by an enlargement of the representations of trained body parts [9]. Our recent study reported functional alterations in the acupuncturist' brain, however, the question whether or not training effects is parallel by allocations of structural changes in acupuncturists' brain remains elusive.

In the current study, we firstly verified the behavioral expertise of acupuncturists. Then, we expected to see structural differences between the professional acupuncturists group and the non-acupuncturist group (NA). Accordingly, a voxel-based morphometry (VBM) technique was used to detect the morphological brain changes between a group of professional acupuncturists (N = 22) and NA (N = 22). Further, we would like to see how training duration corresponds to the structural brain changes, therefore, regression analysis between training duration and VBM differences in acupuncturists was conducted.

To our knowledge, this is the first study focusing on the structural plastic changes in professional acupuncturists. Hopefully, our study can provide primary evidence for tactile-motor plasticity as well as the plasticity in the emotion regulation domain.

Materials and Methods

1. Ethics Statement

All research procedures were approved by the West China Hospital Subcommittee on Human Studies and were conducted in accordance with the Declaration of Helsinki. Written informed consent was obtained after the experimental procedures were fully explained.

2. Subjects

We investigated 44 healthy and right-handed adult volunteers [10]. The experimental group, consisting of 22 licensed professional acupuncturists (mean age = 28.7±1.4 years, 12 males, education 19.3±1.3 years) was compared with a sample of 22 matched NA (mean age = 28.2±2.3 years, 12 males, education 19.4±1.5 years). All acupuncturists attended national medical schools, receiving 5 years of training with basic acupuncture knowledge, passed the national exam and received a license for acupuncture practice. The mean duration of acupuncture training and practice was 81.0±17.2 months. On the other hand, the control group consisted of working staff in a medical school that also received their degree from the medical school but only did office work and had not worked under any clinical conditions in the past four years. They were included in this study because they had not attended any acupuncture lectures or lectures in related fields, had no experience in acupuncture practice or had no exposure to acupuncture manipulation in any available forms before. We also ensured that no participants possessed proficiency in playing instruments. Subjects reported no past or current neurological, psychiatric, or neuropsychological problems, and did not take drugs or illegal medication prior to or during this study. Written informed consent was obtained after the experimental procedures were fully explained.

3. Behavioral Tests

We used three tasks to measure the acupuncturists' behavioral expertise. Specifically, we examined the subjects' tactile discrimination ability for the right index finger and thumb, fine motor skill, and emotion regulation ability. In general, for in all three tests, the subjects were seated comfortably in a quiet room with minimal distraction from the surroundings. After the experimental procedures and requirements of the tasks were explained to the subjects by the same experimenter, the subjects were required to repeat the procedures and demands of the tasks to the experimenter to ensure all details were explicitly comprehended. These tests did not begin until the experimenter was sure that all procedures were precisely understood by all of the participants.

a) Test on tactile discrimination ability. Tactile spatial acuity is a reliable indicator of somatosensory system function. Previous studies have proved that tactile spatial acuity is highly

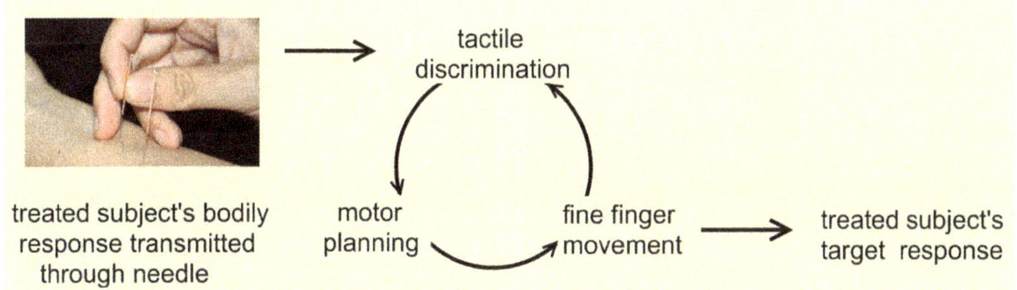

Figure 1. The schematic diagram of tactile-motor procedures during acupuncture manipulation. The schematic diagram for the feedback loop underlying tactile-motor procedures in the process of acupuncture. The patients' concurrent bodily response to each round of needling manipulation is transmitted to acupuncturist through the fine needle. The acupuncturist distinguishes the subtle difference between the actual tactile sensation and the expected one. The tactile discrimination is followed by motor planning procedure in which the next-step plan of method of needling manipulation, frequency and intensity of rotation is generated. Then, the postural configuration from the motor plan is executed as acupuncturist's fine and coordinated finger movement over the needles. This feedback loop is repeated until the target response is obtained.

correlated with subjective tactile perceptual integrity in a broad range of subject populations [11,12,13]. A well-established and reproducible measure of tactile spatial acuity is the psychophysical spatial discrimination threshold (SDT) for the grating orientation discrimination task [12,13,14]. SDT was assessed using Johnson–Van Boven–Phillips domes (Med-Core, St. Louis) at the fingertip [14].

In the current study, we used the grating orientation discrimination task to evaluate the subjects' tactile discrimination ability of the right index finger and thumb. The fingers to be tested were immobilized through double-sided tape affixed to the dorsal aspect of the finger and floor of the fixture to prevent exploratory movements. Grating domes were pressed manually onto the palmar surface of the distal phalanx of the thumb and index finger of the right hand using a spring-loaded apparatus with a spring-loaded force of 1.5 ± 0.2 N, which was adapted following the procedure of a former study [15]. Gratings were applied with the ridges oriented either along or across the long axis of the finger and subjects verbally reported the orientation of the grating as 'along' or 'across'. During this experiment, subjects were blindfolded and seated comfortably. The experimenter was visually cued to manually position [15], then released the gratings to the fingertip and maintained static for 1 second as signaled by a computer-driven timing mechanism [16]. The subsequent experimental block on each finger consisted of 40 trials without feedback. Participants received a 15 s break after every 20 trials, and a 1 min break between fingers. Each trial consisted of two sequential stimulus presentations (inter-stimulus interval, 2 s) with gratings of identical groove width but differing 90° in orientation, i.e. either parallel (vertical) to or transverse (horizontal) to the long axis of the finger. The stimulus order was chosen randomly. Subsequently, for each finger of each subject, dome gratings with progressively finer spatial periods were used until performance was at or below threshold levels (75% correct responses) [15,17,18].The grating sizes yielded the SDTs for two fingers of each individual.

The SDT was the outcome for this task.

b) Test on fine motor skill. An in-house motor task was used in this test to assess the subjects' fine motor skill. The task was designed according to the core kinetic feature of acupuncture manipulation. In the standardized training protocol and acupuncturists' clinical practice, the most basic requirement is that one should rotate the needle quickly and rhythmically, so that therapeutic effects can be optimally elicited [7]. In this sense, in our motor task, the subjects were required to rotate the needle as quickly as possible while making maximal effort to keep the rotation angle of each round within the range of 90°-180°in a pre-determined period, i.e. 30 seconds. A round was defined as from the starting position to the end position where the direction of the rotation changed.

We developed an integrated system enabling on-line recording of needle rotation. An acupuncture needle (2.5 inch in length and 0.25 in diameter) was inserted 2 inches deep into pork. Among all available materials, we chose pork because the resistance delivered to the manipulating hand could best replicate that of the human body. A marker was equipped at the end of the needle to mark the rotation angle for data analysis. A high speed camera (24frames/sec) recorded the whole process of needle rotating. An in-house computer program was developed to calculate the number of rotations for each round, eliminating the rounds whose rotation angles fell out of the required range. Only rounds meeting our criteria were counted. The subject was asked to rotate the needle using the tip of the right index finger and thumb. The palm of the right hand had to stay in that position (almost) vertical to the table surface, but not parallel to the table surface. This needling posture is the most common one in a clinical situation and therefore is the basic needling technique for acupuncturists. No right upper limb parts (e.g. palm, elbow or arm) were allowed to touch the table. Before the task, participants were seated before a table where our system was placed. After the participants adjusted themselves to the most comfortable needling position, they started the process. To ensure the reliability of the measurement, each subject was asked to perform the task three times. For each time, the number of rounds meeting the criteria was counted. The three counts were averaged for each subject. The average number of needle rotations was the outcome for this task.

We evaluated the test-retest reliability of our motor test. The intra-class correlation (ICC), a common measure of test-retest reliability, was employed to assess the stability between multiple measures of the same concept [19,20,21]. The ICC value is between -1.0 to 1.0. An ICC <0.41, from 0.41–0.59, from 0.6–0.75, or >0.75 indicates a poor, fair, good, or excellent reliability respectively [20]. In our study, ICC >0.5 was used as the threshold to determine whether the test is reliable or not according to the previous literature [22]. The SPSS 18.0 was used to compute the ICC.

c) Test on emotion regulation proficiency. Acupuncturists' daily clinical practice naturally leads to empathic pain, which would cause a negative emotional response, such as unpleasantness or distress [23]. There must be a certain central mediating mechanism which helps them cope with adverse daily events and prevents negative emotions from impairing their ability to heal or be of assistance [6]. This test aimed to assess the acupuncturists' emotion regulation proficiency. A unpleasantness rating task used in a previous study was employed [6].

One week before the task, participants filled out a series of self-report dispositional measures, including the situational pain questionnaire (SPQ) that assessed sensitivity to pain [24], the Emotional Contagion Scale(ECS) that measured the susceptibility to others' emotions [25], and the interpersonal reactivity index (IRI) [26]. During the task, all subjects were shown 120 visual stimuli (120 jpeg files). These stimuli consisted of pictures of different body parts of both painful and neutral situations [6]. Pictures were scenarios encountered in daily clinical practice. In half of the stimuli, the body parts were touched by a Q-tip (non-painful situations), and in the other half they were pricked by an acupuncture needle (painful situations). All body parts were chosen to be appropriate acupuncture sites with the assistance of an acupuncture physician with over ten years of clinical experience. The visual stimuli were delivered using the computer program E-prime 2.0 (Psychology Software Tools, Inc.). The sequence of images was randomized. Each image was displayed for 4 seconds, and rating for unpleasantness lasted 2 seconds. Participants were asked to focus on the images shown on the screen and began to score only after the cue for scoring appeared. The screen for scoring read '*How intense is the unpleasantness felt by you now?*'. Participants responded on a 10-point Likert scale ranging from 1 to 10, where 10 referred to the extreme unpleasantness, and 1 referred to no effect.

The ratings for unpleasantness were averaged across neutral and negative stimuli respectively for each subject, rather than variations in body parts that were stimulated. The ratings for both negative and neutral stimuli were the outcomes for this task, since they reliably reflected the subjects' emotion regulation ability [27].

4. MRI Data Acquisition

Imaging data was performed on a 3T Siemens scanner (Allegra; Siemens Medical System) at the Huaxi MR Research Center, West China Hospital of Sichuan University, Chengdu, China. A standard birdcage head coil was used, along with restraining foam pads to minimize head motion and to diminish scanner noise. The axial 3D T1-weighted images were obtained using an MPRAGE sequence with the following parameters: TR = 1900 ms; TE = 2.26 ms; flip angle = 90°; in-plane matrix resolution = 256×256; slices = 176; field of view = 256×256 mm^2; voxel size = 1×1×1 mm^3.

5. Voxel-Based Morphometry

Before analysis, the structural images were examined by a professional radiologist to exclude the possibility of clinically silent lesions for all of the participants. Structural data was analyzed with FSL-VBM, a voxel-based morphometry style analysis [28,29] carried out using FSL4.1 [30] (www.fmrib.ox.ac.uk/fsl/). First, all T1 images were brain-extracted using the brain extracting tool (BET) [31]. Next, tissue-type segmentation was carried out using FMRIB's automated segmentation tool (FAST) V4.1 [32]. The resulting grey-matter partial volume images were then aligned to MNI152 standard space using the affine registration tool FMRIB's Linear Image Registration Tool (FLIRT) [33,34], followed by nonlinear registration using FMRIB's Nonlinear Image Registration Tool (FNIRT) [35], which uses a b-spline representation of the registration warp field [36]. The resulting images were averaged to create a study-specific template, to which the native grey matter (GM) images were then non-linearly re-registered. The registered partial volume images were then modulated (to correct for local expansion or contraction) by dividing by the Jacobian of the warp field.

The modulated segmented images were then smoothed with an isotropic Gaussian kernel with a sigma of 3 mm (analogous to a 7 mm FWHM). Analysis of covariance (ANCOVA) was employed with age, gender, education status effects and total intracranial volume as covariates. Finally, voxel-wise GLM was applied using permutation-based non-parametric testing with 5000 random permutations, correcting for multiple comparisons across space. Results were considered significant at $p<0.01$, corrected for multiple comparisons.

To better identify the anatomical region of the cerebellum, cerebellar cluster localization was determined using the probabilistic atlas [37,38] of the cerebellum with MRIcroN (http://www.cabiatl.com/mricro/mricron/). For display purposes, statistical maps regarding the cerebral regions were superposed on the 'ch2bet' template in MRIcro (http://www.cabiatl.com/mricro/mricro/) and the cerebellar regions were overlaid on a spatially unbiased atlas template of the cerebellum [39] using MRIcroN, following the current consensus in nomenclature [40,41].

6. Regression Analysis

For the regions where acupuncturists showed significantly different gray matter volumes over the controls, the gray matter volumes of these areas were extracted, averaged and regressed against the duration of acupuncture practice. Additionally, to detect the correspondence between central representations and behavioral expertise, the gray matter volumes of these areas were extracted, averaged and regressed against the measurement of behavioral expertise. Results were considered significant at $p<0.05$ (multiple correction using Bonferroni test).

Results

1. Results of Behavioral Tests

a) Results of tactile discrimination ability test. As shown in Table 1, the two sample *t*-test revealed that the acupuncturists had a significantly lower SDT than that of the control group for both fingers, indicating better spatial acuity (*two sample t-test, $p<0.05$ for the index finger and the thumb*). The results verified the acupuncturists' tactile discrimination proficiency.

b) Results of fine motor skill test. The intra-class correlation (ICC) coefficient was used to evaluate the test-retest reliability of our motor test. The ICC was 0.95, better than the 0.5 threshold [22]. This indicates that our test is reliable and provides stable measurement.

Then we evaluated whether acupuncturists outperformer the NA in this test. The results displayed that the acupuncturists achieved 90.1±6.9 rounds of rotations as compared to 46.1±7.5 of non-acupuncturists (*two sample t-test, $p<0.05$*), as shown in Table 1. The results verified that the acupuncturists had better fine motor skills compared to NA.

c) Results of the emotion regulation proficiency test. The analyses of the dispositional measures revealed no differences between the two groups in terms of ECS, SPQ and each sub-domain of IRI scores using a *two sample t-test* (*see Table 2 for detailed p and t values*). The detailed information is summarized in Table 2. Results of the two sample *t*-test showed that unpleasantness ratings for neutral stimuli did not differ between the two groups (*two sample t-test, $p = 0.39$, $t = -0.87$*), which was consistent with previous conclusions [6], whereas for negative stimuli, unpleasantness ratings were significantly lower in the acupuncturists group (Table 2). The results demonstrated that the acupuncturists had better emotion regulation ability than that of the controls.

2. VBM Results

Regional grey matter volume changes were assessed using VBM. Significantly larger grey matter volumes ($p<0.01$) were found in the acupuncturists as compared to NA in a subset of cerebral and cerebellar regions, i.e. the left primary somatosensory cortex (SI), the right lobule V/VI and the bilateral ventral anterior cingulate cortex/the vetral medial prefrontal cortex (vACC/VMPFC) after controlling for potential confounding variables including age, gender effects, level of education and total intracranial volume (shown in Figure 2, Figure 3 and Table 3). Significant grey matter volume (GMV) differences were found exclusively in these regions.

Table 1. Measure of fine motor skill for fingers and spatial discrimination threshold in two groups.

	Experts(n = 22)		NA(n = 22)		two sample t (Experts vs. NA)	
Task	**Mean**	**SD**	**Mean**	**SD**	***p* value**	***t* value**
NoR*	90.1	6.9	46.1	7.5	2.73E-23	20.2501
SDT*(Indext)	0.93	0.23	1.11	0.18	0.0065	−2.8627
SDT*(Thumb)	1.16	0.18	1.33	0.12	6.60E-04	−3.6795

NoR: number of rotations; SDT: spatial discrimination threshold; SD: standard deviation;
***denotes the item that shows significant difference between the two groups (*$p<0.05$*).**

Table 2. Dispositional measurement of empathy and ratings of unpleasantness in two groups.

	Experts(n = 22)		NA(n = 22)		two sample t (Experts vs. NA)	
Task	**Mean**	**SD**	**Mean**	**SD**	**p value**	**t value**
ECS	26.5	3.8	26.6	4.3	0.94	−0.07
SPQ	5.8	0.5	5.6	0.8	0.38	0.89
IRI(PT)	18.4	3.7	18.2	3.1	0.86	0.17
IRI(EC)	21.1	3.2	20.4	3.6	0.45	0.76
IRI(PD)	11.8	3.5	12.5	4.1	0.76	−0.31
IRI(FS)	17.5	4.1	16.9	3.7	0.65	0.46
Unpleasantness*	1.6	0.7	6.1	0.9	1.06E-21	−18.38

ECS: emotional contagion scale; SPQ: situational pain questionnaire; IRI: interpersonal reaction index; PT: perspective taking; EC: empathic concern; PD: personal distress; FS: fantasy; SD: standard deviation;

***denotes the item that shows significant difference between the acupuncturists and NA (*$p<0.05$*).**

3. Results of Regression Analysis

GMV of the left SI and the right V/VI positively correlated with the duration of acupuncture practice (*$p<0.05$, Bonferroni corrected*), after regressing out potential confounding variables of age, gender and level of education in our analysis (Figure 2 and Figure 3). While the correlations/anti-correlations between GMV of left SI, the right V/VI and the bilateral vACC/VMPFC and measurement of behavioral expertise were not found. Specifically, we have done $3 \times 5 = 15$ corrections for regression analysis (3 ROIs vs. duration of acupuncture practice, outcomes for tactile ability test, i.e. SDT for the two fingers, outcomes for motor task and unpleasantness ratings).

Discussion

In the current study, we initiated to investigate the structural brain differences between acupuncturists and NA. Firstly, our behavioral analysis verified the behavioral expertise of acupuncturists in tactile-motor and emotion regulation domains (Table 1 and Table 2). The VBM results showed that the acupuncturist group, as compared to NA, had larger GMV in the left SI, secondary motor areas, i.e. the right V/VI, and the bilateral vACC/VMPFC. Our findings confirmed the notions that any manipulation which produces an enduring change in behavior leaves an anatomic footprint on the brain [42]. We also revealed the positive correlation between the GMV of the left SI (Figure 2) and cerebellar V/VI and the duration of acupuncture practice

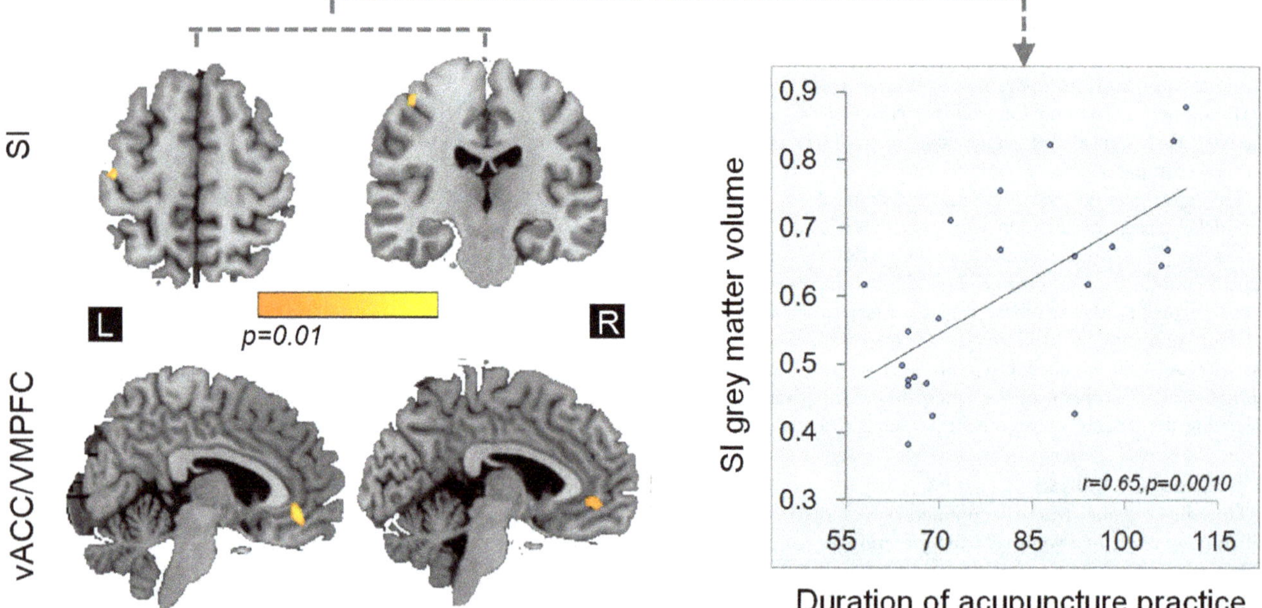

Figure 2. Cerebral VBM differences between groups (*$p<0.01$, corrected*) and regression analysis (*$p<0.05$, Bonferroni corrected*). The GMV differences in cerebral regions between groups. Positive linear correlations were found between GMV in the left SI and the duration of acupuncture practice. All images are shown as (1-p) corrected *p*-value images at the threshold of $p<0.01$, corrected. The corresponding *t* values are provided. The vACC/VMPFC was displayed in the sagittal view, and SI in the axial view (on the left side) and the coronal view (on the right side) using MRIcro. vACC/VMPFC: ventral anterior cingulate cortex/ventral medial prefrontal cortex; primary somatosensory cortex: SI.

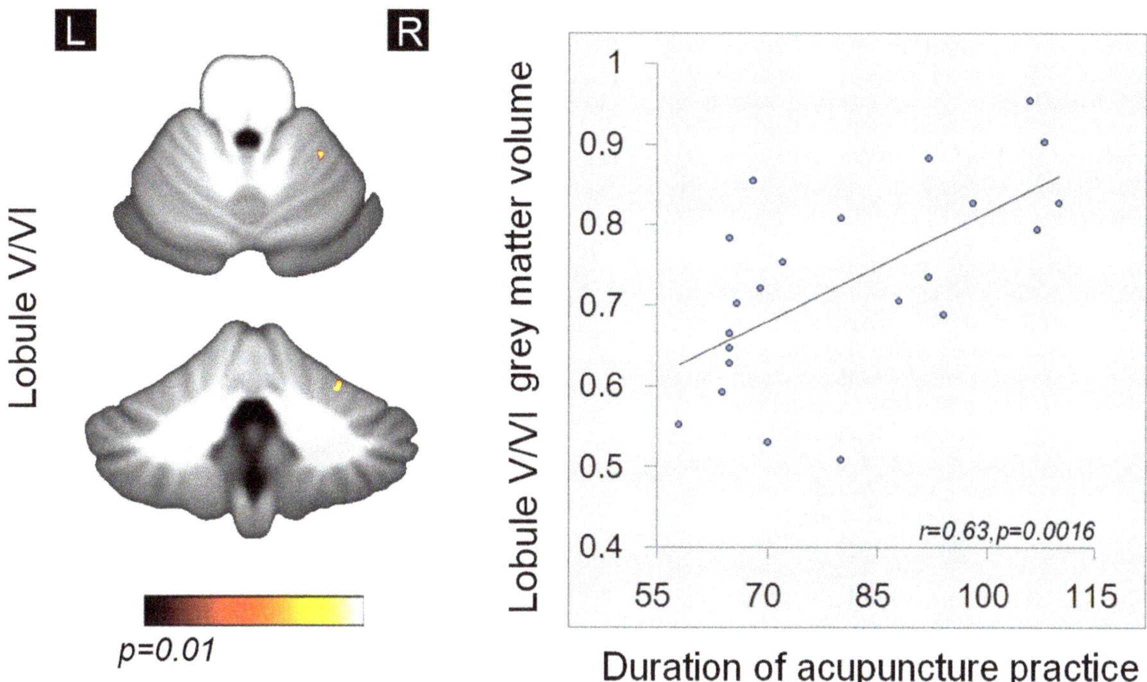

Figure 3. Cerebellar VBM differences between groups (*p*<*0.01, corrected*) and regression analysis (*p*<*0.05, Bonferroni corrected*). The GMV differences in cerebellar regions between groups. Positive linear correlations were found between GMV in the right lobule V/VI and the duration of acupuncture practice. All images are shown as (1-p) corrected *p*-value images at the threshold of *p*<0.01, corrected. The corresponding t values are provided. The Lobule V/VI was displayed in the axial view (the upper figure) and the coronal view (the lower figure) using MRIcroN.

(Figure 3). We suggest that our study may also provide preliminary evidence for neuroanatomical substrates subserving professional acupuncturists' extraordinary skills.

Our study demonstrated larger GMV in the cortical representation of hand in the left SI cortex. This may be linked to acupuncturists' exceptional tactile discrimination ability (Table 1). Indeed, tactile discrimination ability is especially crucial for acupuncturists. Acupuncture aims to elicit unique bodily responses in patients, which is characterized as signified but extremely subtle tightness around the needle and the tactile information is used by acupuncturists to characterize optimal therapeutic effects [7]. However, each round of needle manipulation induces a distinctive bodily response in patients because the patients' concurrent mental state and physical responses to needling are dynamic. In this sense, it is necessary for acupuncturists to decide whether the expected sensation is achieved by carefully discriminating the tactile stimulus delivered to the manipulating digits through the fine needle. The region reported here is known to play an important role in perception of touch [43]. A study applying repetitive transcranial magnetic stimulation over the cortical hand-finger representation of the primary somatosensory cortex revealed a close link between the cortical enlargement and improvement in tactile perception function of the fingers [44], whereas declined tactile perception function was concomitant with shrunken primary somatosensory cortical maps [2]. On one hand, the tactile function is enhanced on the basis of usage [45] and use is a major factor driving plasticity of cortical maps [2]. On the other hand, previous reports further suggested that enrichment in the afferent sensory input could induce cortical morphometry changes in the adult human brain [46]. In our case, the acupuncturists' daily practice exclusively depends on this sensory modality and the function is extensively used [7], which in return also permits enhanced sensory stimulation in this modality. Therefore, we suggest that larger contralateral representations in the primary somatosensory cortex of the right hand may support the acupuncturists' extraordinary ability in perceiving subtle tactile information, eventually facilitating their tactile discrimination ability.

Table 3. Significant grey matter volume differences in the acupuncturists group (*p*<*0.01, corrected*).

	Hemisphere	MNI Coordinates (cluster maxima)			*Peak t-stat*
		x	y	z	
vACC/VMPFC	L	−1	39	−7	6.42
	R	3	47	−7	6.37
SI	L	−44	−20	59	6.53
Lobule V/VI	R	26	−47	−24	6.60

vACC: ventral anterior cingulate cortex; VMPFC: ventral medial prefrontal cortex; SI: primary somatosensory cortex; L, left; R, right.

We reported larger GMV in the right lobule V/VI in acupuncturists (Figure 3 and Table 3), which may be related to acupuncturists' extraordinary motor skills for fingers. The acupuncturists' fine motor skill for fingers is important, since it ultimately determined whether or not optimal clinical outcomes could be achieved. Our behavioral test verified that acupuncture had exceptional fine motor skills (Table 1). The structural changes in this region fits particularly well with the well-established cerebellar involvement in unimanual finger movement control

[47,48]. Specifically, cerebellum has been considered a region largely involved in motor learning [49]. Previous studies using subjects with unimanual finger motor proficiency implicated that skill-relevant functional/structural brain mapping changes occurred in the ipslateral lobule V/VI [50,51]. Therefore, we suggested that the larger GMV of the right lobule V/VI was likely to support the acupuncturists' fine motor skill, in parallel, the structural changes may also serve to facilitate performance retention [1].

The regression analysis demonstrated positive correlation between the GMV of the SI vs. duration of acupuncture practice and the GMV of the right lobule V/VI vs. duration of practice. This is consistent with former observations that long-lasting and exceptional usage of the fingers results in the development of outstanding sensorimotor skills and results in expansions of the cortical finger representations and GMV changes of sensorimotor domain might be developed as a function of time [2]. These also imply that the duration of training was potentially an important variable determining the amount of cortical changes.

Acupuncture procedure substantially involves inflicting painful treatment process to patients to achieve therapeutic effect. Acupuncturists have to be massively exposed themselves to such situations each day during their clinical practice. This painful procedure should naturally induced intensive and prominent aversive empathic responses [6], which would probably lead to anxiety and personal distress [23]. Such response would bias their professional help. But, it seems acupuncturists do not suffer from this, as evidenced significantly lower unpleasantness ratings (Table 2). These differences are not likely to be attributed to depositional or emotion contagion because these personality traits did not differ in the two groups (Table 2). It was also unlikely that this difference was due to attention demands because both groups performed similarly on the continuous performance task. Therefore, we proposed there should be a certain emotion regulation mechanism facilitating acupuncturist. Accordingly, we found a larger GMV in the bilateral vACC/VMPFC in the acupuncturist group in the current study. A number of functional, behavioral, and lesion studies have provided evidence that the region is involved in modulation or inhibition of the emotional response [52,53,54]. Specifically, this region is in association with suppressing or reappraising negative emotional stimuli and with suppressing the influence of negative emotional stimuli on subsequent behavior [55]. Also, a recent report stated that increased GMV in this region was associated with enhanced emotion regulation control performance after long-term meditation training [5]. In contrast, pathological data demonstrated the dysfunction in emotion regulation was largely associated with decreased GMV in this region [56,57]. Taken together, we suggest that larger GMV in the vACC/VMPFC is highly likely to be associated with the acupuncturists' emotion regulation expertise. But, the specific nature of these underlying correlates (e.g., possibly enhanced neuropil, neuronal size, number, and density, size, and/or a particular wiring pattern of neuronal connections in meditators) remains to be established in future studies.

Moreover, no correlation/anti-correlation was found between the GMV of vACC/VMPFC and the duration of acupuncture practice in acupuncturists. Given that emotion regulation was a higher-order cognitive function, we suggested that it was probable that structural underpinnings of this function do not necessarily develop over the same time course with low order sensorimotor functions [58,59].

Conclusions

The present findings demonstrate that long-term acupuncture training occurring in adulthood is associated to structural modifications not randomly distributed, but likely to be related to the specific features of acquired skills. In conclusion, acupuncturists represent a useful group to study human brain structural plasticity in tactile-motor and emotion regulation dimensions. On one hand, we suggest our findings may have ramifications for tactile-motor rehabilitation. On the other hand, our results in emotion regulation domain may serve as a target for our future studies, from which we can understand how modulations of aversive emotions elicited by empathic pain develop in the context of expertise. To a greater extent, we hope that this study may help to understand the behavioral-brain inter-connection, which in return may facilitate occupational skill acquisition [60] and will guide to develop new naturalistic training strategies during adulthood in the future [61].

We understand that a major concern in neuroplasticity research is how developmental origin, training and genetic factor interact with each other, ultimately influencing neuroplasticity. Therefore, we should take cautions when interpreting the current findings, since we cannot exclusively account the differences found in this study to the experience/training alone. To this end, longitudinal experimental design is appropriate to definitively link the structural changes and the factor of use/training. But, our currently available data is not feasible for this purpose. Nevertheless, we are optimistic to suggest the potency of taking our results as the basis for further studies. During the following two years, a series of experiments using longitudinal design, with larger sample size, even with subjects from the same family, are to be carried out, to make stronger inferences about the impact of training *per se*. We do hope to answer this question in the long run.

Acknowledgments

We would like to give special thanks to Dr. Qiyong Gong for his generosity of providing scanner and all available facilities which made the current study possible.

Author Contributions

Conceived and designed the experiments: MHD WQ. Performed the experiments: MHD JBS WQ. Analyzed the data: MHD KY DHY. Contributed reagents/materials/analysis tools: LZ FZ. Wrote the paper: MHD JXL. Contributed to the writing of the manuscript: KMD FRL JT.

References

1. Pascual-Leone A, Amedi A, Fregni F, Merabet LB (2005) The plastic human brain cortex. Annu Rev Neurosci 28: 377–401.
2. Lissek S, Wilimzig C, Stude P, Pleger B, Kalisch T, et al. (2009) Immobilization impairs tactile perception and shrinks somatosensory cortical maps. Curr Bio 19: 837–842.
3. Hänggi J, Koeneke S, Bezzola L, Jäncke L (2010) Structural neuroplasticity in the sensorimotor network of professional female ballet dancers. Hum Brain Mapp 31: 1196–1206.
4. Park IS, Lee KJ, Han JW, Lee NJ, Lee WT, et al. (2009) Experience-dependent plasticity of cerebellar vermis in basketball players. Cerebellum 8: 334–339.
5. Luders E, Toga AW, Lepore N, Gaser C (2009) The underlying anatomical correlates of long-term meditation: larger hippocampal and frontal volumes of gray matter. Neuroimage 45: 672–678.
6. Cheng Y, Lin CP, Liu HL, Hsu YY, Lim KE, et al. (2007) Expertise modulates the perception of pain in others. Curr Bio 17: 1708–1713.
7. Cheng X (2010) Chinese acupuncture and moxibustion; Cheng X, editor. Beijing: Foreign Languages Press.
8. Wolpert DM, Diedrichsen J, Flanagan JR (2011) Principles of sensorimotor learning. Nat Rev Neurosci.

9. May A (2011) Experience-dependent structural plasticity in the adult human brain. Trends Cogn Sci.
10. Oldfield RC (1971) The assessment and analysis of handedness: the Edinburgh inventory. Neuropsychologia 9: 97–113.
11. Johnson KO, Hsiao SS (1992) Neural mechanisms of tactual form and texture perception. Annu Rev Neurosci 15: 227–250.
12. Johnson KO, Phillips JR (1981) Tactile spatial resolution. I. Two-point discrimination, gap detection, grating resolution, and letter recognition. J Neurophysiol 46: 1177–1192.
13. Van Boven RW, Johnson KO (1994) A psychophysical study of the mechanisms of sensory recovery following nerve injury in humans. Brain 117: 149.
14. Sathian K, Zangaladze A (1996) Tactile spatial acuity at the human fingertip and lip. Neurology 46: 1464–1464.
15. Van Boven RW, Ingeholm JE, Beauchamp MS, Bikle PC, Ungerleider LG (2005) Tactile form and location processing in the human brain. Proc Natl Acad Sci USA 102: 12601.
16. Zhang M, Mariola E, Stilla R, Stoesz M, Mao H, et al. (2005) Tactile discrimination of grating orientation: fMRI activation patterns. Hum Brain Mapp 25: 370–377.
17. Goldreich D, Kanics IM (2003) Tactile acuity is enhanced in blindness. J Neurosci 23: 3439–3445.
18. Van Boven RW, Hamilton RH, Kauffman T, Keenan JP, Pascual-Leone A (2000) Tactile spatial resolution in blind Braille readers. Neurology 54: 2230–2236.
19. Bartko JJ (1966) The intraclass correlation coefficient as a measure of reliability. Psychological reports 19: 3–11.
20. McGraw KO, Wong S (1996) Forming inferences about some intraclass correlation coefficients. Psychological methods 1: 30.
21. Shrout PE, Fleiss JL (1979) Intraclass correlations: uses in assessing rater reliability. Psychological bulletin 86: 420.
22. Cicchetti D (2001) The precision of reliability, validity estimates revisited: distinguishing between clinical and statistical significance of sample size requirements. J Clin Exp Neuropsychol 23: 695–700.
23. Hein G, Singer T (2008) I feel how you feel but not always: the empathic brain and its modulation. Curr Opin Neurobiol 18: 153–158.
24. Clark WC, Yang JC (1983) Applications of sensory decision theory to problems in laboratory and clinical pain. In: Melzack R, editor. Pain measurement and assessment. New York: Raven.
25. Doherty RW (1997) The emotional contagion scale: A measure of individual differences. J Nonverbal Behav 21: 131–154.
26. Davis MH (1994) Empathy: A social psychological approach. Madison: Westview Press.
27. Vogt BA (2005) Pain and emotion interactions in subregions of the cingulate gyrus. Nat Rev Neurosci 6: 533–544.
28. Ashburner J, Friston KJ (2000) Voxel-based morphometry–the methods. Neuroimage 11: 805–821.
29. Good CD, Johnsrude IS, Ashburner J, Henson RNA, Fristen K, et al. A voxel-based morphometric study of ageing in 465 normal adult human brains; 2002. IEEE. 16 p.
30. Smith SM, Jenkinson M, Woolrich MW, Beckmann CF, Behrens TEJ, et al. (2004) Advances in functional and structural MR image analysis and implementation as FSL. Neuroimage 23: S208–S219.
31. Smith SM (2002) Fast robust automated brain extraction. Hum Brain Mapp 17: 143–155.
32. Zhang Y, Brady M, Smith S (2001) Segmentation of brain MR images through a hidden Markov random field model and the expectation-maximization algorithm. IEEE T Med Imaging 20: 45–57.
33. Jenkinson M, Bannister P, Brady M, Smith S (2002) Improved optimization for the robust and accurate linear registration and motion correction of brain images. Neuroimage 17: 825–841.
34. Jenkinson M, Smith S (2001) A global optimisation method for robust affine registration of brain images. Med Image Anal 5: 143–156.
35. Andersson JLR, Jenkinson M, Smith S, Andersson J (2007) Non-linear registration, aka spatial normalization. FMRIB technical report TR07JA2: FMRIB Analysis Group of the University of Oxford.
36. Rueckert D, Sonoda LI, Hayes C, Hill DLG, Leach MO, et al. (1999) Nonrigid registration using free-form deformations: application to breast MR images. IEEE T Med Imaging 18: 712–721.
37. Diedrichsen J, Balsters JH, Flavell J, Cussans E, Ramnani N (2009) A probabilistic MR atlas of the human cerebellum. Neuroimage 46: 39–46.
38. Diedrichsen J, Verstynen T, Schlerf J, Wiestler T (2010) Advances in functional imaging of the human cerebellum. Curr Opin Neurol 23: 382.
39. Diedrichsen J (2006) A spatially unbiased atlas template of the human cerebellum. Neuroimage 33: 127–138.
40. Schmahmann JD (2000) MRI atlas of the human cerebellum. San Diego: Academic Press.
41. Larsell O, Jansen J (1972) The comparative anatomy and histology of the cerebellum: the human cerebellum, cerebellar connections, and cerebellar cortex. Minneapolis: University of Minnesota Press.
42. Jäncke L (2009) The plastic human brain. Resto Neurol and Neuros 27: 521–538.
43. Frackowiak RSJ (2004) Human brain function. San Diego: Academic Press.
44. Tegenthoff M, Ragert P, Pleger B, Schwenkreis P, Förster AF, et al. (2005) Improvement of tactile discrimination performance and enlargement of cortical somatosensory maps after 5 Hz rTMS. PLoS Biol 3: e362.
45. Wong M, Gnanakumaran V, Goldreich D (2011) Tactile spatial acuity enhancement in blindness: evidence for experience-dependent mechanisms. J Neurosci 31: 7028.
46. Elbert T, Pantev C, Wienbruch C, Rockstroh B, Taub E (1995) Increased cortical representation of the fingers of the left hand in string players. Science 270: 305.
47. Stoodley CJ, Schmahmann JD (2009) Functional topography in the human cerebellum: a meta-analysis of neuroimaging studies. Neuroimage 44: 489–501.
48. Grodd W, Hülsmann E, Lotze M, Wildgruber D, Erb M (2001) Sensorimotor mapping of the human cerebellum: fMRI evidence of somatotopic organization. Hum Brain Mapp 13: 55–73.
49. Manto MU, Jissendi P (2012) Cerebellum: links between development, developmental disorders and motor learning. Front Neuroanat 6.
50. Koeneke S, Lutz K, Wüstenberg T, Jäncke L (2004) Long-term training affects cerebellar processing in skilled keyboard players. Neuroreport 15: 1279.
51. Franklin DW, Wolpert DM (2011) Computational Mechanisms of Sensorimotor Control. Neuron 72: 425–442.
52. Albert J, López-Martín S, Tapia M, Montoya D, Carretié L (2011) The role of the anterior cingulate cortex in emotional response inhibition. Hum Brain Mapp.
53. Lamm C, Nusbaum HC, Meltzoff AN, Decety J (2007) What are you feeling? Using functional magnetic resonance imaging to assess the modulation of sensory and affective responses during empathy for pain. PloS One 2: e1292.
54. Shackman AJ, Salomons TV, Slagter HA, Fox AS, Winter JJ, et al. (2011) The integration of negative affect, pain and cognitive control in the cingulate cortex. Annu Rev Neurosci 12: 154–167.
55. Quirk GJ, Beer JS (2006) Prefrontal involvement in the regulation of emotion: convergence of rat and human studies. Current opinion in neurobiology 16: 723–727.
56. Drevets WC, Price JL, Simpson JR, Todd RD, Reich T, et al. (1997) Subgenual prefrontal cortex abnormalities in mood disorders. Nature 386: 824–827.
57. Ballmaier M, Toga AW, Blanton RE, Sowell ER, Lavretsky H, et al. (2004) Anterior cingulate, gyrus rectus, and orbitofrontal abnormalities in elderly depressed patients: an MRI-based parcellation of the prefrontal cortex. Am J Psychiat 161: 99–108.
58. Fields RD (2011) Imaging Learning: The Search for a Memory Trace. Neuroscientist 17: 185.
59. Draganski B, May A (2008) Training-induced structural changes in the adult human brain. Behav Brain Res 192: 137–142.
60. Munte TF, Altenmuller E, Jancke L (2002) The musician's brain as a model of neuroplasticity. Nat Rev Neurosci 3: 473–477.
61. Herdener M, Esposito F, di Salle F, Boller C, Hilti CC, et al. (2010) Musical training induces functional plasticity in human hippocampus. J Neurosci 30: 1377.

8

Acupuncture Induces Divergent Alterations of Functional Connectivity within Conventional Frequency Bands: Evidence from MEG Recordings

Youbo You[1,❡], Lijun Bai[1,❡], Ruwei Dai[1], Chongguang Zhong[1], Ting Xue[2], Hu Wang[1], Zhenyu Liu[1], Wenjuan Wei[1], Jie Tian[1,2]*

1 Intelligent Medical Research Center, Institute of Automation, Chinese Academy of Sciences, Beijing, China, **2** Life Science Research Center, School of Electronic Engineering, Xidian University, Xi'an, Shaanxi, China

Abstract

As an ancient Chinese healing modality which has gained increasing popularity in modern society, acupuncture involves stimulation with fine needles inserted into acupoints. Both traditional literature and clinical data indicated that modulation effects largely depend on specific designated acupoints. However, scientific representations of acupoint specificity remain controversial. In the present study, considering the new findings on the sustained effects of acupuncture and its time-varied temporal characteristics, we employed an electrophysiological imaging modality namely magnetoencephalography with a temporal resolution on the order of milliseconds. Taken into account the differential band-limited signal modulations induced by acupuncture, we sought to explore whether or not stimulation at Stomach Meridian 36 (ST36) and a nearby non-meridian point (NAP) would evoke divergent functional connectivity alterations within delta, theta, alpha, beta and gamma bands. Whole-head scanning was performed on 28 healthy participants during an eyes-closed no-task condition both preceding and following acupuncture. Data analysis involved calculation of band-limited power (BLP) followed by pair-wise BLP correlations. Further averaging was conducted to obtain local and remote connectivity. Statistical analyses revealed the increased connection degree of the left temporal cortex within delta (0.5–4 Hz), beta (13–30 Hz) and gamma (30–48 Hz) bands following verum acupuncture. Moreover, we not only validated the closer linkage of the left temporal cortex with the prefrontal and frontal cortices, but further pinpointed that such patterns were more extensively distributed in the ST36 group in the delta and beta bands compared to the restriction only to the delta band for NAP. Psychophysical results for significant pain threshold elevation further confirmed the analgesic effect of acupuncture at ST36. In conclusion, our findings may provide a new perspective to lend support for the specificity of neural expression underlying acupuncture.

Editor: Dante R. Chialvo, National Research & Technology Council, Argentina

Funding: This paper is supported by the Knowledge Innovation Program of the Chinese Academy of Sciences under Grant No. KGCX2-YW-129, the National Natural Science Foundation of China under Grant Nos. 30873462, 30970769, 30970771, 60910006, 81071217, 81171314, the Joint Research Fund for Overseas Chinese Scholars and Scholars in Hong Kong and Macao funder Grant No. 31028010, the Chinese Academy of Sciences Visiting Professorship for Senior International Scientists under Grant No. 2010T2G36, the Fundamental Research Funds for the Central University, Beijing Nova program under Grant No. Z111101054511116, and the National Basic Research Program of China (973 Program) under Grant No. 2011CB707700. The funders had no role in study design, data collection and analysis, decision to publish, or preparation of the manuscript.

Competing Interests: The authors have declared that no competing interests exist.

* E-mail: tian@ieee.org

❡ These authors contributed equally to this work.

Introduction

Acupuncture is one of the most important therapeutic modalities in Traditional Chinese Medicine (TCM), which treats patients by utilizing thin needles inserted into specific anatomical points named acupoints and then twirled manually [1]. Its treatments for postoperative and chemotherapy-induced nausea and vomiting and for postoperative dental pain are promising, and it can also be a beneficial adjunct or alternative treatment for drug addiction, stroke rehabilitation and chronic pain [2,3]. One recent NIH survey in the USA demonstrated the sharply increased percentage of patients visiting acupuncturists from 27.2 per 1000 in 1997 to 79.2 per 1000 in 2007 [4]. In spite of its gaining popularity, however, it remains elusive on the scientific explanation about the neural mechanisms underlying the efficacy of acupuncture, hindering its profound significance in modern medical practice. To unveil the underlying biological mechanism would facilitate better acceptance and integration of this therapeutic modality into the practice of modern medicine.

One of the most highly attention-grabbing controversies focuses on acupoint specificity, which lies in the crucial position of traditional acupuncture theory. Based upon TCM, twirling needles at acupoints can correct imbalances in the flow of *qi* through channels known as meridians, while stimulation at points non-meridian points have little modulation effects [1]. In other words, the clinical effectiveness of acupuncture per se is said to depend on the specific placement of the needles [5]. However, scientific representation on acupoint specificity remains debatable in contemporary biomedical information [2,6]. There are some pioneers, of whom Cho was one of the first, to find that the visual cortex could be activated by peripheral acupuncture at visually associated acupoints other than nearby non-meridian points [7,8]. On the contrary, several recent studies illustrated no significant difference in functional Magnetic Resonance Imaging (fMRI) signal changes in acupuncture whether at vision-related or hearing-related acupoints compared with non-meridian points [9,10]. Further work is therefore needed to elucidate the neurological basis of acupoint specificity so as to promote better acceptance of acupuncture as a viable clinical treatment.

During the last few decades, advances in non-invasive imaging techniques have significantly boosted neuroscience research, among which fMRI has been the dominant tool for exploring brain activity [7,10,11,12,13,14]. Nevertheless, it is limited by its intrinsic nature of indirect assessments on cerebral metabolism and poor temporal resolution due to the protracted hemodynamic response [15]. Therefore, although previous fMRI studies have been of great assistance in spatially identifying function-associated brain regions [8,9,16,17,18], mechanisms underlying acupuncture may be unveiled incompletely considering its prolonged effects and time-varied temporal characteristic [12]. To introduce a more direct measurement of brain activity, as a result, may be of profound significance. Recently, it has been widely acknowledged that electroencephalography (EEG) and magnetoencephalography (MEG) enable us to monitor the dynamic neural activity of the whole brain, through which the electric/magnetic fields induced by the neuronal current flow in the brain are directly measured above the scalp [19,20]. They both have a smaller time scale than fMRI on the order of milliseconds, presenting a much more refined perspective to track the transient neural activity [21]. Besides, since greater amounts of temporal information are being provided, it is more suitable to alternatively investigate from the concept of functional connectivity [22,23,24]. In particular, compared with EEG, MEG has more advantages to assess functional interactivity without distortion of magnetic fields by inhomogeneous conductivity or the need of a reference electrode [25].

The current study was developed to explore whether or not divergent alteration of functional connectivity exists following verum acupuncture (Stomach Meridian 36, ST36) relative to sham acupuncture (non-meridian point, NAP). Since previous electrophysiological investigations have demonstrated differential band-limited signal changes brought about by acupuncture [26,27,28], functional connectivity was sought in the present study with the hypothesis that distinct alteration patterns would be illustrated in response to the verum and sham acupuncture procedure within delta (0.5–4 Hz), theta (4–8 Hz), alpha (8–13 Hz), beta (13–30 Hz) and gamma bands (30–48 Hz).

Materials and Methods

Subjects

In order to reduce the inter-subject difference, 28 Chinese right-handed healthy college students (14 males, 14 females, aged 24.5±1.8 years) selected from a homogeneous group were enrolled in this study. They were all acupuncture naïve. None of them had a history of major medical illness, head trauma, neuropsychiatric disorders, nor did they use any prescription medications within the last month according to a questionnaire they filled out. All subjects gave written, informed consent after the experimental procedures had been fully explained. The research procedures were approved by the Tiantan Hospital Subcommittee on Human Studies and conducted in accordance with the Declaration of Helsinki.

Experimental paradigm

Twenty-eight participants were evenly divided into two groups, being matched by age and gender. Every subject received only once acupuncture stimulation. They were instructed to sit comfortably in a dark and magnetically shielded room with their eyes closed and asked to remain relaxed without engaging in mental tasks.

The experiment consisted of two functional runs. The resting-state run lasted 6 min. Acupuncture in both groups employed the single-block design paradigm, incorporating a 2 min needle manipulation, preceded by a 1 min rest epoch and followed by another 6 min resting scan (needle was kept in place without manipulation). See Fig. 1 for details. The two 6 min data scans were used in the present study. Acupuncture was performed at acupoint ST36 on the right leg, which has been proven to show great efficacy in pain-management in humans [29,30]. It is located four finger breadths below the lower margin of the patella and one finger breadth laterally from the anterior crest of the tibia (arrow pointing to the red dot in Fig. 1). When acupuncture is executed, in classical literature, it is guided by the two classical manipulation procedures named "tonifying" and "reducing" [1]. The former is the reinforcing method of treatment which is performed by a comparatively weak stimulation to increase energy to the body, while the latter is the reducing method conducted by a comparatively strong stimulation to decrease energy. Clinically, the practice difference mainly lies in the fact that "tonifying" is the counter-clockwise rotation of needles while "reducing" is done clockwise [31]. In the present study, a balanced "tonifying and reducing" technique was utilized as twirling the needle clockwise and counter-clockwise equally [11]. Verum acupuncture was delivered using a sterile disposable 38 gauge stainless steel acupuncture needle, 0.2 mm in diameter and 40 mm in length, which was inserted perpendicularly into the skin surface at a depth of 1.5–2.5 cm. Sham acupuncture was exerted with needling at a nearby NAP (2–3 cm apart from ST36, arrow pointing to the green dot), with needle depth (1.5–2.5 cm), stimulation intensity (twirling needle for 2 min at the rate of 60 cycles/min) and manipulation procedure (balanced "tonifying and reducing" technique) all identical to those used in verum acupuncture. The whole procedure was performed by the same experienced and licensed acupuncturist on all participants.

According to TCM, the sensation induced by twirling needles at the acupoints is asserted as "*De-qi*", which is essential to the efficacy of acupuncture [32]. As a concurrent psychophysical analysis, the MGH Acupuncture Sensation Scale (MASS) was utilized in the present study to quantify the subjective "*De-qi*" sensations, including throbbing, aching, soreness, heaviness, fullness, warmth, coolness, numbness, tingling, dull or sharp pain, pressure and one blank row for subjects to add their own observations if the above descriptors did not embody the sensations they experienced during the stimulation [33,34]. The sensation rates ranged from 0 to 10 (0 = no sensation, 1–3 = mild, 4–6 = moderate, 7–8 = strong, 9 = severe and 10 = unbearable sensation). Spreading of any sensation was noted in a binary fashion and coded as follows: 1—spreading reported; 0—spreading not reported. As ST36 is a commonly used acupoint for pain control in clinical practice, we evaluated pain threshold changes as well during the experiment. Pain was induced by modified potassium iontophoresis with gradually increasing anodal currents, which has been accepted as a reliable measurement of pain tolerance [35,36]. The iontophoretic pain generator mainly consists of a computer-controlled constant current source, with the ability to deliver a selected amount of current ranging from 0 to 5.0 mA. Intensity levels were graded in 0.2-mA steps [37]. The

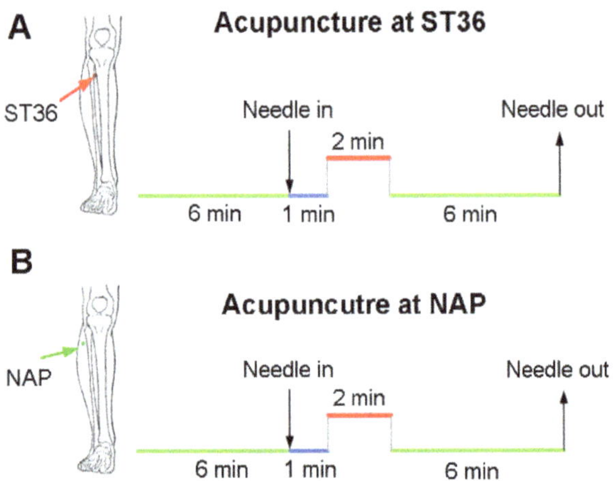

Figure 1. Experimental paradigm. Panel A indicates that acupuncture stimulation was performed at acupoint ST36 on the right leg (Zusanli, arrow pointing to the red dot). Panel B indicates that needling was performed at an adjacent nonacupoint on the right leg (NAP, arrow pointing to the green dot). The red line refers to needle administration, and the blue line represents no acupuncture manipulation but with needles inserted, while the green long line indicates a 6 min resting state or post-stimulus resting state. In this study, the two 6 min resting epochs were employed, while the rest were used for further analysis.

pain threshold was estimated by the current needed to produce pain [38]. Measurements for each subject were taken every 10 min for 60 min separately just before scanning and after the "*De-qi*" questionnaire was completed. The results of 6 scores in each condition were averaged respectively as each subject's pain threshold.

MEG data acquisition

The MEG data were recorded while subjects were comfortably seated inside a magnetically shielded room using a 151-channel whole-head MEG system (CTF Systems Inc., Port Coquitlam, BC, Canada). Average distance between sensors in this system was 3.1 cm. The head position was monitored during the measurement using head position indicator coils. MEG data were recorded at the sample rate of 600 Hz. During the recording, participants were instructed to close their eyes to reduce artifact signals due to eye movements, but remained awake as much as possible. Subjects wore earplugs throughout the experiment to attenuate any sounds heard from outside of the MEG room. The investigator and MEG technician checked the signal on-line and observed the participants using a video monitor. At the beginning and end of each recording, the head position relative to the coordinate system of the helmet was recorded by leading small alternating currents through three head position coils attached to the left and right pre-auricular points and the nasion on the subject's head. If any subject's head moved more than 5 mm during the experiment, data from that subject would be discarded from further analysis. It turns out for all of the participants that the difference between the sensor locations evaluated during the whole experiment was not obvious, confirming a relatively stable head position.

MEG data analysis

A third-order gradient noise reduction (computed with CTF software) was applied on line to the MEG signals. MEG data were then digitally filtered off-line with a band-pass of 0.5–48 Hz and further down sampled to 300 Hz. Subsequently, data were band-passed into the following frequency ranges: delta (0.5–4 Hz), theta (4–8 Hz), alpha (8–13 Hz), beta (13–30 Hz) and gamma bands (30–48 Hz) [39,40]. The 6-min MEG scanning data of each subject before and after acupuncture were selected and split into 6 1-min long epochs respectively. For further off-line processing, the preprocessed MEG data were converted to ASCII files. The following processing was executed for the 6 epochs separately and results were averaged for each subject.

The MEG channels were grouped into 10 regions of interest (ROIs) roughly corresponding to the major cortical areas (frontal, temporal, central, parietal and occipital for each hemisphere). Two of the original 151 channels were not available due to technical problems. Besides, the 9 midline channels were left out of clustering, leaving a total of 140 channels divided over 10 ROIs for further analysis. The band-limited power (BLP) of each channel, defined as the envelope of the band-limited signal, was calculated by first applying the Hilbert transform to the band-limited signal and then taking the absolute value of the resultant complex helical sequence [41]. The BLP signals were thereafter low-pass filtered (cutoff = 8 Hz) to eliminate ringing [42]. With EEG/MEG data, the Hilbert transform has been adopted to estimate power and phase in narrow frequency bands [43,44]. It is a convolution of the data with the kernel $h^{HT} = -1/(\pi t)$, which is equivalent to altering all phases of the original signal components by $\pi/2$. The analytic signal is a complex function given by $y(t) = x(t) + i(h^{HT} * x)(t)$, where x is the original EEG/MEG data of one channel or voxel/equivalent dipole for reconstructed sources and $*$ is the convolution operator [45].

For each frequency band of interest, the pair-wise temporal correlations between the BLP signals were computed using Pearson's correlation. The end result is a $N \times N$ matrix with N equals to 140, where each entry $N_{i,j}$ contains the correlation value for the channels i and j. Results of the 6 epochs were averaged to obtain the mean correlation matrix for each subject both preceding and following acupuncture. Group analysis was carried out by one-sample t-test with the null hypothesis set as there is no significant functional connectivity within or between brain regions. The same items from individual connectivity matrix (with same row index and column index) were taken together for one-sample t-test. After obtaining the P-value for each t-test, false discovery rate (FDR) criterion was then deployed to make the correction for multiple comparisons. The FDR concept was formally described by Benjamini to control the expect proportion of incorrectly rejected null hypotheses [46,47]. It was conducted as follows. Given that there are m hypotheses to be tested $\{H_1^0, H_2^0, \cdots, H_m^0\}$, m_0 are true null hypotheses, the number and identity of which are unknown. The other $m - m_0$ hypotheses are false. Denote the corresponding random vector of test statistics $\{X_1, X_2, \cdots, X_m\}$, and the corresponding P-values $\{P_1, P_2, \cdots, P_m\}$. It was shown that the following procedure controls the FDR at level q: $m_0/m \leq q$ (q was set as 0.05 in our study). Let $p_{(1)} \leq p_{(2)} \leq \cdots \leq p_{(m)}$ be the ordered observed P-values. Define $k = \max\left\{i : p_{(i)} \leq \frac{i}{m} q\right\}$, and reject $H_{(1)}^0 \cdots H_{(k)}^0$ [48]. After FDR procedure, further averaging was carried out to evaluate long distance intra- and inter-hemispheric and short distance local measures both preceding and following acupuncture. The short distance interactivity was computed as the average correlation coefficient between all sensor pairs within one region, while long distance connectivity (8 intrahemispheric: fronto-temporal, fronto-parietal, parieto-occipital and occipito-temporal; 5 interhemispheric: central, frontal, occipital, parietal and temporal) was obtained from sensor pairs where one sensor was in one region, and the other was in another [49,50,51]. Finally, significant alterations induced by acupuncture

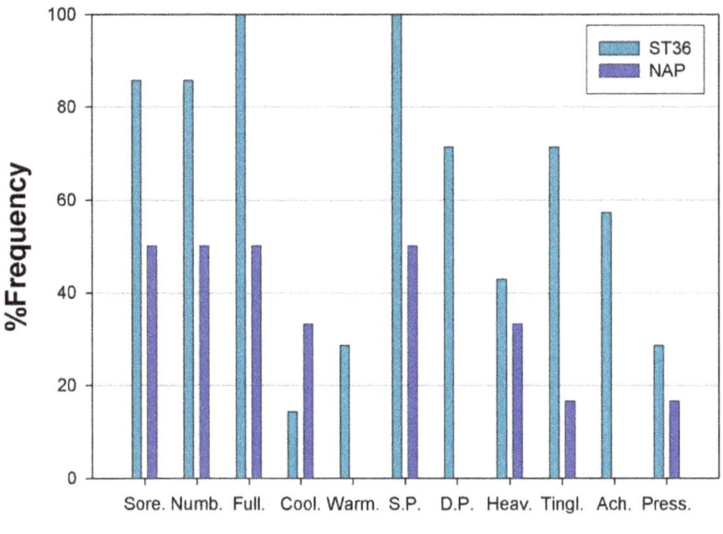
%Frequency
100
80
60
40
20
0
ST36
NAP
Sore. Numb. Full. Cool. Warm. S.P. D.P. Heav. Tingl. Ach. Press.
A

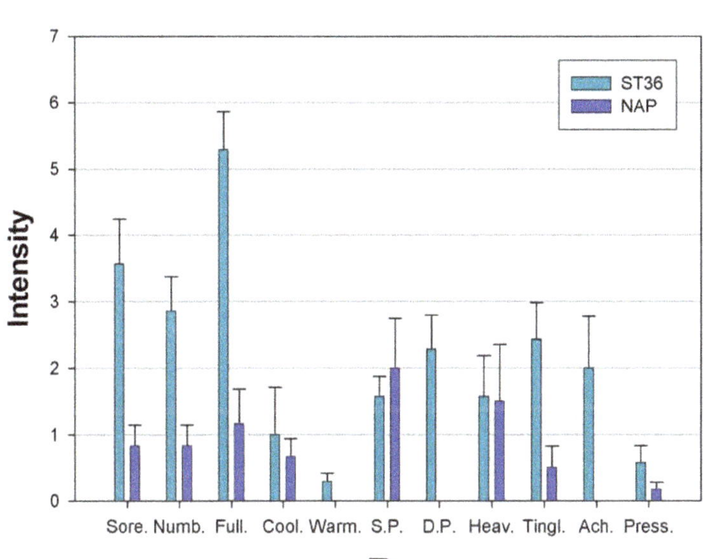
Intensity
7
6
5
4
3
2
1
0
ST36
NAP
Sore. Numb. Full. Cool. Warm. S.P. D.P. Heav. Tingl. Ach. Press.
B

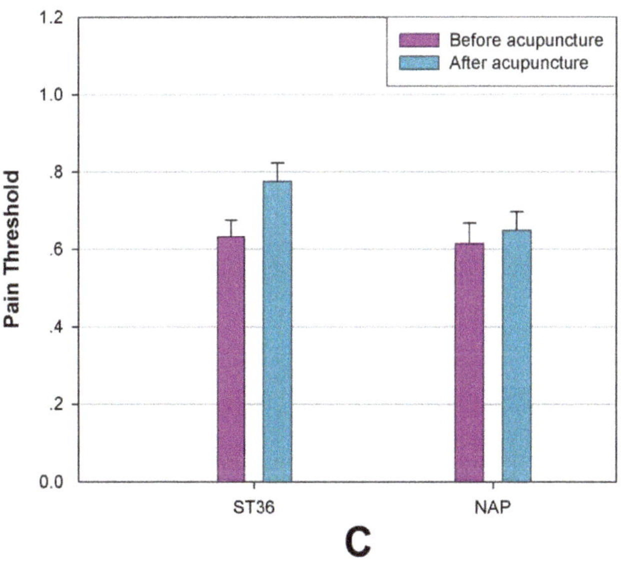
Pain Threshold
1.2
1.0
.8
.6
.4
.2
0.0
Before acupuncture
After acupuncture
ST36
NAP
C

Figure 2. Averaged psychophysical response. A. The percentage of subjects that reported the given sensations. The frequency of aching was found to be greater following acupuncture at ST36. B. The intensity of sensations measured by average score (with standard error bars) on a scale from 0 denoting no sensation to 10 denoting an unbearable sensation. Sore, soreness; Numb, numbness; Full, fullness; Cool, coolness; Warm, warmth; SP, sharp pain; DP, dull pain; Heav, heaviness; Tinl, tingling; Ach, aching; Press, pressure. C. The pain threshold evaluated by average score (with standard error bars) before and after acupuncture at ST36 and NAP. Significant elevation of the pain threshold was observed following acupuncture at ST36.

for either ST36 or NAP group was evaluated for each band by means of a paired *t*-test with threshold at $P<0.05$ in SPSS 17.0 software package for Windows.

Results

Psychophysical responses

The prevalence of subjective "*De-qi*" sensations was expressed as the percentage of individuals in the group who reported the given sensations (Fig. 2A). The intensity was expressed as the average score±standard error (Fig. 2B). No subject opted to add an additional descriptor in the blank row provided. The occurrence frequency of all sensations except coolness was found to be greater during verum acupuncture relative to the sham group. The overall stimulus intensities (mean±SE) were greater for ST36, exhibiting a stronger "*De-qi*" sensation in verum acupuncture. The pain threshold measured for each group per condition was also denoted as the mean±SE. By comparing the pain threshold evaluated preceding and following acupuncture within each group, we illustrated the significant elevation of the pain threshold for acupuncture at ST36 ($P=0.023$, paired *t*-test), while no conspicuous changes were identified for NAP following acupuncture ($P=0.620$, paired *t*-test).

Alteration of functional connectivity

For each condition preceding or following acupuncture, the temporal correlations of band-limited power (BLP) signals were first computed for every pair of MEG channels in each frequency band and then grouped into local and long-distance couplings. The grand averaged local and long-distance couplings for the two conditions in each group were taken in for further statistical analysis.

Among the 5 frequency bands either for verum or sham acupuncture, our results demonstrated dominant enhanced connectivity within the delta band (0.5–4 Hz). As illustrated in Fig. 3 and Table 1, local potentiation of BLP correlations following acupuncture at ST36 was identified over the right frontal ($P=0.005$), right central ($P=0.009$), and left occipital ($P=0.001$) areas, as well as the left ($P=0.0001$) and right ($P=0.007$) temporal regions, none of which could be detected in the NAP group. Although statistical analyses in both groups presented tighter linkage of the right frontal and temporal regions after stimulation (ST36: $P=0.008$; NAP: $P=0.033$), distinct changes in long distance connections were revealed as well. To be specific, left fronto-temporal connectivity was enhanced only for ST36 ($P=0.019$). Elevated connectivity was detected following stimulation at ST36 of the bilateral frontal ($P=0.005$) and temporal ($P=0.007$) regions and the occipito-temporal linkage in both hemispheres (left: $P=0.014$; right: $P=0.020$), while an increased connection was indicated alone in the NAP group between the bilateral central ($P=0.043$) and parietal ($P=0.017$) regions as well as the left parieto-occipital connections ($P=0.048$).

Regarding the beta band (13–30 Hz), both groups displayed a prominently increased left parieto-occipital connection ($P=0.035$ for ST36; $P=0.031$ for NAP). The left fronto-temporal connections for ST36 ($P=0.022$) and local connectivity in the left occipital region for NAP ($P=0.048$) were found to be enhanced following acupuncture. These interaction effects are illustrated schematically in Fig. 4 and Table 2.

As for the gamma band (30–48 Hz), shared patterns of long and short distance interactivity alteration could be detected in both groups to certain extent (Fig. 5 and Table 3). Enhanced connection in the left parieto-occipital (ST36: $P=0.029$; NAP: $P=0.008$) and occipital regions (ST36: $P=0.034$; NAP: $P=0.048$) were illustrated for the two groups. Furthermore, an additional intrahemispheric connection of the left occipito-temporal region was increased following acupuncture in the ST36 group ($P=0.031$) compared with NAP ($P=0.255$).

Additionally, both theta (4–8 Hz) and alpha (8–13 Hz) bands missed significant interaction alterations of functional connectivity

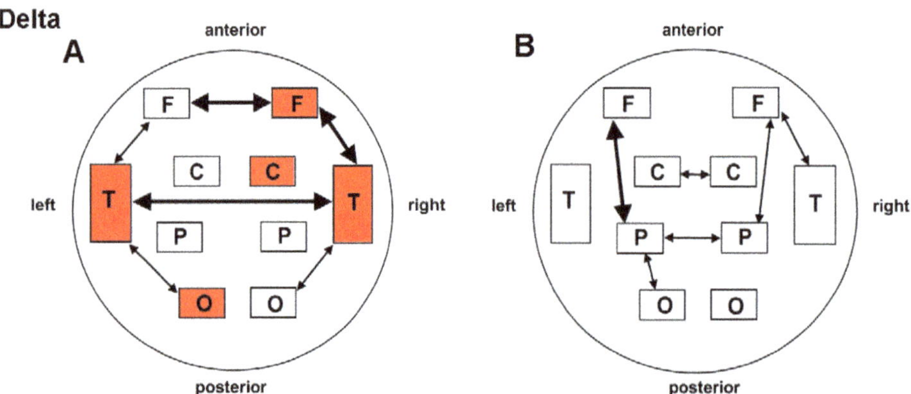

Figure 3. Schematic illustration of BLP correlation alterations for the delta band. A. ST36 group. B. NAP group. Lines correspond to significant changes for the average Band-Limited Power (BLP) correlation induced by acupuncture and squares to significant change in the local BLP correlation (red: local increase in the BLP correlation following acupuncture; thin line: $P<0.05$; thick line: $P<0.01$; significance is based upon a paired *t*-test).

Table 1. Functional connectivity within and between main regions and statistical results in the delta bands for the ST36 and NAP groups.

	Delta							
	Group ST36				Group NAP			
Areas	B_rest	P_rest	*t* value	*P* value	B_rest	P_rest	*t* value	*P* value
LC	0.3902±0.0525	0.4215±0.0612	1.949	0.073	0.4247±0.0864	0.4579±0.0937	1.693	0.114
LF	0.5480±0.1057	0.5908±0.0958	1.961	0.072	0.4953±0.1029	0.5077±0.1127	0.613	0.551
LO	**0.3930±0.0482**	**0.4671±0.0748**	**4.579**	**0.001**	0.4631±0.1203	0.4979±0.1018	1.424	0.178
LP	0.5383±0.0670	0.5721±0.0692	2.063	0.060	0.5481±0.0926	0.5777±0.0996	2.130	0.053
LT	**0.3650±0.0840**	**0.4387±0.0915**	**5.416**	**0.0001**	0.3999±0.0855	0.4204±0.1057	0.904	0.383
RC	**0.3760±0.0801**	**0.4191±0.0730**	**3.055**	**0.009**	0.4287±0.1261	0.4727±0.1038	1.947	0.073
RF	**0.4830±0.1551**	**0.5917±0.1316**	**4.761**	**0.0004**	0.5248±0.1133	0.5546±0.1545	1.088	0.297
RO	0.3940±0.0684	0.4176±0.0475	1.238	0.238	0.4862±0.1740	0.4738±0.4738	−0.539	0.599
RP	0.4592±0.0580	0.4670±0.0869	0.483	0.637	0.4986±0.1353	0.4962±0.1146	−0.341	0.868
RT	**0.3671±0.1044**	**0.4361±0.1276**	**3.063**	**0.009**	0.4110±0.1107	0.4461±0.1150	1.689	0.115
LF_LP	0.1789±0.0533	0.1767±0.0914	−0.119	0.907	**0.1595±0.0910**	**0.2096±0.0645**	**3.131**	**0.008**
LF_LT	**0.2399±0.0568**	**0.2853±0.0521**	**2.670**	**0.019**	0.2373±0.0733	0.2541±0.0757	0.804	0.436
LO_LP	0.2020±0.0617	0.2363±0.0871	1.693	0.114	**0.2528±0.1492**	**0.2926±0.1146**	**2.187**	**0.048**
LO_LT	**0.1451±0.0335**	**0.1965±0.0663**	**2.840**	**0.014**	0.1904±0.0914	0.2037±0.0457	0.562	0.583
RF_RP	0.1428±0.0422	0.1755±0.0995	1.371	0.194	**0.1751±0.1063**	**0.2157±0.0799**	**2.561**	**0.024**
RF_RT	**0.2314±0.0820**	**0.3007±0.1019**	**3.155**	**0.008**	**0.2751±0.0860**	**0.3262±0.1027**	**2.382**	**0.033**
RO_RP	0.1730±0.0445	0.2027±0.0516	1.812	0.093	0.2458±0.1913	0.2522±0.1559	0.301	0.768
RO_RT	**0.1609±0.0445**	**0.2164±0.0595**	**2.653**	**0.020**	0.2049±0.0863	0.2161±0.0593	0.433	0.672
LC_RC	0.1626±0.0428	0.1775±0.0616	0.903	0.383	**0.1789±0.1003**	**0.2322±0.0709**	**2.239**	**0.043**
LF_RF	**0.3104±0.1285**	**0.3755±0.1183**	**3.369**	**0.005**	0.2740±0.0890	0.3067±0.1145	1.169	0.263
LO_RO	0.1637±0.0508	0.1892±0.0763	1.149	0.271	0.2314±0.1829	0.2209±0.1128	−0.436	0.670
LP_RP	0.1516±0.0567	0.1525±0.0748	0.056	0.956	**0.1677±0.1118**	**0.2200±0.0976**	**2.724**	**0.017**
LT_RT	**0.1811±0.0572**	**0.2349±0.0740**	**3.163**	**0.007**	0.2552±0.0961	0.2791±0.1143	1.083	0.298

Significant differences are indicated in bold ($P<0.05$). L = left, R = right. C = central, F = frontal, O = occipital, P = parietal, T = temporal. B_rest, resting data before acupuncture. P_rest, resting data after acupuncture.

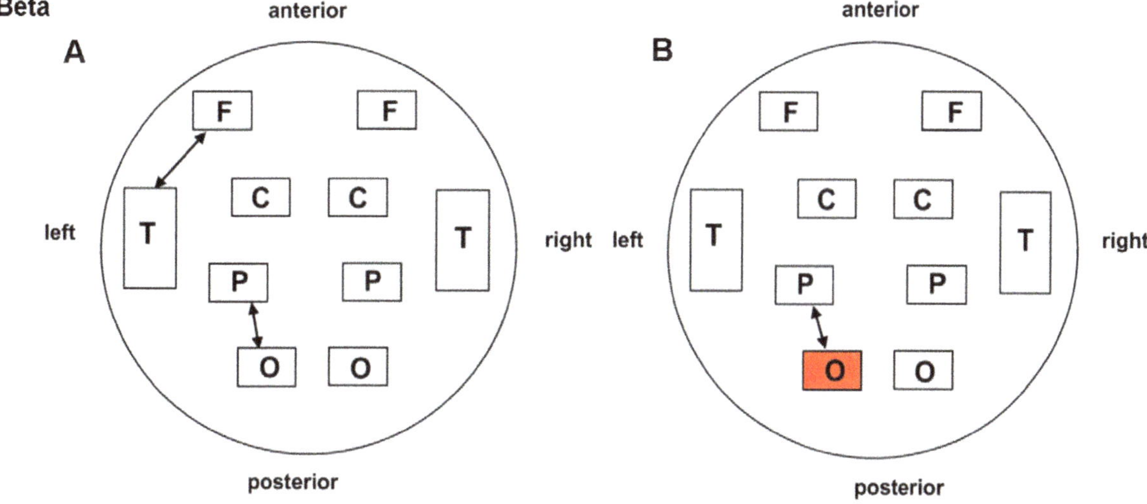

Figure 4. Schematic illustration of BLP correlation alterations for the beta band. A. ST36 group. B. NAP group. Lines correspond to significant changes for the average Band-Limited Power (BLP) correlation induced by acupuncture and squares to significant change in the local BLP correlation (red: local increase in the BLP correlation following acupuncture; thin line: $P<0.05$; thick line: $P<0.01$; significance is based upon a paired *t*-test).

Table 2. Functional connectivity within and between main regions and statistical results in the beta bands for the ST36 and NAP groups.

	Beta							
	Group ST36				**Group NAP**			
Areas	**B_rest**	**P_rest**	***t* value**	***P* value**	**B_rest**	**P_rest**	***t* value**	***P* value**
LC	0.4420±0.0750	0.4431±0.0748	0.074	0.942	0.4373±0.0690	0.4328±0.0872	−0.540	0.598
LF	0.4104±0.0991	0.4186±0.0860	1.381	0.190	0.3898±0.0786	0.3875±0.0811	−0.275	0.788
LO	0.4337±0.0490	0.4480±0.0548	1.658	0.121	**0.4188±0.0631**	**0.4335±0.0778**	**2.183**	**0.048**
LP	0.6715±0.0574	0.6823±0.0673	0.880	0.395	0.6398±0.0604	0.6414±0.0724	0.250	0.806
LT	0.3608±0.0470	0.3586±0.0511	−0.402	0.694	0.3554±0.0674	0.3560±0.0752	0.089	0.931
RC	0.4231±0.0791	0.4164±0.0955	−0.412	0.687	0.4118±0.0675	0.4043±0.0874	−0.677	0.510
RF	0.4822±0.0680	0.4793±0.0670	−0.284	0.781	0.4545±0.0808	0.4492±0.0821	−0.692	0.501
RO	0.4175±0.0582	0.4299±0.0717	1.152	0.270	0.4333±0.0564	0.4456±0.0615	1.609	0.132
RP	0.6959±0.0568	0.6987±0.0479	0.263	0.797	0.6779±0.0503	0.6788±0.0594	0.116	0.909
RT	0.3662±0.0324	0.3645±0.0278	−0.300	0.769	0.3600±0.0638	0.3511±0.0663	−1.303	0.215
LF_LP	0.0865±0.0389	0.1029±0.0505	1.879	0.083	0.0746±0.0371	0.0837±0.0452	1.791	0.097
LF_LT	**0.1382±0.0329**	**0.1537±0.0441**	**2.590**	**0.022**	0.1224±0.0461	0.1308±0.0411	1.803	0.095
LO_LP	**0.2126±0.0565**	**0.2354±0.0652**	**2.358**	**0.035**	**0.1810±0.0579**	**0.2011±0.0702**	**2.412**	**0.031**
LO_LT	0.1598±0.0388	0.1688±0.0474	1.272	0.226	0.1706±0.0617	0.1808±0.0762	1.712	0.111
RF_RP	0.0901±0.0338	0.1088±0.0474	1.834	0.090	0.0842±0.0447	0.0877±0.0473	0.585	0.568
RF_RT	0.1999±0.0407	0.199±0.0424	−0.001	0.999	0.1717±0.0663	0.1714±0.0616	−0.047	0.963
RO_RP	0.2176±0.0527	0.2373±0.0594	2.128	0.053	0.2061±0.0550	0.2182±0.0554	1.671	0.119
RO_RT	0.1539±0.0464	0.1631±0.0453	1.084	0.298	0.1747±0.0519	0.1739±0.0577	−0.089	0.930
LC_RC	0.1361±0.0495	0.1449±0.0605	0.972	0.349	0.1174±0.0435	0.1234±0.0572	0.838	0.417
LF_RF	0.1729±0.0455	0.1865±0.0561	1.791	0.097	0.1460±0.0582	0.1495±0.0572	0.597	0.561
LO_RO	0.1838±0.0530	0.1921±0.0670	0.792	0.443	0.1982±0.0776	0.2124±0.0941	1.614	0.130
LP_RP	0.2224±0.0562	0.2531±0.0755	1.693	0.114	0.2054±0.0504	0.2201±0.0492	1.640	0.125
LT_RT	0.1915±0.0500	0.1837±0.0532	−0.805	0.435	0.1904±0.0539	0.1881±0.0695	−0.303	0.767

Significant differences are indicated in bold ($P<0.05$). L = left, R = right. C = central, F = frontal, O = occipital, P = parietal, T = temporal. B_rest, resting data before acupuncture. P_rest, resting data after acupuncture.

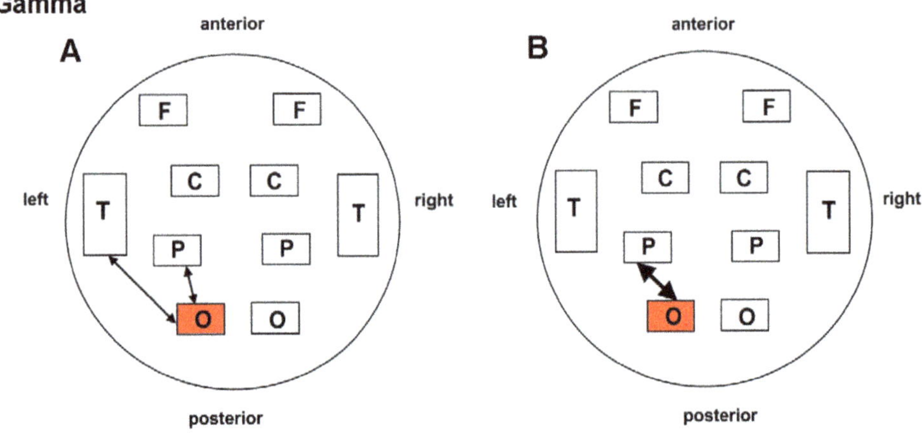

Figure 5. Schematic illustration of BLP correlation alterations for the gamma band. A. ST36 group. B. NAP group. Lines correspond to significant changes for the average Band-Limited Power (BLP) correlation induced by acupuncture and squares to significant change in the local BLP correlation (red: local increase in the BLP correlation following acupuncture; thin line: $P<0.05$; thick line: $P<0.01$; significance is based upon a paired *t*-test).

Table 3. Functional connectivity within and between main regions and statistical results in the gamma bands for the ST36 and NAP groups.

	Gamma							
	Group ST36				**Group NAP**			
Areas	**B_rest**	**P_rest**	***t* value**	***P* value**	**B_rest**	**P_rest**	***t* value**	***P* value**
LC	0.2669±0.0856	0.2473±0.0798	−1.553	0.144	0.2777±0.0880	0.2656±0.0902	−1.584	0.137
LF	0.2187±0.0825	0.2104±0.0660	−0.884	0.393	0.2279±0.0934	0.2244±0.0892	−0.605	0.555
LO	**0.3412±0.0549**	**0.3658±0.0590**	**2.369**	**0.034**	**0.3163±0.0342**	**0.3256±0.0363**	**2.763**	**0.016**
LP	0.4430±0.0723	0.4307±0.0766	−0.886	0.392	0.4486±0.0879	0.4432±0.0883	−0.574	0.576
LT	0.2145±0.0333	0.2232±0.0321	1.850	0.087	0.2131±0.0483	0.2133±0.0454	0.068	0.947
RC	0.2281±0.0739	0.2112±0.0791	−1.672	0.118	0.2396±0.0753	0.2275±0.0789	−1.550	0.145
RF	0.2568±0.0768	0.2578±0.0762	0.109	0.915	0.2640±0.0904	0.2632±0.0797	−0.112	0.913
RO	0.3197±0.0410	0.3144±0.0309	−0.547	0.594	0.3127±0.0388	0.3151±0.0415	0.768	0.456
RP	0.4719±0.0726	0.4598±0.0813	−0.759	0.462	0.4822±0.0734	0.4696±0.0759	−1.279	0.223
RT	0.2260±0.0264	0.2309±0.0297	0.869	0.401	0.2212±0.0428	0.2213±0.0372	0.028	0.978
LF_LP	0.0297±0.0187	0.0331±0.0188	1.319	0.210	0.0338±0.0405	0.0368±0.0368	0.964	0.353
LF_LT	0.0489±0.0209	0.0546±0.0228	1.093	0.079	0.0528±0.0453	0.0558±0.0400	1.086	0.297
LO_LP	**0.1055±0.0176**	**0.1209±0.0266**	**2.460**	**0.029**	**0.0987±0.0332**	**0.1085±0.0317**	**3.099**	**0.008**
LO_LT	**0.0790±0.0198**	**0.0945±0.0255**	**2.411**	**0.031**	0.0768±0.0280	0.0816±0.0257	1.192	0.255
RF_RP	0.0325±0.0160	0.0353±0.0190	0.806	0.435	0.0327±0.0210	0.0315±0.0153	−0.423	0.679
RF_RT	0.0630±0.0219	0.0710±0.0247	1.894	0.081	0.0634±0.0373	0.0660±0.0261	0.452	0.659
RO_RP	0.1098±0.0214	0.1115±0.0212	0.449	0.661	0.1106±0.0280	0.1085±0.0296	−1.169	0.263
RO_RT	0.0734±0.0183	0.0780±0.0184	1.059	0.309	0.0692±0.0209	0.0714±0.0212	1.206	0.249
LC_RC	0.0534±0.0289	0.0488±0.0320	−1.261	0.229	0.0519±0.0317	0.0506±0.0341	−0.327	0.749
LF_RF	0.0639±0.0396	0.0679±0.0386	0.858	0.407	0.0689±0.0695	0.0689±0.0602	−0.002	0.999
LO_RO	0.1084±0.0352	0.1098±0.0330	0.143	0.889	0.0976±0.0381	0.1046±0.0405	1.865	0.085
LP_RP	0.1192±0.0302	0.1210±0.0326	0.319	0.755	0.1176±0.0449	0.1176±0.0393	0.008	0.994
LT_RT	0.0650±0.0245	0.0700±0.0269	1.189	0.256	0.0648±0.0374	0.0634±0.0346	−0.333	0.744

Significant differences are indicated in bold ($P<0.05$). L = left, R = right. C = central, F = frontal, O = occipital, P = parietal, T = temporal. B_rest, resting data before acupuncture. P_rest, resting data after acupuncture.

in the ST36 and NAP groups ($P>0.05$). The overall findings indicated that acupuncture at different designated places may evoke differential alterations of functional connectivity within specific frequency bands.

Discussion

It is noteworthy that when using MEG technology, we should always take into account the question whether the correlation measured between signals at different sensors can be interpreted with physiological interactions between different brain areas. This is the well-known problem of volume conduction effects [52,53]. In other words, nearby MEG sensors have a high probability of capturing activity from common sources, and therefore may show spurious correlation. One possible solution is to estimate correlations between signals from restructured sources rather than from actual recorded signals. Nevertheless, there is to date no reliable way to choose the proper model to unambiguously solve the inverse problem [42,54]. Apart from this, another approach is the adoption of measures of correlation that are not sensitive to volume conduction [55]. However, even this approach may not always be effective [56]. In the present study, we employed a pragmatic approach which has been generally adopted in resting-state MEG investigations, analyzing functional connectivity in sensor space and then grouping the sensor pairs in local and long-distance couplings [49,50,51,53,57]. Although precise correspondence with anatomical localization is to some extent limited, underlying cortical areas are to be considered as indicative since the ROIs are based upon the very extra-cranial position of the MEG sensors [39,50].

Acupuncture-induced modulations on functional connectivity have already been illustrated in previous fMRI investigations [58,59,60]. Given that fMRI is naturally an indirect imaging tool, we attempted to seek whether or not such alterations would be directly observed using an electrophysiological imaging modality, among which MEG being the most suitable for estimating functional connectivity [40,61,62]. The present MEG study was conducted with the objective of exploring the global differences in the interregional functional connectivity induced by acupuncture within delta, theta, alpha, beta and gamma bands.

Although significant alterations for both the verum and sham groups were mainly confined to delta, beta and gamma bands, the functional connectivity within each presented distinct change patterns. One intriguing finding here is the increased degree of connectivity recorded by sensors overlying the left temporal cortex within the delta, theta and gamma bands. Compared to recent fMRI studies in which the temporal gyrus as well as the underlying amygdala and hippocampus were indicated as network hubs following verum acupuncture, with the advantage of MEG we observed that such modulation effects existed specifically within the above-mentioned three bands, among which delta was the most dominant [58,59]. Another thought-provoking result is that in addition to previous investigations which illustrated enhanced interactions of the temporal gyrus with the frontal gyrus and prefrontal cortex following acupuncture either at ST36 or NAP, we further pinpointed that such an effect occurred only in the delta band for sham acupuncture, compared with the additional modulation effect in the beta band of the verum group [60]. Note that both groups presented somewhat shared alteration patterns for beta and gamma bands, mainly comprising of the parietal and occipital regions. This may further implicate the modulation of the resting state network by sham acupuncture [60]. Besides, it is speculated that the shared enhanced couplings may partly support the clinical experience that acupuncture at non-meridian points can also provide partial analgesia in chronic pain [63].

Limitations

To the best of our knowledge, this MEG study is the first to demonstrate the global differences in functional connectivity alterations induced by acupuncture. However, due to the inverse problem currently not to be solved properly, this preliminary research did not involve the source reconstruction. Therefore, we are currently not able to exactly evaluate the anatomical correspondence to the temporal structures, which must be considered as a pitfall. As far as we know, there have been several MEG studies using this methodology which successfully illustrated differential functional connectivity patterns in pathological patients compared with normal control [49,50,51,53]. As a result, although the analysis was conducted at the sensor space, our results to some extent can make a contribution to improving the knowledge about the functional specificity of acupuncture. In the future, to solve the inverse problem will be one of the main research interests so that more specific anatomical information would be dug out by source reconstruction and make further efforts to unveil the neurophysiological mechanism underlying acupuncture.

Acknowledgments

We would like to thank Ying Jiang, Fengbing Wang and Hao Chen for valuable technical assistance in conducting this research.

Author Contributions

Conceived and designed the experiments: YBY LJB RWD. Performed the experiments: YBY CGZ TX. Analyzed the data: YBY LJB CGZ. Contributed reagents/materials/analysis tools: HW ZYL WJW. Wrote the paper: JT.

References

1. Beijing S (1980) Nanjing colleges of traditional Chinese medicine. Essentials of Chinese acupuncture. Beijing, Foreign Language Press.
2. NCDP A (1998) NIH Consensus Conference. Acupuncture. JAMA 280: 1518–1524.
3. Witt CM, Manheimer E, Hammerschlag R, Ludtke R, Lao LX, et al. (2012) How Well Do Randomized Trials Inform Decision Making: Systematic Review Using Comparative Effectiveness Research Measures on Acupuncture for Back Pain. Plos One. DOI:10.1371/journal.pone.0032399.
4. Nahin RL, Statistics NCfH (2009) Costs of complementary and alternative medicine (CAM) and frequency of visits to CAM practitioners: United States, 2007: US Dept. of Health and Human Services, Centers for Disease Control and Prevention, National Center for Health Statistics.
5. Kaptchuk TJ (2002) Acupuncture: theory, efficacy, and practice. Ann Intern Med 136: 374–383.
6. Zhang H, Bian Z, Lin Z (2010) Are acupoints specific for diseases? A systematic review of the randomized controlled trials with sham acupuncture controls. Chin Med. DOI:10.1186/1749-8546-5-1
7. Cho ZH, Chung S, Jones J, Park J, Park H, et al. (1998) New findings of the correlation between acupoints and corresponding brain cortices using functional MRI. Proc Natl Acad Sci U S A 95: 2670–2673.
8. Li G, Cheung RTF, Ma QY, Yang ES (2003) Visual cortical activations on fMRI upon stimulation of the vision-implicated acupoints. Neuroreport 14: 669–673.
9. Wesolowski T, Lotze M, Domin M, Langner S, Lehmann C, et al. (2009) Acupuncture reveals no specific effect on primary auditory cortex: a functional magnetic resonance imaging study. Neuroreport 20: 116–120.
10. Kong J, Kaptchuk TJ, Webb JM, Kong JT, Sasaki Y, et al. (2009) Functional neuroanatomical investigation of vision-related acupuncture point specificity: A multisession fMRI study. Hum Brain Mapp 30: 38–46.
11. Hui KKS, Liu J, Makris N, Gollub RL, Chen AJW (2000) Acupuncture modulates the limbic system and subcortical gray structures of the human brain: evidence from fMRI studies in normal subjects. Hum Brain Mapp 9: 13–25.
12. Bai L, Qin W, Tian J, Liu P, Li LL, et al. (2009) Time-varied characteristics of acupuncture effects in fMRI studies. Hum Brain Mapp 30: 3445–3460.
13. Kwong KK, Belliveau JW, Chesler DA, Goldberg IE, Weisskoff RM, et al. (1992) Dynamic magnetic resonance imaging of human brain activity during primary sensory stimulation. Proc Natl Acad Sci U S A 89: 5675–5679.
14. Ogawa S, Tank DW, Menon R, Ellermann JM, Kim SG, et al. (1992) Intrinsic signal changes accompanying sensory stimulation: functional brain mapping with magnetic resonance imaging. Proc Natl Acad Sci U S A 89: 5951–5955.
15. Brookes MJ, Hale JR, Zumer JM, Stevenson CM, Francis ST, et al. (2011) Measuring functional connectivity using MEG: Methodology and comparison with fcMRI. Neuro Image 56: 1082–1104.
16. Napadow V, Makris N, Liu J, Kettner NW, Kwong KK, et al. (2005) Effects of electroacupuncture versus manual acupuncture on the human brain as measured by fMRI. Hum Brain Mapp 24: 193–205.
17. Yoo SS, Teh EK, Blinder RA, Jolesz FA (2004) Modulation of cerebellar activities by acupuncture stimulation: evidence from fMRI study. NeuroImage 22: 932–940.
18. You Y, Bai L, Xue T, Zhong C, Liu Z, et al. (2011) Differential spatial activity patterns of acupuncture by a machine learning based analysis. Proc SPIE 7965, Medical Imaging 2011. DOI:10.1117/12.877981
19. Fermaglich J (1982) Electric Fields of the Brain: The Neurophysics of EEG. JAMA 247: 1879–1880.
20. Cohen D (1972) Magnetoencephalography: detection of the brain's electrical activity with a superconducting magnetometer. Science 175: 664–666.
21. Hari R, Levanen S, Raij T (2000) Timing of human cortical functions during cognition: role of MEG. Trends Cogn Sci 4: 455–462.
22. Varela F, Lachaux JP, Rodriguez E, Martinerie J (2001) The brainweb: phase synchronization and large-scale integration. Nat Rev Neurosci 2: 229–239.
23. Hampson M, Peterson BS, Skudlarski P, Gatenby JC, Gore JC (2002) Detection of functional connectivity using temporal correlations in MR images. Hum Brain Mapp 15: 247–262.
24. Gross J, Kujala J, Hämäläinen M, Timmermann L, Schnitzler A, et al. (2001) Dynamic imaging of coherent sources: studying neural interactions in the human brain. Proc Natl Acad Sci U S A 98: 694–699.
25. Guevara R, Velazquez JLP, Nenadovic V, Wennberg R, Senjanovi G, et al. (2005) Phase synchronization measurements using electroencephalographic recordings. Neuroinformatics 3: 301–313.
26. Kim MS, Kim HD, Seo HD, Sawada K, Ishida M (2008) The Effect of Acupuncture at the PC-6 on the Electroencephalogram and Electrocardiogram. Am J Chinese Med. DOI: 10.1142/S0192415X08005928.
27. Thomas W, Vitaly N, Norman K, Matti H, Rupali D (2011) Differences in cortical response to acupressure and electroacupuncture stimuli. BMC Neurosci. DOI: 10.1186/1471-2202-12-73.
28. You Y, Bai L, Dai R, Xue T, Zhong C, et al. (2011) Differential neural responses to acupuncture revealed by MEG using wavelet-based time-frequency analysis: A pilot study. Engineering in Medicine and Biology Society, EMBC. DOI: 10.1109/IEMBS.2011.6091794
29. Chen L, Tang J, White P, Sloninsky A, Wender R, et al. (1998) The effect of location of transcutaneous electrical nerve stimulation on postoperative opioid analgesic requirement: acupoint versus nonacupoint stimulation. Anesth Analg 87: 1129–1134.
30. Han JS (2011) Acupuncture analgesia: areas of consensus and controversy. Pain 152: S41–S48.
31. Mayor DF (2007) Clinical introduction to medical acupuncture. Acupunct Med 25: 204–206.
32. Beyens F (1993) Chinese acupuncture and moxibustion. Acupunct Med 11: 105–106.
33. Hui KKS, Liu J, Marina O, Napadow V, Haselgrove C, et al. (2005) The integrated response of the human cerebro-cerebellar and limbic systems to acupuncture stimulation at ST 36 as evidenced by fMRI. NeuroImage 27: 479–496.

34. Kong J, Gollub R, Huang T, Polich G, Napadow V, et al. (2007) Acupuncture de qi, from qualitative history to quantitative measurement. J Altern Complem Med 13: 1059–1070.
35. Voudouris NJ, Peck CL, Coleman G (1989) Conditioned response models of placebo phenomena: further support. Pain 38: 109–116.
36. Voudouris NJ, Peck CL, Coleman G (1990) The role of conditioning and verbal expectancy in the placebo response. Pain 43: 121–128.
37. Johnson M, Stewart J, Humphries S, Chamove A (2011) Marathon runners' reaction to potassium iontophoretic experimental pain: Pain tolerance, pain threshold, coping and self-efficacy. Eur J Pain 16: 767–774.
38. Ulett GA, Han S, Han J (1998) Electroacupuncture: mechanisms and clinical application. Biol Psychiat 44: 129–138.
39. Stoffers D, Bosboom J, Deijen J, Wolters E, Berendse H, et al. (2007) Slowing of oscillatory brain activity is a stable characteristic of Parkinson's disease without dementia. Brain 130: 1847–1860.
40. Douw L, Schoonheim MM, Landi D, van der Meer ML, Geurts JJG, et al. (2011) Cognition is related to resting-state small-world network togology: an magnetoencephalographic stduy. Neuroscience 175: 169–177.
41. Leopold DA, Murayama Y, Logothetis NK (2003) Very slow activity fluctuations in monkey visual cortex: implications for functional brain imaging. Cereb Cortex 13: 422–433.
42. Liu Z, Fukunaga M, De Zwart JA, Duyn JH (2010) Large-scale spontaneous fluctuations and correlations in brain electrical activity observed with magnetoencephalography. Neuroimage 51: 102–111.
43. Breakspear M, Williams LM, Stam CJ (2004) A novel method for the topographic analysis of neural activity reveals formation and dissolution of 'dynamic cell assemblies'. J Comput Neurosci 16: 49–68.
44. Tass P, Fieseler T, Dammers J, Dolan K, Morosan P, et al. (2003) Synchronization tomography: a method for three-dimensional localization of phase synchronized neuronal populations in the human brain using magnetoencephalography. Phys Rev Lett. DOI: 10.1103/PhysRevLett.90.088101 90: 88101.
45. Kiebel SJ, Tallon-Baudry C, Friston KJ (2005) Parametric analysis of oscillatory activity as measured with EEG/MEG. Hum Brain Mapp 26: 170–177.
46. Benjamini Y (2010) Discovering the false discovery rate. J R Statist Soc B 72: 405–416.
47. Benjamini Y, Hochberg Y (1995) Controlling the false discovery rate: a practical and powerful approach to multiple testing. J R Statist Soc B 57: 289–300.
48. Benjamini Y, Yekutieli D (2001) The control of the false discovery rate in multiple testing under dependency. Ann Stat 29: 1165–1188.
49. Stam C, Jones B, Manshanden I, Van Cappellen van Walsum A, Montez T, et al. (2006) Magnetoencephalographic evaluation of resting-state functional connectivity in Alzheimer's disease. Neuroimage 32: 1335–1344.
50. Stoffers D, Bosboom J, Deijen J, Wolters EC, Stam C, et al. (2008) Increased cortico-cortical functional connectivity in early-stage Parkinson's disease: an MEG study. Neuroimage 41: 212–222.
51. Stoffers D, Bosboom JLW, Wolters EC, Stam CJ, Berendse HW (2008) Dopaminergic modulation of cortico-cortical functional connectivity in Parkinson's disease: An MEG study. Exp Neurol 213: 191–195.
52. Stam CJ, de Haan W, Daffertshofer A, Jones BF, Manshanden I, et al. (2009) Graph theoretical analysis of magnetoencephalographic functional connectivity in Alzheimers disease. Brain 132: 213–224.
53. Stam C, De Haan W, Daffertshofer A, Jones B, Manshanden I, et al. (2009) Graph theoretical analysis of magnetoencephalographic functional connectivity in Alzheimer's disease. Brain 132: 213–224.
54. Hadjipapas A, Hillebrand A, Holliday IE, Singh KD, Barnes GR (2005) Assessing interactions of linear and nonlinear neuronal sources using MEG beamformers: a proof of concept. Clin Neurophysiol 116: 1300–1313.
55. Nolte G, Bai O, Wheaton L, Mari Z, Vorbach S, et al. (2004) Identifying true brain interaction from EEG data using the imaginary part of coherency. Clin Neurophysiol 115: 2292–2307.
56. Wheaton LA, Nolte G, Bohlhalter S, Fridman E, Hallett M (2005) Synchronization of parietal and premotor areas during preparation and execution of praxis hand movements. Clin Neurophysiol 116: 1382–1390.
57. Bosboom JLW, Stoffers D, Wolters EC, Stam C, Berendse H (2009) MEG resting state functional connectivity in Parkinson's disease related dementia. J Neural Transm 116: 193–202.
58. Feng Y, Bai L, Ren Y, Wang H, Liu Z, et al. (2011) Investigation of the large-scale functional brain networks modulated by acupuncture. Magn Reson Imaging 29: 958–965.
59. Liu J, Qin W, Guo Q, Sun J, Yuan K, et al. (2011) Divergent neural processes specific to the acute and sustained phases of verum and SHAM acupuncture. J Magn Reson Imaging 33: 33–40.
60. Qin W, Tian J, Bai LJ, Pan XH, Yang L, et al. (2008) FMRI connectivity analysis of acupuncture effects on an amygdala-associated brain network. Mol Pain. DOI:10.1186/1744-8069-4-55.
61. Guevara R, Velazquez JLP, Nenadovic V, Wennberg R, Senjanović G, et al. (2005) Phase synchronization measurements using electroencephalographic recordings. Neuroinformatics 3: 301–313.
62. Stam CJ, Breakspear M, van Walsum AMC, van Dijk BW (2003) Nonlinear synchronization in EEG and whole-head MEG recordings of healthy subjects. Hum Brain Mapp 19: 63–78.
63. Richardson P, Vincent C (1986) Acupuncture for the treatment of pain: A review of evaluative research. Pain 24: 15–40.

9

Manipulation of and Sustained Effects on the Human Brain Induced by Different Modalities of Acupuncture: An fMRI Study

**Yin Jiang[1,2,3], Hong Wang[4], Zhenyu Liu[5], Yuru Dong[4], Yue Dong[2], Xiaohui Xiang[1,2,3], Lijun Bai[5], Jie Tian[5], Liuzhen Wu[1,2,3], Jisheng Han[1,2,3], Cailian Cui[1,2,3]*

1 Neuroscience Research Institute, Peking University, Beijing, China, **2** Department of Neurobiology, School of Basic Medical Sciences, Peking University, Beijing, China, **3** Key Laboratory of Neuroscience, The Ministry of Education and Ministry of Public Health, Beijing, China, **4** Department of Magnetic Resonance, General Hospital of Armed Police Forces, Beijing, China, **5** Institute of Automation, Chinese Academy of Sciences, Beijing, China

Abstract

The javascript:void(0)manipulation and sustained effects of acupuncture have been investigated in multiple studies, but several findings are inconsistent with one another. One possible explanation for these discrepancies is that different modalities of acupuncture were utilized in these studies. In the present study, we investigated both the manipulation and sustained effects of acupuncture in different modalities, including manual acupuncture (MA), electroacupuncture (EA) and transcutaneous electrical acupoint stimulation (TEAS). MA, EA, TEAS and sensory control stimulation were applied to 18 healthy subjects, and combined block-designed and resting-state fMRI scans were performed. In analyzing these data, the block-designed datasets were used to assess the manipulation effect by employing a modified general linear model. The data from the resting states, before and after stimulation, were used to explore the brain networks involved in the sustained effect. The results showed that the two 1-min stimulation periods produced similar activation patterns in the sensory control with positive activation in the sensorimotor areas and negative activation in the default mode areas. Although similar patterns could be detected in the first stimulation period in MA, EA and TEAS, no positive activation result was observed in the second stimulation period, and EA showed a more extensive deactivation compared to MA and TEAS. Additionally, all three of the modalities of acupuncture stimulation could increase the instinct brain network in rest. A more secure and spatially extended connectivity of the default mode network was observed following MA and EA, and TEAS specifically increased the functional connectivity in the sensorimotor network. The present study suggested that different brain mechanisms might be recruited in different acupuncture modalities. In addition, the findings from our work could provide methodological information for further research into the mechanism of acupuncture.

Editor: Wang Zhan, University of Maryland, College Park, United States of America

Funding: This work was supported by the National Basic Research Program of China (2007CB512501, 2013CB531905, 2009CB522003). The funders had no role in study design, data collection and analysis, decision to publish, or preparation of the manuscript. No additional external funding was received for this study.

Competing Interests: The authors have declared that no competing interests exist.

* E-mail: clcui@bjmu.edu.cn

Introduction

Acupuncture is a traditional Chinese treatment that has been used in the Orient for thousands of years and is now gaining widespread acceptance as an alternative and complementary treatment in modern medicine [1]. In addition to traditional manual acupuncture (MA), new acupuncture modalities, such as electroacupuncture (EA) and transcutaneous electrical acupoint stimulation (TEAS), are gaining in popularity.

Unlike MA, which uses manual needling at specific acupoints to achieve a therapeutic effect, in EA, electrical pulses are delivered on the needles inserted into the acupoints, and in TEAS, electrical pulses are delivered on the skin of the acupoints via electrode. There is solid evidence that both EA and TEAS have treatment effects on pain [2,3] and substance abuse [4,5] in both humans and animal models. In addition, Zhang et al. recently reported that TEAS could increase the success rate for women undergoing embryo transfer [6] and also had the potential to improve autistic behavior in children [7]. Compared to MA, EA is more effective in pain relief [8,9], and the precision of the simulation parameters ensures high reproducibility for therapeutic effects and research. Additionally, EA without manual manipulation of the needles also saves labor. TEAS has been shown to be as effective as EA in analgesia [10], and with training for nurses and patients, it can be performed even without an acupuncturist. Furthermore, the non-invasiveness of the procedure makes it more acceptable to patients.

Previous studies in animals have shown that acupuncture stimulation could facilitate the release of specific neuropeptides in the central nervous system and elicit profound physiological effects [11]. However, the exploration of acupuncture mechanisms in the human brain was limited by lack of noninvasive methods until the recent development of imaging techniques, particularly functional magnetic resonance imaging (fMRI). Research has mainly focused on two acupuncture effects: the manipulation and sustained effects. A block-designed method has mostly been used for detecting the manipulation effect of acupuncture, and it has generally been accepted that acupuncture deactivates the limbic system and activates sensorimotor areas [12,13,14,15,16,17]. Resting-state connectivity has mostly been used to investigate the sustained effect of acupuncture, and increased functional connectivity in the resting brain network following acupuncture has been observed in many studies [18,19,20,21,22]. However, only one modality of acupuncture was utilized in these works, and varied results were often reported [23]. It is reasonable to wonder whether different modalities of acupuncture could induce different brain activity responses. To the best of our knowledge, only a small number of studies attempted to compare the manipulation effect induced by MA and EA [24,25,26], and the brain activation patterns observed in these studies seemed inconsistent. We hypothesize that these discrepancies may be due to small sample sizes and less powerful statistical thresholds.

The aim of the present study is to investigate both the manipulation and sustained effects induced by three popularly utilized acupuncture modalities, namely, MA, EA and TEAS. We used block-designed datasets combined with a modified general linear model (GLM) analysis [27] to observe the manipulation effect. Data from the resting states before and after stimulation were also collected to detect the sustained effect of acupuncture. On the basis of former studies, the default mode network (DMN) and the sensorimotor network (SMN) could be modulated by acupuncture [18,21,28]; thus, our exploration of the sustained effect focused on these two networks.

Materials and Methods

Subjects

Eighteen healthy, right-handed participants naïve to acupuncture (9 male, mean age-22 years, range-19 to 27) were enrolled in this experiment. Prior to the commencement of the experiment, all subjects signed an informed consent agreement regarding the purpose, procedure and potential risks of this study and were free to withdraw from the experiment at any time. All research procedures were approved by the ethical committee of Peking University.

Experiment Procedures

At the beginning of the experiments, subjects were told that there were four modalities in the acupuncture treatment and that the purpose of our research was to use fMRI to determine how the modalities changed brain functions. All subjects were recruited to participate in four fMRI scanning sessions, and in each session, the subjects received only one type of stimulation: MA, EA, TEAS or a sensory control. The four sessions were randomized and separated by a minimum of one week.

Acupuncture was performed at acupoint ST-36 on the left leg (Zusanli, located in the tibialis anterior muscle) and was performed by the same experienced and licensed acupuncturist. The needles used in the MA and EA sessions were sterile, disposable, stainless-steel acupuncture needles, which would not distort MR images, measuring 0.22 mm in diameter and 40 mm in length. The needle was inserted in ST-36 with a depth of 1.5–2.5 cm. In the MA session, stimulation was delivered by twisting the needle at 1–2 Hz. In the EA session, in addition to one needle in ST-36, another needle was shallowly inserted (less than 1 cm depth) to a non-acupoint proximal to ST-36. The same locations were attached with electrode slices to the skin surface in the TEAS session. Current was delivered by HANS (Han's acupoint nerve stimulator, model LH-202H, Neuroscience Research Institute, Peking University, Beijing, China) with a frequency of 2 Hz in both the EA and TEAS sessions. The current intensity for each subject was adjusted to a maximal but comfortable level (2.16±0.20 mA for EA and 23.73±1.71 mA for TEAS). Manual tapping with a 5.88 von Frey monofilament over ST-36 with a 1–2 Hz frequency was utilized in the sensory control session, which is a maneuver that has often been chosen as a control stimulation in acupuncture studies [24,29]. In all sessions, no sharp pain feeling was allowed.

Functional scanning was incorporated with three independent runs in each session. Two rest runs, each lasting 6 min, were separated by a 5.5 min block-designed run and a 5 min stimulation period (Fig. 1). During the scanning, subjects lay supine on the scanner bed, wearing ear plugs to suppress scanner noise and with the head immobilized by cushioned supports. They were instructed to keep their eyes closed and their minds clear and to remain awake. In addition, the feelings of *deqi* were collected at the end of the session, including soreness, numbness, fullness, heaviness and dull pain. Subjects were asked to rate each component of the *deqi* feeling they had experienced during the stimulation period using a visual analog scale (VAS) ranging from 0 (none) to 100 (max).

fMRI Data Acquisition

Functional images were acquired on a Siemens 3T whole-body scanner with a standard whole head coil. Blood oxygenation level-dependent (BOLD) functional imaging was conducted using a T2*-weighted single-shot, gradient-recalled echo planar imaging (EPI) sequence (TE = 30 ms, TR = 2 s, flip angle = 90°, FOV = 250 mm×250 mm). Twenty-nine axial sections, each measuring 4 mm in thickness with 1-mm inter-slices, were collected to encompass the whole cerebrum and cerebellum. Prior to the functional run in the first session, high-resolution structural images of each subject were acquired using a 3D T1-weighted sequence (TR/TE = 2.7s/3.19 ms, FOV = 256 mm×256 mm, flip angle = 7°, slice thickness = 1 mm).

fMRI Data Analysis

SPM5 software (Wellcome Department of Cognitive Neurology, London, UK) and Group ICA of the fMRI Toolbox (GIFT, http://icatb.sourceforge.net/) were used for the fMRI data analysis. For each run, all the functional images were first realigned to the first one. The image data were further processed with spatial normalization based on the Montreal Neurological Institute (MNI) template and resampled at 2 mm×2 mm×2 mm and spatially smoothed thereafter using a Gaussian Kernel with 6 mm full-width at half maximum (FWHM). Then these data were filtered to reduce the effect of low-frequency drift and high-frequency noise by using a band-pass filter (0.01–0.08 Hz).

To investigate the manipulation effect, GLM was used to analyze the block-designed data. Because the sustained effect of acupuncture has been shown to exist even after a very short period (1 min) of acupuncture stimulation [27], we utilized a modified GLM design matrix that separated different conditions across each subject with regressors coded for the difference between the baseline (BL) and the stimulation period (S1 and S2) (Fig. 1). Further statistical analyses were performed at both the individual level and the group level. In the individual analysis, two *t*-contrasts were defined as S1 minus BL and S2 minus BL. The resulting statistical maps indicated the voxel-wise signal changes for a specific stimulation condition relative to the baseline. These maps from each subject were later used to generate the group map using one sample *t*-test. Statistical significance was thresholded at cluster-level FDR corrected to $P<0.05$, with a cluster size of no less than 15 voxels.

To investigate the sustained effects of acupuncture, independent component analysis (ICA) was used to analyze the rest datasets.

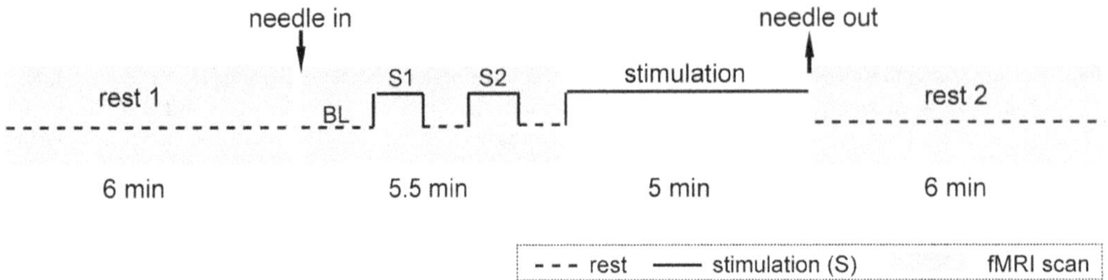

Figure 1. Experimental paradigm. Functional scanning incorporated with three independent runs: two rest runs (rest 1 and rest 2), each lasting 6 min, were separated by a 5.5 min block-designed run and a 5 min stimulation period. The block-designed scanning included two cycles, 1 min stimulation (S1 and S2) and a 1 min rest epoch, preceded by a 1.5 min rest period as baseline (BL). Immediately after the block-designed run, the same modality of stimulation was continued for 5 min without scanning.

Using the Informax ICA algorithm, the smoothed rest data were separated into 40 independent components, and the number was estimated by minimum description length criteria. The DMN or SMN component was identified by spatially sorting the entire components with the corresponding mask [30]. Next, for each subject, the best-fit component was extracted from each individual run. One sample t-test with a significant level of voxel-level FDR corrected to $P<0.05$ was used to examine the group maps for the DMN and SMN, and these maps were made into masks for later comparisons. Paired *t*-tests were performed to determine the differences in the spatial extant of DMN/SMN between rest 1 versus rest 2 for each modality of stimulation, thresholded at voxel-wise of $P<0.001$ uncorrected with 15 continuous voxels within the masks.

Results

General Results of Experimental Performance

Sixteen of eighteen consenting volunteers completed the study, and two withdrew. In the functional data processing, data with head movements exceeding 1 mm on any axis or with a head rotation greater than 1° were excluded. In the final cohort, the block-designed datasets included 15 subjects for sensory control, 14 for MA, 15 for EA and 15 for TEAS. Meanwhile, there were 16 subjects for sensory control, 15 for MA, 15 for EA and 14 for TEAS in the rest datasets.

The percentage of the subjects who reported *deqi* feelings, including soreness, numbness, fullness, heaviness and dull pain, varied among different types of stimulation (Fig. 2). Compared to sensory control ($F_{3,295} = 19.00$, $P<0.001$), EA and MA showed higher fullness and heaviness reports. Stronger soreness and numbness feelings were specifically reported in MA and TEAS, respectively, and there were no differences in dull pain (Fig. 2B). The mean intensities of all sensations were also compared, and significant higher mean *deqi* scores were observed in MA and EA, compared to the sensory control ($F_{3,62} = 7.252$, $P<0.001$) (Fig. 2C).

Results of the Manipulation Effect

Group results during stimulation on ST-36 included two *t*-contrasts, S1 vs. BL and S2 vs. BL. For sensory control, both S1 and S2 produced signal increases in the sensorimotor area, prefrontal cortex and the cerebellum, and decreased BOLD signals were observed in the precuneus and the precentral gyrus. In addition to these areas, the insula, anterolateral prefrontal cortex, striatum and the middle temporal gyrus showed positive activation during S1 (Table 1). During MA on ST-36, S1 also increased the BOLD responses in the sensorimotor area, the anterolateral prefrontal cortex and the middle temporal gyrus. However, there was neither positive nor negative activation during S2 (Table 2). EA only activated the insula and the cerebellum in S1 but produced extensive signal decreases in the sensorimotor area, the limbic system, and other cortical regions such as the prefrontal cortex, superior temporal gyrus and the precuneus during S2 (Table 3). For TEAS, in addition to similar activations as in the sensory control, the premotor cortex, the thalamus and the parahippocampal gyrus showed specific signal changes in S1. There was no positive activation above the statistical threshold in S2, and deactivations were observed in the premotor area and the precuneus (Table 4).

Results of the Sustained Effect

The group maps of the DMN in the resting state consistently demonstrated spatial distribution with the DMN mask (Fig.S1A), including in the posterior cingulate, precuneus, medial prefrontal cortex and the inferior parietal lobule. Increased connectivity of this network was observed in the precuneus, middle occipital gyrus, temporal gyrus and the premotor cortex following MA stimulation. Additionally, the middle occipital gyrus, fusiform gyrus and the cerebellum also showed increased connectivity in EA. Decreased connectivity was found in the superior temporal gyrus following MA, in the inferior parietal lobule following EA and in the cuneus after EA and TEAS. There was no connectivity change in the sensory control (Table 5 and Fig. 3).

The group maps of the SMN during rest were also consistently spatially distributed with a predefined mask (Fig.S1B) and included the pre- and post-central gyrus, supplemental motor area and the secondary somatosensory area. MA, EA and the sensory control showed decreased connectivity in this network. Decreases were observed in the primary somatosensory area and the premotor cortex after MA, in the cuneus after EA, in the premotor cortex and the supplementary motor area after sensory control. However, TEAS predominantly increased connectivity in several regions, including the primary somatosensory area, the premotor cortex, the dorsal anterior cingulate cortex, the supplementary motor area, the superior temporal and the parietal lobule (Table 6 and Fig. 4).

Discussion

Although the manipulation effect of acupuncture on human brain activity has been studied for a long time, most of these studies have used block-designed datasets with typical GLM contrast analysis [15,17,24,31]. However, it is well-known that the sustained effects of acupuncture could last for a long period of time after removing the needles [27,32,33]. Thus, the typical GLM analysis with block-design is inappropriate for identifying the

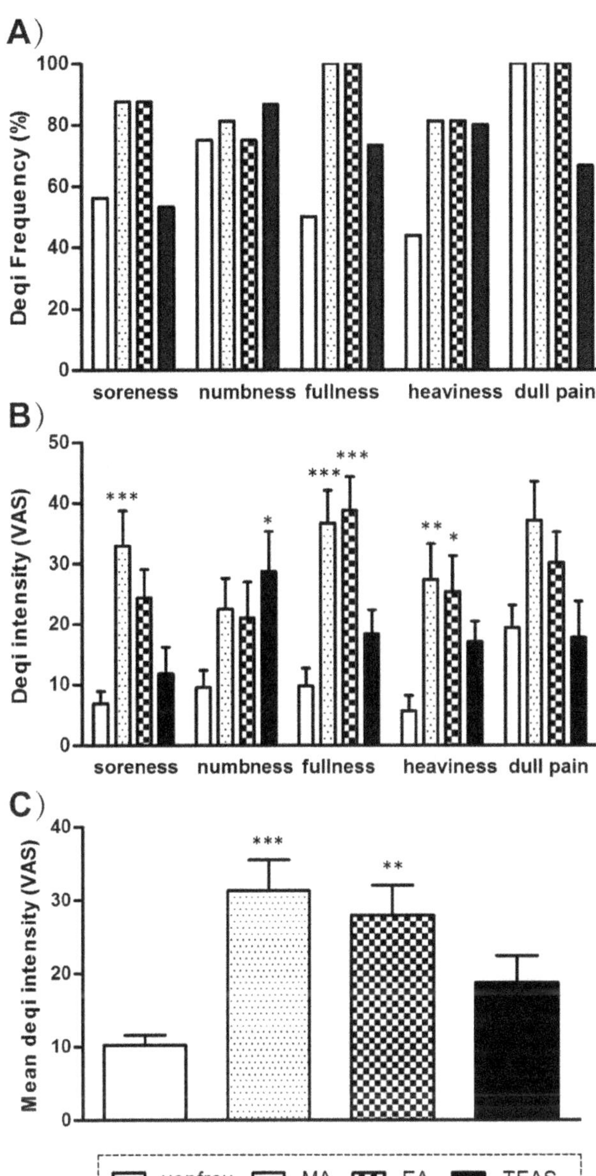

Figure 2. Reports of *deqi* sensations. A) The percentage of subjects who reported having experienced the feelings of *deqi*. B) The intensity of reported sensations measured by an average score (mean±SEM), tested with VAS from 0 to 100. Two-way ANOVA with Bonferroni post-tests were used. C) The mean intensity of all sensations, one-way ANOVA with Tukey's multiple comparison tests were used. *, $P<0.05$, **, $P<0.01$, ***, $P<0.001$ compared to the sensory control.

manipulation effect on human brain activity from acupuncture. In the present study, only the 1.5 min rest period before stimulation was defined as the baseline (Fig. 1), and a modified GLM design matrix was used [27]. Thus, the manipulation effect can be observed without baseline contamination from other rest periods after acupuncture.

In our study, the sensory control stimulation induced similar brain activation during S1 and S2. The BOLD signal increases were mainly distributed in the sensory-motor areas and the lateral prefrontal cortex. The negative activation was observed in DMN (Table 1). These findings were mostly reported by other studies using 5.88 von Frey monofilaments as sensory controls [14,24,33]. In addition, the activation during S1 was more widespread than during S2, which could be attributed to habituation, a progressive decrease in the physiological response to a repeating stimulus that is neither rewarding nor harmful [34]. In contrast, for MA, EA and TEAS, group results during S1 and S2 displayed distinct patterns of activation. Similar positive activation in the sensory-motor area was observed during S1, but the BOLD responses during S2 trended to a negative activation pattern. In Table 2–4, no positive activation could be found in each of the three types of acupuncture stimulation during S2, and EA produced predominantly negative BOLD responses in brain regions, including the sensory-motor areas, the limbic system and other cortical gyri. It is in keeping with the findings that acupuncture stimulation evokes deactivation in the limbic-paralimbic-neocortical network [12,13]. Although MA and TEAS exhibited absent or reduced deactivation during this period, we did observe sub-thresholded decreases in BOLD signal changes. Studies using a less strict level of significance also observed a trend of deactivation instead of activation during the S2 period in the MA group [27]. For pain-relief, EA has been shown to be more effective than MA, and TEAS was equally effective as EA [8,9]. Furthermore, Napadow et al. reported that EA induced more widespread fMRI signal changes than MA when a traditional GLM with block design was used [24]. The current findings indicate that, inconsistent with the sensory habituation in the control, the manipulation effect of all the three modalities of acupuncture stimulation was an early somatosensory activation with later cortical-subcortical deactivation, and EA produced more obvious deactivation than MA and TEAS.

Recently, more studies have paid close attention to the sustained after-effects of acupuncture by comparing the resting state connectivity before and after acupuncture. To the best of our knowledge, most of these studies used short periods of stimulation of less than 6 min [20,21,22,35], which does not fully model the clinical effect produced by relatively longer periods of acupuncture [3]. An early study from our research group revealed a time-curve for the analgesic effect of MA in healthy human beings, and the skin pain threshold started to increase after approximately 10 min of treatment [36]. For this reason, 5 more minutes of stimulation were added after the block to make our model more appropriate for the explanation of the mechanism of potential acupuncture treatment effects.

Interestingly, in the present study, the resting state network following TEAS stimulation displayed a different pattern of connectivity changes than MA and EA. As shown in Table 5 and Fig. 3, the modulating effect of MA and EA is predominantly through the DMN, whereas a more secure and spatially extended connectivity of the SMN was specifically detected in the post-TEAS rest (Table 6 and Fig. 4). Similar increased connectivity between the DMN with other brain regions including the temporal, occipital and frontal cortex were also reported in other studies using MA [21,28,37] and EA [38]. This modulatory effect is speculated to be potent in treating diseases with dysfunctional DMN, such as pain, substance abuse and Alzheimer's disease [39,40,41,42,43]. Additionally, a recent study reported that although EA had a better analgesic effect than MA, a sustained effect was better produced by MA [9], which might explain the more extended increased connectivity in cortical regions induced by MA in our work. To the best of our knowledge, there has been little research investigating the sustained effect following TEAS, and in this study, we first discovered this specific SMN modulating effect. Dhond et al. reported that MA could also increase the functional connectivity in SMN in several regions by acupuncture in PC-6, but the predominant changes were still focused on the

Table 1. Regions of activation for group analysis of sensory control in different stimulation periods.

region	side	stimulation 1 vs. baseline					stimulation 2 vs. baseline				
		t value	coordinate (MNI)			voxels	t value	coordinate (MNI)			voxels
			x	y	z			x	y	z	
positive activation (stimulation>baseline)											
primary and secondary somatosensory area	L	7.09	−56	−24	24	835	6.83	−56	18	30	1091
	R	7.19	60	−28	30	1009	7.28	52	−42	58	1001
insula	R	6.62	32	−2	16	145					
lateral prefrontal cortex	L	4.90	−48	12	16	71	6.51	−42	8	26	532
	R	6.49	54	10	32	624	8.26	46	16	2	231
anterolateral prefrontal cortex	L	4.47	−38	28	6	72					
	R	5.46	40	44	0	155					
middle temporal gyrus	R	5.23	54	−62	2	129					
striatum	R	8.20	20	−14	−8	48					
cerebellum	L	8.06	−22	−66	−44	860	7.48	−22	−72	−50	474
	R	5.06	14	−74	−46	71					
negative activation (stimulation<baseline)											
precuneus	L	−5.77	−16	−96	25	453	−7.22	10	−60	22	360
	R	−5.34	20	−95	25	299					
precentral gyrus	L	−5.64	−26	−30	64	220	−6.89	−28	−16	72	98
	R	−4.50	42	−26	56	77					

L, left; R, right.

DMN [21]. Recently, long-term transcutaneous electrical nerve stimulation (TENS) was shown to be effective in reorganizing the motor cortex in a neurologically intact human, which highlights the potential benefit of sensory training by TENS as a useful complementary therapy in neurorehabilitation [44]. Thus, we surmised that TEAS might be specifically sensitive in the SMN, and this transcutaneous acupuncture might be more suitable for treating diseases with sensory dysfunction. It is notable that our recent work showed that when the stimulation period lasts 30 min, in addition to the SMN modulatory effect, TEAS could also increase the functional connectivity in the DMN [18]. This finding indicated that the effect of acupuncture may have been dependent on the duration of the stimulation and that the treatment time should be considered to be an important factor for studies on the mechanisms of acupuncture.

The sensations of *deqi* were different in the three modalities of acupuncture stimulation; MA and EA produced stronger *deqi* sensations of fullness and heaviness than did the control (Fig. 2), and stronger soreness was also reported in MA. Interestingly, unlike MA and EA, TEAS specifically induced more reports of numbness. Because the *deqi* sensation is considered to be related to the clinical efficacy in traditional Chinese medicine [45,46], our results suggested that different types of acupuncture treatment, especially the transcutaneous and invasive acupuncture, might have varied treatment effects, and further studies are required to support this speculation. Moreover, no difference was observed in

Table 2. Regions of activation for group analysis of MA in different stimulation periods.

region	side	stimulation 1 vs. baseline				
		t value	coordinate (MNI)			voxels
			x	y	z	
positive activation (stimulation>baseline)						
primary and secondary somatosensory area	L	6.23	−48	−26	38	443
	R	8.48	58	−22	26	665
anterolateral prefrontal cortex	R	6.38	42	56	10	95
middle temporal gyrus	R	6.81	52	−52	−4	176
negative deactivation (stimulation<baseline)						
no regions above threshold						

L, left; R, right. There was no statistically significant region in comparison of 'stimulation 2 vs. baseline'.

Table 3. Regions of activation for group analysis of EA in different stimulation periods.

region	side	stimulation 1 vs. baseline					stimulation 2 vs. baseline				
		t value	coordinate (MNI)			voxels	t value	coordinate (MNI)			voxels
			x	y	z			x	y	z	
positive activation (stimulation>baseline)											
insula	R	4.68	48	8	0	129					
cerebellum	L	6.52	−16	−68	−44	143					
negative activation (stimulation<baseline)											
postcentral gyrus	L						−6.62	−12	-46	64	460
parahippocampal gyrus	R						−6.33	14	−12	−24	186
superior temporal gyrus	R						−5.38	54	−58	16	135
supplementary motor area	L						−4.64	−4	−18	66	90
premotor cortex	R						−6.22	22	2	68	87
precuneus	R						−6.20	4	−54	46	209
medial prefrontal cortex	R						−5.94	6	52	50	101
dorsal anterior cingulate cortex	L,R						−4.89	6	10	34	193

L, left; R, right.

dull pain sensation between the acupuncture and control groups, which confirmed *deqi* as a multiple-feeling sensation more than only pain [24,47].

Several limitations in this study should be noted. Although we observed differences among different acupuncture modalities in *deqi* sensation and in the effects on brain activities by using fMRI, less information about autonomic response was collected (for

Table 4. Regions of activation for group analysis of TEAS in different stimulation periods.

region	side	stimulation 1 vs. baseline					stimulation 2 vs. baseline				
		t value	coordinate (MNI)			voxels	t value	coordinate (MNI)			voxels
			x	y	z			x	y	z	
positive activation (stimulation>baseline)											
primary and secondary somatosensory area	L	6.64	−48	−40	26	544					
	R	7.87	68	−22	28	591					
postcentral gyrus	R	5.26	12	−48	74	107					
supplementary motor area	R	6.01	8	−20	68	92					
anterolateral prefrontal cortex	L	5.00	−38	46	−12	112					
	R	5.52	42	42	−10	145					
middle temporal gyrus	R	5.07	−52	−58	4	62					
thalamus	R	5.73	16	−14	−4	727					
striatum	L	4.69	−24	2	20	118					
cerebellum	L	6.36	−30	−62	−48	88					
	R	5.27	26	−66	−26	88					
negative activation (stimulation<baseline)											
precentral gyrus	R	−5.82	38	−16	64	202					
premotor cortex	L						−5.87	−22	12	70	188
	R						−6.68	32	10	64	257
parahippocampal gyrus	L	−5.37	−20	−8	−30	87					
	R	−5.45	30	−20	−26	200					
precuneus	L						−4.71	−8	−64	58	285
	R						−5.25	4	−46	48	90

L, left; R, right.

Table 5. Brain regions in the DMN modulated by different modalities of acupuncture.

		MA					EA					TEAS				
Region	**side**	**t value**	**coordinate (MNI)**			**voxels**	**t value**	**coordinate (MNI)**			**voxels**	**t value**	**coordinate (MNI)**			**voxels**
			x	**y**	**z**			**x**	**y**	**z**			**x**	**y**	**z**	
Rest 1<Rest 2																
premotor cortex	R	5.91	50	0	40	22										
middle temporal gyrus	L	4.82	−42	−54	12	19										
superior temporal gyrus	L	5.49	−62	−56	14	15										
middle occipital gyrus	L	5.89	−24	−86	−8	34	5.84	−20	−96	2	71					
fusiform gyrus	R						4.87	30	−38	−24	23					
precuneus	R	6.08	2	−70	38	50										
cerebellum	L						5.40	−8	−40	−24	16					
	R						5.29	2	−58	−18	29					
Rest 1>Rest 2																
superior temporal gyrus	R	−6.28	48	−20	4	28										
inferior parietal lobule	L						−4.87	−52	−42	56	21					
Cuneus	L											−4.50	−12	−104	4	28
	R						−6.39	10	−80	26	48					

L, left; R, right. There was no statistically significant region in comparison of 'sensory control'.

instance, heart rate and skin conductance). Napadow et al. recently reported that different brain responses underling MA stimulation may be related to differential autonomic outflows and may result from heterogeneity in evoked sensations [29]. In addition, a recent report by Florian et al. provided an insight into the linkage of the *deqi* sensation, autonomic responses and the potential of therapeutic effect [48]. Thus, it is possible that the differences in brain activity changes induced by different acupuncture modalities might also have a relationship with the autonomic responses. To study this possibility further, combined fMRI and autonomic response measurements are needed. It also should be noted that the present study focused primarily on changes in brain activity induced by acupuncture in healthy subjects and could only provide clues in exploring the mechanisms of acupuncture treatment. Further studies in patients would provide more convincing evidence of the differences among these modalities of acupuncture. Also, the significant threshold of the paired-*t* test was without FDR corrected, further researches with large sample size may conquer this limitation.

In summary, the current study suggests that although different modalities of acupuncture could be clinically effective, the underlining mechanisms might be varied, and acupuncture in differential modalities might have treatment potentials for specific dysfunctions. In addition, the findings of our research could supply

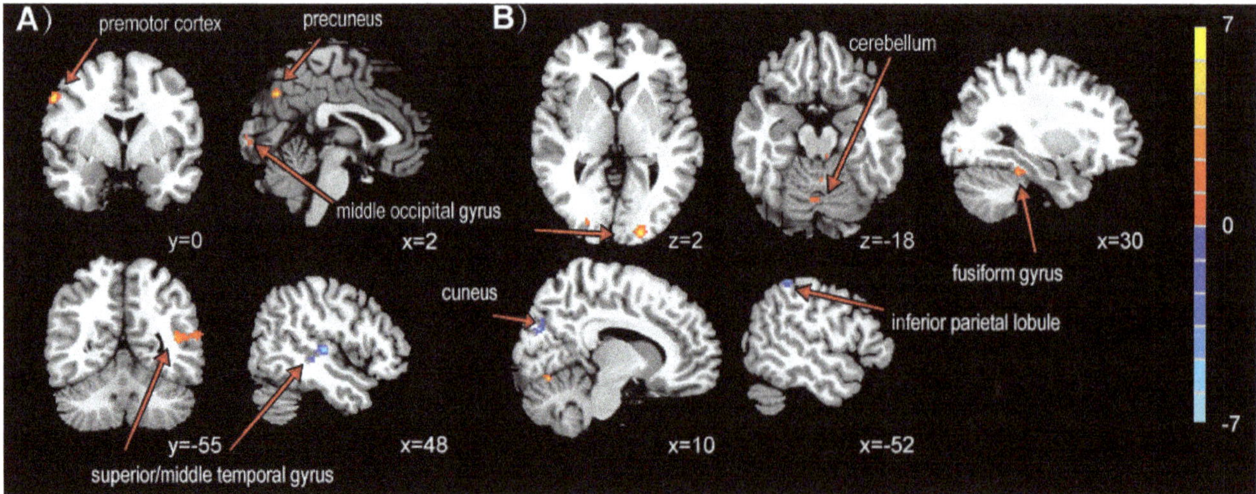

Figure 3. Changes in functional connectivity of the DMN following MA (A) or EA (B). Using paired *t*-test. The threshold of display was set to voxel-wise $P<0.001$ uncorrected with at least 15 contiguous voxels. The colored bar indicates T-values. The group maps for the DMN before and after MA/EA stimulation were shown in Fig.S1.A.

Table 6. Brain regions in the SMN modulated by different modalities of acupuncture.

		sensory control					MA					EA					TEAS				
Region	side	t value	coordinate (MNI)			voxels	t value	coordinate (MNI)			voxels	t value	coordinate (MNI)			voxels	t value	coordinate (MNI)			voxels
			x	y	z			x	y	z			x	y	z			x	y	z	
Rest 1<Rest 2																					
primary somatosensory area	L																6.09	−36	−34	60	102
	R																5.17	22	−34	66	102
premotor cortex	L																4.91	−30	−16	68	19
dorsal anterior cingulate cortex/ supplementary motor area	R																7.88	10	−4	46	243
superior temporal gyrus	R																5.57	36	−52	−22	28
superior parietal lobule	R																4.14	22	−12	70	11
Rest 1>Rest 2																					
primary somatosensory area	R						−5.49	42	−24	64	53										
premotor cortex	L						−6.27	−48	−12	46	21										
	R	−5.15	64	−6	34	20															
supplementary motor area	R	−4.64	4	8	62	18															
Cuneus	L											−5.25	−16	−80	16	19					

L, left; R, right.

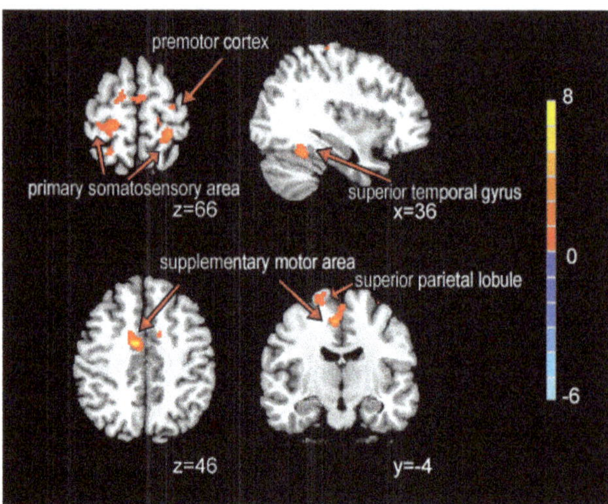

Figure 4. Changes in functional connectivity of the SMN following TEAS. Using paired *t*-test. The threshold of display was set to voxel-wise $P<0.001$ uncorrected, with at least 15 contiguous voxels. The colored bar indicates T-values. The group maps for the SMN before and after TEAS were shown in Fig.S1.B.

methodological information for further studies examining the mechanism of acupuncture.

Supporting Information

Figure S1 Group maps for the DMN and the SMN, before and after acupuncture stimulation. The best-fit components were selected by using the templates of the DMN and SMN shown in the right line of the graph. The group results of (A) the DMN and (B) the SMN components decomposed by ICA included the pre-MA rest/post-MA rest, the pre-EA rest/post-EA rest and the pre-TEAS rest/post-TEAS rest. The threshold of one sample *t*-test was set as FDR corrected, $P<0.05$, with at least 10 continuous voxels in all group statistics. Color bar indicates T-values.
(DOC)

Author Contributions

Conceived and designed the experiments: YJ CLC JSH. Performed the experiments: YJ YRD YD HW XHX LZW. Analyzed the data: YJ ZYL LJB JT. Contributed reagents/materials/analysis tools: HW. Wrote the paper: YJ CLC.

References

1. NIH Consensus Conference (1998) Acupuncture. 1518–1524.
2. Xiang X, Jiang Y, Ni Y, Fan M, Shen F, et al. (2012) Catechol-O-methyltransferase polymorphisms do not play a significant role in pain perception in male Chinese Han population. Physiol Genomics 44: 318–328.
3. Han JS (2011) Acupuncture analgesia: Areas of consensus and controversy. Pain 152: 41–48.
4. Cui CL, Wu LZ, Luo F (2008) Acupuncture for the treatment of drug addiction. Neurochem Res 33: 2013–2022.
5. Unterrainer AF, Friedrich C, Krenn MH, Piotrowski WP, Golaszewski SM, et al. (2010) Postoperative and preincisional electrical nerve stimulation TENS reduce postoperative opioid requirement after major spinal surgery. J Neurosurg Anesthesiol 22: 1–5.
6. Zhang R, Feng XJ, Guan Q, Cui W, Zheng Y, et al. (2011) Increase of success rate for women undergoing embryo transfer by transcutaneous electrical acupoint stimulation: a prospective randomized placebo-controlled study. Fertil Steril 96: 912–916.
7. Zhang R, Jia MX, Zhang JS, Xu XJ, Shou XJ, et al. (2012) Transcutaneous electrical acupoint stimulation in children with autism and its impact on plasma levels of arginine-vasopressin and oxytocin: a prospective single-blinded controlled study. Res Dev Disabil 33: 1136–1146.
8. Ulett GA, Han S, Han JS (1998) Electroacupuncture: mechanisms and clinical application. Biol Psychiatry 44: 129–138.
9. Schliessbach J, van der Klift E, Arendt-Nielsen L, Curatolo M, Streitberger K (2011) The effect of brief electrical and manual acupuncture stimulation on mechanical experimental pain. Pain Med 12: 268–275.
10. Wang JQ, Mao L, Han JS (1992) Comparison of the antinociceptive effects induced by electroacupuncture and transcutaneous electrical nerve stimulation in the rat. Int J Neurosci 65: 117–129.
11. Han JS (2003) Acupuncture: neuropeptide release produced by electrical stimulation of different frequencies. Trends Neurosci 26: 17–22.
12. Hui KK, Marina O, Liu J, Rosen BR, Kwong KK (2010) Acupuncture, the limbic system, and the anticorrelated networks of the brain. Auton Neurosci.
13. Fang J, Jin Z, Wang Y, Li K, Kong J, et al. (2009) The salient characteristics of the central effects of acupuncture needling: limbic-paralimbic-neocortical network modulation. Hum Brain Mapp 30: 1196–1206.
14. Hui KK, Liu J, Marina O, Napadow V, Haselgrove C, et al. (2005) The integrated response of the human cerebro-cerebellar and limbic systems to acupuncture stimulation at ST 36 as evidenced by fMRI. Neuroimage 27: 479–496.
15. Zhang WT, Jin Z, Cui GH, Zhang KL, Zhang L, et al. (2003) Relations between brain network activation and analgesic effect induced by low vs. high frequency electrical acupoint stimulation in different subjects: a functional magnetic resonance imaging study. Brain Res 982: 168–178.
16. Wu MT, Sheen JM, Chuang KH, Yang P, Chin SL, et al. (2002) Neuronal specificity of acupuncture response: a fMRI study with electroacupuncture. Neuroimage 16: 1028–1037.
17. Hui KK, Liu J, Makris N, Gollub RL, Chen AJ, et al. (2000) Acupuncture modulates the limbic system and subcortical gray structures of the human brain: evidence from fMRI studies in normal subjects. Hum Brain Mapp 9: 13–25.
18. Jiang Y, Hao Y, Zhang Y, Liu J, Wang X, et al. (2012) Thirty minute transcutaneous electric acupoint stimulation modulates resting state brain activities: A perfusion and BOLD fMRI study. Brain Res.
19. Liu B, Chen J, Wang J, Liu X, Duan X, et al. (2012) Altered Small-World Efficiency of Brain Functional Networks in Acupuncture at ST36: A Functional MRI Study. PLoS One 7: e39342.
20. Bai L, Qin W, Tian J, Dong M, Pan X, et al. (2009) Acupuncture modulates spontaneous activities in the anticorrelated resting brain networks. Brain Res 1279: 37–49.
21. Dhond RP, Yeh C, Park K, Kettner N, Napadow V (2008) Acupuncture modulates resting state connectivity in default and sensorimotor brain networks. Pain 136: 407–418.
22. Qin W, Tian J, Bai L, Pan X, Yang L, et al. (2008) FMRI connectivity analysis of acupuncture effects on an amygdala-associated brain network. Mol Pain 4: 55.
23. Huang W, Pach D, Napadow V, Park K, Long X, et al. (2012) Characterizing acupuncture stimuli using brain imaging with FMRI - a systematic review and meta-analysis of the literature. PLoS One 7: e32960.
24. Napadow V, Makris N, Liu J, Kettner NW, Kwong KK, et al. (2005) Effects of electroacupuncture versus manual acupuncture on the human brain as measured by fMRI. Hum Brain Mapp 24: 193–205.
25. Li G, Cheung RT, Ma QY, Yang ES (2003) Visual cortical activations on fMRI upon stimulation of the vision-implicated acupoints. Neuroreport 14: 669–673.
26. Kong J, Ma L, Gollub RL, Wei J, Yang X, et al. (2002) A pilot study of functional magnetic resonance imaging of the brain during manual and electroacupuncture stimulation of acupuncture point (LI-4 Hegu) in normal subjects reveals differential brain activation between methods. J Altern Complement Med 8: 411–419.
27. Bai L, Qin W, Tian J, Liu P, Li L, et al. (2009) Time-varied characteristics of acupuncture effects in fMRI studies. Hum Brain Mapp 30: 3445–3460.
28. Hui KKS, Marina O, Claunch JD, Nixon EE, Fang J, et al. (2009) Acupuncture mobilizes the brain's default mode and its anti-correlated network in healthy subjects. Brain Research 1287: 84–103.
29. Napadow V, Lee J, Kim J, Cina S, Maeda Y, et al. (2012) Brain correlates of phasic autonomic response to acupuncture stimulation: An event-related fMRI study. Hum Brain Mapp.
30. Franco AR, Pritchard A, Calhoun VD, Mayer AR (2009) Interrater and intermethod reliability of default mode network selection. Hum Brain Mapp 30: 2293–2303.

31. Napadow V, Dhond R, Park K, Kim J, Makris N, et al. (2009) Time-variant fMRI activity in the brainstem and higher structures in response to acupuncture. Neuroimage 47: 289–301.
32. Price DD, Rafii A, Watkins LR, Buckingham B (1984) A psychophysical analysis of acupuncture analgesia. Pain 19: 27–42.
33. Napadow V, Dhond RP, Kim J, LaCount L, Vangel M, et al. (2009) Brain encoding of acupuncture sensation–coupling on-line rating with fMRI. Neuroimage 47: 1055–1065.
34. Thompson RF, Spencer WA (1966) Habituation: a model phenomenon for the study of neuronal substrates of behavior. Psychol Rev 73: 16–43.
35. Liu J, Qin W, Guo Q, Sun J, Yuan K, et al. (2010) Distinct brain networks for time-varied characteristics of acupuncture. Neurosci Lett 468: 353–358.
36. Research Group Of Acupuncture Anesthesia PMC (1973) The effect of acupuncture on the human skin pain threshold.: Chin Med J. 151–157.
37. Zhong C, Bai L, Dai R, Xue T, Wang H, et al. (2011) Modulatory effects of acupuncture on resting-state networks: A functional MRI study combining independent component analysis and multivariate granger causality analysis. J Magn Reson Imaging.
38. Liu P, Zhang Y, Zhou G, Yuan K, Qin W, et al. (2009) Partial correlation investigation on the default mode network involved in acupuncture: an fMRI study. Neurosci Lett 462: 183–187.
39. Zyloney CE, Jensen K, Polich G, Loiotile RE, Cheetham A, et al. (2010) Imaging the functional connectivity of the Periaqueductal Gray during genuine and sham electroacupuncture treatment. Mol Pain 6: 80.
40. Zhang Y, Tian J, Yuan K, Liu P, Zhuo L, et al. (2011) Distinct resting-state brain activities in heroin-dependent individuals. Brain Res 1402: 46–53.
41. Ma N, Liu Y, Fu XM, Li N, Wang CX, et al. (2011) Abnormal brain default-mode network functional connectivity in drug addicts. PLoS One 6: e16560.
42. Baliki MN, Geha PY, Apkarian AV, Chialvo DR (2008) Beyond feeling: chronic pain hurts the brain, disrupting the default-mode network dynamics. J Neurosci 28: 1398–1403.
43. Wang Z, Nie B, Li D, Zhao Z, Han Y, et al. (2012) Effect of acupuncture in mild cognitive impairment and Alzheimer disease: a functional MRI study. PLoS One 7: e42730.
44. Meesen RL, Cuypers K, Rothwell JC, Swinnen SP, Levin O (2011) The effect of long-term TENS on persistent neuroplastic changes in the human cerebral cortex. Hum Brain Mapp 32: 872–882.
45. Cheng X (1997) Chinese Acupuncture and Moxibustion.
46. Hui KK, Sporko TN, Vangel MG, Li M, Fang J, et al. (2011) Perception of Deqi by Chinese and American acupuncturists: a pilot survey. Chin Med 6: 2.
47. Kong J, Gollub R, Huang T, Polich G, Napadow V, et al. (2007) Acupuncture de qi, from qualitative history to quantitative measurement. J Altern Complement Med 13: 1059–1070.
48. Beissner F, Deichmann R, Henke C, Bar KJ (2011) Acupuncture - Deep pain with an autonomic dimension? Neuroimage.

10

Proteomic Response to Acupuncture Treatment in Spontaneously Hypertensive Rats

Xinsheng Lai[1 9], Jiayou Wang[2*9], Neel R. Nabar[3], Sanqiang Pan[4], Chunzhi Tang[1], Yong Huang[5], Mufeng Hao[2], Zhonghua Yang[2], Chunmei Ma[2], Jin Zhang[2], Helen Chew[3], Zhenquan He[2], Junjun Yang[1], Baogui Su[4], Jian Zhang[6], Jun Liang[3], Kevin B. Sneed[7], Shu-Feng Zhou[3*]

1 Department of Acupuncture and Moxibustion, School of Acupuncture and Moxibustion, Guangzhou University of Chinese Medicine, Guangzhou, China, **2** Department of Human Anatomy, School of Fundamental Medical Sciences, Guangzhou University of Chinese Medicine, Guangzhou, China, **3** Department of Pharmaceutical Sciences, College of Pharmacy, University of South Florida, Tampa, Florida, United States of America, **4** Department of Human Anatomy, School of Medicine, Jinan University, Guangzhou, China, **5** Department of Acupuncture and Moxibustion, School of Chinese Medicine, Southern Medical University, Guangzhou, China, **6** Department of Surgery, The Third Hospital of Nanchang, Nanchang, Jiangxi, China, **7** Department of Pharmacotherapeutics and Clinical Research, College of Pharmacy, University of South Florida, Tampa, Florida, United States of America

Abstract

Previous animal and clinical studies have shown that acupuncture is an effective alternative treatment in the management of hypertension, but the mechanism is unclear. This study investigated the proteomic response in the nervous system to treatment at the Taichong (LR3) acupoint in spontaneously hypertensive rats (SHRs). Unanesthetized rats were subject to 5-min daily acupuncture treatment for 7 days. Blood pressure was monitored over 7 days. After euthanasia on the 7th day, rat medullas were dissected, homogenized, and subject to 2D gel electrophoresis and MALDI-TOF analysis. The results indicate that blood pressure stabilized after the 5th day of acupuncture, and compared with non-acupoint treatment, Taichong-acupunctured rat's systolic pressure was reduced significantly ($P<0.01$), though not enough to bring blood pressure down to normal levels. The different treatment groups also showed differential protein expression: the 2D images revealed 571 ± 15 proteins in normal SD rats' medulla, 576 ± 31 proteins in SHR's medulla, 597 ± 44 proteins in medulla of SHR after acupuncturing Taichong, and 616 ± 18 proteins in medulla of SHR after acupuncturing non-acupoint. In the medulla of Taichong group, compared with non-acupoint group, seven proteins were down-regulated: heat shock protein-90, synapsin-1, pyruvate kinase isozyme, NAD-dependent deacetylase sirtuin-2, protein kinase C inhibitor protein 1, ubiquitin hydrolase isozyme L1, and myelin basic protein. Six proteins were up-regulated: glutamate dehydrogenase 1, aldehyde dehydrogenase 2, glutathione *S*-transferase M5, Rho GDP dissociation inhibitor 1, DJ-1 protein and superoxide dismutase. The altered expression of several proteins by acupuncture has been confirmed by ELISA, Western blot and qRT-PCR assays. The results indicate an increase in antioxidant enzymes in the medulla of the SHRs subject to acupuncture, which may provide partial explanation for the antihypertensive effect of acupuncture. Further studies are warranted to investigate the role of oxidative stress modulation by acupuncture in the treatment of hypertension.

Editor: Jianping Ye, Pennington Biomedical Research Center, United States of America

Funding: The authors appreciate the support by the National 973 program of China (Grant No. 2006CB504505), the Natural Science Foundation of China (Grant No. 90709027), and University of South Florida College of Pharmacy Startup Fund. The funders had no role in study design, data collection and analysis, decision to publish, or preparation of the manuscript.

Competing Interests: The authors have declared that no competing interests exist.

* E-mail: szhou@health.usf.edu (SFZ); xmishu@126.com (JW)

9 These authors contributed equally to this work.

Introduction

Hypertension is a multifactorial condition characterized by systolic blood pressure (SBP) of $\geq$140 mmHg or diastolic blood pressure (DBP) of $\geq$90 mmHg [1,2]. Currently, estimates for the number of people worldwide affected by hypertension exceed 1 billion [3], including at least 76.4 million American adults $\geq$20 years of age (i.e. about one out of three U.S. adults is affected based on data from the 2005–2006 National Health and Nutrition Examination Survey) [4]. The prevalence of hypertension is almost the same between men and women in America. In 2010, hypertension raised a cost of $76.6 billion in health care services, medications, and missed days of work in the United States [5]. Despite the recent increase in public awareness of hypertension, only 78% of hypertensive patients were aware of their condition; 68% were using antihypertensive drugs; and 64% of those treated had their blood pressure controlled [4]. It has been projected that an additional 27 million American people could suffer from hypertension, a 9.9% increase in prevalence from 2010 [6]. Chronic hypertension is a major causative factor of morbidity and mortality, as uncontrolled hypertension can contribute to myocardial infarction, stroke, congestive heart failure, and renal failure. The overall death rate resulting from hypertension was 18.3 in the United States in 2008 [4]. Major barriers to successful conventional pharmacological treatment include side effects, out-of-pocket expenses, noncompliance of patients and improper dosage/regimen.

Acupuncture provides an alternative treatment approach to hypertension and has been a critical constituent of traditional Chinese Medicine (TCM) for the past 2,500 years [7,8]. More recently, the practice of acupuncture has become prevalent in the United States, with over 2 million Americans reporting recent use of acupuncture [9]. In TCM, acupuncture theory is based on the premise that energy (called "Qi") goes along determined pathways or meridians within the body and is responsible for maintaining good health by providing homeostatic regulation of vital body function [10]. In TCM, diseases are believed to result from imbalances and disturbances in the flow of "Qi" within the body, thus acupuncture consists of treatments by insertion and manipulation of needles at specific anatomic locations (acupoints) in the body with the intent of regulating the energy flow and restoring that balance. In acupuncture, the placement of needles into the body is dictated by the location of meridians, thought to mark patterns of energy flow throughout the human body in TCM [10]. Acupuncture has been widely used to manage musculokeletal pains, nausea secondary to surgery and chemotherapy, and other diseases.

A number of animal and clinical studies have reported the efficacy of acupuncture in reducing hypertension [11,12,13,14]. Although there is some discrepancy between the reports, the majority of them indicate that acupuncture of traditional acupoints causes a significant decrease in blood pressure, while acupuncture at sham points does not [11]. However, the long-term effect and elucidation of the mechanisms through which acupuncture lowers blood pressure has not been reported. On a systemic level, studies have suggested the involvement of plasma renin, aldosterone, and angiotensin II activity [15,16,17,18]. The involvement of increased sodium excretion [19], as well as changes in plasma norepinephrine, serotonin, and endorphin levels have also been implicated [20,21,22].

Although many studies have looked at the systemic effect of acupuncture on hypertension, less research has been conducted on the response to acupuncture at proteomic and cellular/subcellular levels. We hypothesize that acupuncture at proper acupoints will result in differential protein expression compared to acupuncture at sham points. Additionally, as hypertension is a multifactorial condition and acupuncture results in a multitude of *in vivo* changes, we believe that acupuncture will lower blood pressure through modulation of multiple biochemical and molecular pathways. This study is the first to examine the proteomic response in the medulla of rats to acupuncture at the LR3 point compared to stimulation at a sham-acupuncture site in spontaneously hypertensive rats (SHRs). Now rats are a well accepted animal model for acupuncture studies because both rats and humans share a number of anatomical and genomic features. A large number of published acupuncture studies use rats as the experimental model [23,24,25].

Materials and Methods

Ethics Statement

All animal experiments were conducted at the Laboratory Animal Center of Guangzhou University of Chinese Medicine, Guangzhou, China. The procedure was approved by the Ethics Committee of Guangzhou University of Chinese Medicine, Guangzhou, China [permit No.: SYXK (Yue) 2008-0085].

Chemicals and Reagents

Chemicals and materials used for our proteomic study, including urea, CHAPS detergent, dithiothreitol (DTT), 2-mercaptoethanol, bio-lyte3/10, bromophenol blue, mineral oil, filter paper wicks, immobilized pH gradient (IPG) ready strip (11 cm, pH 5–8), 12.5% Tris-HCl, 1.5 M Tris-HCl (pH 8.8), iodoacetamide, ready prep overlay agarose, 10 × Tris/glycine/SDS buffer, precision plus unstained standard, and SYPRO® Ruby protein gel stain were purchased from Bio-Rad Co. (Hercules, CA). Thiouea, protease inhibitor cocktail and a matrix solution of α-cyano-4-hydroxycinnamic acid in acetonitrile/methanol were purchased from Sigma-Aldrich Inc. (St Louis, MO). For matrix-assisted laser desorption/ionization time-of-flight (MALDI-TOF) mass spectrometry (MS) experiments, pure trypsinogen was obtained from Shanghai Sangon Biotech Co. Ltd (Shanghai, China). For enzyme immunoassay experiments, reagent kits for measuring rat glutathione *S*-transferase M5 (GSTM5), aldehyde dehydrogenase 2 (ALDH2), and protein kinase C (PKC) were purchased from R&D Systems Inc. (Minneapolis, MN).

Animals

Due to supply shortage in China, we could not get Wistar Kyoto rats during our experimental period. Based on literature reports, Sprague Dawley (SD) rats have been used as the normotensive controls for spontaneously hypertensive rats [26,27]. In fact, SD rats are originally derived from Wistar Kyoto rats with minor physiological and biochemical differences.

A total of 54 9-week-old male SHRs weighing 180–200 g and body weight-matched 18 SD rats were obtained from Beijing Vital River Laboratory Animals Co. Ltd (Beijing, China). They were housed at a controlled ambient temperature of 22–25°C with 55±5% relative humidity and a 12 hr light/12 hr dark cycle (lights on at 8:00 AM) at the Laboratory Animal Center of Guangzhou University of Chinese Medicine, Guangzhou, China. The animals were given food and water *ad libitum* for 3 days, and were acclimatized to handling by the researchers and BP-measuring conditions for 1 week prior to acupuncture treatments. After measuring BP, the SHRs (BP≥140 mmHg) were randomly divided into three groups: the Taichong group (n = 18) was treated with acupuncture at the LR3 acupoint, the non-acupoint group (n = 18) was treated at non-acupoints, and the model group (n = 18) was untreated throughout the duration of the experiment. Body weight-matched SD rats with normal BP (normal group) were used as comparative control and were untreated throughout the duration of the experiment (n = 18).

Acupuncture Treatment

In one group of the SHRs, acupuncture was performed at bilateral Taichong points (LR3) located between the 1st and the 2nd metatarsal of dorsal foot; while in non-acupoint group acupuncture was done at bilateral non-acupoint located at the fossa between the 3rd and 4th metatarsal of dorsal foot (Figure 1). The locations for sham vs nonsham acupoints are based on the anatomic locations in TCM that have been mapped to rats by other researchers [28,29,30]. Two researchers, a technician and a trained acupuncturist (Dr Jiayou Wang), completed the acupuncture procedure in Taichong group and non-acupoint groups. The acupuncture procedure was performed on a heated table; and the technician and acupuncturist were seated across from one another. Each unanesthetized rat was placed headfirst into a homemade black restraint cone (similar to the pastry bags used by bakers) so that the anterior portion rats' body was firmly in the cone, while the posterior portion was exposed. A zip tie was used to secure the restraint cone around the rats' bodies, while the technician fixed the rats' hind legs in place. The acupuncturist then bi-laterally inserted the acupuncture needle 3 mm deep into the appropriate location. The needle was twisted 180 degrees at a rate of 80±5

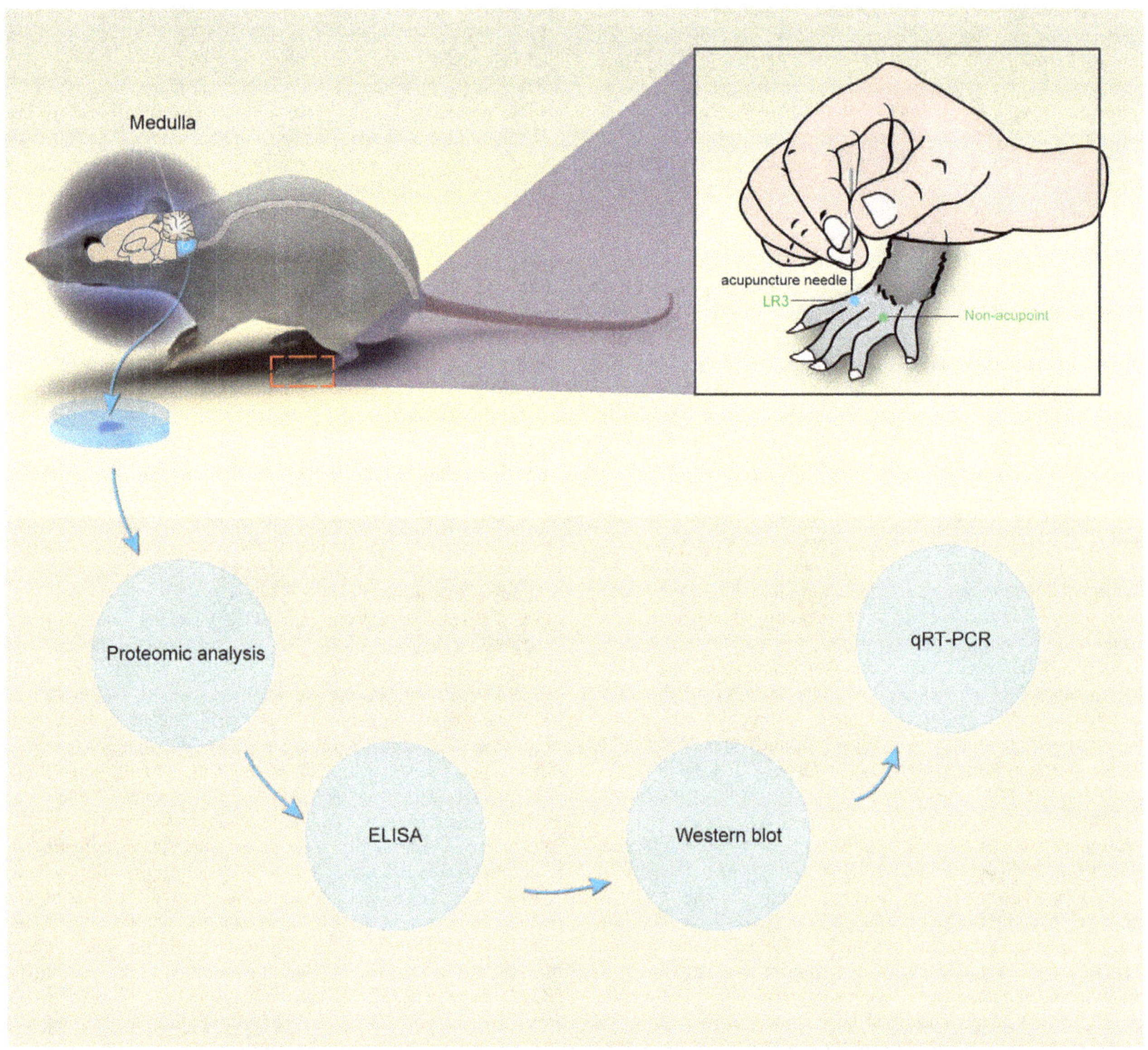

Figure 1. The Taichong (LR3) point and non-acupoint in hypertensive rats.

times per min. Acupuncture treatment was given daily (5 min per treatment) for 7 days. The acupuncture procedure was carried out with extremely gentle operation to avoid any unnecessary stimulus and stress to the rats.

Measurement of Blood Pressure

Blood pressure measurements were performed by two experienced technicians directly after acupuncture. SBP was measured non-invasively by the tailcuff method after at least a 5-min resting period using the BP-6A blood pressure measuring system from Chengdu TME Technology Co. Ltd (Chengdu, China). Immediately after acupuncture treatment, each rat was gently placed into restraint cones and their tails were fixed using the rat-tail fixing facility. The ventral portion of each rat was placed on the heat pad, while the BP measurement cuffs were put in place. Once a batch of 6 rats was in place, SBP was recorded by the pulse recording sensor facility following a 5-min warm-up period. Ten preliminary cycles (10×1.5 min) were performed to allow the rats to adapt to the rat-tail fixing facility. After the preliminary cycles, 5 cycles were recorded at each time point without intervention. To ensure accuracy and reproducibility, the rats were trained for 1 week prior to the experiment, and measurements were taken at the same time each day. During experiments, all animals were handled with extreme caution to minimize stress to the rats. Two BP-6A measuring systems were used so that blood pressure measurements could be done concurrently with acupuncture.

Tissue Preparation

The animals were anesthetized with an overdose of sodium phenobarbital (50 mg/kg body weight) by intraperitoneal injection on the 7th day after starting the acupuncture treatment and perfused intracardially with 50 ml physiological saline. The brain capsule was removed carefully and the medulla quickly dissected and collected. The medulla was preserved using liquid nitrogen until analysis. Twelve medullas (three medullas per group) were used to run the 2D gel assay. Each medulla was added in 700 ml buffer containing 7 mol/L urea, 2 mol/L thiourea, 2% CHAPS, 1% Triton X-100, 1% cocktail, and ultrasonicated for 5 sec three times. The mixture was centrifuged at 1,500 *g* for 10 min, and the supernatants were collected.

Two Dimensional (2D) Gel Running

A tube gel running system was used for first-dimensional running with 100 mmol/L sodium hydroxide, cathode buffer, 10 mmol/L phosphoric acid, and anode buffer. Pre-cast carrier ampholyte tube gels (pH 5–8, 11 cm) were prefocused with a maximum of 1,500 V and 110 μA per tube. The protein samples of 160 μg were loaded into the tube gels and focused for 17 hr and 30 min to reach 18,000 Vh.

The gels were extruded from the tubes after completion of focusing and were incubated in premixed Tris acetate equilibration buffer with 0.01% bromphenol blue and 50 mmol/L dithiothreitol for 2 min before loading onto pre-cast 50 mmol/L dithiothreitol for 2 min before loading onto pre-cast 10% homogeneous, 200×200 mm slab gels. The upper running buffer contained 0.2 mol/L Tris base and 0.2 mol/L Tricine. The system was run with a maximum of 500 V and 20,000 mW per gel.

The gel slabs were fixed in 10% methanol and 7% acetic acid for 30 min. The fixed solution was removed, and 500 ml of SYPRO® Ruby gel stain was added to each gel and incubated on a gently continuous rocker at room temperature for 16 hr.

Image Analysis

The gel images were obtained with Typhoon9200 scanner (GE Healthcare Co., Piscataway, NJ). Imagesaster 6.0 2D software was used for matching and quantitative analysis of the protein spots on the gels. The average gel was constructed as a representative gel for the three medulla samples taken from each group of rats. The average mode of background subtraction was used for normalization of intensity volume that represents protein concentration or amount on each spot. The average gel was then used for determination of the existence of difference of protein expression levels between each group.

Matrix Assisted Laser Desorption/ionization Time-of-flight (MALDI-TOF) and Data Analysis

Tryptic digests were analyzed using 2 separate instruments, an electrospray Q-TOF-2 mass spectrometer coupled with capillary high-performance liquid chromatography and MALDI Ultraflex TOF-TOF (Bruker Daltonics Inc., Fremont, CA). Protein identification from the tandem mass spectrometry (MS/MS) data was done by searching the National Center for Biotechnology Information nonredundant database with the GPS software, to search and identify proteins in the MASCOT database.

Quantitative Reverse Transcription-polymerase Chain Reaction (qRT-PCR)

Twenty four medullas (six medullas from each group) were used to run the qRT-PCR. The medulla was homogenized in 400 μL of TRIzol reagent (Invitrogen, Grand Island, NY). To avoid contamination with genomic DNA, the RNA samples were treated with RNase-free DNase (Promega, Madison, WI). Reverse transcription was performed using M-MLV reverse transcriptase (Promega, Madison, WI).

The 18srRNA gene (112 bp, F: 5′-CCTGGATACCGCAGCTAGGA; R: 5′-GCGGCGCAATACGAATGCCCC), synapsin I gene (160 bp, F: 5′-ATGGGCAAGGTCAAGGTAGA; R: 5′-ATGTCCTCATGTAGGCCTTGT) and myelin basic protein genes (152 bp, F: 5′-AACGCAGGGACGAAACTT; R: 5′-CCAAGAACAGTAGGTGCTTCT) were tested in this study. Real-time RT-PCRs were carried out using an ABI PRISM® 7500 Sequence Detection System (Applied Biosystems, Carlsbad, CA) and the SYBR Green PCR Master Mix kit (Toyobo Co. Ltd., Osaka, Japan). The expression of the target genes was assessed in relation to a housekeeping gene (18 srRNA) using the comparative (2-ΔΔCT) method in each sample. Fold differences against average values of SD rats were calculated.

Western Blotting Assay

Twelve medullas (three medullas from each group) were used to run the Western blotting assay. The medulla was homogenized in the lysis buffer (0.05 mol/L Tris-HCl at pH 7.4, 0.15 mol/L NaCl, 0.001 mol/L EDTA, 0.001 mol/L EGTA,1% Triton X-100, and 1% cocktail) using an ultrasound homogenizer at 50 Hz. The lysate was then centrifuged at 12, 000×*g* for 10 min. The protein concentration of the supernatant was measured with the Bradford protein assay. The supernatant was heated in the 5 × SDS sample buffer at 95°C for 10 min. An aliquot of 30 μg of the sample was loaded into a 10% polyacrylanide gel and separated at 120 V. Subsequently, proteins on the gel were transferred to PVDF membrane. The membrane was incubated with synapsin-1 antibody (1:1,000, Sigma-Aldrich, St Louis, MO), or myelin basic protein antibody (1:1,200, Sigma-Aldrich, St Louis, MO) overnight at 4°C, rinsed with TBST buffer, and then incubated with anti-rabbit IgG (1:5,000 Dako, Glostrup, Denmark) or anti-mouse IgG (1:4,000 Dako, Glostrup, Denmark) for 1 hr at room temperature. The immune complexes were detected by ECL and exposed to X-ray film.

Enzyme-linked Immunosorbent Assay (ELISA)

Twenty four (six medullas from each group) were used to carry out the ELISA. The medulla was ultrasonicated in PBS (pH7.4) and centrifuged at 1,000×*g* for 25 min; the supernatants were collected. The tissues were manipulated according to the instructions of the commercially available kits.

Statistical Analysis

Data analysis was conducted by either t test or one-way analysis of variance (ANOVA). Statistical significance was considered only when $P<0.05$.

Results

Effect of Acupuncture on Systolic Pressure in SHRs

Due to the acclimation period, the rats did not experience excess stress during the acupuncture treatment. Before acupuncture, the SBP of Taichong group, and the non-acupoint group and model group were insignificantly different ($P>0.05$), but significantly higher than the normal rats. On the 1st day after starting the acupuncture treatment, the SBP between the Taichong group, the non-acupoint group and model group were insignificantly different ($P>0.05$). On the 2nd day after acupuncture, compared with the model group and non-acupoint group, the SBP of Taichong group was significantly decreased ($P<0.01$, Figure 2). On the 3rd day after acupuncture, compared with Taichong group, the SBP of the non-acupoint group was significantly higher, suggesting that the acupuncture at non-acupoint may serve as a stimulus, resulting in a significantly increased SBP in rats. On the 4th day after acupuncture, the SBP among Taichong, non-acupoint and model groups were insignificantly different ($P>0.05$). On the 5th day of acupuncture, compared with non-acupoint, Taichong group's SBP reduced significantly ($P<0.01$). On the 6th

or 7th day after acupuncture, compared with the model group and non-acupoint group, Taichong group's SBP were significantly lower ($P<0.01$, Figure 2), suggesting acupuncture at Taichong points begin to stabilize the blood pressure since the 5th day after acupuncture. In the model, Taichong and non-acupoint groups, the SBP values were significantly higher than the normal group ($P<0.01$) over the experiment period, suggested that acupuncture at Taichong or non-acupoint were unable to reduce the systolic pressure to normal levels in this study.

The results of between-day comparison in each group are as follows: compared with the 1st day, the SBP of Taichong group decreased significantly on the 2nd day ($P<0.01$); but on the 3rd and 4th day, the SBP was increased again ($P>0.05$), and then began to decrease at the 5th day ($P<0.01$), until the 6th and 7th day, at which point the level of SBP remained stable ($P<0.01$, Figure 2), suggesting that acupuncture at Taichong point begin to stabilize the blood pressure level since the 5th day. Non-acupoint group's SBP were insignificantly altered in any time period ($P>0.05$). Compared with the 3rd day, the model rats' SBP was significantly increased on the 6th day ($P<0.01$); compared with the 4th day, model group's SBP was also significantly increased on the 6th day and the 7th days ($P<0.01$), suggesting that SBP of model group was rising. Rats in the normal group had stable and normal SBP over the experiment period ($P>0.05$).

Differential Protein Expression Profiles in Different Groups of Rats

The 2-DE image of rat medulla in each group is shown in Figure 3. In this study, 2-DE images revealed 571±15 proteins in normal SD rats' medulla, 576±31 proteins in SHR's medulla, 597±44 proteins in the medulla of SHRs after acupuncturing Taichong, and 616±18 proteins in the medulla of SHRs after acupuncturing non-acupoint (for Venn diagrams, see Figure 4). Compared with model group, 70±15 proteins were found differentially expressed in the medulla from Taichong group (expression ratio of protein was >2 folds, Table 1); 39±7 proteins were found differentially expressed in medulla oblongata from non-acupoint group (expression ratio of protein was >2 fold); and 59±12 proteins were found differentially expressed in medulla oblongata from normal group (expression ratio of protein was >2 fold). However, after artificial comparative analysis, it was found that there were only 23 protein spots all showing differential expression on 2-D gels among 4 groups.

Identification of Differentially Expressed Proteins in Different Groups of Rats

In this study, 23 protein spots were cut and proteins identified from 2D gel and MALDI-TOP MS (Figure 4). Among these spots, 22 proteins were identified by MALDI-TOP MS, with 14 of which being functional proteins and further analyzed (Table 2 & Table 3). The latter group of proteins included spots 69, 148, 273, 274, 306, 485, 497, 571, 603, 605–1, 605–2, 683, 739, and 754.

In the medulla of the Taichong group, compared with model group, six proteins were significantly down-regulated: synapsin-1, myelin basic protein (MBP), pyruvate kinase isozyme, protein kinase C inhibitor protein 1 (KCIP-1), electron transfer flavinprotein subunit-α (α-ETF), and NAD-dependent deacetylase sirtuin-2 (SIRT2). Six proteins were up-regulated: glutamate dehydrogenase 1 (GLUD1), ALDH2, GSTM5, superoxide dismutase (SOD), Rho GDP dissociation inhibitor 1 (ARHGDIA), and DJ-1 protein (Table 4).

In the medulla of non-acupoint group, compared with model group, only one protein was down-regulated: electron transfer flavoprotein; but three proteins were up-regulated: heat shock protein 90 (HSP90), ubiquitin hydrolase isozyme L1 (UCHL1) and DJ-1 protein (Table 4).

In the medulla of Taichong group, compared with non-acupoint group, seven proteins were down-regulated: HSP90, synapsin-1, pyruvate kinase isozyme, SIRT2, KCIP-1, UCHL1, and MBP. Six proteins were up-regulated: GLUD1, ALDH2, GSTM5, ARHGDIA, DJ-1 protein and SOD.

In the medulla of model group, compared with normal group, five proteins were down-regulated: GLUD1, GSTM5, ALDH2, UCHL1 and SOD. Seven proteins were up-regulated: HSP90, synapsin-1, pyruvate kinase isozymes, SIRT2, α-EFT, KCIP-1, and MBP (Table 4).

In the medulla of Taichong group, compared with normal group, two proteins were down-regulated: UCHL1 and MBP. Four proteins were up-regulated: HSP90, ARHGDIA, DJ-1 protein and SOD.

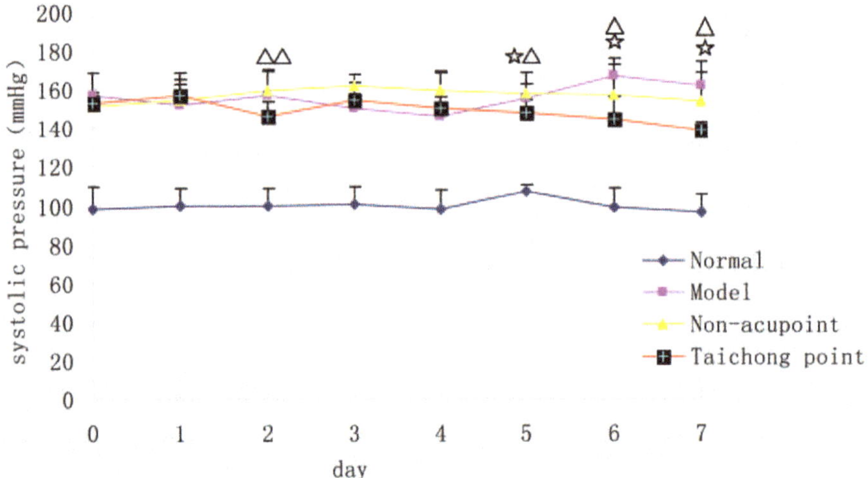

Figure 2. Effect of acupuncture on systolic pressure in 4 groups of rats. $^{\triangle\triangle}P<0.01$, the 1st vs. 2nd day in Taichong group; $^{☆\triangle}P<0.01$, Taichong group vs. non-acupoint, the 1st vs. 5th day in Taichong group; $^{\triangle}P<0.01$, Taichong group vs. model group, the 1st vs. 6th or 7th day in Taichong group; $^{☆}P<0.01$, the 4th vs. 6th or 7th day in model group.

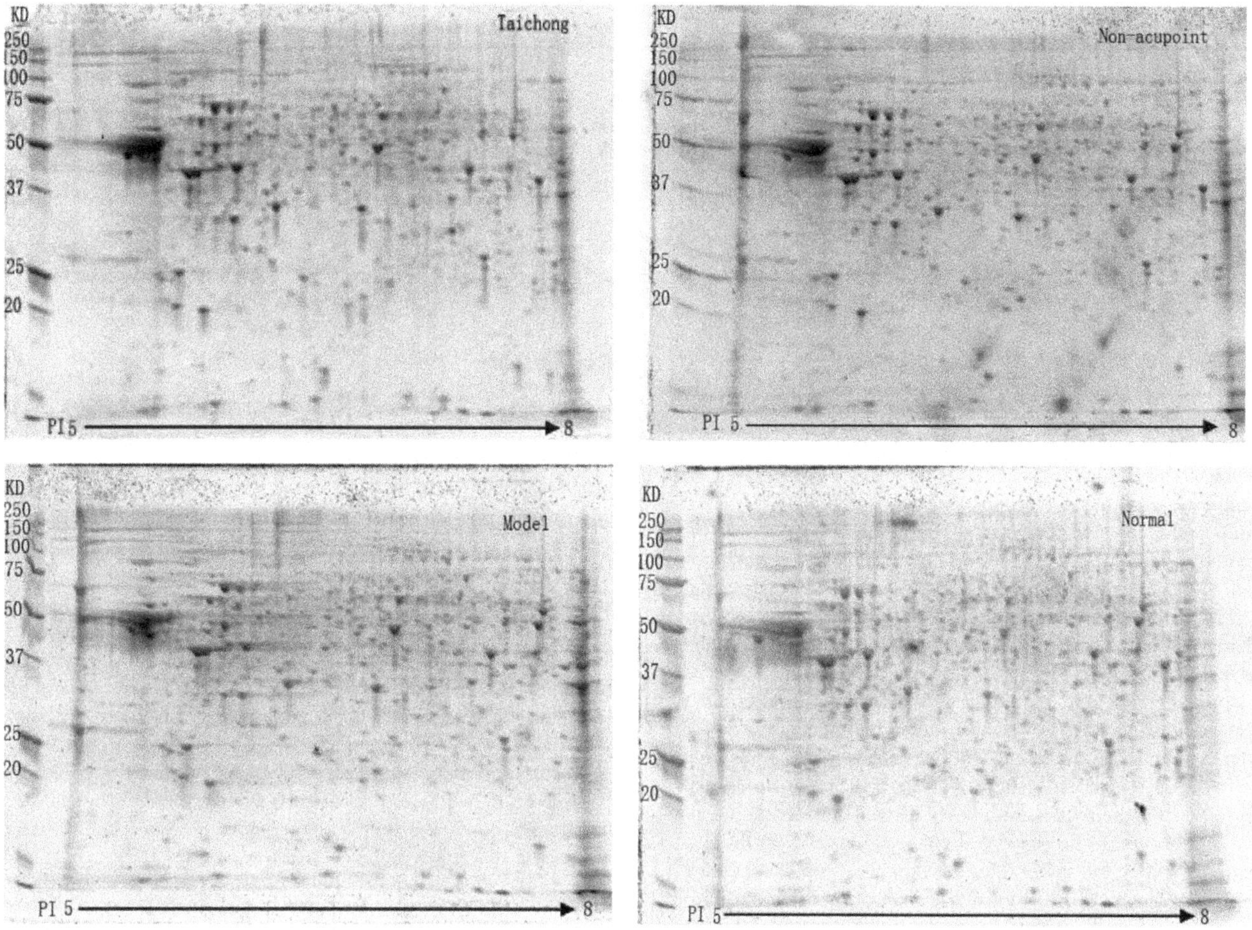

Figure 3. Protein profiles of rat medulla obtained over different pI ranges.

In the medulla of non-acupoint group, compared with the normal group, four proteins were down -regulated: GLUD1, ALDH2, GSTM5 and SOD; six proteins were up-regulated: HSP90, synapsin-1, SIRT2, KCIP-1, DJ-1 and MBP (Table 4).

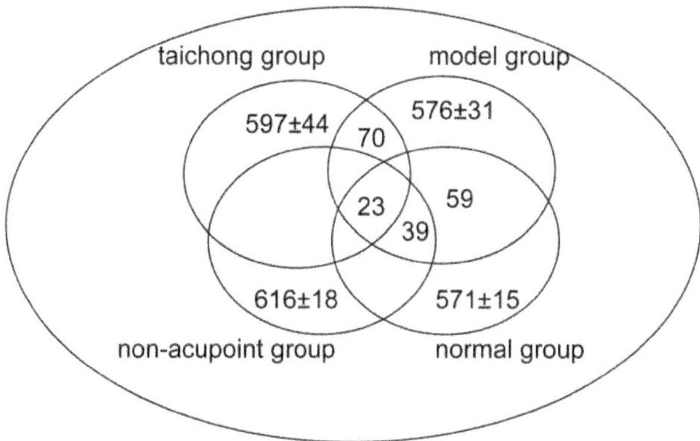

Figure 4. Venn diagrams. A, the differentially expressed protein spots by four groups; and B. the identified proteins by 2D gel ± MALDI-TOP MS/MS.

Data from qRT-PCR, ELISA and Western Blotting Assays

To further verify the reliability of the proteomic analysis, the expression of synapsin I and MBP at protein and mRNA levels were analyzed by Western blot and qRT-PCR, respectively. In addition, the GSTM5, ALDH2 and PKC levels in medullas were determined by ELISA.

Our Western blot analysis revealed that synapsin I was significantly increased in SHRs compared to age-matched normotensive SD rats, and remained unchanged after acupuncture treatment at non-acupoint but was down-regulated after acupuncture treatment at Taichong point (Figure 5). MBP was also significantly increased in 9-week-old SHRs compared to age-matched normotensive SD rats, and remained unchanged after acupuncture treatment at non-acupoint but was down-regulated after acupuncture treatment at Taichong point.

Our qRT-PCR assay revealed that synapsin I was up-regulated in 9-week-old SHRs compared to age-matched normotensive SD rats, and remained unchanged after acupuncture treatment at non-acupoint but were down-regulated after acupuncture treatment at Taichong point (Figure 6). The mRNA of MBP was down-regulated in SHRs compared to age-matched normotensive SD rats, and remained unchanged after acupuncture treatment at non-acupoint but were up-regulated after acupuncture treatment at Taichong point.

The results of synapsin I by Western blot and qRT-PCR assays were consistent with those from 2D gel analysis. Although

Table 1. Number of differentially expressed proteins compared to the model group.

Group	No. of protein spots identified by image 2D software (between 2 groups)	No. of protein spots identified by artificial comparative analysis (among 4 groups)	No. of proteins identified by MALDI-TOP MS/MS
Normal	59±12	23	22
Taichong	70±15	23	22
Non-acupoint	39±7	23	22

the results of MBP by Western blot assay were consistent with those by 2-D gel analysis, but were opposite to those from qRT-PCR.

Our ELISA results of GSTM5 and ALDH2 are consistent with the results of 2D gel (Figure 7). In the medulla of model group, compared with normal group, the expression of GSTM5 was significantly down-regulated ($P<0.01$). After acupuncture treatment, the expression of GSTM5 in the medulla of Taichong group were significantly up-regulated ($P<0.01$); but the expression of GSTM5 in the medulla of non-acupoint group has no significant change compared to the model group ($P>0.01$), but lower than the normal group ($P<0.01$).

In the medulla model group, compared with normal group, the expression of ALDH2 was significantly down-regulated ($P<0.01$). After acupuncture treatment, the expression of ALDH2 in the medulla of Taichong group were significantly up-regulated ($P<0.01$), but the expression of ALDH2 in the medulla of non-acupoint group has no significant change compared to the model group ($P>0.01$), but lower than the normal group ($P<0.01$).

The expression of PKC in the medulla of model group has no significant change compared to the normal group ($P>0.01$). After acupuncture treatment, the expression of PKC in the medulla of Taichong group was the lowest compared to the model, normal, and non-acupoint group, but did not achieve statistical significance ($P>0.01$) (data not shown).

Discussion

Although there has been some discordance as to the efficacy of acupuncture in hypertension [13,15,31], our results indicate that acupuncture at the Taichong (LR3) acupoint does alleviate high blood pressure due to essential hypertension, though this treatment alone is not able to bring blood pressure down to normal levels. When discussing the efficacy of acupuncture as a treatment for hypertension, it is important to distinguish between the short-term and long-term effect of acupuncture on hypertension. Our study, like most others, reports the short-term effect of acupuncture (directly following treatment) on blood pressure. Due to the proteomic nature of our study and the necessary euthanasia of the rats, the long-term effect of acupuncture on blood pressure regrettably could not be studied.

There are remarkable gender differences in many physiological parameters in health and disease. To avoid the interfering effect of female sex hormones on blood pressure, we have chosen male animals in this study. Studies have revealed sex hormones play a role in the regulation of blood pressure and development of hypertension [32]. The prevalence of hypertension is predicted to increase more among women than men. When rats were fed with an 8% NaCl diet, female rats became less hypertensive than male rats [32], which suggests that female sex hormones protect against the development of hypertension.

As stabilization of blood pressure in the Taichong group takes 5 days, the lag time between acupuncture treatment and stabiliza-

Table 2. Differentially expressed proteins among 4 groups of rats.

Spot num.	Swiss-Prot Accession NO.	Protein name	Protein Score C.I.%/ Total Ion Score C.I.%	Sequence Coverage %	Major function
1	IPI00231023	Synapsin-1	100/100	28	Adjust release of neurotransmitters
2	IPI00607210	MBP	100/100	90	Form medulla sheath
3	IPI00324893	KCIP-1	100/100	55	Signal transduction
4	IPI00205332	α-ETF	100/100	51	Regulate oxidative stress
5	IPI00562798	SIRT2	100/100	31	Oxidative phosphorylation
6	IPI00324633	GLUD1	100/100	44	Amino acid oxidation; chaperones
7	IPI00197770	ALDH2	100/100	31	Regulate oxidizing reaction
8	IPI00208636	GSTM5	100/100	31	Anti-oxidative stress
9	IPI00231643	SOD	100/100	52	Anti-oxidative stress
10	IPI00196994	ARHGDIA	100/100	56	Revascularization
11	IPI00212523	DJ-1	100/100	56	Oxidative stress
12	IPI00210566	HSP90-α	100/100	34	Amino acid oxidation; chaperones
13	IPI00231929	Pyruvate kinase isozyme	100/100	40	Protein catabolism
14	IPI00204375	UCHL1	100/100	51	Protein catabolism

Table 3. The expression of protein spots in the medulla of four different groups of rats.

Spot	Protein	% Volume (mean ± SD)			
		Model	Taichong point	Non-acupoint	Normal
1	Synapsin-1	0.574±0.004*	0.119±0.007#	0.673±0.006	0.179±0.003■
2	MBP	1.24±0.036*	0.119±0.033#▼	1.32±0.033	0.683±0.127■
3	KCIP-1	0.747±0.038*	0.148±0.012#	0.665±0.059	0.116±0.001■
4	α-ETF	0.044±0.005*	0.014±0.004	0.014±0.004▲	0.023±0.005
5	SIRT2	0.275±0.011*	0.086±0.011#	0.27±0.021	0.09±0.001■
6	GLUD1	0.021±0.001*	0.037±0.004#	0.022±0.002	0.039±0.001■
7	ALDH2	0.08±0.007*	0.180±0.005#	0.084±0.006	0.187±0.006■
8	GSTM5	0.109±0.011*	0.155±0.003#	0.107±0.018	0.147±0.008■
9	SOD	0.074±0.012*	0.223±0.017#▼	0.077±0.008	0.169±0.006■
10	ARHGDIA	0.122±0.005*	0.242±0.025#▼	0.025±0.004	0.024±0.02
11	DJ-1	0.046±0.004	0.283±0.031#▼	0.124±0.029▲	0.031±0.009■
12	HSP90-α	0.571±0.056	0.637±0.046▼	0.776±0.051▲	0.226±0.019■
13	Pyruvate kinase isozyme	0.185±0.029*	0.067±0.017#	0.145±0.045	0.076±0.019
14	UCHL1	0.148±0.007	0.156±0.006#▼	0.37±0.051▲	0.354±0.019

*$P<0.01$, model group vs. Taichong point group or normal group;
#$P<0.01$, Taichong group vs. non-acupoint group;
▼$P<0.01$, Taichong group vs. normal group;
▲$P<0.01$, non-acupoint group vs. model group; and ■$P<0.01$, non-acupoint group vs. normal group.

Table 4. Relative protein expression among four different groups of rats.

Protein	Up/Down-regulation			
	Model vs. Normal	Taichong vs. Model	Taichong vs. Non-Acupoint	Non-Acupoint vs. Model
Oxidative Stress				
α-EFT	↑	↓	T	↓
HSP90-α	↑	T	↓	↑
SOD	↓	↑	↑	T
DJ-1	T	↑	↑	↑
GSTM5	↓	↑	↑	T
ALDH2	↓	↑	↑	T
GLUD1	↓	↑	↑	T
Neurotransmitter Release				
Synapsin-1	↑	↓	↓	T
Revascularization				
ARHGDIA	T	↑	↑	T
Protein Catabolism				
Pyruvate kinase isozyme	↑	↓	↓	T
UCHL1	↓	T	↓	↑
Oxidative Phosphorylation				
SIRT2	↑	↓	↓	T
Medullary Sheath				
MBP	↑	↓	↓	T
Signal Transduction				
KCIP-1	↑	↓	↓	T

↑: up-regulated; ↓: down-regulated; T: unchanged.

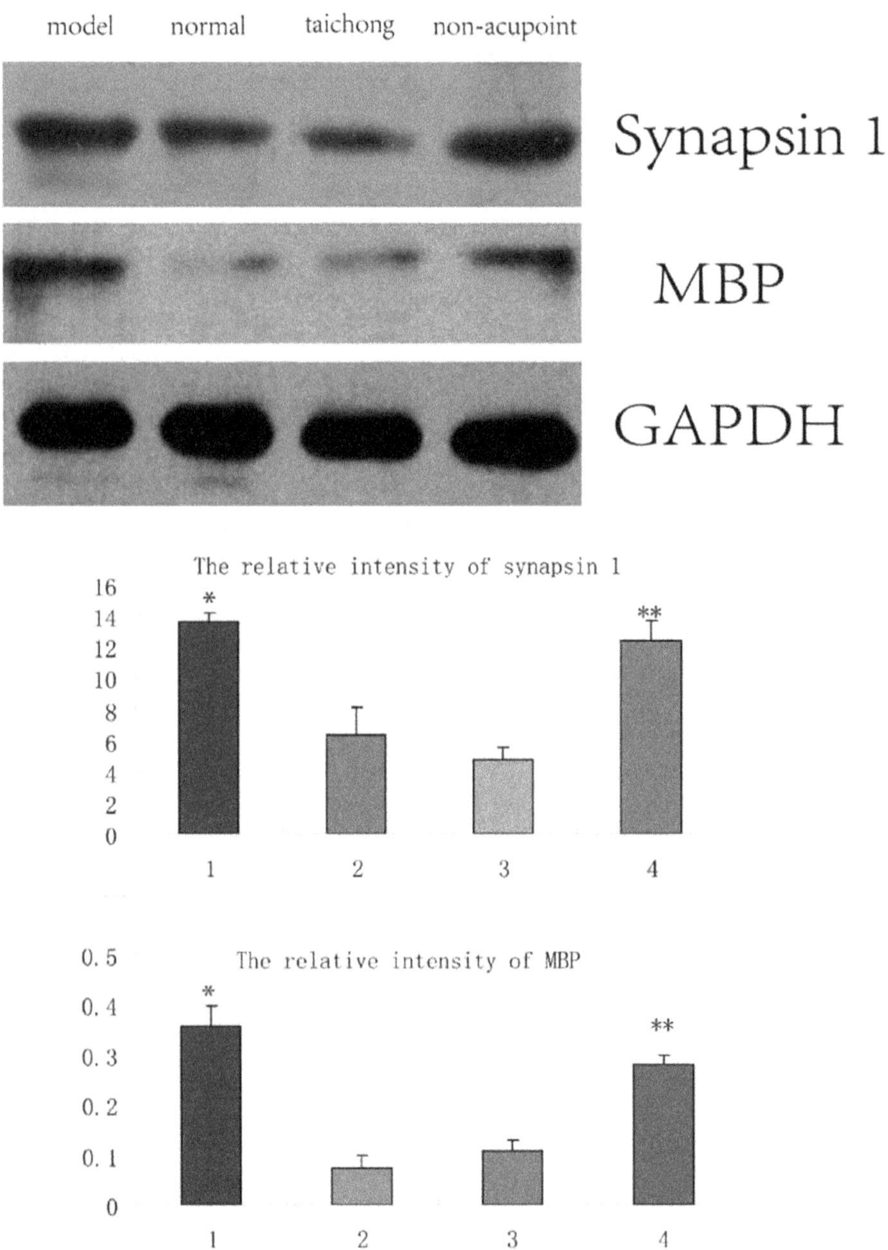

Figure 5. Blots of Western blot assays for synapsin-1 and myelin basic protein (MBP) in the medulla of SHRs. $^{*}P<0.05$; $^{**}P<0.01$.

tion of blood pressure suggests activation of specific metabolic pathways, causing changes at the protein expression level that contribute to the alteration at the cellular level. Changes at the cellular level eventually induce reduction in blood pressure at the systemic level. Analysis of the effects of acupuncture at the Taichong point in SHRs reveals a complex scenario of dramatic changes in abundance of various cellular proteins. Analysis of the fourteen statistically significant differentially proteins between the groups provided insights into the potential mechanisms through which acupuncture may reduce hypertension. As acupuncture is a general treatment with "pleiotropic" responses, the simultaneous activation of multiple therapeutic mechanisms is expected. The results are in accordance with our belief that multiple mechanisms play a role in alleviation of hypertension. Due to the complexity and underlying discord relating to the pathogenic factors associated with essential hypertension, this discussion will address the major changes in the proteomic/peptidomic analysis and how they may tie in with the incomplete reversal of hypertension pathogenesis in SHRs. The potential mechanisms involved include: reduction of oxidative stress, sympathetic modulation via synapsin-1, as well as NO level modulation.

As shown in Table 2 & Figure 3, protein expression in the model SHR rats is significantly different from those of normal (non-SHR) rats. The proteomic response that contributes to the SHR phenotype and reduction of hypertension in Taichong-needled rats includes the modulation of seven proteins related to oxidative stress, including SOD, ALDH2, GSTM5, GLUD1, protein DJ-1, HSP90α, and α-ETF. Many studies have reported the involvement of oxidative stress in hypertension, but questions have been raised as to whether oxidative stress causes hyperten-

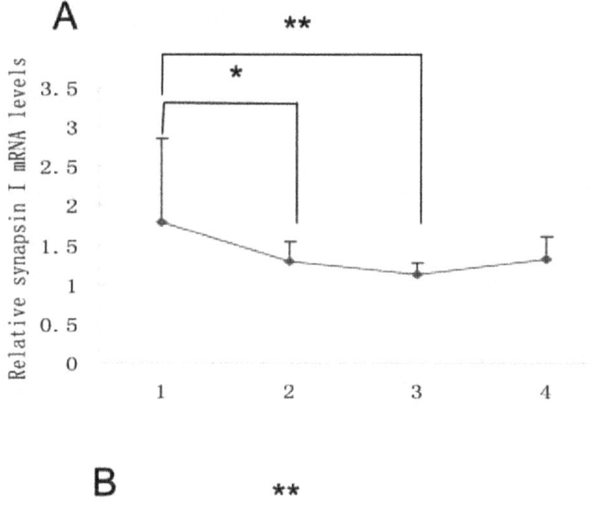

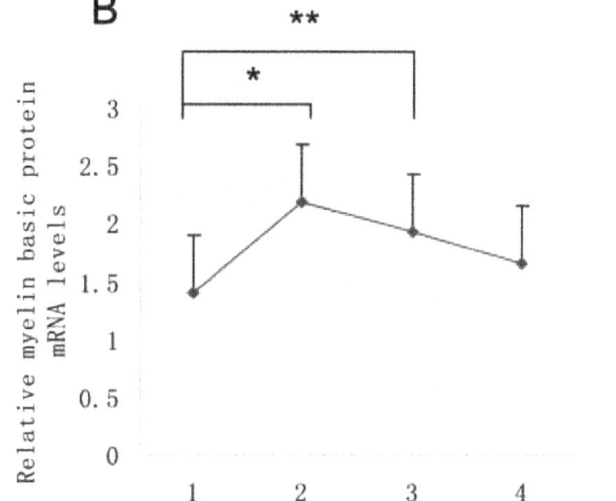

Figure 6. Blots of qRT-PCR assays for the mRNA levels of synapsin-1 and myelin basic protein (MBP) genes in the medulla of SHRs. Lane 1, model group; lane 2, normal group; lane 3, Taichong group; and lane 4, non-acupoint group. $^{*}P<0.05$; $^{**}P<0.01$.

sion, or if hypertension causes oxidative stress: a "chicken or egg" scenario. Oxidative stress results in the formation of reactive oxygen species (ROS), which are present in low levels in normal cells and functions and play an important role in vascular biology in regards to cell signaling and vascular contraction-relaxation. Delano et al. and other authors [33,34,35,36] reported that oxidative stress might be a more global condition not only confined to vascular tissues, and more recently a number of reports have been published relating to the modulatory effect of ROS on hypertension in the brain.

Of these proteins, SOD, ALDH2, GSTM5, DJ-1 and GLUD1 were up-regulated, while electron α-ETF and HSP90α are down-regulated with Taichong treatment when compared to the model SHR rats. SOD, a protein involved in the dismutation of the superoxide anion into oxygen and hydrogen peroxide, is an important antioxidant defense in most cells. GSTM5 is involved in the conjugation of reduced glutathione to a wide number of exogenous and endogenous hydrophobic electrophiles, resulting in the detoxification of many oxidative stress proteins. GLUD1, primarily a mitochondrial matric enzyme, is involved in oxidative deamination and ammonia detoxification. ALDH2, another mitochondrial protein, functions to catalyze the oxidation of aldehydes and is also necessary for the bioactivation of organic nitrates, which are molecules with high vasodilator potency. The DJ-1 protein protects against oxidative stress and hydrogen peroxide based cell death, especially in neurons. HSP90α is a heat shock protein that promotes structural maintenance cell cycle control, and signal transduction, especially during stressful conditions; while α-ETF is a mitochondrial matrix protein that functions as a primary electron acceptor for primary dehydrogenase.

While the proteomic response of oxidative stress proteins demonstrates a complex, interweaved modulation, the predominant up-regulation of enzymes involved in ROS removal suggest an overall decrease in oxidative stress levels intracellularly due to acupuncture. The two oxidative stress related proteins down-regulated in response to acupuncture, HSP90α and α-ETF, play a major role when stressful conditions present, so reduction of oxidative stress should result in the down-regulation of these proteins. Furthermore, many other studies have linked acupuncture with a reduction in oxidative stress [37,38]. ROS have many effects intracellularly as they function in signal transduction. This is the first report to implicate oxidative stress reduction as a possible mechanism of the therapeutic effect of acupuncture in hypertension. Acupuncture at the Taichong point changes the protein expression such that it reverses the changes seen in the proteomics analysis of SHR model compared to the normal rat, moving SHR rats back towards a normal protein expression as it related to hypertension. Additionally, it is interesting to note that multiple mitochondrial proteins have modulated protein levels after acupuncture treatment; additional research must be done to determine if mitochondrial function is in any way linked to the alleviation of hypertension due to acupuncture.

An up-regulation of oxidative stress enzymes and a decrease of oxidative stress may have multiple effects through which blood pressure is modulated. An increase in ROS in the rostral ventrolateral medulla (RVLM) contributes to the neural pathogenesis of hypertension [39]. In the RVLM, Nox-induced ROS initiate a forward loop in cross-activation of different receptors and between Nox and mitochondrial ROS [40]. Thus, a decrease in ROS due to acupuncture may oppose this pathogenic mechanism of hypertension. Additionally, the caudal ventrolateral medulla (CVLM) provides inhibitory input to the RVLM of the brain. A lack of these inhibitory inputs is believed to in part play a role in the neuropathogenesis of hypertension [41]. The increase in oxidative stress seen in hypertension could affect the frequency of these inhibitory inputs, thus the reduction of oxidative stress seen in acupuncture may provide a mechanism through with CVLM inhibitory input to the RVLM is augmented. In addition, paraventricular nucleus (PVN) of the hypothalamus plays a major role in autonomic and neuroendocrine regulation of blood pressure and body fluid homeostasis [42]. Functional studies have demonstrated the involvement of PVN in the control of fluid electrolyte homeostasis, feeding behavior, cardiovascular regulation, and stress adaptation [42]. It is unclear whether acupuncture affects the regulatory function of these regions through modulation of ROS.

It is technically difficult to oblate specific nuclei from the rat medulla and to collect enough samples for our proteomic and biochemical analysis. Since multiple regions/nuclei of the medulla are involved in blood pressure regulation, we collected the whole medulla for our study. To examine whether the proteins located in specific nuclei of the medulla are related to blood pressure modification by acupuncture, we have conducted a preliminary immunohistochemical study and shown altered MBP and synapsin I expression in some specific regions (e.g. NTS and RVLM) of SHR medulla (data not shown). Further studies are ongoing to

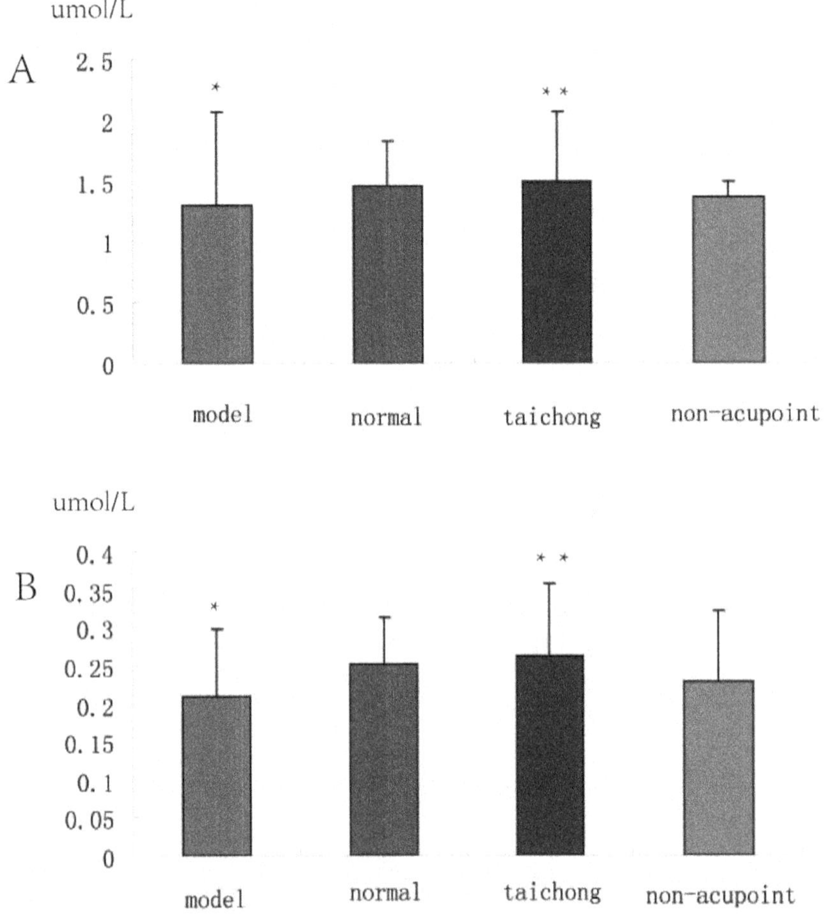

Figure 7. Content of glutathione *S*-transferase M5 and aldehyde dehydrogenase 2 in rat medulla by ELISA.

investigate which nuclei and what types of neurons and glial cells are involved in the proteomic responses to acupuncture in SHRs.

We would like to state that this study does not provide direct evidence for the involvement of oxidative stress reduction in hypertension. Our results show a strong correlation between acupuncture treatments, upregulation of antioxidant enzymes, and reduction of hypertension. In the future, our laboratory will conduct long term studies to generate direct evidence of this involvement.

ALDH2, an enzyme involved in the activation of NO compounds, plays a role in the bioactivation of multiple drugs used for heart failure, such as glyceryl trinitrate and pentaerythritol tetranitrate. Although acupuncture does not directly lower blood pressure to normal level in SHRs, the resulting up-regulation of ALDH2 suggests that it could be used as a complementary treatment to modern medicine to increase the efficacy of certain nitric oxide based drugs. Additionally, hypertension has been shown to result in decreases of endothelial and neuronal nitric oxide synthase (eNOS & nNOS), while acupuncture has been shown to stop the reduction of nNOS and eNOS in SHRs [43,44,45]. The increased levels of nNOS as a result of hypertension directly affect NO levels, which is a potent vasodilator, further supporting our hypothesis that acupuncture modulates hypertension through multiple, simultaneously acting pathways.

The synapsins are a family of phosphoproteins present in neurotransmitter vesicles that are essential to normal neurotransmitter release at the synaptic cleft. Studies have shown that double knockout (synapsin-1 and synapsin-2) mice have a lower basal blood pressure than normal mice, and additional studies from the same group showed that the same double knockout mice did not respond with progressive hypertension to treatment with cyclosporine A as is normally seen in mice, indicating that the synapsins play an integral role in control of blood pressure [46]. As shown from our proteomic panel, synapsin-1 is significantly down-regulated in the Taichong group when compared to the model group. Down-regulation of synapsin could be another parallel avenue through which acupuncture helps control hypertension in SHRs.

Currently, there are no globally accepted biomarkers that readily differentiate between acupuncture at acupoints and acupuncture at a sham location. One of the biggest issues facing acupuncture research is the lack of a reliable method to determine if acupuncture was properly administered. Identification of reliable biomarker(s) for acupuncture would be a powerful tool for researchers to validate the efficacy of acupuncture treatments and optimize acupuncture regimen. Although the modulation of the medullar levels of oxidative stress enzymes cannot be used as a clinical biomarker for acupuncture, it may be useful for validation of acupuncture in animal studies. Adaptation of these changes in specific protein levels in the plasma, urine, or other easily accessible samples, is the next step in development and validation of these alterations as potential biomarkers for acupuncture. Other reports [37,38] have corroborated our results on a much smaller scale, showing acupuncture does in fact up-regulate SOD and glutamate dehydrogenase, however, our complete proteomic expression panel is a more useful and accurate measure of successful acupuncture as the proteomic response is available for more proteins.

In this study, the Western blot analysis revealed that the expression of synapsin I remained unchanged after acupuncture treatment at non-acupoint but was down-regulated after acupuncture treatment at Taichong point (see Figure 5). In contrast, MBP remained unchanged after acupuncture treatment at non-acupoint but was up-regulated after acupuncture treatment at Taichong point. Western blot analysis can provide useful semi-quantitative data on protein expression. However, this commonly used assay can easily generate inconsistence of protein expression data given that most proteins are subject to degradation and modification by a number of factors.

In this study, we have observed some inconsistent expression data of individual proteins/genes when distinct techniques/assays are used. For example, although the results of MBP by Western blot assay were consistent with those by qRT-PCR, but were opposite to those from the 2-D gel analysis. Unlike Western blot and 2D gel assays, RT-PCR assays can generate quantitative data of gene expression at mRNA levels. Theoretically, the expression data of a specific gene at both protein and mRNA levels should be consistent. However, these data may be inconsistent due to the following reasons: a) mRNA is unstable and fragile; b) mRNA can be modified and thus its translation into the protein can be altered; and c) transcription and translation are regulated by a number of epigenetic and genetic factors and these two processes can be uncoupled under some conditions.

The clinical implication of our current study is unclear but may implicate the potential use of antioxidants in hypertension management. Potential sources of excessive ROS in hypertension include nicotinamide adenine dinucleotide phosphate (NADPH) oxidase, mitochondria, cyclooxygenase 1 and 2, cytochrome P450 epoxygenase, xanthine oxidase, endothelium-derived NO synthase, and transition metals [47]. A number of epidemiological and clinical data suggests that antioxidant-rich diets or natural antioxidants reduce blood pressure and cardiovascular risk [48,49], and animal studies have also shown the antihypertensive activity of antioxidants [50,51]. However, the majority of randomized clinical studies using natural antioxidants including include vitamins A, C and E, L-arginine, flavanoids, and mitochondria-targeted agents (coenzyme Q10, acetyl-L-carnitine, and α-lipoic acid have given disappointing or conflicting results [47]. Further mechanistic studies are needed to elucidate the role of ROS in the pathogenesis of hypertension and if proper use of antioxidants in combination of conventional antihypertensive agents benefits hypertensive patients.

Our current study focused on the "acute" effect over 1 week and identification of proteomic responses for the short-term effect of acupuncture on hypertension. From that point of view, we thought it to be less important to measure SBP before acupuncture each day, and focus more on the proteomic responses through which changes occur. We knew that to study the proteomic response to acupuncture, the rats would be sacrificed shortly after the experiment. Thus, it would be difficult to completely study the long term (e.g. >1 month) effect and sustainability of acupuncture on hypertension. In the future, we would be interested in performing studies to unfold the long-term effect of acupuncture on hypertension.

In conclusion, this study is the first to report the complete protein expression profile of acupuncture on SHRs, and has shown the potential involvement of oxidative stress as a partial mechanism in reduction of blood pressure by acupuncture therapy. Further studies are warranted to investigate the role of oxidative stress modulation by acupuncture in the treatment of hypertension.

Author Contributions

Conceived and designed the experiments: XL JW NRN BS KBS SFZ JY. Performed the experiments: JW SP CT YH MH ZY CM Jin Zhang ZH. Analyzed the data: XL NRN CM HC JL Jian Zhang. Contributed reagents/materials/analysis tools: JW XL CM SFZ. Wrote the paper: NRN SFZ.

References

1. Bertoia ML, Waring ME, Gupta PS, Roberts MB, Eaton CB (2011) Implications of new hypertension guidelines in the United States. Hypertension 58: 361–366.
2. Chobanian AV, Bakris GL, Black HR, Cushman WC, Green LA, et al. (2003) Seventh report of the Joint National Committee on Prevention, Detection, Evaluation, and Treatment of High Blood Pressure. Hypertension 42: 1206–1252.
3. Kearney PM, Whelton M, Reynolds K, Muntner P, Whelton PK, et al. (2005) Global burden of hypertension: analysis of worldwide data. Lancet 365: 217–223.
4. Roger VL, Go AS, Lloyd-Jones DM, Benjamin EJ, Berry JD, et al. (2012) Heart disease and stroke statistics - 2012 Update: a report from the American Heart Association. Circulation 125: e2–e220.
5. Lloyd-Jones D, Adams RJ, Brown TM, Carnethon M, Dai S, et al. (2010) Heart disease and stroke statistics - 2010 update: a report from the American Heart Association. Circulation 121: e46–e215.
6. Heidenreich PA, Trogdon JG, Khavjou OA, Butler J, Dracup K, et al. (2011) Forecasting the future of cardiovascular disease in the United States: a policy statement from the American Heart Association. Circulation 123: 933–944.
7. Kim LW, Zhu J (2010) Acupuncture for essential hypertension. Altern Ther Health Med 16: 18–29.
8. Kaplan NM (2006) Acupuncture for hypertension: can 2500 years come to an end? Hypertension 48: 815.
9. Burke A, Upchurch DM, Dye C, Chyu L (2006) Acupuncture use in the United States: findings from the National Health Interview Survey. J Altern Complement Med 12: 639–648.
10. Cantwell SL (2010) Traditional Chinese veterinary medicine: the mechanism and management of acupuncture for chronic pain. Top Companion Anim Med 25: 53–58.
11. Yin C, Seo B, Park HJ, Cho M, Jung W, et al. (2007) Acupuncture, a promising adjunctive therapy for essential hypertension: a double-blind, randomized, controlled trial. Neurol Res 29 Suppl 1: S98–103.
12. Park JM, Shin AS, Park SU, Sohn IS, Jung WS, et al. (2010) The acute effect of acupuncture on endothelial dysfunction in patients with hypertension: a pilot, randomized, double-blind, placebo-controlled crossover trial. J Altern Complement Med 16: 883–888.
13. Sugioka K, Mao W, Woods J, Mueller RA (1977) An unsuccessful attempt to treat hypertension with acupuncture. Am J Chin Med (Gard City N Y) 5: 39–44.
14. Kalish LA, Buczynski B, Connell P, Gemmel A, Goertz C, et al. (2004) Stop Hypertension with the Acupuncture Research Program (SHARP): clinical trial design and screening results. Control Clin Trials 25: 76–103.
15. Huang H, Liang S (1992) Acupuncture at otoacupoint heart for treatment of vascular hypertension. J Tradit Chin Med 12: 133–136.
16. Chiu YJ, Chi A, Reid IA (1997) Cardiovascular and endocrine effects of acupuncture in hypertensive patients. Clin Exp Hypertens 19: 1047–1063.
17. Akhmedov TI, Vasil'ev Iu M, Masliaeva LV (1993) [The hemodynamic and neurohumoral correlates of the changes in the status of hypertension patients under the influence of acupuncture]. Ter Arkh 65: 22–24.
18. Anshelevich Iu V, Merson MA, Afanas'eva GA (1985) [Serum aldosterone level in patients with hypertension during treatment by acupuncture]. Ter Arkh 57: 42–45.
19. Yao T (1993) Acupuncture and somatic nerve stimulation: mechanism underlying effects on cardiovascular and renal activities. Scand J Rehabil Med Suppl 29: 7–18.
20. Li P, Sun FY, Zhang AZ (1983) The effect of acupuncture on blood pressure: the interrelation of sympathetic activity and endogenous opioid peptides. Acupunct Electrother Res 8: 45–56.
21. Zhou Y, Wang Y, Fang Z, Xia C, Liu B, et al. (1995) [Influence of acupuncture on blood pressure, contents of NE, DA and 5-HT of SHR and the interrelation between blood pressure and whole blood viscosity]. Zhen Ci Yan Jiu 20: 55–61.
22. Bobkova AS, Gaponiuk P, Korovkina EG, Sherkovina T, Leonova MV (1991) [The effect of acupuncture on endocrine regulation in hypertensive patients]. Vopr Kurortol Fizioter Lech Fiz Kult: 29–32.

23. Zhang Y, Meng X, Li A, Xin J, Berman BM, et al. (2011) Acupuncture alleviates the affective dimension of pain in a rat model of inflammatory hyperalgesia. Neurochem Res 36: 2104–2110.
24. Meng X, Zhang Y, Li A, Xin J, Lao L, et al. (2011) The effects of opioid receptor antagonists on electroacupuncture-produced anti-allodynia/hyperalgesia in rats with paclitaxel-evoked peripheral neuropathy. Brain Res 1414: 58–65.
25. Fei W, Tian de R, Tso P, Han JS (2011) Arcuate nucleus of hypothalamus is involved in mediating the satiety effect of electroacupuncture in obese rats. Peptides 32: 2394–2399.
26. Benter IF, Yousif MH, Al-Saleh FM, Raghupathy R, Chappell MC, et al. (2011) Angiotensin-(1–7) blockade attenuates captopril- or hydralazine-induced cardiovascular protection in spontaneously hypertensive rats treated with NG-nitro-L-arginine methyl ester. J Cardiovasc Pharmacol 57: 559–567.
27. Christe ME, Rodgers RL (1994) Altered glucose and fatty acid oxidation in hearts of the spontaneously hypertensive rat. J Mol Cell Cardiol 26: 1371–1375.
28. Friedemann T, Shen X, Bereiter-Hahn J, Schwarz W (2011) Regulation of the cardiovascular function by CO(2) laser stimulation in anesthetized rats. Lasers Med Sci.
29. Huang XK, Zhuo LS, Ren LY, Liu QY, Zhu Y (2008) [Effect of electroacupuncture of "Hegu" (LI 4)-"Taichong" (LR 3) on colonic nitric oxide synthase and glutathione peroxidase activity and nitric oxide content in depression rats]. Zhen Ci Yan Jiu 33: 183–185.
30. Duan DM, Tu Y, Chen LP (2008) [Effects of electroacupuncture at different acupoint groups on behavior activity and p-CREB expression in hippocampus in the rat of depression]. Zhongguo Zhen Jiu 28: 369–373.
31. Macklin EA, Wayne PM, Kalish LA, Valaskatgis P, Thompson J, et al. (2006) Stop Hypertension with the Acupuncture Research Program (SHARP): results of a randomized, controlled clinical trial. Hypertension. United States. 838–845.
32. Pimenta E (2012) Hypertension in women. Hypertens Res 35: 148–152.
33. Paravicini TM, Touyz RM (2008) NADPH oxidases, reactive oxygen species, and hypertension: clinical implications and therapeutic possibilities. Diabetes Care. United States. S170–180.
34. Peterson JR, Sharma RV, Davisson RL (2006) Reactive oxygen species in the neuropathogenesis of hypertension. Curr Hypertens Rep 8: 232–241.
35. Harrison DG, Gongora MC (2009) Oxidative stress and hypertension. Med Clin North Am. United States. 621–635.
36. DeLano FA, Balete R, Schmid-Schonbein GW (2005) Control of oxidative stress in microcirculation of spontaneously hypertensive rats. Am J Physiol Heart Circ Physiol. United States. H805–812.
37. Liu CZ, Yu JC, Zhang XZ, Fu WW, Wang T, et al. (2006) Acupuncture prevents cognitive deficits and oxidative stress in cerebral multi-infarction rats. Neurosci Lett. Ireland. 45–50.
38. Yu YP, Ju WP, Li ZG, Wang DZ, Wang YC, et al. (2010) Acupuncture inhibits oxidative stress and rotational behavior in 6-hydroxydopamine lesioned rat. Brain Res. Netherlands: 2010 Elsevier B.V. 58–65.
39. Kishi T, Hirooka Y, Kimura Y, Ito K, Shimokawa H, et al. (2004) Increased reactive oxygen species in rostral ventrolateral medulla contribute to neural mechanisms of hypertension in stroke-prone spontaneously hypertensive rats. Circulation. United States. 2357–2362.
40. Datla SR, Griendling KK (2010) Reactive oxygen species, NADPH oxidases, and hypertension. Hypertension. United States. 325–330.
41. Colombari E, Sato MA, Cravo SL, Bergamaschi CT, Campos RR, Jr., et al. (2001) Role of the medulla oblongata in hypertension. Hypertension 38: 549–554.
42. Stocker SD, Osborn JL, Carmichael SP (2008) Forebrain osmotic regulation of the sympathetic nervous system. Clin Exp Pharmacol Physiol 35: 695–700.
43. Kim DD, Pica AM, Duran RG, Duran WN (2006) Acupuncture reduces experimental renovascular hypertension through mechanisms involving nitric oxide synthases. Microcirculation 13: 577–585.
44. Hwang HS, Kim YS, Ryu YH, Lee JE, Lee YS, et al. (2008) Electroacupuncture delays hypertension development through enhancing NO/NOS activity in spontaneously hypertensive rats. Evid Based Complement Alternat Med 2011: 1–7.
45. Huang YL, Fan MX, Wang J, Li L, Lu N, et al. (2005) Effects of acupuncture on nNOS and iNOS expression in the rostral ventrolateral medulla of stress-induced hypertensive rats. Acupunct Electrother Res 30: 263–273.
46. Zhang W, Li JL, Hosaka M, Janz R, Shelton JM, et al. (2000) Cyclosporine A-induced hypertension involves synapsin in renal sensory nerve endings. Proc Natl Acad Sci U S A 97: 9765–9770.
47. Kizhakekuttu TJ, Widlansky ME (2010) Natural antioxidants and hypertension: promise and challenges. Cardiovasc Ther 28: e20–32.
48. Engelhard YN, Gazer B, Paran E (2006) Natural antioxidants from tomato extract reduce blood pressure in patients with grade-1 hypertension: a double-blind, placebo-controlled pilot study. Am Heart J 151: 100.
49. Boshtam M, Rafiei M, Sadeghi K, Sarraf-Zadegan N (2002) Vitamin E can reduce blood pressure in mild hypertensives. Int J Vitam Nutr Res 72: 309–314.
50. Perez-Vizcaino F, Duarte J, Jimenez R, Santos-Buelga C, Osuna A (2009) Antihypertensive effects of the flavonoid quercetin. Pharmacol Rep 61: 67–75.
51. Kumar A, Kaur H, Devi P, Mohan V (2009) Role of coenzyme Q10 (CoQ10) in cardiac disease, hypertension and Meniere-like syndrome. Pharmacol Ther 124: 259–268.

11

Acupuncture Enhances the Synaptic Dopamine Availability to Improve Motor Function in a Mouse Model of Parkinson's Disease

Seung-Nam Kim[1,2], Ah-Reum Doo[1], Ji-Yeun Park[1], Hyungjin Bae[1], Younbyoung Chae[1], Insop Shim[1], Hyangsook Lee[1], Woongjoon Moon[1]*, Hyejung Lee[1], Hi-Joon Park[1]*

1 Studies of Translational Acupuncture Research, Acupuncture and Meridian Science Research Center, Kyung Hee University, Seoul, Republic of Korea, **2** Department of Oriental Medical Science, Kyung Hee University, Seoul, Republic of Korea

Abstract

Parkinson's disease (PD) is caused by the selective loss of dopaminergic neurons in the substantia nigra (SN) and the depletion of striatal dopamine (DA). Acupuncture, as an alternative therapy for PD, has beneficial effects in both PD patients and PD animal models, although the underlying mechanisms therein remain uncertain. The present study investigated whether acupuncture treatment affected dopamine neurotransmission in a PD mouse model using 1-methyl-4-phenyl-1,2,3,6-tetrahydropyridine (MPTP). We found that acupuncture treatment at acupoint GB34 improved motor function with accompanying dopaminergic neuron protection against MPTP but did not restore striatal dopamine depletion. Instead, acupuncture treatment increased dopamine release that in turn, may lead to the enhancement of dopamine availability in the synaptic cleft. Moreover, acupuncture treatment mitigated MPTP-induced abnormal postsynaptic changes, suggesting that acupuncture treatment may increase postsynaptic dopamine neurotransmission and facilitate the normalization of basal ganglia activity. These results suggest that the acupuncture-induced enhancement of synaptic dopamine availability may play a critical role in motor function improvement against MPTP.

Editor: Huaibin Cai, National Institute of Health, United States of America

Funding: This work was supported by the National Research Foundation of Korea (NRF) grant funded by the Korea government (MEST) [2010-0008834 and 2005-0049404]. The funders had no role in study design, data collection and analysis, decision to publish, or preparation of the manuscript.

Competing Interests: The authors have declared that no competing interests exist.

* E-mail: acufind@khu.ac.kr (H-JP); wm9306@naver.com (WM)

Introduction

Dopaminergic system dysfunction is implicated in a wide variety of neurological disorders, including Parkinson's disease (PD). PD is characterized by the selective loss of dopaminergic neurons in the substantia nigra (SN) and a depletion of striatal dopamine (DA), and dopamine depletion in PD leads to abnormal changes of basal ganglia activity that in turn, result in an inability to control voluntary movement [1]. Dopamine replacement therapies remain the most effective clinical option for PD patients despite the occasionally severe side effects [2].

Recent studies from several laboratories including ours have shown that acupuncture has a beneficial effect in rodent models of PD [3,4,5]. In both the 6-hydroxydopamine (6-OHDA) lesioned rat and 1-methyl-4-phenyl-1,2,3,6-tetrahydropyridine (MPTP) lesioned mouse, acupuncture has proven to be neuroprotective. We have demonstrated that acupuncture rescues dopaminergic neurons by increasing the expressions of trkB [5], cycolphilin A [3], and Akt [6] and by decreasing the inflammation in the substantia nigra [7]. Acupuncture has also been shown to reduce the oxidative stress in the substantia nigra and striatum [8,9]. However, the underlying mechanisms of acupuncture on the improvement of motor dysfunction in PD models are not well understood.

Given the critical role of dopamine and the importance in the neuroplasticity of the impaired basal ganglia on regulating motor function in PD, we hypothesized that acupuncture improves the motor deficits by modulating dopaminergic neurotransmission in the striatum, and thus ameliorating the abnormal postsynaptic changes induced by dopamine depletion in mouse Parkinsonian model. Thus, in the present study, we compared the effects of acupuncture on the motor function and dopaminergic neuron survival with sham acupuncture (the same acupuncture stimulation was given to a control point) in mouse Parkinsonian model. The changes in the expressions of the phosphorylated DARPP-32 and FosB as well as the dopamine contents, dopamine efflux, and turnover ratios were measured to investigate the role of acupuncture against the changes induced by dopamine depletion in the striatum.

Materials and Methods

Animals and MPTP intoxication

All experiments were approved by the Kyung Hee University Animal Care Committee for animal welfare [KHUASP(SE)-09-046] and were maintained in strict accordance with Guidelines of the NIH and Korean Academy of Medical Sciences. Twelve-week-old male C57BL/6 mice (Central Lab. Animal Inc., Seoul, Republic of Korea), weighing 23–26 g each, were used in all of the experiments. The mice were divided into Control, MPTP (MPTP only), MPTP with acupuncture treatment at acupoint GB34

(MPTP+AP), and MPTP with sham acupuncture at a control point (MPTP+CP) groups. The mice in all of the MPTP groups (MPTP, MPTP+AP, and MPTP+CP groups) received an intraperitoneal injection of MPTP-HCl (30 mg/kg of free base; Sigma-Aldrich, St. Louis, MO, USA) in saline at 24-h intervals for five consecutive days. The mice in the Control group were injected with saline instead of MPTP (Fig. 1B).

Acupuncture treatment

Two hours after each MPTP injection, acupuncture stimulation was performed at an acupoint GB34 (MPTP+AP group) or at a control point (MPTP+CP group) (Fig. 1A). After the final MPTP injection, acupuncture stimulation continued daily for seven days (total 12 days). In order to rule out the non-specific effects of acupuncture, we used the sham acupuncture group in which the same acupuncture stimulation was given to the control point. Acupoint GB34 has been used to treat movement disorders in traditional East Asian medicine [10], and also studied on the relation with motor function in recent neuroimaging studies [11,12]. Since we previously found that acupoint GB34 exerted the highest neuroprotective effect among several candidate acupoints (GB34, SI3, BL62, and ST36) using the same MPTP protocol [3], GB34 was chosen for the present study. It is located at the point of the intersection of lines from the anterior border to the head of the fibula [13,14]. The control point was set at a point that was approximately 3 mm to the lateral side of the tail on the gluteus muscle (Fig. 1C, D). The mice were lightly immobilised to minimize the restraint stress. Acupuncture needles (15 mm in length, 0.20 mm in diameter; Haeng-lim-seo-weon Acuneedle Co., Seoul, Republic of Korea) were bilaterally inserted to a depth of 3 mm at GB34 or the control point, turned at a rate of two spins per second for 15 seconds, and then immediately removed. All mice in all groups were also gently immobilized by holding their necks with the head in an upright position for 15 seconds, to give the same immobilization stress as the acupuncture group.

Behavioural test

A rotarod instrument (MED associates Inc., St. Albans, VT, USA) was used to simultaneously record the latency to fall of five mice. The overall rod performance (ORP) method was used, as previously described [15]. On day seven after the last MPTP or saline injection, the mice were pre-trained three times with 1-h intervals on an accelerating rod speed mode. The time on the rod was recorded with a maximum of 240 seconds for successive rotational speeds (16, 20, 24, 28, and 32 rpm), and the ORP score was calculated by the trapezoidal method [16]. All assessors were blinded to the expected results and experimental groups.

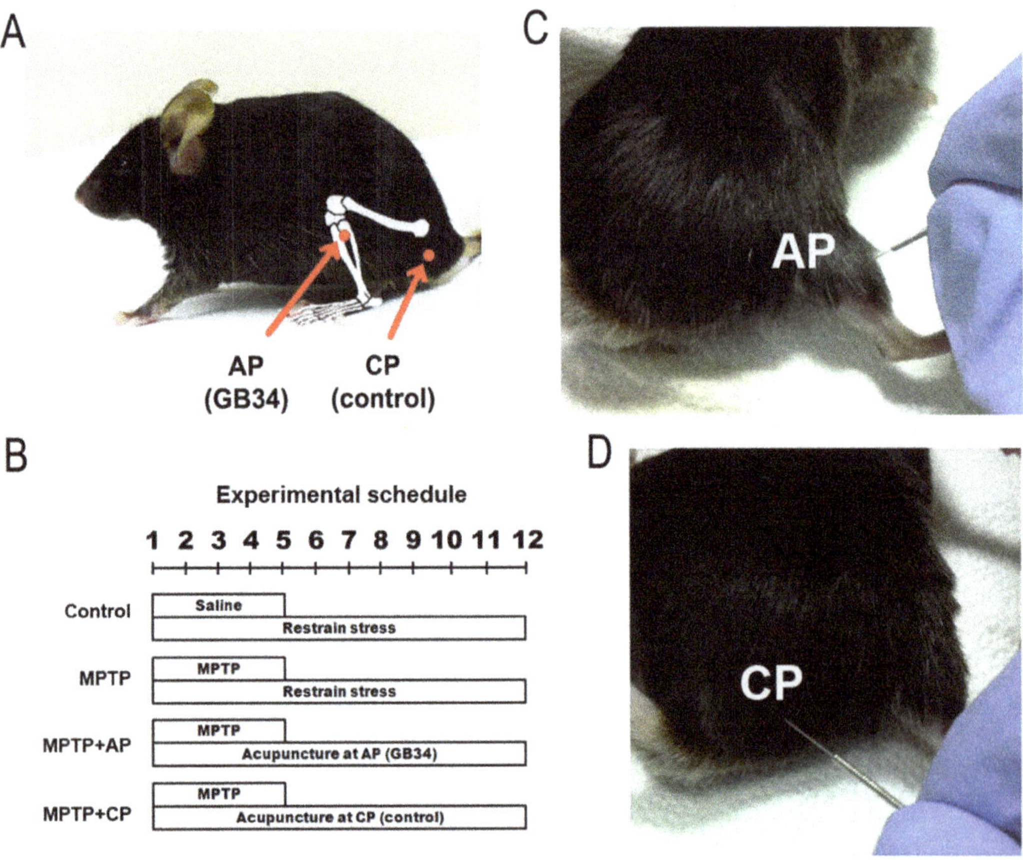

Figure 1. Acupuncture treatment and experimental procedure. (A) The point location of acupuncture treatment (red circle). 'AP (GB34)' refers to acupoint GB34. 'CP' (control point) refers to control point. (B) Experimental schedule. Mice in the MPTP, MPTP+AP, and MPTP+CP groups were treated with 30 mg/kg of MPTP for five consecutive days, unless Control group were treated with saline instead of MPTP. Acupuncture treatment was performed at acupoint GB34 (MPTP+AP) or a control point (MPTP+CP) once a day for 12 consecutive days after the first MPTP administration. (C, D) Photographs of acupuncture treatment at GB34 (C) and control point (D). The mice were immobilised by holding their neck. Acupuncture needles were inserted, turned at a rate of two spins per second for 15 seconds, and then immediately removed.

Immunohistochemistry

On day seven after the last MPTP or saline injection, the mice were transcardially perfused with 4% paraformaldehyde in a 0.2 M phosphate buffer. Free-floating sections encompassing the entire midbrain and striatum (40 μm thickness). Tissues, which are between AP −3.08~−3.28 mm from bregma for midbrain and between AP +0.38~+0.98 mm from bregma for striatum in accordance with the atlas of the mouse brain [17], were selected for analysis. The selected tissues were removed, fixed, and cryoprotected. An immunohistochemistry method was performed, as previously described [18,19]. After incubation with 3% H_2O_2 in a 0.05 M phosphate-buffered saline, the sections were blocked with 1% BSA and normal goat serum. The sections were incubated overnight at room temperature in primary antibodies: rabbit tyrosine hydroxylase (TH, 1:1,000; Santa Cruz Biotechnology, Santa Cruz, CA, USA), dopamine transporter (DAT, 1:500; Millipore Co., Billerica, MA, USA), Thr-34-phospho-DARPP-32 (1:500; Abcam Inc., Cambridge, MA, USA), and FosB (1:500; Cell Signalling Technology, Danvers, MA, USA). The tissue sections were incubated with biotinylated anti-rabbit IgG (Vector Laboratories, Inc., Burlingame, CA, USA) for 1 h at room temperature, incubated with ABC reagent (Vector Laboratories Inc., Burlingame, CA, USA) for 1 h at room temperature, and incubated for 2 min in 0.02% diaminobenzidine and 0.003% hydrogen peroxide in 1 M Tris-buffered saline (pH 7.5). After the reaction, the tissue sections were mounted on gelatin-coated slides, dried, dehydrated, and covered. For Nissl double staining, 0.5% Cresyl violet solution was used for 5 min before mounting.

Image analysis

For stereological analysis of dopaminergic neuron cell counting, TH- and Nissl-positive cells in the substantia nigra pars compacta (SNpc) were counted bilaterally in five continuous 40 μm thickness immunostained mesencephalic sections at the level between AP −3.08~−3.28 mm from bregma (accordance with atlas of the mice brain) using a Zeiss Axioscope 2 (Zeiss, Jena, Germany) and an attached StereoInvestigator system (MicroBrightfield, VT, USA). Stereological methods were used to analyze total volume of the SNpc using optical fractionator (StereoInvestigator system; MicroBrightfield, VT, USA). After counting, the SNpc nuclei were reconstructed serially and their volume calculated with Stereo-Investigator software. The optical fractionator stereological probe was used to determine neuronal count in the SNpc in sections stained for both Nissl and TH. For dopaminergic fiber analysis, pictures of the striatum were taken using a bright-field microscope (BX51; Olympus, Tokyo, Japan). Immunoreactive optical densities were calculated using Image Pro software (version 6.0 for Windows; Media Cybernetics Inc., Bethesda, MD, USA). To correct for background differences, the optical density of the corpus callosum of each brain tissue was selected and used for normalization. p-DARPP-32 and FosB counts were performed by sampling a 500 μm wide by 350 μm high area where 1 mm distant from the vertical center of the brain and under the corpus callosum.

In vivo microdialysis

The mice were anaesthetised with an anaesthetic solution containing tiletamine/zolazepam 30 mg/kg (Zoletile; Virbac, France) and xylazine 10 mg/kg (Rompun; Bayer, Korea). An intracerebral guide cannula (MBR-5; BASi, USA) was stereotaxically implanted into the striatum (AP +0.1; ML +0.2; DV −0.2 from bregma), and coordinates are in accordance with atlas of the mice brain. Acrylic cement (GC Corporation) was used for fixation of the guide cannulas. Then the mice were placed individual home cage 24 h for recovery from surgery. On the day of the experiment, a microdialysis probe (MBR-2-5, 0.24 mm diameter, 2 mm membrane length, cut-off 38 KDa; BASi, USA) was inserted through the guide cannula. The probes were connected to a microinjection syringe pump (CMA/Microdialysis) and filtered Ringer's solution (145 mM NaCl, 3 mM KCl, 1 mM $MgCl_2$, 1.2 mM $CaCl_2$, pH 7.4) perfused the probes at a flow rate of 1 μl/min. After insertion of the probes, samples were collected during 20-min throughout the experimental period. And total 220-min samples were collected. The experiment was performed under normal light conditions in an undisturbed room. The dialysates were stored at −80°C until DA determination with high-performance liquid chromatography (HPLC).

High performance liquid chromatography (HPLC) analysis

The tissue contents of the neurotransmitters were measured using HPLC (Waters Co., Milford, MA, USA) in combination with an electrochemical detecting system (ESA Coulochem III detection system, range 100 nA, potential −100 mV to +320 mV; ESA Inc., Chelmsford, MA, USA). Mice were sacrificed on day seven after the last MPTP or saline injection, and the striatum of each mouse was rapidly dissected, frozen in liquid nitrogen, and stored at −72°C until assayed. These brain striatum tissues were homogenized in 300 μl of 0.1% perchloric acid. The resultant homogenates were centrifuged for 20 minutes at 1000× g at 4°C. The supernatant was filtered through a 0.22 μm membrane, and an aliquot (15 μl in volume) of the resulting solution was injected into the HPLC pump. Chromatographic separation was performed using a C18 reverse-phase column (150 mm×3.9 mm, 4 μm; Waters Co., Milford, MA, USA), and data analyses were performed using computer software (Empower; Waters Co., Milford, MA, USA). The mobile phase, which had a pH of 3.2, consisted of 150 mM sodium phosphate monobasic monohydrate, 1.85 mM octanesulfonic acid, 0.05 mM EDTA, 0.01% triethylamine, 4% methanol, and 6% acetonitrile. DA, 3,4, dihydroxyphenylacetic acid (DOPAC), homovanillic acid (HVA), and serotonin standards were prepared in 0.1% perchloric acid (Sigma-Aldrich, St. Louis, MO, USA). Each concentration was adjusted with respect to the standard and quantified from a standard curve. The levels of DA, DOPAC, HVA, and serotonin were calculated as nanograms per microgram of total protein.

Data analysis

All procedures, assessments, and analyses were performed in a blinded manner to minimise the observer bias. The SPSS, version 17.0 (SPSS Inc., Chicago, IL, USA), was used for statistical procedures. All data are expressed as the mean ± SEM. A statistical analysis was performed using one-way ANOVA followed by a post-hoc Newman-Keuls test. The effect of acupuncture stimulation on dopamine efflux was determined by two-way ANOVA analysis with repeated measures over time followed by Bonferroni's post-hoc test. In all of the analyses, differences were considered to be statistically significant at $P<0.05$.

Results

Acupuncture treatment at GB34 improved motor function and prevented dopaminergic neuron degeneration against MPTP

Previously, we reported that GB34 exerted the highest neuroprotective effect among several candidate acupoints in a mice Parkinsonian model [3,8]. In this study, we first examined whether this acupoint was indeed critical for the effects of acupuncture against MPTP. Acupuncture treatment was performed at GB34 (MPTP+AP group) or the control point (MPTP+CP group) once a day for 12 consecutive days after the first MPTP administration (Fig. 1). Acupuncture treatment at GB34 induced a significant improvement of motor function against MPTP, whereas acupuncture treatment at the control point had no effect. Mice in the MPTP group showed significantly lower overall rod performance (ORP) scores (4901.3±501.9) in comparison to mice in the Control group (6347.7±272.2, $P<0.05$). Mice in the MPTP+AP group showed significantly higher ORP scores (6148.7±178.0) in comparison to mice in the MPTP group ($P<0.05$). The ORP scores were not statistically different between the MPTP and MPTP+CP groups (5217.7±251.6, Fig. 2E).

Also, a significant recovery of TH-positive cell numbers in the MPTP+AP group was observed. The MPTP group had significantly fewer TH-positive neurons in the SN (2536.83±626.06) in comparison to those observed in the Control group (5309.90±461.48, $P<0.01$); however, the MPTP+AP group had significantly more TH-positive neurons in the SN (4233.34±405.72) in comparison to those observed in the MPTP group ($P<0.05$). There was no statistical difference between the MPTP and the MPTP+CP groups (2140.07±543.33, Figs. 2A, B, D). To further support TH-positive cell count result, we also performed Nissl-positive cell counts (supplementary figure S2). Consistent with TH-positive cell counts, MPTP caused a considerable loss of Nissl-positive cells in the substantia nigra pars compacta (SNc), while acupuncture treatment led to a significant recovery of Nissl-positive cell numbers in the SNc against MPTP. In the striatum, acupuncture treatment also showed similar protection of dopaminergic fibers against MPTP toxicity (65.61±2.85% vs. 90.14±2.47% of Control group, $P<0.001$, Figs. 2C, F). These results demonstrate that acupuncture treatment at a specific acupoint (GB34), but not at a control point, significantly alleviated MPTP-induced motor dysfunction and dopaminergic neuron degeneration.

Since all of our above results display that acupuncture on control point did not produce any effects, we did not use the MPTP+CP group in the following experiments to minimize the number of animals.

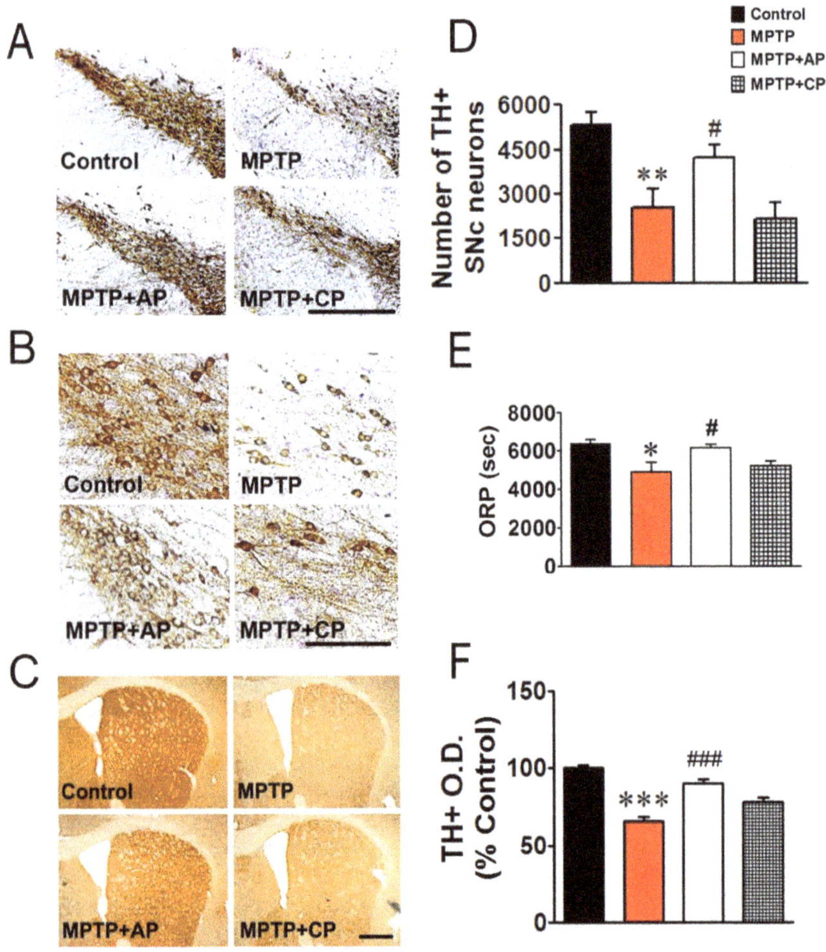

Figure 2. The behavioural and neuroprotective effects of acupuncture treatment at GB34 in MPTP mice. (A, B) Immunohistochemical staining for TH-positive and Nissl-positive dopaminergic neurons in the substantia nigra in a low magnification (A, scale bar: 300 μm) and in a higher magnification (B, scale bar: 100 μm). (C) Immunohistochemical staining for TH-positive dopaminergic fibers in the striatum. (Scale bar: 500 μm.) (D) Bar graph of TH-positive cell counts in the substantia nigra of each group. (E) Bar graph of the overall rod performance (ORP) scores of each group. (F) Bar graph of optical density of TH-positive fibers in the striatum of each group (n = 7–10 per group). A significant recovery of TH-positive cell numbers and fibers in the MPTP+AP group was observed. Also, acupuncture treatment at GB34 significantly improved motor function against MPTP. Data are normalized to the Control group. *$P<0.05$, **$P<0.01$ and ***$P<0.001$ versus Control group, #$P<0.05$ and ###$P<0.001$ versus MPTP group via one-way ANOVA followed by a Newman-Keuls test.

Acupuncture treatment at GB34 increased dopamine turnover ratios in the striatum

To examine any possible effect of acupuncture treatment on the dopaminergic system, the levels of striatal DA and its metabolites, DOPAC and HVA, were measured using HPLC. In this analysis, the levels of serotonin in the same brain were measured for internal control. In Figure 3, HPLC analysis revealed that MPTP administration induced a significant 80% depletion in striatal dopamine levels in both the MPTP and MPTP+AP groups in comparison to the Control group (95.7±10.5 vs. 22.1±4.4 ng/mg protein, $P<0.001$, Fig. 3A), whereas serotonin levels were not statistically different among the groups (43.0±6.0 vs. 39.3±1.3 ng/mg protein, $P>0.05$, Fig. 3E). There were no significant differences in striatal dopamine levels between the MPTP and MPTP+AP groups (22.1±4.4 vs. 24.4±4.7 ng/mg protein, Fig. 3A); however, there was a significant increase in HVA in the MPTP+AP group in comparison to that observed in the MPTP group (2.7±0.3 vs. 4.4±0.5 ng/mg protein, $P<0.05$, Fig. 3A). Moreover, there were significant increases in dopamine turnover ratios (DOPAC/DA, HVA/DA, and DOPAC+HVA/DA) in the MPTP+AP group (25.3±3.5, 23.6±5.1, and 48.9±8.1) in comparison to both the MPTP (14.7±1.2, $P<0.01$; 13.5±1.5 and 28.2±2.6, $P<0.05$ each) and Control groups (10.9±2.2, 7.5±0.5, and 18.4±2.3, $P<0.01$ each, Figs. 3B, C, D).

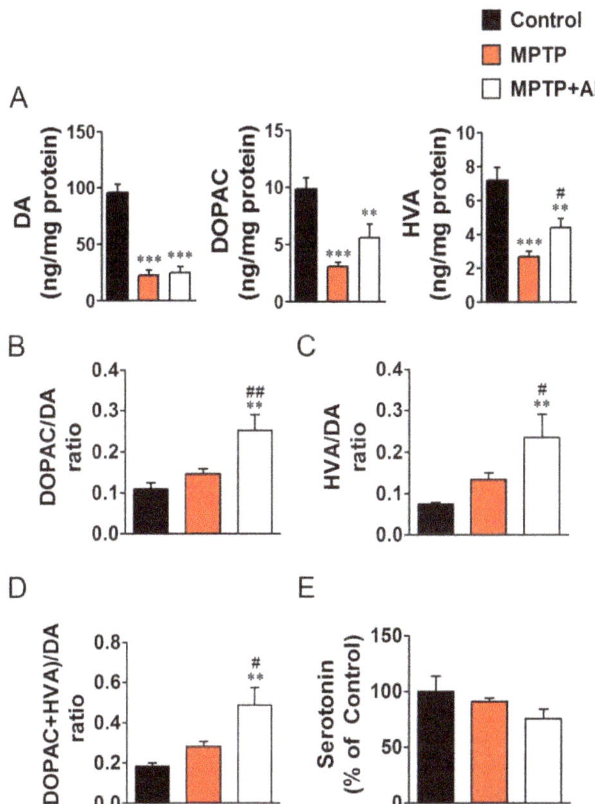

Figure 3. Tissue dopamine contents and its turnover ratios in the striatum of each group. (A) Contents of dopamine and its metabolates, DOPAC and HVA, in the striatum of each group (n = 8 per group). (B) DOPAC/DA, (C) HVA/DA, and (D) (DOPAC plus HVA)/DA turnover ratio of each group (n = 8 per group). (E) Serotonin levels of each group (n = 8 per group). MPTP administration induced a significant decrease in the dopamine and its metabolates levels, whereas acupuncture treatment at GB34 significantly increased the dopamine turnover ratio. **$P<0.01$ and ***$P<0.001$ compared to Control, #$P<0.05$ and ##$P<0.01$ compared to MPTP group, one-way ANOVA, followed by Newman-Keuls test.

Since acupuncture treatment improved motor function (Fig. 2E) but did not restore striatal dopamine level (Fig. 3A), we further investigated whether acupuncture treatment modulates dopamine release in the striatum. Using microdialysis-HPLC method, extracellular dopamine levels in the striatum of Control, MPTP, and MPTP+AP mice were measured after acupuncture stimulation. We found that, only in the striatum of MPTP+AP mice, acupuncture stimulation significantly increased dopamine efflux at time point 20 min ($P<0.001$). Dopamine efflux was six-fold higher in MPTP+AP group than in MPTP group ($P<0.001$, Fig. 4). However, dopamine efflux was not altered both in the striatum of Control and MPTP mice at all time points. These results indicate that acupuncture treatment at GB34 did not restore the MPTP-induced depletion of total striatal dopamine but significantly increased dopamine release in the striatum, which may result in improvement of motor fun'ction in this model of PD.

Acupuncture treatment at GB34 mitigated MPTP-induced increases in the phosphorylation of DARPP-32 and the expression of FosB

Striatal dopamine depletion causes compensatory changes in postsynaptic medium spiny neurons through the hyperactivation of 3′-5′-cyclic adenosine monophosphate (cAMP) signalling [20], which is mediated by dopamine- and cAMP-regulated phospho-

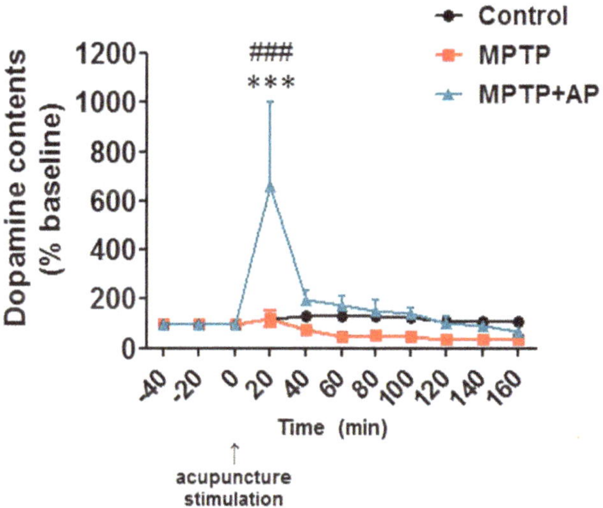

Figure 4. Time courses of dopamine (DA) efflux levels in the striatum. Data presented are mean ± SEM. On the day of the behavioral test (on day 12 after the first saline (Control group) or MPTP (MPTP group and MPTP+AP group) injection), extracellular DA levels in the striatum of Control, MPTP, and MPTP+AP mice were measured after a single acupuncture stimulation using microdialysis-HPLC method. Since MPTP+AP mice already received 11 day's acupuncture treatment before the final acupuncture stimulation, MPTP+AP mice received in total 12 day's acupuncture treatment, whereas Control and MPTP mice received only a single acupuncture treatment. At 20 min after acupuncture stimulation, only MPTP+AP group showed an increase in dopamine efflux. The increase in dopamine efflux was returned to its basal level at 120 min after acupuncture stimulation. Data are normalized to the baseline data of each group. The effect of acupuncture stimulation on dopamine efflux was determined by two-way ANOVA analysis with repeated measures over time followed by Bonferroni's post-hoc test. *** $P<0.001$ versus Control group and ### $P<0.001$ versus MPTP group.

protein of 32 kDa (DARPP-32) [21]. Therefore, we examined MPTP-induced postsynaptic changes using immunohistochemical staining for phospho-DARPP-32 at Thr34. MPTP administration induced a significant increase in the phosphorylation of DARPP-32 at Thr34 in the MPTP group (162.7±16.5% of Control group) in comparison to the Control group (100.0±12.2% of Control group, $P<0.001$). Acupuncture treatment at GB34 significantly mitigated the increased phosphorylation of DARPP-32 at Thr34 in the MPTP+AP group (107.8±9.1% of Control group, $P<0.001$, Figs. 5A, B).

In addition, we looked for another change in postsynaptic markers of dopamine depletion in the striatum. Because MPTP administration is known to upregulate expression of immediate early gene, FosB [22,23,24], we also examined changes of FosB expression in the striatum. Consistent with previous reports, MPTP administration induced a significant increase in FosB expression in the MPTP group (130.7±11.2% of Control group) in comparison to the Control group (100.0±4.1% of Control group, $P<0.05$). Acupuncture treatment at GB34 significantly reduced the MPTP-induced increase of FosB expression in the MPTP+AP group (83.2±8.3% of Control group, $P<0.001$, Figs. 6A, B). These results demonstrate that MPTP-induced increases in the phosphorylation of DARPP-32 and the expression of FosB were mitigated by acupuncture treatment at GB34, suggesting that the acupuncture treatment may normalize MPTP-induced abnormal postsynaptic changes.

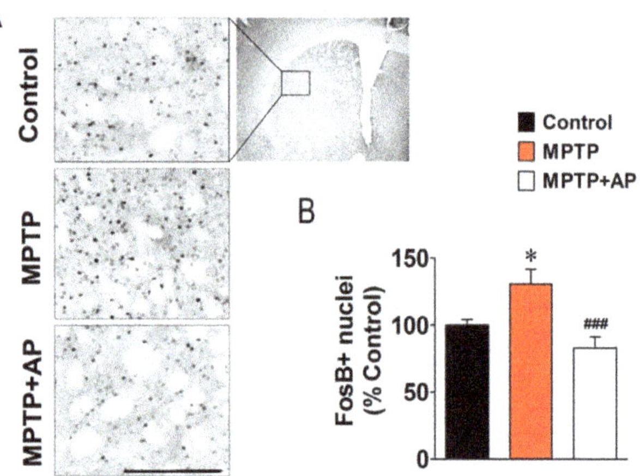

Figure 6. Changes in the expression of FosB by MPTP and acupuncture treatment at GB34. (A) Representative images of immunohistochemical staining for FosB. (Scale bars: 100 μm.) The top-right panel shows a transverse section of the striatum. The box represents the analysed area. (B) Bar graph of striatal FosB-positive nuclei counts (n = 12 per group). Data are normalized to the Control group. MPTP administration increased FosB expression, whereas acupuncture treatment at GB34 reduced the MPTP-induced increase of FosB expression. *$P<0.05$ versus Control group and ###$P<0.001$ versus MPTP group via one-way ANOVA followed by a Newman-Keuls test.

Discussion

The present study demonstrates that acupuncture treatment improved motor function against MPTP most likely through an enhancement of dopamine availability in the synaptic cleft rather than the restoration of the levels of total striatal dopamine.

We found that only acupuncture treatment at GB34, but not at control point significantly improved motor function and prevented dopaminergic neuron degeneration against MPTP (Fig. 2), suggesting that the stimulating a specific point is important to produce the benefits of acupuncture. We also found that acupuncture treatment at GB34 alleviated MPTP-induced motor dysfunction and dopaminergic neuron degeneration, and increased dopamine turnover ratios but did not restore the levels of total striatal dopamine (Figs. 2, 3). It has been suggested that increases in DOPAC/DA and HVA/DA ratios in the striatum reflect an increased metabolism and release of dopamine [25]. Therefore, the observed increases in relative HVA concentrations and increases in DOPAC/DA and HVA/DA ratios following acupuncture treatment in MPTP-intoxicated mice (Fig. 3) suggest that acupuncture may induce an increased rate of dopamine metabolism in the protected dopaminergic neurons with an accompanying increase in dopamine release from dopaminergic terminals. Indeed, we found that acupuncture stimulation significantly increased dopamine release only in MPTP+AP group, but not in Control and MPTP groups (Fig. 4). Some studies displayed that MPTP administration increased the dopamine turnover ratio as a compensatory mechanism with the impairment of motor function [26,27]. In our study, MPTP group also showed mild increase of turnover ratios, but not statistically different with the Control group. However, the animals with the improvement of motor function after acupuncture enhanced dopamine turnover ratios much more significantly than MPTP group. Recently, we reported that acupuncture can restore MPTP-induced impairment of phosphatidylinositol 3-kinase (PI3K)/Akt cell survival pathway, and PI3K/Akt signalling mediates both acupuncture-induced dopaminergic neuron protection and motor function improvement [6]. Given LY294002, a specific inhibitor of PI3K, concomitantly blocked both acupuncture-induced dopaminergic neuron protection and motor function improvement [6], there seems to be a strong correlation between acupuncture-induced neuroprotection and motor function improvement. Therefore, our previous [6] and the present (Figs. 2, 3, 4) results raise one possibility that the acupuncture-induced

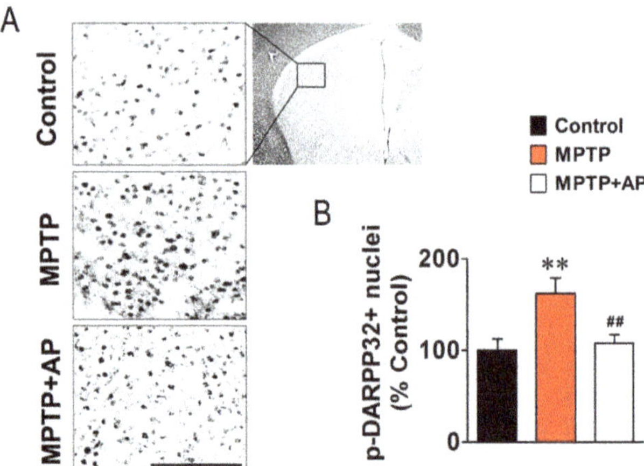

Figure 5. Changes in the phosphorylation state of DARPP-32 by MPTP and acupuncture treatment at GB34. (A) Representative images of immunohistochemical staining for phospho-DARPP-32 at Thr34. (Scale bars: 100 μm.) The top-right panel shows a transverse section of the striatum. The box represents the analysed area. (B) Bar graph of striatal phospho-DARPP-32-positive signal counts (n = 12 per group). Data are normalized to the Control group. MPTP administration induced a significant increase in the phosphorylation of DARPP-32 at Thr34, whereas acupuncture treatment at GB34 significantly mitigated the increased phosphorylation of DARPP-32 at Thr34. **$P<0.01$ versus Control group and ##$P<0.01$ versus MPTP group via one-way ANOVA followed by a Newman-Keuls test.

dopaminergic neuronal protection may lead to increase in dopamine efflux from the surviving dopaminergic neurons, which in turn may result in improved motor function without necessitating restoration of the striatal dopamine content. There are several studies suggesting that the striatal dopamine content is not necessarily correlated with the improvement of motor function [28,29,30]. It is well known that dopamine transporter (DAT) density also plays a role in dopamine transmission by modulating dopamine reuptake. Thus, additionally, we performed the immunohistochemical detection of DAT in the striatum to observe the involvement of DAT. Intriguingly, we observed that there were no significant differences in DAT expression levels between MPTP and MPTP+AP groups (Supplementary Fig. S1), whereas MPTP-induced reduction of TH expression in the adjacent striatum was significantly restored after acupuncture treatment (Fig. 2D), which might result in the increases in DOPAC/DA and HVA/DA ratios in the striatum. However, whether the changes in DAT density participate in the improvement of motor function needs further investigation.

Taken together, our results suggest that acupuncture treatment at GB34 ameliorates MPTP-induced motor dysfunction most likely through an enhancement of dopamine availability in the synaptic cleft rather than the restoration of the levels of total striatal dopamine. Alternatively, the acupuncture-induced protection of dopaminergic neurons shown in our study may result in the maintenance of the functional integrity of the SNr, thereby compensating for striatal dopamine depletion. Because, there are several showing that the substantia nigra pars compacta dopaminergic neurons release dopamine not only from the striatal terminal fibres but also from the dendrite network to the substantia nigra pars reticulata (SNr) [31,32]. The basal ganglia output structure also may participate in the improvement of motor function induced by acupuncture as Jia et al. suggested [30,33]. However, to clarify the relationship between our results and above hypothesis needs to be further exploration.

MPTP-induced striatal dopamine depletion induces postsynaptic abnormalities [22,34]. Therefore, if an acupuncture-induced increase in synaptic dopamine availability (or dopamine neurotransmission) can compensate for the MPTP-induced depletion of absolute dopamine levels in the synaptic cleft, a normalization of MPTP-induced postsynaptic abnormalities may occur. Because MPTP-induced postsynaptic changes are often measured by changes in FosB expression [22,23,24] and FosB expression is regulated by DARPP-32 signalling [20], we examined MPTP-induced postsynaptic changes of phospho-DARPP-32 at Thr34 and FosB using immunohistochemistry. Consistent with previous reports [22,23,24], MPTP intoxication increased FosB expression in the striatum (Fig. 6). We also found an increase in the phosphorylation of DARPP-32 after MPTP intoxication (Fig. 5). Considering the report that 6-hydroxydopamine did not alter the phosphorylation levels of DARPP-32 [35], our result suggests that MPTP-induced DARPP-32 signalling may differ from 6-OHDA-induced DARPP-32 signalling. More importantly, acupuncture treatment significantly reduced MPTP-induced increases in the phosphorylation of DARPP-32 and the expression of FosB (Figs. 5, 6). These results demonstrate that acupuncture treatment mitigated MPTP-induced abnormal postsynaptic changes, suggesting that acupuncture treatment may increase postsynaptic dopamine neurotransmission and facilitate the normalization of basal ganglia activity.

In conclusion, our results suggest that increased dopamine release after acupuncture treatment at GB34 may lead to an enhancement of dopamine availability in the synaptic cleft that in turn, may play an essential role in motor function improvement

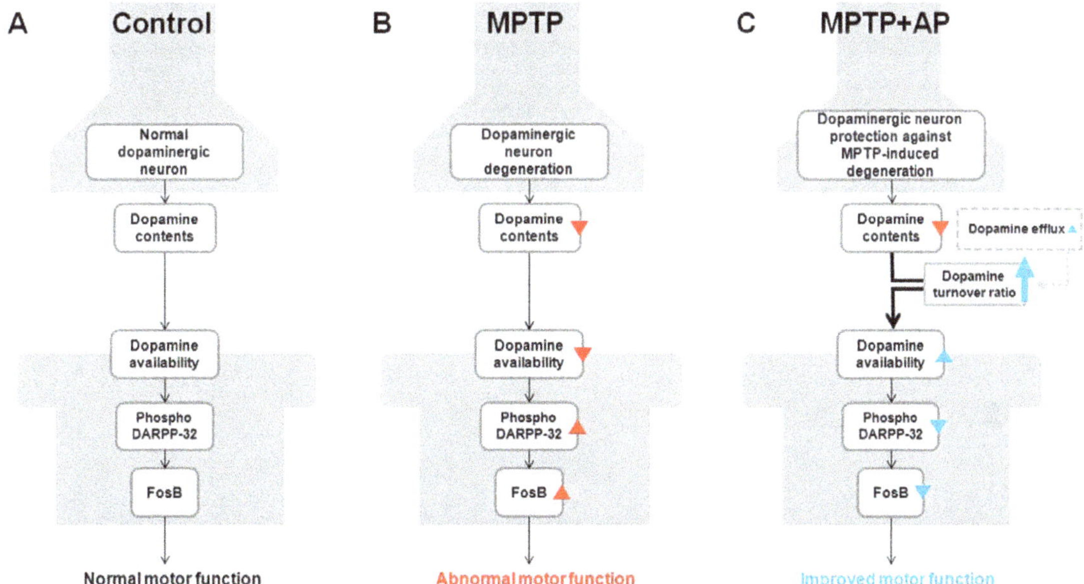

Figure 7. Schematic representation of the effect of acupuncture on dopamine availability and the concomitant postsynaptic response. (A) Normal condition (Control group). (B) MPTP lesioning (MPTP group). (C) Acupuncture treatment at GB34 following MPTP lesioning (MPTP+AP group). Striatal dopamine depletion caused by MPTP-induced dopaminergic denervation leads to abnormally high levels of Thr34-phosphorylated DARPP-32 and the consequent upregulation of FosB in the striatum, which, in turn, may result in abnormal motor function (B). Acupuncture treatment at GB34 following MPTP lesioning alleviated MPTP-induced denervation of dopaminergic neurons but did not restore the levels of total striatal dopamine; however, acupuncture treatment increased dopamine availability likely through increased dopamine release, which, in turn, may lead to the normalization of postsynaptic abnormalities. Therefore, we propose that acupuncture treatment at GB34 improved motor function against MPTP most likely through an enhancement of dopamine availability in the synaptic cleft.

against MPTP (Fig. 7). From a clinical point of view, one of the major issues in the treatment of PD is how to reduce the adverse effects of L-DOPA. Indeed, various attempts have been made to find a new clinical therapy that can decrease the adverse effects of L-DOPA and increase its efficacy [36]. Our finding that acupuncture improved motor function without necessitating striatal dopamine refilling suggests that acupuncture treatment can be complementary to dopamine replacement therapy. Therefore, we expect that the elucidation of the underlying mechanisms of acupuncture may contribute to the development of novel clinical strategies for the treatment of PD.

Supporting Information

Figure S1 Dopamine transporter (DAT) expression in the striatum of each group. Immunochemistry was performed to detect DAT (1:1000, Millipore, USA) positive dopaminergic fibers in the striatum. (A) Immunohistochemical staining for DAT-positive dopaminergic fibers in the striatum. (Scale bars: 500 μm.) (B) Bar graph of DAT-positive optical density of fibers in the striatum of each group (n = 7–10 per group). MPTP group showed significant decrease in DAT expression compared to Control, and MPTP+AP group did not alter the decrease. Data are normalized to the Control group. *** $P<0.001$ versus Control group via one-way ANOVA followed by a Newman-Keuls test.
(DOC)

Figure S2 Nissl staining in the substantia nigra pars compacta. For Nissl staining, the substantia nigra tissues were stained with 0.5% cresyl violet, and unbiased stereological counts were made. (A) Representative images of Nissl stained neurons in the substantia nigra of each group. Red lines mark the boundaries of the substantia nigra pars compacta (SNc). (B) Bar graph of Nissl stained neuron counts in the SNc of each group (n = 4 per group). Consistent with TH-positive cell counts, a significant recovery of Nissl-positive cell numbers in MPTP+AP group was observed. Data are normalized to the Control group. *$P<0.05$ versus Control group, and #$P<0.05$ versus MPTP group via one-way ANOVA followed by a Newman-Keuls test.
(DOC)

Author Contributions

Conceived and designed the experiments: H-JP WM. Performed the experiments: S-NK A-RD J-YP HB. Analyzed the data: S-NK IS HL YC HL WM H-JP. Wrote the paper: S-NK WM H-JP. Designed research: H-JP WM. Performed research: S-NK A-RD J-YP HB.

References

1. Fahn S (2003) Description of Parkinson's disease as a clinical syndrome. Ann N Y Acad Sci 991: 1–14.
2. Mouradian MM, Juncos JL, Serrati C, Fabbrini G, Palmeri S, et al. (1987) Exercise and the antiparkinsonian response to levodopa. Clin Neuropharmacol 10: 351–355.
3. Jeon S, Kim YJ, Kim ST, Moon W, Chae Y, et al. (2008) Proteomic analysis of the neuroprotective mechanisms of acupuncture treatment in a Parkinson's disease mouse model. Proteomics 8: 4822–4832.
4. Liang XB, Luo Y, Liu XY, Lu J, Li FQ, et al. (2003) Electro-acupuncture improves behavior and upregulates GDNF mRNA in MFB transected rats. Neuroreport 14: 1177–1181.
5. Park HJ, Lim S, Joo WS, Yin CS, Lee HS, et al. (2003) Acupuncture prevents 6-hydroxydopamine-induced neuronal death in the nigrostriatal dopaminergic system in the rat Parkinson's disease model. Exp Neurol 180: 93–98.
6. Kim S-N, Kim S-T, Doo A-R, Park J-Y, Moon W, et al. (2011) The phosphatidylinositol 3-kinase/Akt signalling pathway mediates acupuncture-induced improvements in a mouse model of Parkinson's disease. Int J Neurosci (in press).
7. Kang JM, Park HJ, Choi YG, Choe IH, Park JH, et al. (2007) Acupuncture inhibits microglial activation and inflammatory events in the MPTP-induced mouse model. Brain Res 1131: 211–219.
8. Kim ST, Moon W, Chae Y, Kim YJ, Lee H, et al. (2009) The effect of electroaucpuncture for 1-methyl-4-phenyl-1,2,3,6-tetrahydropyridine-induced proteomic changes in the mouse striatum. J Physiol Sci 60: 27–34.
9. Yu YP, Ju WP, Li ZG, Wang DZ, Wang YC, et al. (2010) Acupuncture inhibits oxidative stress and rotational behavior in 6-hydroxydopamine lesioned rat. Brain Res 1336: 58–65.
10. Liangyue D, Yijun G, Shuhui H, Xiaoping J, Yang L, et al. (2004) Chinese Acupuncture and Moxibustion. Beijing: Foreign Language Press.
11. Jeun SS, Kim JS, Kim BS, Park SD, Lim EC, et al. (2005) Acupuncture stimulation for motor cortex activities: a 3T fMRI study. Am J Chin Med 33: 573–578.
12. Na BJ, Jahng GH, Park SU, Jung WS, Moon SK, et al. (2009) An fMRI study of neuronal specificity of an acupoint: electroacupuncture stimulation of Yanglingquan (GB34) and its sham point. Neurosci Lett 464: 1–5.
13. World.Health.Organization (2008) WHO Standard Acupuncture Point Locations in the Western Pacific Region. Manila: WHO Regional Office for the Western Pacific.
14. Yin CS, Jeong HS, Park HJ, Baik Y, Yoon MH, et al. (2008) A proposed transpositional acupoint system in a mouse and rat model. Res Vet Sci 84: 159–165.
15. Rozas G, Lopez-Martin E, Guerra MJ, Labandeira-Garcia JL (1998) The overall rod performance test in the MPTP-treated-mouse model of Parkinsonism. J Neurosci Methods 83: 165–175.
16. Rozas G, Guerra MJ, Labandeira-Garcia JL (1997) An automated rotarod method for quantitative drug-free evaluation of overall motor deficits in rat models of parkinsonism. Brain Res Brain Res Protoc 2: 75–84.
17. Keith BJ, Franklin GP (2008) The Mouse Brain in Stereotaxic Coordinates. California: Academic.
18. Hirsch EC, Faucheux BA (1998) Iron metabolism and Parkinson's disease. Mov Disord 13 Suppl 1: 39–45.
19. Hirsch EC, Hunot S, Damier P, Faucheux B (1998) Glial cells and inflammation in Parkinson's disease: a role in neurodegeneration? Ann Neurol 44: S115–120.
20. Santini E, Valjent E, Fisone G (2008) Parkinson's disease: levodopa-induced dyskinesia and signal transduction. FEBS J 275: 1392–1399.
21. Greengard P, Allen PB, Nairn AC (1999) Beyond the dopamine receptor: the DARPP-32/protein phosphatase-1 cascade. Neuron 23: 435–447.
22. Crocker SJ, Smith PD, Jackson-Lewis V, Lamba WR, Hayley SP, et al. (2003) Inhibition of calpains prevents neuronal and behavioral deficits in an MPTP mouse model of Parkinson's disease. J Neurosci 23: 4081–4091.
23. Mount MP, Lira A, Grimes D, Smith PD, Faucher S, et al. (2007) Involvement of interferon-gamma in microglial-mediated loss of dopaminergic neurons. J Neurosci 27: 3328–3337.
24. Smith PD, Crocker SJ, Jackson-Lewis V, Jordan-Sciutto KL, Hayley S, et al. (2003) Cyclin-dependent kinase 5 is a mediator of dopaminergic neuron loss in a mouse model of Parkinson's disease. Proc Natl Acad Sci U S A 100: 13650–13655.
25. Nishi A, Kuroiwa M, Miller DB, O'Callaghan JP, Bateup HS, et al. (2008) Distinct roles of PDE4 and PDE10A in the regulation of cAMP/PKA signaling in the striatum. J Neurosci 28: 10460–10471.
26. Petzinger GM, Walsh JP, Akopian G, Hogg E, Abernathy A, et al. (2007) Effects of treadmill exercise on dopaminergic transmission in the 1-methyl-4-phenyl-1,2,3,6-tetrahydropyridine-lesioned mouse model of basal ganglia injury. J Neurosci 27: 5291–5300.
27. Vuckovic MG, Wood RI, Holschneider DP, Abernathy A, Togasaki DM, et al. (2008) Memory, mood, dopamine, and serotonin in the 1-methyl-4-phenyl-1,2,3,6-tetrahydropyridine-lesioned mouse model of basal ganglia injury. Neurobiol Dis 32: 319–327.
28. Gash DM, Zhang Z, Ovadia A, Cass WA, Yi A, et al. (1996) Functional recovery in parkinsonian monkeys treated with GDNF. Nature 380: 252–255.
29. Tseng JL, Baetge EE, Zurn AD, Aebischer P (1997) GDNF reduces drug-induced rotational behavior after medial forebrain bundle transection by a mechanism not involving striatal dopamine. J Neurosci 17: 325–333.
30. Jia J, Li B, Sun ZL, Yu F, Wang X, et al. (2010) Electro-acupuncture stimulation acts on the basal ganglia output pathway to ameliorate motor impairment in Parkinsonian model rats. Behav Neurosci 124: 305–310.
31. Robertson GS, Robertson HA (1989) Evidence that L-dopa-induced rotational behavior is dependent on both striatal and nigral mechanisms. J Neurosci 9: 3326–3331.
32. Cheramy A, Leviel V, Glowinski J (1981) Dendritic release of dopamine in the substantia nigra. Nature 289: 537–542.
33. Jia J, Sun Z, Li B, Pan Y, Wang H, et al. (2009) Electro-acupuncture stimulation improves motor disorders in Parkinsonian rats. Behav Brain Res 205: 214–218.
34. Andersson M, Hilbertson A, Cenci MA (1999) Striatal fosB expression is causally linked with l-DOPA-induced abnormal involuntary movements and the associated upregulation of striatal prodynorphin mRNA in a rat model of Parkinson's disease. Neurobiol Dis 6: 461–474.

35. Picconi B, Centonze D, Hakansson K, Bernardi G, Greengard P, et al. (2003) Loss of bidirectional striatal synaptic plasticity in L-DOPA-induced dyskinesia. Nat Neurosci 6: 501–506.

36. Antonini A, Tolosa E, Mizuno Y, Yamamoto M, Poewe WH (2009) A reassessment of risks and benefits of dopamine agonists in Parkinson's disease. Lancet Neurol 8: 929–937.

12

Acupuncture Promotes Angiogenesis after Myocardial Ischemia through H3K9 Acetylation Regulation at VEGF Gene

Shu-Ping Fu[1,☯], Su-Yun He[1,☯], Bin Xu[1], Chen-Jun Hu[3], Sheng-Feng Lu[1], Wei-Xing Shen[1], Yan Huang[1], Hao Hong[1], Qian Li[1], Ning Wang[1], Xuan-Liang Liu[1], Fanrong Liang[2]*, Bing-Mei Zhu[1]*

1 Key Laboratory of Acupuncture and Medicine Research of Ministry of Education, Nanjing University of Chinese Medicine, Nanjing, Jiangsu, China, **2** School of Acupuncture and Tuina, Chengdu University of Traditional Chinese Medicine, Chengdu, Sichuan, China, **3** School of Information Technology, Nanjing University of Chinese Medicine, Nanjing, Jiangsu, China

Abstract

Background: Acupuncture exerts cardioprotective effects on several types of cardiac injuries, especially myocardial ischemia (MI), but the mechanisms have not yet been well elucidated. Angiogenesis mediated by VEGF gene expression and its modification through histone acetylation has been considered a target in treating myocardial ischemia. This study aims to exam whether modulation of angiogenesis through H3K9 acetylation regulation at VEGF gene is one possible cardioprotective mechanism of acupuncture.

Results: We generated rat MI models by ligating the left anterior descending coronary artery and applied electroacupuncture (EA) treatment at the Neiguan (PC6) acupoint. Our results showed that acupuncture reversed the S-T segment change, reduced Q-wave area, decreased CK, CK-MB, LDH levels, mitigated myocardial remodeling, and promoted microvessel formation in the MI heart. RNA-seq analysis showed that VEGF-induced angiogenesis signaling was involved in the modulation of EA. Western blot results verified that the protein expressions of VEGF, Ras, phospho-p44/42 MAPK, phospho-p38 MAPK, phospho-SAPK/JNK and Akt, were all elevated significantly by EA treatment in the MI heart. Furthermore, increased H3K9 acetylation was also observed according with the VEGF. ChIP assay confirmed that EA treatment could notably stimulate the recruitment of H3K9ace at the VEGF promoter.

Conclusions: Our study demonstrates for the first time that acupuncture can effectively up-regulate VEGF expression through H3K9 acetylation modification directly at the VEGF promoter and hence activate VEGF-induced angiogenesis in rat MI models. We employed high throughput sequencing in this study and, for the first time, generated genome-wide gene expression profiles both in the rat MI model and in acupuncture treatment.

Editor: Meijing Wang, Indiana University School of Medicine, United States of America

Funding: This work was supported by grants from the national basic research program of China (973 program, No. 2012CB518501), the National Natural Science Foundation of China (No. 81273838), the Natural Science Foundation of the Jiangsu Hager Education Institutions of China (No. 12KJB360005), the Natural Science Foundation of the Jiangsu Province of China (No. BK20130956) and the Scientific and Technological Innovation Group of "Qinglan-Project" of Jiangsu Province. The funders had no role in study design, data collection and analysis, decision to publish, or preparation of the manuscript.

Competing Interests: The authors have declared that no competing interests exist.

* E-mail: 0001170@cdutcm.edu.cn (FL); zhubm64@hotmail.com (BMZ)

☯ These authors contributed equally to this work.

Background

Acupuncture, the most well-known complementary and alternative medical approach, has been applied to prevent and cure diseases, including angina[1], palpitation [2], stroke [3], and dysfunction of the left cardiac function in coronary heart disease (CHD) [4] for more than 3000 years. Past records indicate that needling at Neiguan (PC6) acupoint exerts cardioprotective effects on several kinds of ischemic heart injuries, including cardiac surgery, myocardial ischemia-reperfusion, and acute myocardial ischemia by improving hemodynamics, microcirculation and energy metabolism, as well as decreasing susceptibility to ventricular tachycardia [5–13].

Angiogenesis is the generation and expansion of blood vessels from a preexisting vascular network under endogenous or exogenous stimuli and can be used as a therapeutic target for myocardial ischemia. Myocardial function relies on sufficient blood supply and the normal capillary/myocardial fiber ratio of 1:1 (one capillary to one myocardial fiber) in an adult heart. In the case of hypoxia, angiogenesis is triggered by insufficient blood supply [14,15]. Vascular endothelial growth factor (VEGF), one of angiogenic factors, is involved in all phases of angiogenesis, including generation of angiogenic vascular sprout, stabilization of immature neovascular sprout, and maturation of physiological angiogenesis [14]. In ischemic areas, VEGF expression can increase up to 30 times in a few minutes by the accumulation of hypoxia-inducible factor-1 (HIF-1), which activates VEGF transcription by binding to the hypoxia response element (HRE) on the VEGF promoter [16]. However, in the absence of VEGF, the emerging neovascular sprout is destabilized and eventually regresses due to the lack of VEGF signals [17]. All above evidence indicates that VEGF plays an important role in stimulating both physiological and pathological angiogenesis.

In order to investigate whether acupuncture at the PC6 acupoint can regulate VEGF expression and angiogenesis, as well as the mechanism of gene regulation by acupuncture, we generate rat MI models by ligating the left anterior descending coronary artery and applying electroacupuncture (EA) treatment at the PC6 acupoint. In the present study, we demonstrated for the first time that acupuncture can effectively up-regulate VEGF expression through H3K9 acetylation modification directly at the VEGF promoter and hence contribute to angiogenesis in the rat MI model. Our results suggest that post-translation histone modification plays a role in the cardioprotective effects of EA following MI injury.

Materials and Methods

Antibodies and reagents

Antibodies for VEGF, alpha-smooth muscle actin (α-SMA), and Histone H3 were purchased from Abcam (Cambridge, UK). Antibody for CD34 was obtained from Santa Cruz Biotechnology (Santa Cruz, CA, USA). Antibodies for Acetyl-Histone H3 (Lys9) (H3K9ace), Ras, Akt GAPDH and Phospho-MAPK family antibody sampler kit, were obtained from Cell Signaling. Dynabeads protein A was obtained from Invitrogen. Supersignal west pico chemiluminescent substrate was purchased from Pierce (Rockford, IL). Truseq RNA sample prep kit-v2, Truseq DNA sample prep kit-PCR box, c-BOT Multiplex re-hybridization plate and Truseq Sbs kit V3 were all purchased from Illumina.

Animals and grouping

Adult male Sprague Dawley (SD) rats (250–300 g), supplied by the Experimental Animal Center of Nanjing University of Chinese Medicine, were used for this study. All rats were fasted (with free access to water) for 24 h before surgical operation and randomized into control, control+EA (CEA), MI and EA groups. The study was approved by the Institutional Animal Care and Use Committee of Nanjing University of Chinese Medicine, and all procedures were conducted in accordance with the guidelines of the National Institutes of Health Animal Care and Use Committee.

In vivo MI

The rat MI model was created after thoracotomy by applying permanent ligation of the left anterior descending coronary artery (LAD) as described previously [18]. Rats were anaesthetized by inhalation of 5% isoflurane and maintained with 2% isoflurane in a mixture of 70% N2O and 30% O2, then subjected to a tracheal cannula, carotid artery intubation, and thoracotomy between the 3rd and 4th intercostal spaces on the left side of the chest along the sternum, and permanent LAD ligation. In the control group, the same procedure was performed except for the LAD ligation. Blood pressure and ECG were monitored throughout the operation.

Electrocardiogram (ECG) recording of electrode resettlement

To evaluate situation of myocardial ischemia we monitored chest lead of rats. ECG was continuously monitored before, during, and after myocardial ischemia by the use of a computerized PowerLab system (ADInstruments, Australia). For recording ECG of the anterior precordial lead V3–V4, rats were anaesthetized by inhalation of isoflurane as mentioned above, two stainless steel electrodes were placed beneath the skin close and to the left of the xiphoid-process and the dorsal neck, respectively. The reference electrode was placed beneath the skin of the right hindlimb. The areas of Q-wave in ECG [width(s) × voltage (mv)] was recruited as an index of ischemia, and were compared statistically in each group on day 1, day 2, and day 7 after surgery. In addition, the S-T segment of ECG elevated over 100 μV from the baseline was recruited as an index of ischemia. ΔS-T value, the absolute value of S-T segment above and below baseline of each group before surgery and 7 days after surgery, were compared statistically.

EA intervention

As previously described, bilateral PC6 which were located at a point 1.5 cm proximal to the palm crease just above the median nerve [12]. Two acupuncture needles (Gauge-28, 0.5 cm) were separately inserted into each acupoint located on each upper limb, and an electrical current was provided to the needles through an electrical stimulator with a stimulus isolation unit (Han Acuten, WQ1002F, Beijing, China) with parameters of 2/15 Hz at an intensity level of 1 mA, for a total stimulation period of 20 minutes (Fig. S5). The acupuncture needle, 15 mm long and 0.3 mm in diameter, was inserted 2–3 mm into the subcutis. Rats in EA and CEA groups were put under anesthesia after MI or sham operation and were applied EA treatment once a day, for a total of 7 days. Rats were then euthanized with intravenous injections of high-dose pentobarbitone, and cardiac tissues were harvested for morphological or molecular analyses.

Myocardial enzyme analysis

Five milliliters of blood was collected from the jugular vein with a procoagulant on day 1, day 2, and day 7 after surgery and centrifuged (10,000 g, 10 minutes, 4°C). Serum was extracted and analyzed for creatine kinase (CK), creatine kinase-MB (CK-MB), and lactate dehydrogenase (LDH) levels with a biochemistry analyzer.

Histological analysis and Immunofluorescence staining

After sacrificing the rats via intravenous injection of high-dose pentobarbitone at the end of the 7-day EA treatment, cardiac tissues and sections were prepared from the paraffin-embedded hearts. The sections from the apex, mid-left ventricle (LV), and base were stained with H&E and Masson's trichrome according to the manufacturer's protocols (Sigma). Images were acquired using a light microscope (Nikon, Japan). The area of infarction and the total area of LV were traced manually and measured using Image J software (National Institutes of Health Bethesda, MD). Scar size was then measured according to the reference [19].

To assess the angiogenesis, sections of the heart were used for CD34, α-SMA and VEGF immunohistochemistry. Circulating endothelial progenitor cells (cEPCs) were identified by CD34 antibody, smooth muscle cells were identified by α-SMA, and endothelial cells were identified by VEGF. Tissue sections were placed at 70°C for 30 min and subsequently immersed in xylene and ethanol at decreasing concentrations. Slides were then washed in distilled water. After one hour of blocking with the buffer solution, sections were incubated overnight at 4°C with CD34 (1: 200, Abcam), α-SMA (1:500, Abcam), or VEGF (1: 200, Abcam). After rinsing in PBS, slides were then incubated with the appropriate Alexa 568 Goat anti mouse secondary antibody (1:400, Invitrogen) or Alexa 488 Goat anti rabbit secondary antibody (1:400, Invitrogen) for two hours at room temperature; DAPI was then used to stain the nucleus. Sections were mounted with anti-fade fluorescence mounting medium (Dako, Denmark). Images were acquired using a fluorescent microscope at a constant exposure. Approximately 20 randomized fields of each tissue sections, taken at the mid plane of each heart, and containing infarct and border regions, were counted for the stained number of cells. The total numbers of VEGF$^+$, CD34$^+$, α-SMA$^+$ cells from each group were calculated and normalized to the number of DAPI$^+$ cells with Image J software.

RNA-Seq and computational analysis for RNA-seq data

At the end of the 7-day EA treatment, total RNA was extracted by Trizol reagent (Invitrogen) from the harvested hearts. For RNA-Seq, RNA samples were prepared according to the TruSeq RNA Sample Preparation v2 protocol, and the DNA libraries were applied to the cluster generation and sequencing using c-BOT Multiplex re-hybridization plate and Truseq Sbs kit V3. Sequencing was performed using Illumina Hiseq 2000 (Illumina, USA).

After sequencing with HiSeq 2000 (Illumina), raw fastq files were extracted from Illumina BCL using the Illumina CASAVA program. The single-end reads of biological triplicates obtained from each sample were aligned to the rat reference genome (UCSC rn4 assembly) using the TopHat program [20,21]. The Cufflinks program was used to assemble individual transcripts from RNA-seq reads that have been aligned to the genome and to qualify the expression level of each transcript. Differential transcripts expression analysis was performed with the Cuffdiff program. The gene's functional annotation and pathway were analyzed using the DAVID Bioinformatics Resources [22]. The raw data have been deposited onto NCBI'S Read Archhive (SRA) database and the accession number is GSE54132.

Western blot

The cardiac tissues were obtained 7 days post-surgery and lyses with RIPA buffer supplemented with a protease inhibitor cocktail. Protein concentrations were determined using the BCA protein assay (Pierce). Equivalent amounts of protein (30 μg/lane) were resolved electrophoretically by SDS-polyacrylamide gels (10%) and transferred onto PVDF membranes. Nonspecific reactivity was blocked in 5% BSA in TBST (10 mM Tris-HCl, pH 7.5, 150 mM NaCl, 1% Tween-20) for one hour. Membranes were incubated with anti-VEGF (1:1000), anti-H3K9ace (1:1000), anti-Histone H3 (1:1000), Akt(1:1000), Ras(1:1000), Phospho-p44/42 MAPK (1:1000), Phospho-p38 MAPK (1:1000), Phospho-SAPK-JNK(1:1000), and GAPDH (1:3000) overnight at 4°C, followed by incubation with secondary antibodies for one hour at room

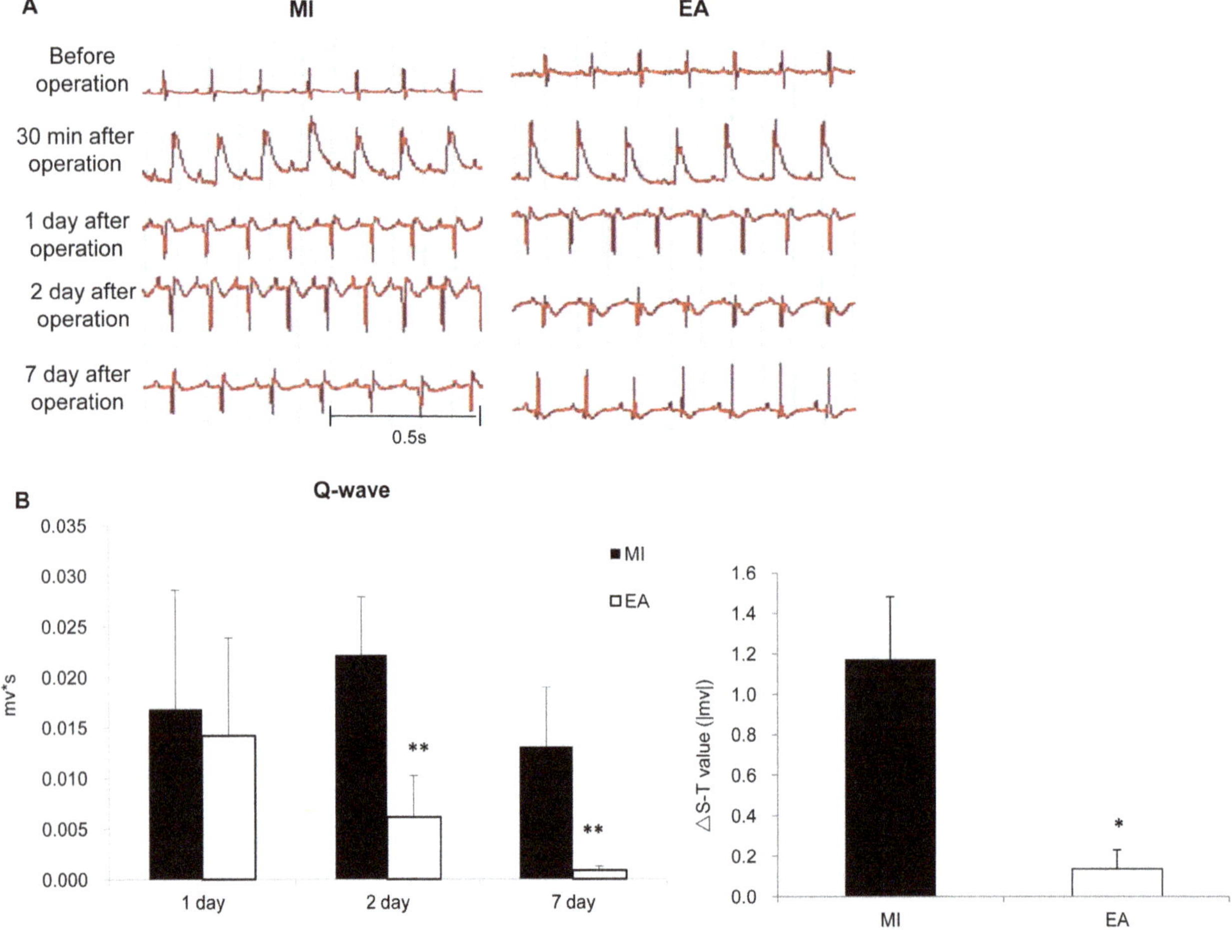

Figure 1. Effects of EA treatment on ECG recording of MI heart. ECG was continuously monitored before, during and after myocardial ischemia. A. Representative ECG recording in anterior precordial lead V3-V4. B. Quantification of Q-wave area value and ΔS-T value in each group. Data were expressed as means ± SD, n = 10, $^{**}P<0.01$ *vs* MI.

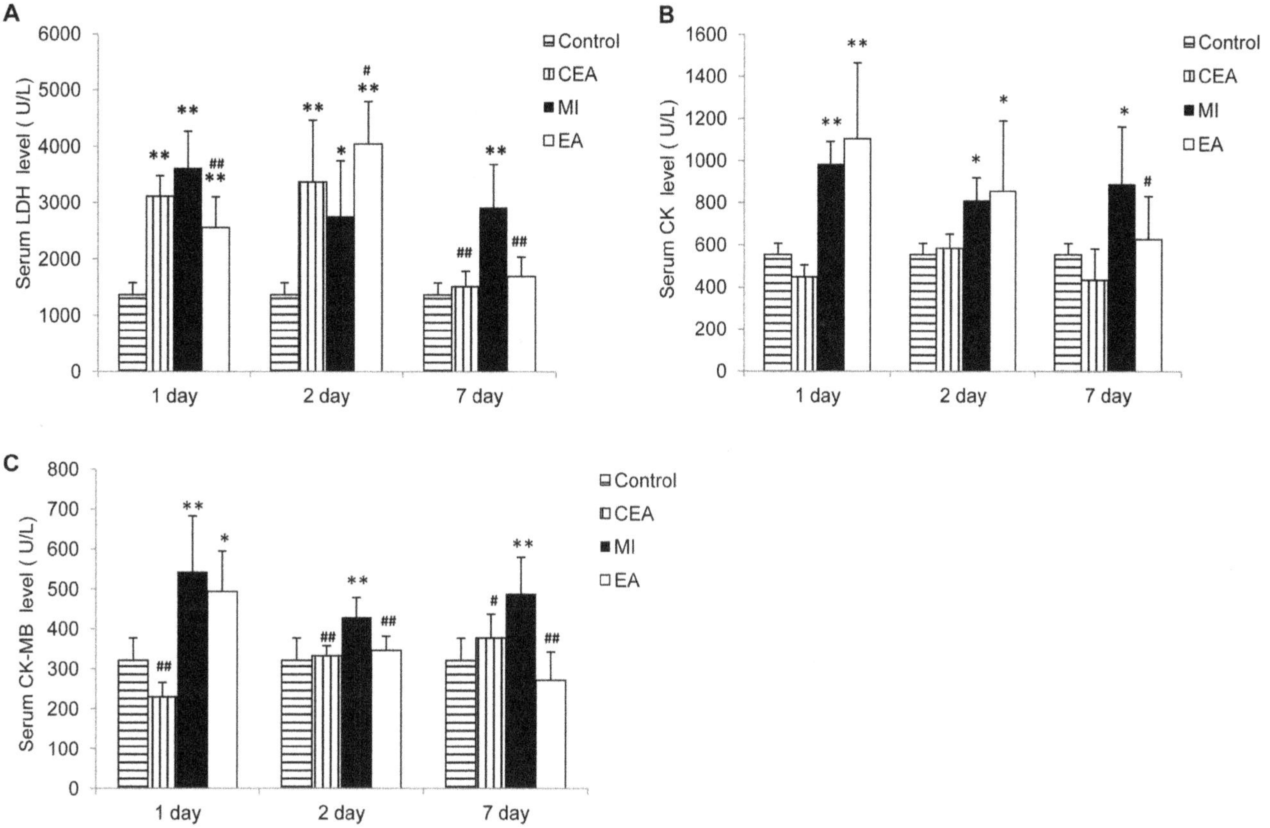

Figure 2. Effects of EA treatment on myocardial enzymes release of MI hearts. Serum was extracts and analyzed for LDH (A), CK (B) and CK-MB (C) levels by biochemistry analyzer on the 1st, 2nd and 7th day after operation. Data were expressed as means ± SD, n = 10, **P<0.01, *P<0.05 vs. Control, $^{\#\#}$ P<0.01, $^{\#}$ P<0.01vs MI.

temperature. Proteins were visualized by using the supersignal west pico chemiluminescent substrate (Pierce).

Chromatin immunoprecipitation (ChIP) assay

To determine histone modifications in the VEGF promoter region, chromatin immunoprecipitation (ChIP) assay was carried out [23]. In brief, the protein-chromatin lysate was fragmented to a length between 200 and 1,000 bp by sonication (Diagenode). The chromatin was precleaned by incubating with Dynabeads protein A and immunoprecipitated with rotation; at 4°C overnight with the antibody against anti-H3K9ace (1:50). The precipitated chromatin was then harvested by Dynabeads protein A and eluted in buffer after a series of washes. The ChIP DNA was eluted and purified by phenol/chloroform method, to reach a final volume of 50 µl. 2 µL of the ChIP DNA was subjected to quantitative analysis by real-time PCR (qPCR). Primers were designed to amplify the promoter region between 500 bp upstream and 1000 bp downstream of TTS at the VEGF gene. The primer sequences are as follows: rat VEGF -485 to -317: forward 5′-CGTAACTTGGGCGAGCCG -3′: and reverse 5′-CGTAACTTGGGCGAGCCG -3′

rat VEGF −403 to −124: forward 5′-GTGTGTCTGGGTA-TAGTGTG-3′ and reverse 5′-GCCACTACTGCGAAATA-GAAA-3′

rat VEGF -68 to +126: forward 5′- GTTTCCA-CAGGTCGTCTC -3′ and reverse 5′- GGGGAGTATGCT-TATCTG -3′

rat VEGF +666 to +928: forward 5′-TGAGTCAAGAGGA-CAGAGAG-3′and reverse 5′-ATTAC-CAGGCCTCTTCTTCC-3′

Fold enrichment in the binding of H3K9ace to VEGF promoter regions in each immunoprecipitation was normalized to the indicated histone binding level in its corresponding input DNA. Two independent ChIP experiments were performed for each analysis, and qPCR was performed twice for each of the ChIP DNA sample. The standard deviation among the experiments did not exceed 10% of the average values. The average values were graphed to demonstrate the relative percent of occupancy.

Statistical analysis

Data were presented as means ± standard deviation (SD). Statistics analysis was performed using SPSS 18.0; multiple group comparisons were made by ANOVA and two group comparison was determined using unpaired 2-tailed Student's t test. P<0.05 was considered statistically significant.

Results

EA at PC6 protected rat heart from MI injury

To investigate protective effects of EA on ischemic injury induced by MI, we first observed the ECG's Q wave area, ST segment, myocardial damage, and myocardial enzyme levels. Our results showed that the diastolic and systolic blood pressure were both decreased after ligation (Fig.S1), the ST segment was noticeably elevated in both MI and EA groups in 30 min, and

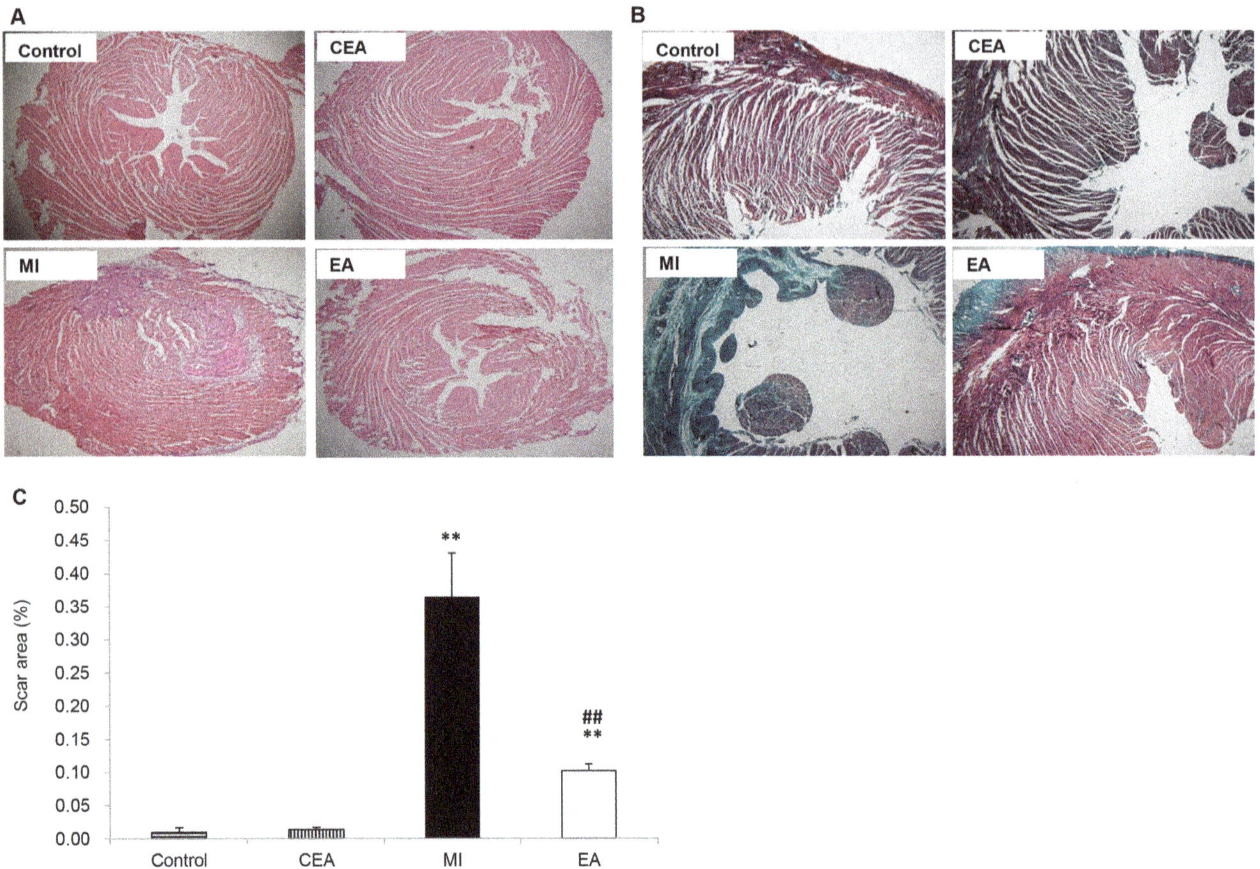

Figure 3. Evaluation of myocardial remodeling. A. Representative image of hematoxylin and eosin (H&E) staining of each group. B. Representative image of Masson's trichrome staining of each group, scale bar, 100 μm. C. Relative quantification of scar size. Data were showed as means ± SD, n = 5, *P<0.01 vs. Control, $^{\#}$ P<0.01vs MI.

the representative necrotic Q-waves were appeared 1 day after operation, indicating the success of the MI model (Fig.1A). Q waves on the 2nd day after operation was deeper than on the 1st day, and was relieved on the 7th day in MI group. However in the EA group, Q-wave areas were significantly decreased the on 2nd and 7th day after operation compared with the MI group. At the same time, we observed that the ΔS-T values were also significantly decreased in the EA group compared with the MI group ($P<0.01$) (Fig.1A and B). The levels of enzymes, which reflect acute myocardial injury, were measured from peripheral blood serum of the rats. Concentrations of LDH, CK, and CK-MB significantly increased in the MI model group from the 1st day through the 7 days after operation. In the EA group, the enzymes concentrations decreased significantly to the level of the control group on the 7th day after operation, and MI induced elevation of CK-MB was alleviated by EA at PC6 early on the 2nd day after operation (Fig.2A, 2B, 2C). Additionally, EA applied on the control rats did not affect most of the enzymes except LDH, which was increased on the 1st and 2nd day after operation and went back to the normal level on 7th day. Meanwhile, rat survival rate in the EA group was also improved compared with the MI model group (Fig.S2). Moreover, the extent of myocardial damage and remodeling was assessed by H&E and Masson's trichrome staining (Fig.3A, 3B, S3 and S4). In the control group and CEA group, myocardial cells and fibers showed integrate structure without inflammatory cell infiltration and swelling. The ischemic heart in the MI group displayed myocardial fiber fracture, edema, and degeneration, as well as a small amount of necrosis, infiltration of inflammatory cells, and fibrosis. EA significantly reduced cardiac tissue damage compared with the MI group; myocardial cell structure was reserved with decreased edema and degeneration of myocardial fibers. Statistical analysis showed that the infarct scar area was decreased from 36.46% to 10.21% in the EA group compared to the MI group ($P<0.001$) (Fig.3C).

Genome-wide profiling of gene expression under EA treatment on MI heart in rats

After we confirmed the cardioprotective effect of EA on MI injury, we further investigated its possible mechanisms. RNA-seq by next generation sequencing was used to identify the rat genome-wide alterations after MI and EA treatment (The raw data shown in GEO with the number GSE54132). Following MI, we saw at least a two-fold increase in the expression of 1023 genes and a similar decrease in the expression of 1139 genes. Interestingly, EA treatment reversed some of the gene expression changes induced by MI; 343 out of 1023 genes whose expressions decreased in the MI group were increased, and 144 out of 1139 genes whose expressions increased in the MI group were decreased post-EA treatment. In addition to these co-regulated genes, other gene expression levels that were not influenced by MI were also regulated by EA (Fig 4A and 4B). Pathway analysis indicated that these co-regulated genes were mainly involved in the calcium signaling pathway, cardiomyopathy related pathways, and cancer

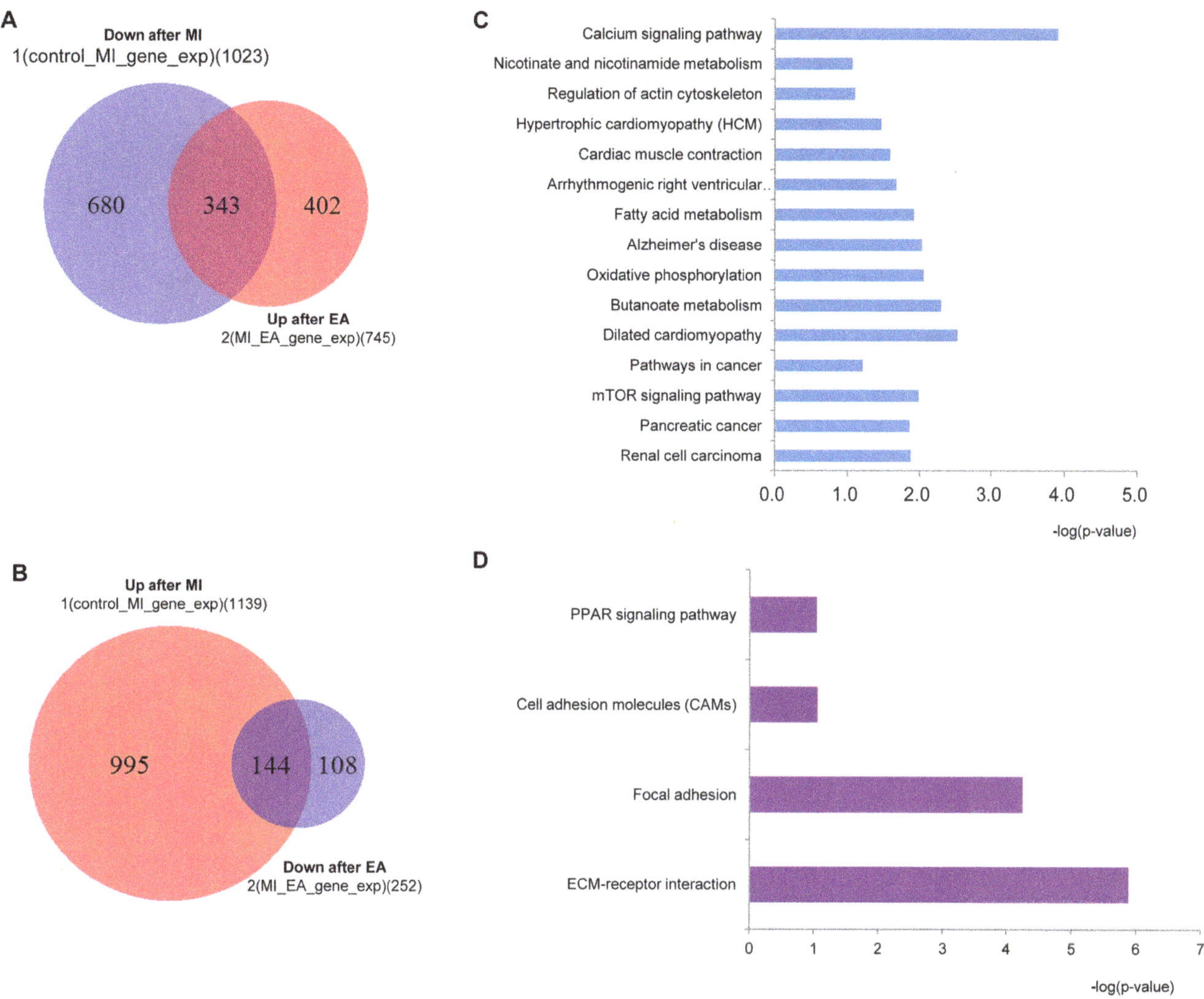

Figure 4. Genome-wide association study results. At the end of EA treatment for 7 days, the total RNA was extracted from the harvested hearts for RNA-Seq analysis. A and B, Venn diagrams of regulated gene numbers by MI and EA treatment. A. Overlapped area represents increased gene number (343) in EA group but decreased in MI group; B. Overlapped area represents decreased gene number (144) in EA group but increased in MI group. C. The top 15 pathways of these genes involved in the 343 genes in A; D. Major pathways of the 144 genes shown in B.

Table 1. VEGF signaling related gene expressions (FPKM).

gene	Control	MI	EA	MI/Control	EA/MI
Vegfb	92.28	52.72	154.27	0.57	2.93
Vegfa	26.28	12.61	26.49	0.48	2.10
Rassf3	3.59	1.40	58.19	0.39	16.22
Map3k13	4.43	1.92	6.78	0.43	3.52
Akt2	70.30	35.712	63.50	0.51	1.78
Aktip	17.43	9.47	18.00	0.54	1.90
Mapk1	25.24	11.01	24.03	0.44	2.18
Mapkapk2	75.60	51.93	155.46	0.69	3.00
Mapkbp1	0.76	0.58	1.20	0.77	2.06
Mapk3	74.65	58.19	81.67	0.78	1.40

related pathways (Fig 4C and 4D), such as VEGF, an angiogenic factor, and VEGF-activated signaling component, including Ras, Akt and MAPK family members, decreased in the MI group, but significantly increased in the EA group (Table 1).

EA at PC6 promoted angiogenesis in ischemic myocardium through activation of VEGF signaling

To verify that angiogenesis is a possible mechanism in the EA-induced myocardioprotective effect; angiogenic responses were examined by immunofluorescence staining of CD34, α-SMA and VEGF. CD34-, α-SMA- and VEGF- positive cells were presented to the circulating endothelial progenitor cells (cEPCs), vascular smooth muscle cells, and endothelial cells, respectively. As shown in Fig.5A and 5C, EA treatment caused a marked increase in CD34-positive cEPCs, suggesting increased vessel density in EA-treated hearts compared with the MI group ($P<0.01$). In the border and center regions of the infarct zone, α-SMA positive vascular density staining was observed, indicating that EA

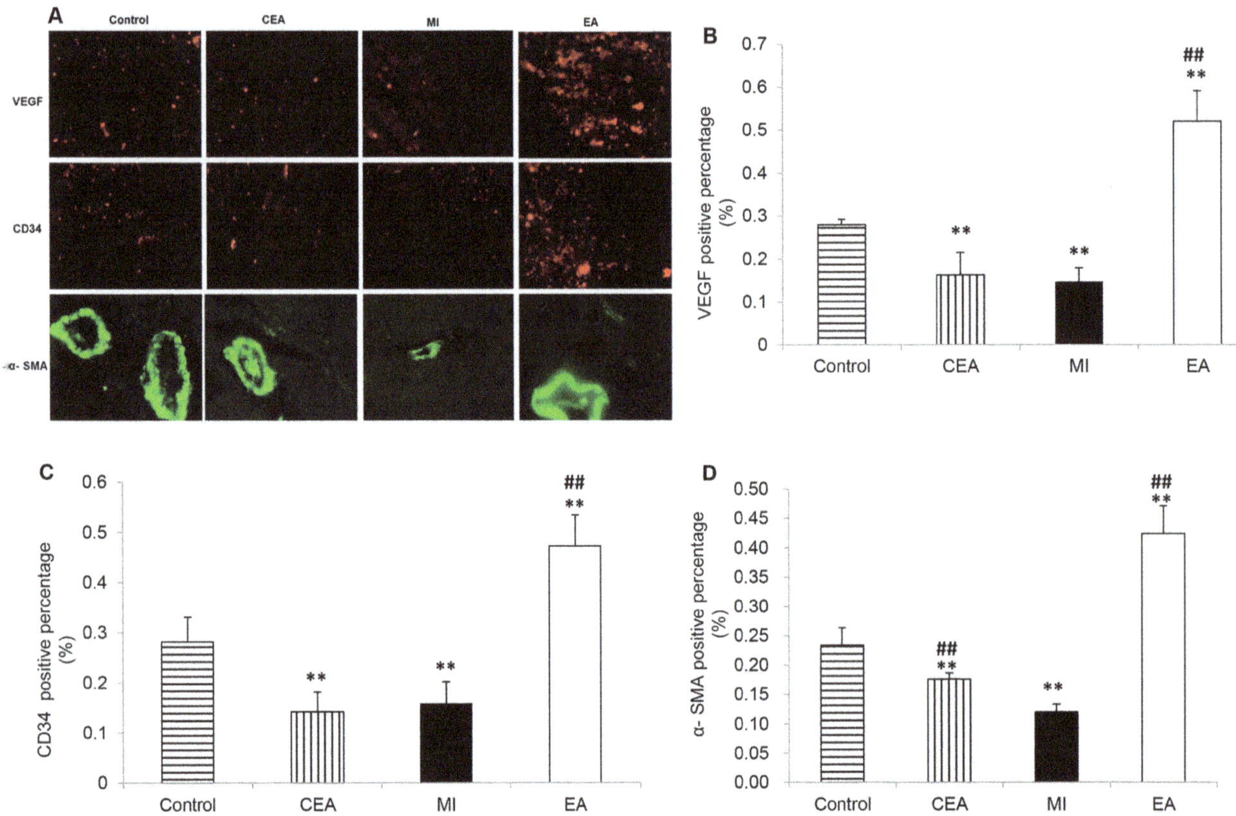

Figure 5. Effect of EA treatment on angiogenesis in MI hearts. A. Representative immunofluorescence staining images of VEGF (red), CD34 (red) and α-SMA (green) in each group, scale bars, 100 μm. B to D, Quantitative analysis of VEGF-positive, CD34-positive and α-SMA–positive percentages. Data were shown as means ± SD, n = 5, **P<0.01 vs. Control, $^{\#\#}$ P<0.01vs MI.

treatment significantly increased α-SMA positive ratio compared with the MI group (Fig.5A and 5D). Likewise, we also observed a significant increase in VEGF-positive staining after treatment with EA, whereas in the center and border regions of the MI heart VEGF protein level markedly decreased (P<0.01) (Fig.5A and 5B), suggesting that VEGF-induced angiogenesis is involved in the EA treatment. Western blot results showed that VEGF protein expression was decreased obviously, accompanying with the decrease of Ras, phospho-p44/42 MAPK, phospho-p38 MAPK, phospho-SAPK/JNK and Akt proteins in the MI group. In contrast, EA treatment inhibited MI induced decrease of these proteins; the phospho-p44/42 MAPK and phospho-p38 MAPK expression were even overexpressed compared with the control group. Surprisingly, in CEA group, the expressions of VEGF, phospho-p44/42 MAPK and phospho-p38 MAPK were also decreased, meanwhile phospho-SAPK/JNK and Akt expressions were significantly increased. (Fig.6A, 6B, 6D)

Elevation of VEGF are regulated directly by H3K9 acetylation

After we validated that VEGF was related to EA-induced angiogenesis, we further explored the mechanism underlying the EA-induced increase of VEGF expression. Western blot results showed that acetylation level of H3K9, an epigenetic marker, was altered according to the expression level of VEGF. The expression of H3K9ace in myocardium decreased in the MI group and the CEA group but increased significantly after EA treatment (P<0.01), which corresponded with the changes in VEGF (Fig.6B, 6D). ChIP assay was then applied to study transcriptional and epigenetic regulation during EA-induced angiogenesis. We measured H3K9ace chromatin occupancy at the VEGF promoter region in the infarct myocardial zone (Fig.7). Our results indicated that H3K9ace occupancy at −500 bp to +200 bp region was augmented prominently by EA treatment (P<0.01), suggesting a direct modification of H3K9 acetylation at the VEGF gene. Thus this mechanism might be a major contributor to angiogenesis in ischemic myocardium and the cardioprotective effect of acupuncture.

Discussion

In light of the theory of Chinese medicine, the use of PC6 in acupuncture is generally advised for the treatment of symptoms of heart and chest diseases, such as palpitation, chest distress, and thoracalgia, nausea, gastralgia, and vomiting. Recently, acupuncture at the PC6 acupoint has been reported to attenuate cardiac injury, such as correcting arrhythmia, reducing apoptosis, and decreasing myocardial enzymes and infarction [9–12], which were induced by acute myocardial ischemia. However, the mechanism underlying the protective effects of acupuncture on MI remains unclear.

In order to investigate the effects of acupuncture on MI when the ischemia was in progress instead of stable stage and to explore the epigenetic modification on the MI with or without EA treatment, which should occur before the pathologic changes are stable, we first generated rat MI models by LAD ligation and applied EA intervention to the MI rats. We evaluated myocardial

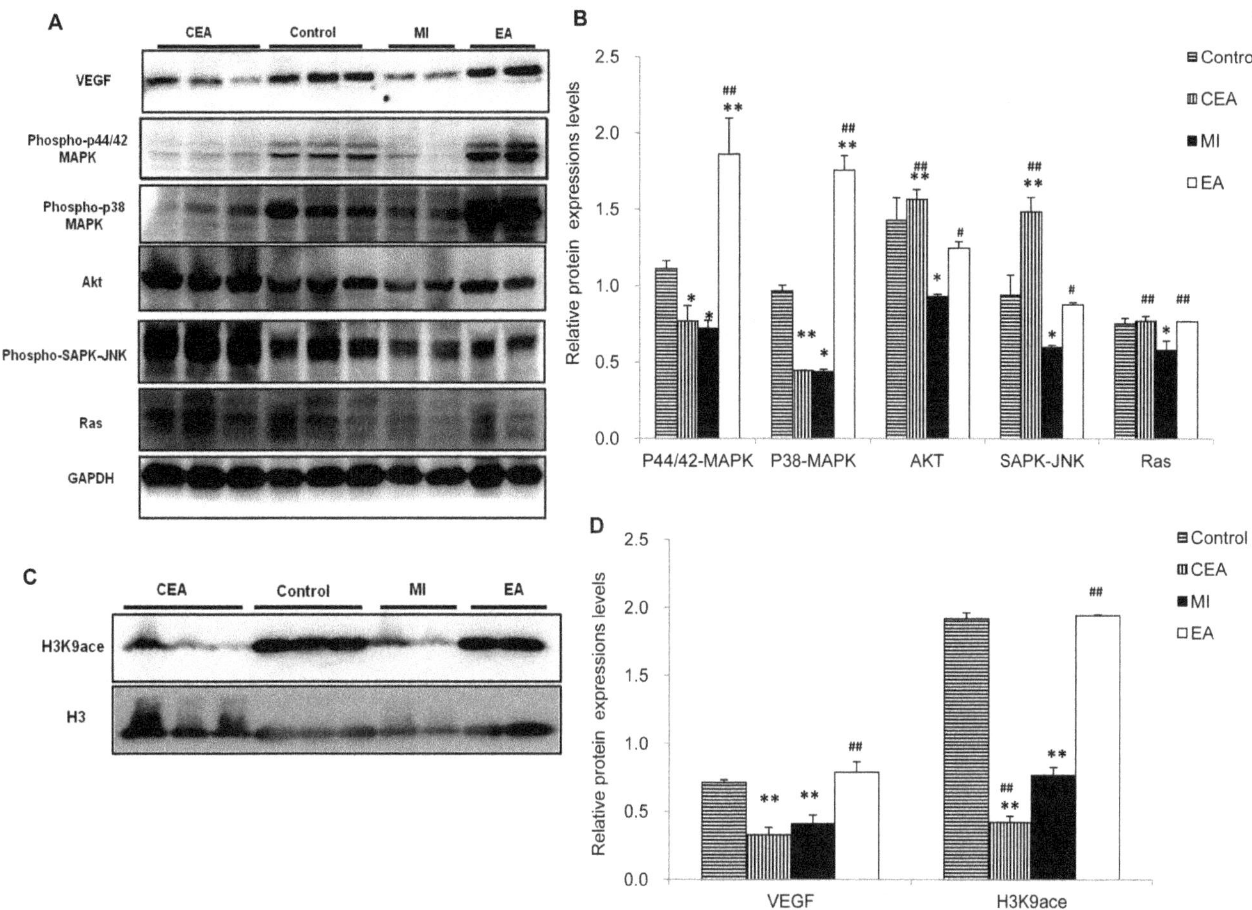

Figure 6. Detection of protein expressions related to VEGF-induced angiogenesis and H3K9 acetylation level. A and C. Representative western blot results of VEGF signaling proteins and H3K9ace in each group. B and D. Quantitative analysis of VEGF signaling proteins and H3K9 ace. Data were showed as means ± SD (n = 4~6), *P<0.05, **P<0.01 vs. Control, # P<0.05, # # P<0.01 vs. MI.

injury by noting ECG's ST segment changes, Q-waves, myocardial enzyme levels, and myocardial histologist. The results suggested that EA treatment decreased ST segment change and Q-wave area, reduced the release of CK, LDH, and CK-MB from the necrosis heart tissue, and alleviated myocardial remodeling. These findings were consistent with previous studies [9–12].

After confirming the cardioprotective effect of acupuncture on MI, we explore its possible mechanisms. Genome-wide expression profiles of rats subjected to MI operation and EA treatment were acquired by RNA-seq. According to our RAN-seq data, EA treatment was able to reverse some MI-induced gene expression changes. Pathway analysis indicated that these genes were mainly involved in the calcium signaling pathway, cardiomyopathy related pathways, and the angiogenesis pathway, which was the main interest of this study. Our data indicated a marked increase in VEGF genes expression as a result of EA treatment. Angiogenesis is known as an adaptive response to tissue hypoxia in ischemic myocardial areas, and it is considered a target in treating ischemic diseases, including myocardial ischemia [14], [24]. Acupuncture treatment has also proven to alleviate ischemic symptoms in other types of ischemic diseases via promoting angiogenesis [25,26]. In the present study, angiogenic responses in ischemic myocardial tissues were examined. Recruitment of cEPCs, as well as proliferation and survival of endothelial cells and vascular smooth muscle cells were necessary for the formation of vascular sprout and lumen. Usually, the high number or density of these cells is indicative of angiogenesis [14]. Our results showed that promoting angiogenesis in ischemic myocardial tissues could be a possible mechanism of the cardioprotective effects of acupuncture in MI cases. Our quantitative analyses for VEGF protein expression levels further confirmed this hypothesis. VEGF-triggered signaling pathways have been well studied. As Cao summarized[27], Ras-Raf-MEK-MAPK is an important cascade for VEGF-induced angiogenesis. Additionally, Akt signaling in endothelial cells also plays critical role in regulating multiple critical steps in angiogenesis, including endothelial cell survival, migration, and capillary-like structure formation[28]. Our genome-wide RNA-seq analysis detected that in accordance with VEGF expression, the expressions of Ras, Akt and several MAPK family members were down-regulated in MI condition and up-regulated by EA treatment (Table 1). Western blot results also showed that VEGF induced Ras-p44/42 MAPK signaling, p38 MAPK signaling, p-JNK signaling and Akt signaling were all activated by EA treatment in MI heart.

Surprisingly and interestingly, the EA treatment on the control rats resulted in reduced expression of VEGF, accompanying with attenuated phospho-p44/42 MAPK and phospho-p38 MAPK expressions. These changes did not induce any pathological phenotypes even these proteins were as low as that in the MI rats. This might be due to a compensatory mechanism by elevating

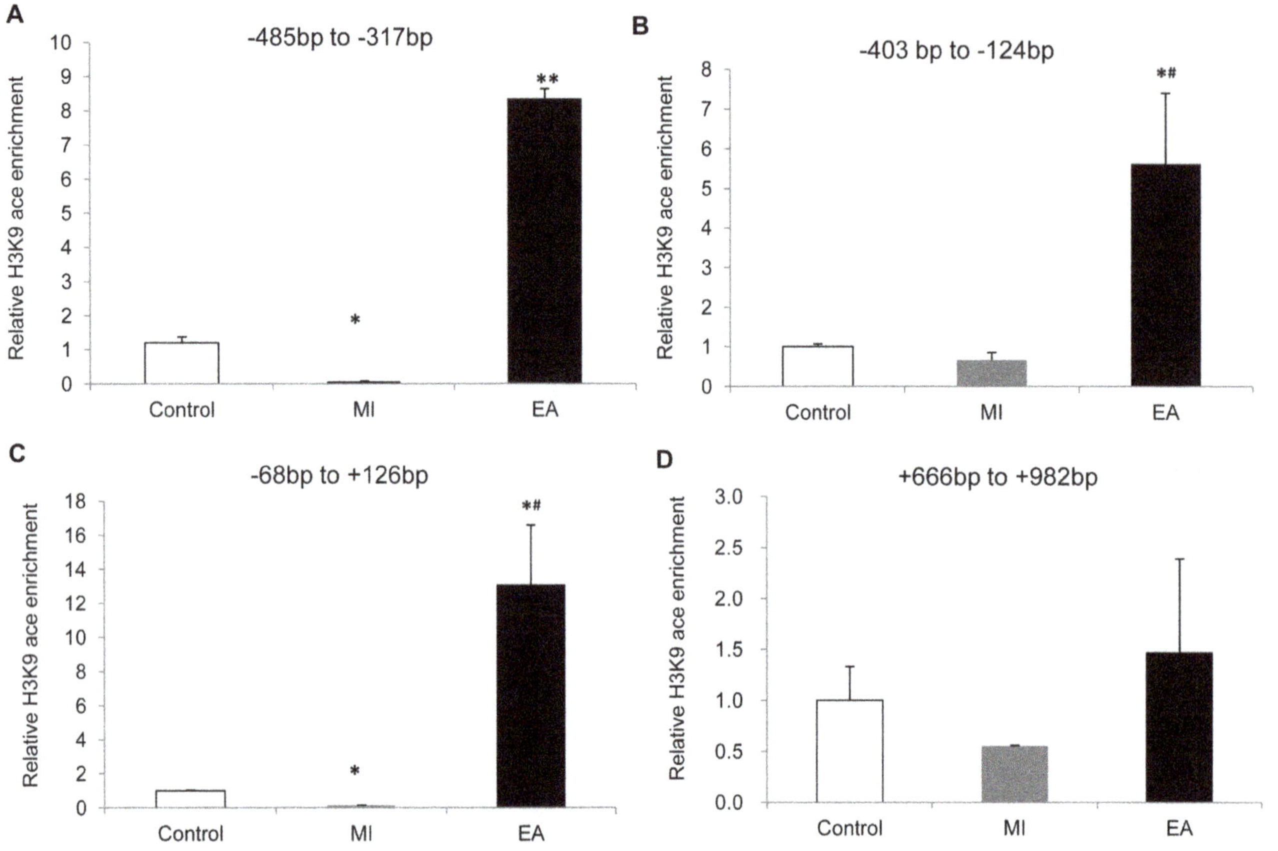

Figure 7. ChIP assay analyses for the enrichment of acetylated H3K9 on the VEGF promoter. For quantitative ChIP analysis, chromatin was extracted from hearts of each group and precipitated with antibodies against H3K9ace. Quantitative PCR was performed to amplify VEGF promoter regions. Results were normalized with respect to input and nonspecific IgG results by using formula [2-(△ Ct) specific antibody/2-(△ Ct) nonspecific IgG], where △Cp is the Cp (immunoprecipitated DNA)- Cp(input) and Cp is the cycle where the threshold is crossed. The bps on the top of each figure shows positions of upstream (+) or downstream (−) of transcription start site on VEGF promoter region (TSS). Data were showed as means ± SD, n=4, *P<0.05, **P<0.01 vs. Control, # P<0.01vs MI.

other essential proteins such as Akt and SAPK/JNK, whose signals were much stronger than that in EA group (Figure 6A, B). This compensation did not occur in the ischemic hearts.

To further explore the mechanism underlying the EA-induced increase of VEGF expression, DNA transcriptional and epigenetic regulations during EA-induced angiogenesis were subjected to measurement. Gene expression depends on chromatin structure, which in turn relies on epigenetic modification of histone. In principle, hyperacetylated and decondensed chromatin facilitate gene transcription, whereas nontranscriptionally active regions are often, although not exclusively, hypoacetylated or hypermethylated [29]. Hypoxia induced increase in VEGF expression has been well accepted, and it has recently been found to increase H3K9 acetylation at the VEGF promoters as well [30]. In this study, we found that the alteration of H3K9 acetylation level was consistent with the expression of VEGF. The expression of H3K9ace in ischemic myocardium decreased, but EA treatment could drastically increase its level, along with the retrieval of the VEGF protein. ChIP assay results indicated that H3K9ace occupancy at several regions of VEGF promoter was all increased by MI, and the augmentation of H3K9ace occupancy was prominently magnified by EA treatment. All these data confirmed that acupuncture at PC6 regulates the VEGF expression directly through H3K9 acetylation. Similarly, a decreased level of acetylation of H3K9 was observed in EA treated control rats (Figure 6C, D), suggesting a strong candidate for mediating the decrease of VEGF, phospho-p44/42 MAPK and phospho-p38 MAPK expressions. It indicated that pre-treatment of electro-acupuncture might be a stimulation to initiate a protective effect on ischemic hearts, similar as an ischemic preconditioning [31–33]. A further study for this hypothesis might be of significance.

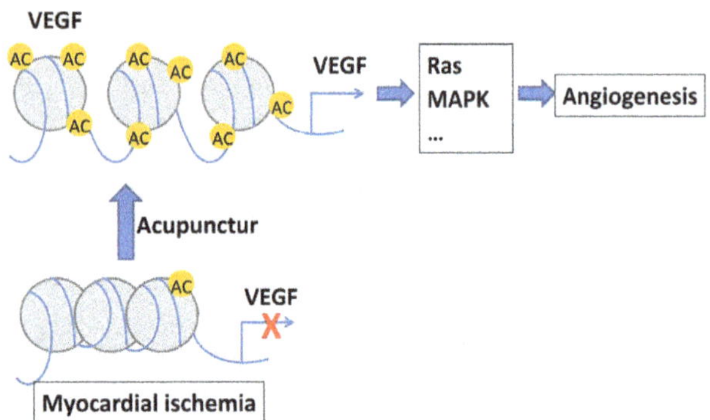

Figure 8. Scheme of a possible mechanism for EA on myocardial ischemia through VEGF signaling.

Conclusions

In summary, our data indicate that acupuncture exerts a cardioprotective effect in MI rats by promoting angiogenesis, which is mediated through H3K9 acetylation modification directly at the VEGF promoter (Fig.8). We also present evidence that histone modification plays a role in the cardioprotective effects of EA upon MI injury, and H3K9 acetylation can be a therapeutic target for EA or cardioprotective medicines following myocardial ischemia, although additional molecular experiments may be needed to verify its therapeutic potentials. In addition, our study provides, for the first time, informative genome-wide profiles of gene expressions in MI injury and electroacupuncture treatment that can be used in future studies. Further ChIP-seq analyses will be employed to investigate genome-wide H3K9ace modification and other epigenetic marks that could regulate gene expressions in the EA treatment of MI cases.

Supporting Information

Figure S1 Blood pressure change after ligation of LAD. During the operation, rats blood pressure were monitored by the carotid artery intubation, data were expressed as means ± SD (n = 10), ** $P<0.01$ *vs.* before operation. A. Carotid artery diastolic; B. systolic blood pressure.
(TIF)

Figure S2 Survival rate of rats in each group. The survival number of each group was recorded very day after operation, and the survival rate of each group was calculated with the formula: (survival rat number/the total rat number) ×100%. Data were expressed as means ± SD, n = 10~32, significantly compared $P<0.001$, EA group vs. MI group.
(TIF)

Figure S3 Representative Hematoxylin and Eosin (H&E) staining results of each group. Cardiac tissues were collected at the end of EA treatment for 7 days, and prepared for H&E staining. The sections from the apex (a to d, 40 magnification), mid-left ventricle (e to h, 40 magnification), and the ventricular wall (i to p, 200 magnification) were shown.
(TIF)

Figure S4 Representative Masson's trichrome staining results of each group. Cardiac tissues were collected at the end of EA treatment for 7 days, and prepared for Masson's trichrome staining. The sections showed the results by different amplifications (a to d, 40 magnification, e to h, 100 magnification,i to l, 200 magnification, m to p, 400 magnification).
(TIF)

Figure S5 Schematic diagram of rats under the EA treatment on PC6.
(TIF)

Acknowledgments

We thank WX LIU (University of Pennsylvania School of Veterinary Medicine) for editing of English.

Author Contributions

Conceived and designed the experiments: BMZ FL BX. Performed the experiments: SPF SYH SFL WXS YH HH QL NW XLL. Analyzed the data: SYH NW. Wrote the paper: BMZ SPF. Performed computational analysis for RNA-seq: CJH.

References

1. Xu FH, Wang JM (2005) [Clinical observation on acupuncture combined with medication for intractable angina pectoris]. Zhongguo Zhen Jiu 25: 89–91.
2. Hu J (2008) Acupuncture treatment of palpitation. J Tradit Chin Med 28: 228–230.
3. Zhang F, Wu Y, Jia J (2011) Electro-acupuncture can alleviate the cerebral oedema of rat after ischemia. Brain Inj 25: 895–900.
4. Meng J (2004) The effects of acupuncture in treatment of coronary heart diseases. J Tradit Chin Med 24: 16–19.
5. Ni X, Xie Y, Wang Q, Zhong H, Chen M, et al. (2012) Cardioprotective effect of transcutaneous electric acupoint stimulation in the pediatric cardiac patients: a randomized controlled clinical trial. Paediatr Anaesth 22: 805–811.
6. Yang L, Yang J, Wang Q, Chen M, Lu Z, et al. (2010) Cardioprotective effects of electroacupuncture pretreatment on patients undergoing heart valve replacement surgery: a randomized controlled trial. Ann Thorac Surg 89: 781–786.
7. Zhang H, Liu L, Huang G, Zhou L, Wu W, et al. (2009) Protective effect of electroacupuncture at the Neiguan point in a rabbit model of myocardial ischemia-reperfusion injury. Can J Cardiol 25: 359–363.
8. Wang SB, Chen SP, Gao YH, Luo MF, Liu JL (2008) Effects of electroacupuncture on cardiac and gastric activities in acute myocardial ischemia rats. World J Gastroenterol 14: 6496–6502.
9. Gao J, Zhang L, Wang Y, Lu B, Cui H, et al. (2008) Antiarrhythmic effect of acupuncture pretreatment in rats subjected to simulative global ischemia and reperfusion—involvement of adenylate cyclase, protein kinase A, and L-type Ca2+ channel. J Physiol Sci 58: 389–396.
10. Lujan HL, Kramer VJ, DiCarlo SE (2007) Electroacupuncture decreases the susceptibility to ventricular tachycardia in conscious rats by reducing cardiac metabolic demand. Am J Physiol Heart Circ Physiol 292: H2550–2555.
11. Gao J, Fu W, Jin Z, Yu X (2006) A preliminary study on the cardioprotection of acupuncture pretreatment in rats with ischemia and reperfusion: involvement of cardiac beta-adrenoceptors. J Physiol Sci 56: 275–279.
12. Tsou MT, Huang CH, Chiu JH (2004) Electroacupuncture on PC6 (Neiguan) attenuates ischemia/reperfusion injury in rat hearts. Am J Chin Med 32: 951–965.
13. Tjen ALSC, Li P, Longhurst JC (2003) Prolonged inhibition of rostral ventral lateral medullary premotor sympathetic neurons by electroacupuncture in cats. Auton Neurosci 106: 119–131.
14. Lorier G, Tourino C, Kalil RA (2011) Coronary angiogenesis as an endogenous response to myocardial ischemia in adults. Arq Bras Cardiol 97: e140–148.
15. Ferrara N, Kerbel RS (2005) Angiogenesis as a therapeutic target. Nature 438: 967–974.
16. Pugh CW, Ratcliffe PJ (2003) Regulation of angiogenesis by hypoxia: role of the HIF system. Nat Med 9: 677–684.
17. Jain RK (2003) Molecular regulation of vessel maturation. Nat Med 9: 685–693.
18. Tseng A, Stabila J, McGonnigal B, Yano N, Yang MJ, et al. (2010) Effect of disruption of Akt-1 of lin(−)c-kit(+) stem cells on myocardial performance in infarcted heart. Cardiovasc Res 87: 704–712.
19. Cheng K, Li TS, Malliaras K, Davis DR, Zhang Y, et al. (2010) Magnetic targeting enhances engraftment and functional benefit of iron-labeled cardiosphere-derived cells in myocardial infarction. Circ Res 106: 1570–1581.
20. Trapnell C, Pachter L, Salzberg SL (2009) TopHat: discovering splice junctions with RNA-Seq. Bioinformatics 25: 1105–1111.
21. Trapnell C, Roberts A, Goff L, Pertea G, Kim D, et al. (2012) Differential gene and transcript expression analysis of RNA-seq experiments with TopHat and Cufflinks. Nat Protoc 7: 562–578.
22. Huang da W, Sherman BT, Lempicki RA (2009) Systematic and integrative analysis of large gene lists using DAVID bioinformatics resources. Nat Protoc 4: 44–57.
23. Dasgupta P, Chellappan SP (2007) Chromatin immunoprecipitation assays: molecular analysis of chromatin modification and gene regulation. Methods Mol Biol 383: 135–152.
24. Henry TD, Annex BH, McKendall GR, Azrin MA, Lopez JJ, et al. (2003) The VIVA trial: Vascular endothelial growth factor in Ischemia for Vascular Angiogenesis. Circulation 107: 1359–1365.
25. Park SI, Sunwoo YY, Jung YJ, Chang WC, Park MS, et al. (2012) Therapeutic Effects of Acupuncture through Enhancement of Functional Angiogenesis and Granulogenesis in Rat Wound Healing. Evid Based Complement Alternat Med 2012: 464586.
26. Du Y, Shi L, Li J, Xiong J, Li B, et al. (2011) Angiogenesis and improved cerebral blood flow in the ischemic boundary area were detected after electroacupuncture treatment to rats with ischemic stroke. Neurol Res 33: 101–107.
27. Cao Y (2010) Wake-up call for endothelial cells. Blood 115: 2336–2337.
28. Shiojima I, Walsh K (2002) Role of Akt signaling in vascular homeostasis and angiogenesis. Circ Res 90: 1243–1250.
29. Jenuwein T, Allis CD (2001) Translating the histone code. Science 293: 1074–1080.

30. Lu Y, Chu A, Turker MS, Glazer PM (2011) Hypoxia-induced epigenetic regulation and silencing of the BRCA1 promoter. Mol Cell Biol 31: 3339–3350.
31. Sun XC, Xian XH, Li WB, Li L, Yan CZ, et al. (2010) Activation of p38 MAPK participates in brain ischemic tolerance induced by limb ischemic preconditioning by up-regulating HSP 70. Exp Neurol 224: 347–355.
32. Zhang J, Bian HJ, Li XX, Liu XB, Sun JP, et al. (2010) ERK-MAPK signaling opposes rho-kinase to reduce cardiomyocyte apoptosis in heart ischemic preconditioning. Mol Med 16: 307–315.
33. Zhao L, Liu X, Liang J, Han S, Wang Y, et al. (2013) Phosphorylation of p38 MAPK mediates hypoxic preconditioning-induced neuroprotection against cerebral ischemic injury via mitochondria translocation of Bcl-xL in mice. Brain Res 1503: 78–88.

13

Impact of Including Korean Randomized Controlled Trials in Cochrane Reviews of Acupuncture

Kun Hyung Kim[1], Jae Cheol Kong[2], Jun-Yong Choi[3], Tae-Young Choi[4], Byung-Cheul Shin[5], Steve McDonald[6], Myeong Soo Lee[4]*

1 Department of Acupuncture and Moxibustion Medicine, Korean Medicine Hospital, Yangsan, South Korea, **2** Department of Rehabilitation Medicine, College of Korean Medicine, Wonkwang University, Iksan, South Korea, **3** Department of Korean Medical Science, School of Korean Medicine, Pusan National University, Yangsan, South Korea, **4** Medical Research Division, Korea Institute of Oriental Medicine, Daejeon, South Korea, **5** Department of Rehabilitation Medicine, School of Korean Medicine, Pusan National University, Yangsan, South Korea, **6** Australasian Cochrane Centre, School of Public Health and Preventive Medicine, Monash University, Melbourne, Victoria, Australia

Abstract

Objective: Acupuncture is commonly practiced in Korea and is regularly evaluated in clinical trials. Although many Cochrane reviews of acupuncture include searches of both English and Chinese databases, there is no information on the value of searching Korean databases. This study aimed to investigate the impact of searching Korean databasesand journals for trials eligible for inclusion in existing Cochrane acupuncture reviews.

Methods: We searched 12 Korean databases and seven Korean journals to identify randomised trials meeting the inclusion criteria for acupuncture reviews in the *Cochrane Database of Systematic Reviews*. We compared risk of bias assessments of the Korean trials with the trials included in the Cochrane acupuncture reviews. Where possible, we added data from the Korean trials to the existing meta-analyses in the relevant Cochrane review and conducted sensitivity analyses to test the robustness of the results.

Results: Sixteen Korean trials (742 participants) met the inclusion criteria for eight Cochrane acupuncture reviews (125 trials; 13,041 participants). Inclusion of the Korean trials provided data for 20% of existing meta-analyses (24 out of 120). Inclusion of the Korean trials did not change the direction of effect in any of the existing meta-analyses. The effect size and heterogeneity remained mostly unchanged. In only one meta-analysis did the significance change. Compared to the studies included in the Cochrane acupuncture reviews, the risk of bias in the Korean trials was higher in terms of outcome assessor blinding and allocation concealment.

Conclusions: Many Korean studies contributed additional data to the existing meta-analyses in Cochrane acupuncture reviews. Although inclusion of these studies did not alter the results of the meta-analyses, comprehensive searches of the literature are important to avoid potential language bias. The identification and inclusion of eligible Korean trials should be considered for reviews of acupuncture.

Editor: Neil R. Smalheiser, University of Illinois-Chicago, United States of America

Funding: Myeong Soo Lee and Tae-Young Choi were supported by Korea Institute of Oriental Medicine (C12080 and K12130). The funders had no role in study design, data collection and analysis, decision to publish, or preparation of the manuscript.

Competing Interests: The authors have declared that no competing interests exist.

* E-mail: drmslee@gmail.com

Background

Systematic reviews and meta-analyses of the best available evidence can inform decision-making in clinical practice, guide further research, and lead to the efficient allocation of resources [1]. The *Cochrane Database of Systematic Reviews* (*CDSR*) is regarded as a significant and reliable resource of systematic reviews of the effects of a broad range of healthcare interventions in both conventional and complementary medicine. The reputation of Cochrane reviews is based on their comprehensive search strategies, periodical updates and rigorous analytic methods [2].

Acupuncture is a therapeutic intervention that has traditionally been used in East Asian regions, such as China, Korea, Japan, and Vietnam, and one that more recently, has been increasingly accepted and popularized in Western societies. Many controlled clinical trials of acupuncture are widely available in medical databases (e.g., MEDLINE). At the same time, there are also many studies that are indexed in less widely available local databases that include languages other than English as the primary language [3,4,5,6].

When preparing Cochrane reviews, it is strongly recommended that review authorssearch at least three databases that use English as the principal language (i.e., EMBASE, MEDLINE and CENTRAL) and conduct extensive literature searches that cover all relevant languages to avoid publication, language, and citation biases [7]. An empirical study revealed that language bias derived from language-restricted search strategies, or from ignorance of certain databases that employ languages other than English, has been known to significantly affect the results of systematic reviews in complementary and alternative medicine (CAM) [8]. This study showed that systematic reviews of CAM resulted in 63% smaller effect estimates when only English studies were included compared to those without any restriction on thelanguage of included studies. However, in that study, most of the CAM trials in languages other than English (LOE) were published in European countries that had evaluated CAM interventions other than acupuncture. Thus, the impact of language bias due to the omission of papers from Asian databases when evaluating the evidence about effects of acupuncture still remains largely unknown.

In Cochrane acupuncture reviews, the decision to search databases of languages other than English seems to depend, at least partly, on individual review authors and the topic-related Cochrane Review Groups (CRGs). As a result, the search strategies of many Cochrane reviews of acupuncture are characterized by considerable heterogeneity [9]. A previous study found that the number of databases searched varied among Cochrane acupuncture reviews, with only two out of ten reviews searching Chinese databases [4]. Another study revealed that 26 out of 65 Cochrane acupuncture reviews and protocols searched Chinese language databases [9]. Both studies emphasized the inclusion of Chinese databases to prevent bias associated with the exclusion of controlled trials reported in languages other than English.

While the importance of including Chinese databases in Cochrane systematic reviews of acupuncture is highlighted, the potential influence upon Cochrane or non-Cochrane acupuncture reviews of controlled trials in East Asian databases, other than those in Chinese, remains largely unknown. In our pilot study using the January 2011 issue of CDSR, 59 Cochrane reviews and protocols that regarded acupuncture as a primary intervention were identified [10]. The number of Cochrane reviews or protocols that included at least one Chinese database in their search was significantly higher (44 out of 59) than those in the study of Lui et al., [9] whereas the number that included at least one Korean database search was much smaller (4 out of 59). Although the number of Cochrane acupuncture reviews and protocols that include Chinese databases in the search is increasing, the lack of relevant database searches using languages other than English or Chinese still increases the susceptibility of these searches to the risk of language bias. Currently, there is no information on the influence of Korean papers reported in the Korean language upon Cochrane acupuncture reviews. To minimize potential language bias and ensure that comprehensive searchesare used to update Cochrane acupuncture reviews in future, the value of additional searching of Korean databases needs to be tested and its potential influence explored.

Study objective

This study aimed to investigate whether the inclusion of searches of Korean databases might alter the results of Cochrane acupuncture reviews. We were also interested in any additional information that might be brought out by the hypothetical inclusion of Korean databases in the existing Cochrane acupuncture reviews.

Methods

Eligibility criteria

Randomized controlled trials (RCTs) written in Korean or English and indexed in Korean databases were eligible for this study. We decided not to include Korean RCTs written in English and indexed in English databases, because these studies might already have been identified as potentially eligible RCTs and thus could not serve the purpose of this study.

RCTs of patients with any particular health problems or diseases that corresponded to existing Cochrane acupuncture reviews were eligible. RCTs of healthy individuals were excluded.

Parallel group or crossover RCTs that involved any type of acupuncture point stimulation as treatment interventions, such as needle acupuncture, acupressure, device-involved acupuncture point stimulation (i.e., wrist band application) were deemed eligible. RCTs that employed moxibustion (a heat stimulation on acupuncture points using herbal preparations containing *Artemisia vulgaris*) [11] as a primary treatment intervention were excluded because we defined minimum criteria of acupuncture to involve a mechanical stimulation of predefined points (i.e., meridian points, Ashi points or local trigger points). RCTs providing *pharmacopuncture* (i.e., herbal injectionon acupuncture points) as a treatment intervention were only included if the Cochrane review clearly mentioned the inclusion of these studies or included these studies in the results. Otherwise, those studies were excluded.

Searching methods and study-review selection process

For the initial selection of relevant Cochrane acupuncture reviews, the July 2011 issue of CDSR was searched using the term "acupuncture." Reviews that considered acupuncture as a primary intervention were eligible for this study. Protocols and reviews that included acupuncture as one of various interventions were excluded. The topics of Cochrane reviews were screened and selected to identify whether the condition in the review related to

Table 1. Search terms used and journals searched.

Search terms used	
Acupuncture related	Acupuncture OR acupressure OR acupoint OR meridian OR acup*
Design related	Random OR control OR group OR divide
Journals searched	Journal of Korean Acupuncture and Moxibustion Society
	Korean Journal of Acupuncture (formerly the Journal of Korean AM-Meridian & Pointology Society)
	Journal of Pharmacopuncture
	Journal of Oriental Rehabilitation Medicine
	Journal of Korea CHUNA Manual Medicine for Spine & Nerves
	Journal of Korean Oriental Medicine
	Journal of Korean Oriental Internal Medicine

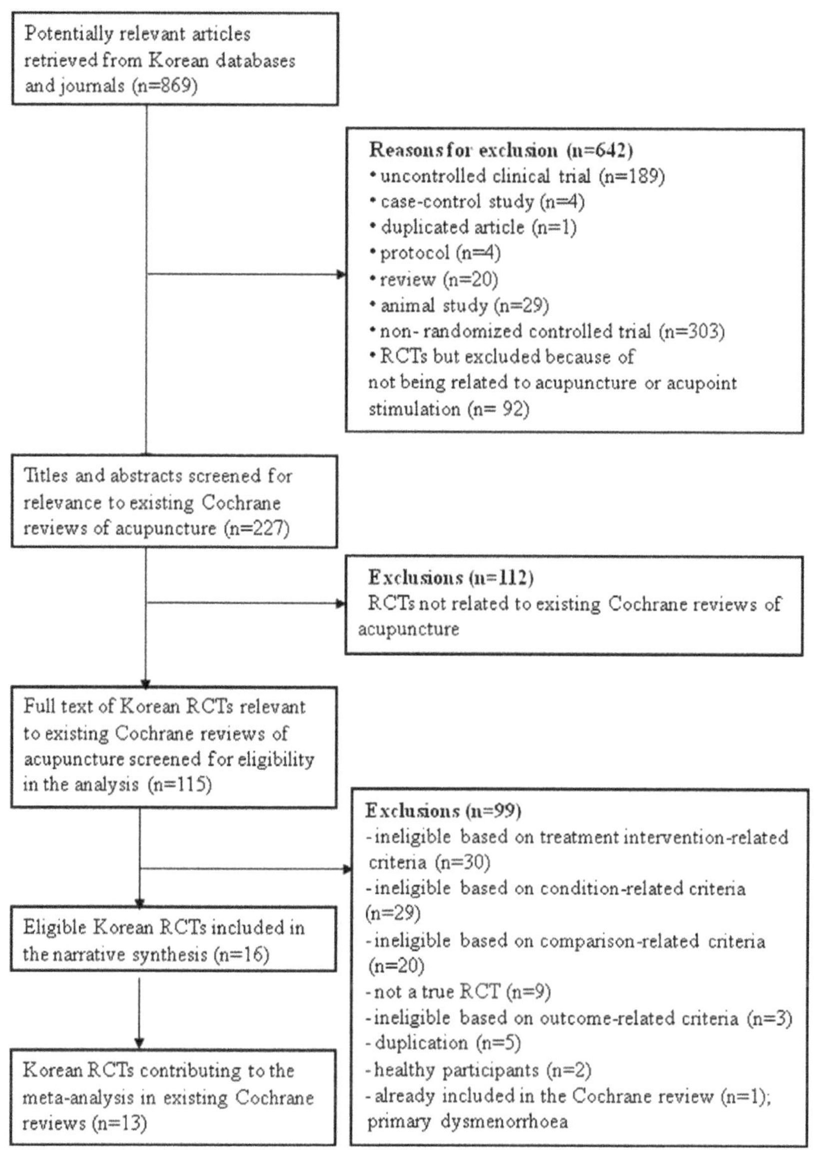
Potentially relevant articles retrieved from Korean databases and journals (n=869)
Reasons for exclusion (n=642)
• uncontrolled clinical trial (n=189)
• case-control study (n=4)
• duplicated article (n=1)
• protocol (n=4)
• review (n=20)
• animal study (n=29)
• non-randomized controlled trial (n=303)
• RCTs but excluded because of not being related to acupuncture or acupoint stimulation (n= 92)
Titles and abstracts screened for relevance to existing Cochrane reviews of acupuncture (n=227)
Exclusions (n=112)
RCTs not related to existing Cochrane reviews of acupuncture
Full text of Korean RCTs relevant to existing Cochrane reviews of acupuncture screened for eligibility in the analysis (n=115)
Exclusions (n=99)
- ineligible based on treatment intervention-related criteria (n=30)
- ineligible based on condition-related criteria (n=29)
- ineligible based on comparison-related criteria (n=20)
- not a true RCT (n=9)
- ineligible based on outcome-related criteria (n=3)
- duplication (n=5)
- healthy participants (n=2)
- already included in the Cochrane review (n=1); primary dysmenorrhoea
Eligible Korean RCTs included in the narrative synthesis (n=16)
Korean RCTs contributing to the meta-analysis in existing Cochrane reviews (n=13)

Figure 1. Flowchart of trial selection process. RCT = randomized controlled trial.

those in the Korean RCTs. The texts of relevant Cochrane reviews were read in full for further analysis.

As for identifying the Korean RCTs that were able to be matched with the topics of published Cochrane acupuncture reviews, one author (JCK) conducted searches of controlled clinical trialsof acupuncture in 12 Korean academic portal databases (i.e., NANET, RISS4U, KISS, DBpia, KMbase, KoreaMed, KISTI, NDSL, OASIS, Dlibrary, KoreanTK, and RICHIS) from the time of their inception to July 2011. Unpublished theses and dissertations were also searched. In most Korean electronic databases, only simple Boolean searches were available. As not all Korean journals related to acupuncture are registered in the Korean academic portal databases, studies recorded electronically on the websites of seven acupuncture-related journals were also searched to ensure completeness of the search process. Since some Cochrane reviews included quasi-randomized trials, and because our experience showed that Korean RCTs did not always clearly demonstrate in the titles or abstracts that they were randomized, we included studies whose methods of randomization seemed doubtful at an initial screening phase. A list of search terms and journals searched is provided in Table 1.

For the initial selection of Korean RCTs, one author (JCK) examined the titles and abstracts obtained from the initial search and selected all potentially relevant studies. At this stage, only explicitly unrelated studies, including animal studies, surveys, narrative reviews, and case reports that could be identified by titles and abstracts, were excluded.

Titles and abstracts of screened studies were examined to check whether the topics corresponded to those of existing Cochrane reviews. Korean RCTs that did not match the topics of existing Cochrane reviews were discarded. The same author performed all the aforementioned study-selection processes.

The full texts of selected studies were then reviewed independently by three pairs of reviewers (KHK-JYC, BCS-JCK, and MSL-TYC) matched according to their clinical specializations. The purpose of this step was to select RCTs that met the specific eligibility criteria for each Cochrane review and to conduct the

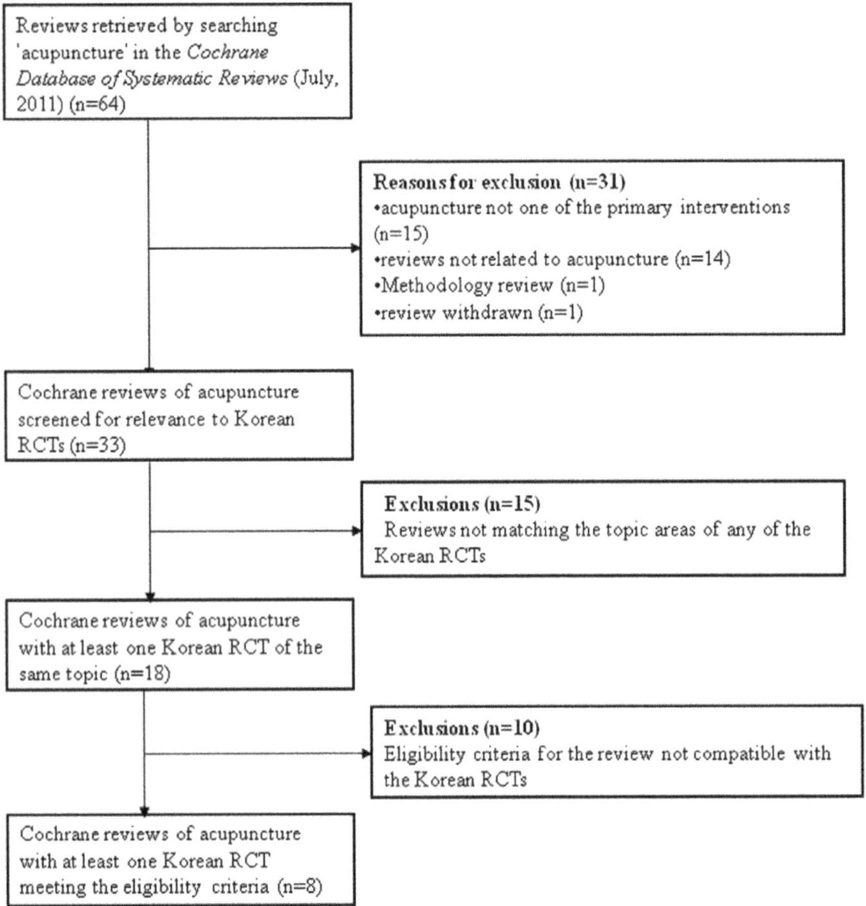
Reviews retrieved by searching 'acupuncture' in the Cochrane Database of Systematic Reviews (July, 2011) (n=64)
Reasons for exclusion (n=31)
•acupuncture not one of the primary interventions (n=15)
•reviews not related to acupuncture (n=14)
•Methodology review (n=1)
•review withdrawn (n=1)
Cochrane reviews of acupuncture screened for relevance to Korean RCTs (n=33)
Exclusions (n=15)
Reviews not matching the topic areas of any of the Korean RCTs
Cochrane reviews of acupuncture with at least one Korean RCT of the same topic (n=18)
Exclusions (n=10)
Eligibility criteria for the review not compatible with the Korean RCTs
Cochrane reviews of acupuncture with at least one Korean RCT meeting the eligibility criteria (n=8)

Figure 2. Flowchart of review selection process. RCT = randomized controlled trial.

assessment of the risk of bias. The entire data extraction, excluding assessment of the risk of bias, was conducted by two authors independently. No attempt was made to conceal the names of the authors, institutions, or journals that published the original studies. We attempted to resolve any disagreements among the authors by convening monthly whole-group discussions over a period of six months, producing as great a degree of consensus as possible.

Data extraction

Data extraction of eligible Korean RCTs was performed as follows: general trial information (year of publication, sample size); assessment of the risk of bias using the same criteria describedin the corresponding Cochrane review; trial outcomes as defined by the relevant Cochrane review. For reviews of low back pain trials, the Cochrane Back Group criteria were used to assess methodological quality [12]. Otherwise, risk of bias was assessed according to the Cochrane Handbook [13]. General information about trials already included in the relevant Cochrane acupuncture reviews were also extracted and compared to those of eligible Korean RCTs, to determine whether there were any trends showing differences in trial characteristics. The frequency of each database searched in Cochrane acupuncture reviews was counted to produce a descriptive summary.

Comparison between Korean RCTs and studies included in the Cochrane reviews in regard to methodological quality

Similar to previous research , assessment of the risk of bias was conducted for two domains (i.e., allocation concealment and assessor blinding) in order to enable comparison between Korean RCTs and studies included in the Cochrane reviews with respect to their methodological quality [7]. Previous research has found that inadequately performed allocation concealment and assessor blinding significantly overestimate the effects of study interventions [14,15]. The number of trials showing low versus high or unclear risk of bias in the two domains was compared.

Data pooling and sensitivity analysis

To identify whether newly included Korean RCTs influenced the previous results of the Cochrane acupuncture reviews, sensitivity analyses were performed for augmented and new meta-analyses. The original RevMan files for each Cochrane review were downloaded from *The Cochrane Library* (www.thecochranelibrary.com). We defined a meta-analysis as the effect estimation of pairwise comparison for a certain outcome using statistical pooling of at least two sets of study data, regardless of whether total or subtotal estimation was calculated [2]. Augmented meta-analyses were defined as those with at least two alreadyexisting studiesplus at least one Korean study. New meta-analyses were defined as those having at least two studies after the

Table 2. Screening results for potentially eligible Korean RCTs for relevant Cochrane reviews.

Cochrane review topics	No language restriction	Number of Korean Studies		
		At screening	Excluded	Eligible
Included (n = 8)				
Low back pain	Yes	21	16	5
Shoulder pain	Yes	13	10	3
Preventing postoperative nausea and vomiting	Yes	4	2	2
Insomnia	Unclear	4	2	2
Tension-type headache	Unclear	3	2	1
Primary dysmenorrhoea	Yes	6	5	1
Neck disorders	Yes	9	8	1
Cancer pain in adults	Yes	1	0	1
Excluded (n = 10)				
Lateral elbow pain	Yes	3	3	0
Stroke rehabilitation	Unclear	27	27	0
Dysphagia in acute stroke*	No	1	1	0
Induction of labor	Yes	1	1	0
Smoking cessation	Unclear	1	1	0
Pain management in labor	Yes	1	1	0
Rheumatoid arthritis**	No	1	1	0
Chemotherapy-induced nausea and vomiting	Yes	1	1	0
Peripheral OA	Yes	17	17	0
Bell's palsy	Yes	12	12	0

*: Studies reported in English and Chinese were searched.
**: Studies reported in English and French were searched.

inclusion of the Korean studies. The number of augmented meta-analyses, of new meta-analyses and of forest plots with a single Korean study after the inclusion of studies from Korean databases was recorded.

Differences in the size and direction of effect estimates before and after the inclusion of the Korean RCTs were investigated. For augmented meta-analyses, changes of statistical heterogeneity presented by I^2 scores were also compared. I^2 scores of 25 percent, 50 percent and 75 percent were regarded as corresponding to low, moderate, and high levels of heterogeneity. Any change in the heterogeneity level in the augmented meta-analyses (e.g., from low to moderate) was considered as a significant change of heterogeneity. Where available, a sensitivity analysis was also performed to identify whether the inclusion of the Korean RCTs altered funnel plot asymmetry of the meta-analysis. For effect size estimation, the decision to use a fixed-effect or a random-effects model was made according to the methods in each Cochrane review. When this was not clearly mentioned in the relevant Cochrane review, the random-effects model was preferred, taking account of the possible clinical heterogeneity that may have been attributable to the inclusion of Korean RCTs. The standardized mean difference (SMD) was used for continuous outcomes and risk ratio (RR) for dichotomous outcomes, respectively.

Statistical analysis

Statistical analyses were performed using the SAS statistical package, version 9.1.3 (SAS Inc., Cary, NC, USA), and a two-sided p-value less than 0.05 was regarded as the level of statistical significance. Differences of general characteristics between trials in the Cochrane reviews and those in the Korean RCTs were tested using the chi-square test for dichotomous variables and t tests for continuous variables. Sensitivity analysis was performed using the RevMan software, version 5.1 (The Nordic Cochrane Centre, Copenhagen, Denmark).

Results

A total of 869 articles were identified by the initial search of the Korean databases. (Additional searches of seven Korean acupuncture-related journals did not yield any new articles.) Of these, 642 clearly ineligible articles were excluded after screening the titles and abstracts. From among the remaining 227 potential studies, trials that did not match with topics of published Cochrane acupuncture reviews were further excluded (n = 112). The remaining 115 potentially relevant trials from Korean databases were examined in full, to investigate whether they met the eligibility criteria of the 18 topic-relevant Cochrane acupuncture reviews; this yielded a total of 16 studies (742 participants) that were eligible in eight Cochrane reviews (125 trials; 13,041 participants) (See the flowchart Figure 1 and 2, Table 2). Brief reasons for exclusion of Korean RCTs at this stage are provided in supporting information (Table S2).

The search term "acupuncture" in the *Cochrane Database of Systematic Reviews* (Issue 7, July 2011) yielded 64 reviews. Of these, 31 reviews were excluded for the following reasons: acupuncture was one of the treatment interventions but not the primary intervention (n = 15); reviews were not related to acupuncture (n = 14); methodology review (n = 1); review withdrawn (n = 1).

The relevance of the remaining 33 Cochrane reviews to the diseases or conditions investigated in the Korean RCTs was examined. Fifteen Cochrane acupuncture reviews did not match any Korean RCTs at the screening phase. Topics of excluded reviews included: chronic asthma, breech presentations, schizophrenia, acute strokes, cocaine dependence, irritable bowel syndrome, glaucoma, vascular dementia, restless leg syndrome, migraine prophylaxis, depression, uterine fibrosis, epilepsy, traumatic brain injury and attention deficit hyperactivity disorders. As a result, 18 Cochrane reviews that had at least one Korean study with the same topic were identified. Further investigation revealed that 10 reviews did not have any eligible Korean RCTs and were thus excluded from the analysis, leaving eight Cochrane reviews for this analysis.

The 16 hypothetically eligible Korean RCTs usedneedle acupuncture (n = 12), acupressure (n = 2), and transcutaneous electrical acupoint stimulation (n = 2) as treatment interventions. Diseases or conditions covered by Korean RCTs included low back pain (n = 5), shoulder pain (n = 3), insomnia (n = 2), prevention of postoperative nausea and vomiting (n = 2), tension-type headaches (n = 1), primary dysmenorrhea (n = 1), cancer pain in adults (n = 1), and neck disorders (n = 1). Eleven (69%) of the 16 Korean RCTs were published in acupuncture or traditional Korean medicine (TKM) journals (Table 3).

Summary characteristics of the 16 Korean RCTs are provided in supporting information (Table S1) and should contribute to future updates of the eight Cochrane reviews being investigated in this study. Compared to the component studies included in the Cochrane acupuncture reviews, the risk of bias in the Korean trials was higher in terms of outcome assessor blinding and allocation concealment although the difference did not reach statistical significance in terms of allocation concealment (Table 4).

Databases searched in the eight Cochrane acupuncture reviews are illustrated in Table 5. The most frequently searched databases were MEDLINE, EMBASE and CENTRAL. The number of reviews that included searches of Chinese and Japanese databases was four and one respectively. One review searched both Chinese and Japanese databases. None of the eight reviews documented attempts to search Korean databases.

Six of the eight Cochrane acupuncture reviews reported that no language restriction had been imposed (Table 2). Two reviews did not mention whether language restrictions had occurred, [16,17] although one of these included Chinese database searching [16]. The language of publication of trials already included in the eight Cochrane acupuncture reviews consisted of English (n = 102), Chinese (n = 12), Japanese (n = 7), German (n = 2), Norwegian (n = 1), and Polish (n = 1).

Among 120 meta-analyses in the eight Cochrane reviews, the inclusion of the 16 Korean RCTs contributed to 24 existing meta-analyses, seven new meta-analyses and 50 new forest plots containing a single Korean RCT (Table 6). Inclusion of the Korean trials did not change the direction of effect in any of the existing meta-analyses. In the 24 meta-analyses augmented by the inclusion of Korean RCTs, the effect estimates became more beneficial in 13 meta-analyses, less beneficial in fourand did not change in the remaining six. For the outcome of side effects in the Cochrane low back pain review, no effect estimates were possible, although the result of the relevant Korean trial was combined into existing forest plot. Twelve out of the 13 meta-analyses in which the effect estimate became more beneficial showed a change in favor of the intervention of less than four percentage points. The remaining one meta-analysis showed 207% beneficial effects towards treatment interventions compared to no treatment in the reviews of insomnia [16]. However, heterogeneity significantly

Table 3. Characteristics of RCTs already included in the Cochrane reviews and the hypothetically eligible Korean RCTs.

	Trials in the Cochrane reviews (n = 125)	Korean studies (n = 16)
Total number of participants in trials	13,041	742
Mean (SD)	105 (134)	46(19)
Median (Range)	68 (10–1265)	48 (12–86)
Number of studies in different conditions*		
Low back pain	35 (2861)	5 (226)
Neck disorders	10 (661)	3 (43)
Shoulder pain	9 (525)	3 (205)
Tension type headache	11 (2317)	1 (32)
Primary dysmenorrhea	10 (1025)	1 (47)
PONV	40 (4858)	2 (126)
Insomnia	7 (590)	2 (52)
Cancer pain in adults	3 (204)	1 (11)
Journal fields		
Acupuncture/TKM	-	11
Nursing/Physiotherapy	-	2
Conventional medicine	-	2
PhD thesis	-	1

RCTs: randomized controlled trials.
SD: standard deviation.
PONV: postoperative nausea and vomiting.
TKM: traditional Korean medicine.
*Values are provided as number of trials and (total number of participants).

Table 4. Methodological quality of trials included in the eight topic-matched Cochrane reviews and the corresponding16 Korean studies.

	Trials in the Cochrane reviews (n = 125)	Korean studies (n = 16)	P*
Adequate concealment of allocation			0.1192
Yes	34 (27.2%)	1 (6.2%)	
No/Unclear	91 (72.8%)	15 (93.8%)	
Outcome assessor blinding			0.0136
Yes	75 (60%)	4 (25%)	
No/Unclear	50 (40%)	12 (75%)	

*Fisher's exact test.
Values are presented as number (%).

increased (from zero to 95%). In the four meta-analyses which became less beneficial after the inclusion of Korean RCTs, the percentage change of effect estimates ranged between 1% and 25%. In only one meta-analysis did the significance change (RR 0.78, [0.59, 1.02] $I^2 = 37\%$ to RR 0.76 [0.59, 0.98] $I^2 = 37\%$) in one Cochrane review [18].

Three out of the 7 new meta-analyses (of low back pain) showed significant effect estimates in favor of the treatment interventions. All of newly generated meta-analyses showed less than 15% heterogeneity.

Five of the eight Cochrane reviews had an additional 50 single-study forest plots after the inclusion of Korean RCTs. Among these, seven forestplots showed significant between-group differences. 90% (45 out of 50) of single-study forest plots belonged to the review of shoulder pain [19].

There was only one Cochrane acupuncture review that had a meta-analysis with at least 10 studies after the inclusion of Korean RCTs [18]. However, inclusion of the Korean RCTs did not change the funnel plot asymmetry.

Table 5. Frequency of each database searched in the eight topic-matched Cochrane acupuncture reviews.

	Number of reviews, n (%)
English databases	
MEDLINE	8 (100.0)
EMBASE	7 (87.5)
CENTRAL	7 (87.5)
Cochrane Review Group specialized register	3 (37.5)
CINAHL	3 (37.5)
AMED	3 (37.5)
PsycInfo	2 (25.0)
Specialist acupuncture database	1 (12.5)
Other databases	7 (87.5)
East Asian databases	
Chinese databases	4 (50.0)
Japanese databases	1 (12.5)
Korean databases	0 (0.0)

Effect estimates and 95% confidence intervals of meta-analyses and single-study forest plots generated after the inclusion of Korean trials are provided in supporting information (Table S3, S4 and S5).

Discussion

To the best of our knowledge, this is the first study that has evaluated the impact of including studies in individual languages on the existing results of Cochrane reviews. Hypothetical eligibility testing of the Korean literature using the same eligibility criteria as that used for selected Cochrane acupuncture reviews found a noticeable number of Korean RCTs that could have been included in the Cochrane reviews, had Korean databases been searched as part of the review process. In most cases, the inclusion of Korean RCTs did not change the result of the meta-analyses. Korean RCTs identified from the Korean databases added, at most, two studies with a small number of participants, in any of the individual forest plots. Nevertheless, a considerable number of new analyses became available by inclusion of Korean RCTs, suggesting that new information could be gained by inclusion of Korean databases in the search methods of Cochrane acupuncture reviews.

Risk of bias in the 16 hypothetically eligible Korean RCTs was higher in the domain of outcome assessor blinding and allocation concealment. Whether trials in languages other than English

Table 6. Changes of meta-analysis after the inclusion of 16 Korean RCTs in relevant eight topic-matched Cochrane reviews.

	Numbers
Meta-analyses before inclusion of Korean RCTs	120
Meta-analyses augmented by Korean RCTs	24
New Meta-analyses after the inclusion of Korean RCTs	7
Forest-plots newly generated with a single Korean RCT	50
Meta-analyses augmented by Korean RCTs	24
Direction of effect changed	0
Effect size changed	1
Significance changed	1
Heterogeneity changed	2

(LOE) that have a higher risk of bias should be included in evidence synthesis or not remains controversial. This is because studies with high risk of bias could be associated with exaggerated effect estimates [20]. However, previous empirical studies have suggested that there is no evidence of significant differences in terms of methodological quality between trials in English and those in LOE [21,22]. Systematic searches for eligible studies regardless of the language of publication are recommended since a core component of systematic reviews is to ensure their validity and comprehensiveness [8,23]. Given the controversy, one reasonable option would be to perform sensitivity analysis based on the trial quality and publication language. None of the Cochrane acupuncture reviews considered in our study conducted a sensitivity analysis according to publication language (i.e., trials reported in English versus LOE trials). Only one review attempted to perform a sensitivity analysis based on the publication country, but it failed to do so because of the paucity of component studies [16]. Four out of eight reviews attempted to perform sensitivity analysis based on the quality of trials, [16,19,24,25] but only one was successful, again due to the paucity of component studies in the other three reviews [16,24,25]. From the viewpoint of Korean trialists, more attention should be devoted to maintaining methodological rigor, minimizing risk of bias, and adhering to the high quality of trial reporting guidelines (i.e., CONSORT) to maximize the potential benefit of including Korean RCTs in systematic reviews. Editors of Korean domestic journals should guide trial authors toward fulfilling all of the relevant reporting items of CONSORT in order to improve the reporting quality. Empirical evidence indicates that published Korean RCTs in conventional medicine show low adherence to the CONSORT guidelines [26]. Low adherence to these guidelines was also found in a traditional Chinese medical journal [27]. Collaborative efforts among Korean researchers and journal editors to improve methodological and reporting quality may bring about the inclusion of Korean RCTs in future Cochrane reviews of acupuncture.

Inclusion of Korean RCTs seemed unlikely to contribute sufficiently to the number of included trials for sensitivity analysis in any of the included Cochrane reviews. In future Cochrane reviews of acupuncture, as well as those analyzing healthcare interventions which have been performed in various cultural contexts and countries, sensitivity analyses of the inclusion of trials in English may be a reasonable option to assess whether language-restrictive analyses makes a difference to the robustness of review results compared to language-inclusive ones, as well as to secure both the comprehensiveness of the trial search process and the reliability of the evidence. No language restriction was declared in six of the eight Cochrane reviews. However, the language of publication included in those Cochrane reviews was mostly English. Our findings correspond to those of a previous study showing that only half of the 159 meta-analyses that reported language-inclusive searches had located studies published in languages other than English [7]. Possible reasons might be poor participation of Korean authors in the conduct of Cochrane acupuncture reviews. In our pilot study, only four Korean authors were found to have participated in Cochrane acupuncture reviews in the January 2011 issue of CDSR [10]. Low awareness among international researchers about research activity, as well as the clinical practice of acupuncture in Korea, might also have played a role in the omission of Korean literature from current evidence syntheses. Appropriate training and education for enhancing the participation of Korean researchers in Cochrane acupuncture reviews will contribute to increasing the inclusion of Korean literature in future evidence syntheses.

Methods to improve accessibility of Korean literature for international researchers should also be investigated. We are aware that controlled clinical trials of acupuncture in the Korean literature are being registered in the Cochrane Central Register of Controlled Trials (CENTRAL) by Korean researchers and the Cochrane CAM Field. This will accelerate the identification of Korean RCTs and the testing of their eligibility, thus reducing the potential risk of language bias and maximizing completeness of current and future evidence of acupuncture available in CDSR. Collaborative efforts for incorporating local evidence into Cochrane reviews, such as those being made by the Chinese Cochrane Center and CONSORT groups to improve the quality of reporting in RCTs published in Chinese languages, [28] are needed between Korean and international researchers to overcome the incompleteness of the search strategies addressed in this study.

A relatively large number of Korean RCTs did not satisfy the eligibility criteria of existing Cochrane acupuncture reviews and were excluded from the analysis. A substantial number of Korean RCTs employed different comparisons, different styles of acupuncture, and different outcomes from those in the Cochrane reviews, hence they were ultimately excluded from the reviews. This might be partly due to the existence of research questions and priorities among Korean acupuncture researchers that are different from those of Cochrane acupuncture reviewers, although in the context of Korea, no information is available for the research priorities relating to acupuncture. A recent survey showed that practice characteristics and research priorities of practitioners of traditional acupuncture were different in China and Europe [29]. Acupuncture is a complex intervention, in which the whole process of patient consultation and therapeutic interaction comprises overall effectiveness, and these are significantly influenced by cultural and societal backgrounds [30,31]. Competing local priorities for research and research interests of those involved in trials might be different in different countries. This might partly explain the high rate of exclusion from the Cochrane reviews of Korean studies, due to ineligible comparison (i.e., comparing two different acupuncture techniques). Future research focusing on factors that potentially determine the research questions and trial designs in the field of acupuncture research in the Korean situation might be helpful in explaining gaps between evidence generated in Korea and evidence generated by Cochrane systematic reviews, reflecting current variability in the field of acupuncture research and practice.

Differences between the findings of this study and previous research

Previous research has assessed whether language-inclusive meta-analyses make a difference to the results compared to language-restrictive ones, by conducting sensitivity analyses for trials reported in languages other than English [7,23]. In one study, only meta-analyses which had included trials reported in both English and LOE were collected [7]. One major weakness of this approach is that review authors assume that meta-analyses being analyzed had included all relevant LOE trials by comprehensive and adequate search methods, which was clearly not the case in our findings. Although our study included only a limited number of Cochrane reviews and Korean RCTs in terms of a specific intervention (i.e., acupuncture), it showed that even Cochrane reviews with language-inclusive searches had omitted a certain proportion of eligible LOE RCTs. This means that the impact of LOE trials might have been underestimated in previous research studies that only included given study sets in meta-analyses [7]. Based on our findings, we suggest that Cochrane reviews of acupuncture should pay more attention to develop adequate methods to access and identify LOE trials. Future research that evaluates the impact of language bias should also consider the risk of omission of LOE trials when using already included study sets in meta-analyses, unless searches of hypothetically eligible studies could be performed by the researchers themselves.

Strengths of this study

First, to the best of our knowledge, the largest number of Korean databases and relevant acupuncture journals published in Korean were searched for this study. Future Cochrane acupuncture reviews and protocols might refer to this study for developing search strategies that include Korean literature. Second, study summaries and information on excluded studies are available in supporting information (Table S1 and S2) for existing and future Cochrane review authors, thus making this study more informative for concerned researchers. A summary of 16 hypothetically eligible Korean RCTs found in this study is provided and could be directly integrated into forthcoming updates of existing Cochrane acupuncture reviews. Third, we have tried to develop the data set of acupuncture RCTs published in Korean literature, which could be periodically updated and used as an important source of building regional data sets for Korean acupuncture RCTs. We also suggest future collaborative activity for incorporating evidence of acupuncture in Korean literature covered by this study into CENTRAL, one of the most important databases for systematic reviews.

Limitations of this study

Limitations of this study should be discussed. First, search terms used in this study for locating controlled acupuncture trials in Korean literature might not be optimal. To the best of our knowledge, however, there is no standard search filter for the most efficient identification of RCTs in Korean databases. We attempted to overcome this weakness by extensively searching all relevant electronic databases and performing ancillary searches in related journals. To address this limitation, development of sensitivity-maximizing search filters for Korean RCTs is needed. Second, only a small number of Korean RCTs were eligible in this analysis. However, we tried to screen all relevant studies in several Korean databases by methods stated above; thus, we believe we have used the most representative set of acupuncture trials reported in Korean databases. Third, initial searching and screening for relevant Korean studies was performed by only one assessor since the process was labor-intensive and research resources did not extend to independent screening. Instead, three pairs of two independent researchers at the post-screening stage selected eligible RCTs, assessed the risk of bias, and extracted data. Fourth, only published Cochrane reviews were screened for this analysis. Current ongoing protocols and registered review titles that might be relevant to Korean RCTs were not considered in the analysis. Thus, the results of this study might be outdated when reviews are completed and updated in the near future. Continuous efforts, regional and international research activities, and research funding are needed to maintain an up-to-date body of evidence for the practice of acupuncture in Korea and for the incorporation of such evidence into CDSR. Lastly, only Cochrane reviews that considered acupuncture as a primary treatment intervention were included in this study. Hence, the impact of inclusion of Korean RCTs on existing Cochrane reviewsfor other health-related fields might not be fully assessed.

Conclusions

Inclusion of Korean databases in the search methods for Cochrane systematic reviews of acupuncture can add valuable information to enhance current evidence of the use of acupuncture in relevant clinical fields. Inclusion of Korean RCTs should be considered for any Cochrane reviews in preparation and for future revisions and periodic updates of existing Cochrane acupuncture reviews.

Supporting Information

Table S1 Summary characteristics and risk of bias of included 16 Korean studies.
(DOC)

Table S2 Characteristics of 99 excluded Korean studies.
(DOC)

Table S3 Seven new meta-analyses after the inclusion of Korean trials.
(DOC)

Table S4 24 augmented meta-analyses after the inclusion of Korean trials.
(DOC)

Table S5 50 Single-study forest plots generated by the inclusion of Korean studies.
(DOC)

Acknowledgments

The authors especially thank Miranda Cumpston to help authors obtain statistical data of Cochrane acupuncture reviews.

Author Contributions

Conceived and designed the experiments: KHK SM. Performed the experiments: KHK JCK JYC TYC. Analyzed the data: KHK JCK JYC TYC BCS SM MSL. Contributed reagents/materials/analysis tools: JCK TYC SM. Wrote the paper: KHK.

References

1. Egger M, Davey Smith G, O'Rourke K (2001) Rationale, potentials and promise of systematic reviews. In: Egger M, Davey Smith G, Altman DG, editors. Systematic Reviews in Health Care: Meta-Analysis in Context. London: BMJ Books. pp 23–42.
2. Davey J, Turner RM, Clarke MJ, Higgins JPT (2011) Characteristics of meta-analyses and their component studies in the Cochrane Database of Systematic Reviews: a cross-sectional, descriptive analysis. BMC Med Res Methodol 11: 160. Available: http://www.biomedcentral.com/1471-2288/1411/1160. Acessed 2012 July 2.
3. Kim YS, Jun H, Chae Y, Park HJ, Kim BH, et al. (2005) The practice of Korean medicine: an overview of clinical trials in acupuncture. Evid Based Complement Alternat Med 2: 325–352. Available: http://www.ncbi.nlm.nih.gov/pmc/articles/PMC1193543/?tool=pubmed. Accessed 2012 July 2.
4. Sood A, Sood D, Bauer BA, Ebbert JO (2005) Cochrane systematic reviews in acupuncture: methodological diversity in database searching. J Altern Complement Med 11: 719–722.
5. Tsukayama H, Yamashita H (2002) Systematic review of clinical trials on acupuncture in the Japanese literature. Clinical acupuncture and oriental medicine 3: 105–113.
6. Kong JC, Lee MS, Shin BC (2009) Randomized clinical trials on acupuncture in Korean literature: a systematic review. Evid Based Complement Alternat Med 6: 41–48. Available: http://www.ncbi.nlm.nih.gov/pmc/articles/PMC2644266/?tool=pubmed. Accessed Acessed 2012 July 2.
7. Jüni P, Holenstein F, Sterne J, Bartlett C, Egger M (2002) Direction and impact of language bias in meta-analyses of controlled trials: empirical study. Int J Epidemiol 31: 115–123.

8. Pham B, Klassen TP, Lawson ML, Moher D (2005) Language of publication restrictions in systematic reviews gave different results depending on whether the intervention was conventional or complementary. J Clin Epidemiol 58: 769–796.
9. Lui S, Smith EJ, Terplan M (2010) Heterogeneity in search strategies among Cochrane acupuncture reviews: is there room for improvement? Acupunct Med 28: 149–153.
10. Kim KH, Noh SH, Lee MS, Yang GY, Shin BC, et al. (2011) Current evidence of acupuncture in the Cochrane Database of Systematic Reviews: an Overview. Journal of Korean Acupuncture & Moxibustion Society 28: 57–64.
11. WorldHealthOrganizationWesternPacificRegion (2007) WHO International Standard Terminologies on Traditional Medicine in the Western Pacific Region. Manilla, Phlippine: World Health Organization Western Pacific. 251 p. Available: http://www.wpro.who.int/publications/docs/WHOIST_226JUNE_FINAL.pdf. Acessed 2012 July 2.
12. Furlan AD, vanTulder MW, Cherkin DC, Tsukayama H, Lao L, et al. (2005) Acupuncture and dry-needling for low back pain. Cochrane Database Syst Rev: CD001351. Available: http://onlinelibrary.wiley.com/doi/10.1002/14651858.CD001351.pub2/abstract. Acessed 2012 July 2.
13. Higgins JPT, Altman DG, Sterne JAC (2011) Chapter 8: Assessing risk of bias in included studies. In: Higgins JPT, Green S, editors. Cochrane Handbook for Systematic Reviews of Interventions Version 5.1.0 (updated March 2011).The Cochrane Collaboration. Available: http://www.cochrane-handbook.org. Accessed 2 July 2012.
14. Hróbjartsson A, Thomsen AS, Emanuelsson F, Tendal B, Hilden J, et al. (2012) Observer bias in randomised clinical trials with binary outcomes: systematic review of trials with both blinded and non-blinded outcome assessors. BMJ 344: e1119. Available: http://www.bmj.com/content/344/bmj.e1119?view=long&pmid=22371859. Acessed 2012 July 2.
15. Schulz KF, Grimes DA (2002) Allocation concealment in randomised trials: defending against deciphering. Lancet 359: 614–618.
16. Cheuk DK, Yeung WF, Chung KF, Wong V (2007) Acupuncture for insomnia. Cochrane Database Syst Rev: CD005472. Available: http://onlinelibrary.wiley.com/doi/005410.001002/14651858.CD14005472.pub14651852/abstract. Acessed 2012 July 2.
17. Linde K, Allais G, Brinkhaus B, Manheimer E, Vickers A, et al. (2009) Acupuncture for tension-type headache. Cochrane Database Syst Rev: CD007587. Available: http://www.ncbi.nlm.nih.gov/pmc/articles/PMC3099266/?tool=pubmed. Acessed 2012 July 2.
18. Lee A, Fan LTY (2009) Stimulation of the wrist acupuncture point P6 for preventing postoperative nausea and vomiting. Cochrane Database Syst Rev: CD003281. Available: http://onlinelibrary.wiley.com/doi/003210.001002/14651858.CD14003281.pub14651853/abstract. Acessed 2012 July 2.
19. Green S, Buchbinder R, Hetrick S (2005) Acupuncture for shoulder pain. Cochrane Database Syst Rev: CD005319. Available: http://onlinelibrary.wiley.com/doi/005310.001002/14651858.CD14005319/abstract. Acessed 2012 July 2.
20. Egger M, Juni P, Bartlett C, Holenstein F, Sterne J (2003) How important are comprehensive literature searches and the assessment of trial quality in systematic reviews? Empirical study. Health Technol Assess 7: 1–76. Available: http://www.hta.ac.uk/execsumm/summ701.htm. Acessed 2012 July 2.
21. Klassen TP, Pham B, Lawson ML, Moher D (2005) For randomized controlled trials, the quality of reports of complementary and alternative medicine was as good as reports of conventional medicine. J Clin Epidemiol 58: 763–768.
22. Moher D, Fortin P, Jadad AR, Jüni P, Klassen T, et al. (1996) Completeness of reporting of trials published in languages other than English: implications for conduct and reporting of systematic reviews. Lancet 347: 363–366.
23. Egger M, Zellweger-Zähner T, Schneider M, Junker C, Lengeler C, et al. (1997) Language bias in randomised controlled trials published in English and German. Lancet 350: 326–329.
24. Paley CA, Johnson MI, Tashani OA, Bagnall AM (2011) Acupuncture for cancer pain in adults. Cochrane Database Syst Rev: CD007753. Available: http://onlinelibrary.wiley.com/doi/10.1002/14651858.CD007753.pub2/abstract. Accessed 2012 Sept 14.
25. Smith CA, Zhu XS, He L, Song J (2011) Acupuncture for dysmenorrhoea. Cochrane Database Syst Rev: CD007854. Available: http://onlinelibrary.wiley.com/doi/10.1002/14651858.CD007854.pub2/abstract. Accessed 2012 Sept 14.
26. Hwang YE, Lee KW, Hwang IH, Kim SY (2008) The quality of reporting of randomized controlled trials in Korean medical journals indexed in KoreaMed: survey of items of the revised CONSORT statement. J Korean Acad Fam Med 29: 276–282.
27. Wang G, Mao B, Xiong ZY, Fan T, Chen XD, et al. (2007) The quality of reporting of randomized controlled trials of traditional Chinese medicine: a survey of 13 randomly selected journals from mainland China. Clin Ther 29: 1456–1467.
28. MacPherson H, Altman DG (2009) Improving the quality of reporting acupuncture interventions: describing the collaboration between STRICTA, CONSORT and the Chinese Cochrane Centre. J Evid Based Med 2: 57–60.
29. Robinson N, Lorenc A, Ding W, Jia J, Bovey M, et al. (2012) Exploring practice characteristics and research priorities of practitioners of traditional acupuncture in China and the EU-A survey. J Ethnopharmacol 140: 604–613.
30. Birch S, Lewith G (2008) Chap 2: Acupuncture research: the story so far. In: MacPherson H, Hammerschlag R, Lewith G, Schnyer R, editors. Acupuncture Research: Strategies for Establishing an Evidence Base. London: Churchill Livingstone. pp 15–35.
31. Paterson C, Dieppe P (2005) Characteristics and incidental (placebo) effects in complex interventions such as acupuncture. BMJ 330: 1202–1205.

14

A Systematic Review of Comparative Efficacy of Treatments and Controls for Depression

Arif Khan[1,2]*, James Faucett[1], Pesach Lichtenberg[3], Irving Kirsch[4,5], Walter A. Brown[6,7]

1 Northwest Clinical Research Center, Bellevue, Washington, United States of America, **2** Department of Psychiatry, Duke University Medical School, Durham, North Carolina, United States of America, **3** Herzog Hospital, and the School of Medicine of the Hebrew University, Department of Psychiatry, Jerusalem, Israel, **4** Program in Placebo Studies, Beth Israel Deaconess Medical Center, Harvard Medical School, Boston, Massachusetts, United States of America, **5** University of Plymouth, Plymouth, United Kingdom, **6** Department of Psychiatry and Human Behavior, Brown University, Providence, Rhode Island, United States of America, **7** Department of Psychiatry, Tufts University, Boston, Massachusetts, United States of America

Abstract

Background: Although previous meta-analyses have examined effects of antidepressants, psychotherapy, and alternative therapies for depression, the efficacy of these treatments alone and in combination has not been systematically compared. We hypothesized that the differences between approved depression treatments and controls would be small.

Methods and Findings: The authors first reviewed data from Food and Drug Administration Summary Basis of Approval reports of 62 pivotal antidepressant trials consisting of data from 13,802 depressed patients. This was followed by a systematic review of data from 115 published trials evaluating efficacy of psychotherapies and alternative therapies for depression. The published depression trials consisted of 10,310 depressed patients. We assessed the percentage symptom reduction experienced by the patients based on treatment assignment. Overall, antidepressants led to greater symptom reduction compared to placebo among both unpublished FDA data and published trials ($F = 38.5$, $df = 239$, $p < 0.001$). In the published trials we noted that the magnitude of symptom reduction with active depression treatments compared to controls was significantly larger when raters evaluating treatment effects were un-blinded compared to the trials with blinded raters ($F = 2.17$, $df = 313$, $p < 0.05$). In the blinded trials, the combination of antidepressants and psychotherapy provided a slight advantage over antidepressants ($p = 0.027$) and psychotherapy ($p = 0.022$) alone. The magnitude of symptom reduction was greater with psychotherapies compared to placebo ($p = 0.019$), treatment-as-usual ($p = 0.012$) and waiting-list ($p < 0.001$). Differences were not seen with psychotherapy compared to antidepressants, alternative therapies or active intervention controls.

Conclusions: In conclusion, the combination of psychotherapy and antidepressants for depression may provide a slight advantage whereas antidepressants alone and psychotherapy alone are not significantly different from alternative therapies or active intervention controls. These data suggest that type of treatment offered is less important than getting depressed patients involved in an active therapeutic program. Future research should consider whether certain patient profiles might justify a specific treatment modality.

Editor: Christian Holscher, University of Ulster, United Kingdom

Funding: The authors have no support or funding to report.

Competing Interests: The authors have declared that no competing interests exist.

* E-mail: akhan@nwcrc.net

Introduction

A number of recent articles have emphasized the inability of antidepressant medication to consistently demonstrate superiority to placebo pills [1–4]. Approximately half of clinical trials fail to differentiate active treatments from controls, and mean differences between drug and placebo on the Hamilton Rating Scale for Depression are small [2,5]. This phenomenon has sparked considerable concern and criticism from the popular media, clinicians and researchers [6,7].

Psychotherapies for depression have also come under scrutiny for their inability to demonstrate substantial superiority to various treatment controls as opposed to waiting-list (no treatment) controls [8]. Similarly, although alternative therapies such as acupuncture and exercise have shown promise in individual published studies [9,10], the profile is less impressive according to independent reviews such as Cochrane Reviews [11,12] and those conducted by the National Institute for Health and Clinical Excellence [13].

Given this level of ambiguity, it is unclear if pharmacological treatments are any better or worse than psychotherapies or if psychotherapies are any better than non-traditional treatments such as exercise and acupuncture. Thus, we undertook to critically evaluate relative efficacy among the various treatments for depression along with control procedures, including placebo pills.

To provide a relatively unbiased perspective of the response to treatments for depression, we used as an anchor the clinical trial data from pivotal antidepressant trials that had been submitted to the United States Food and Drug Administration (FDA) during the drug approval process. Because drug companies are required to submit information on all of the trials they conducted, these data should be free of publication and author bias [3]. Furthermore, these trials all contain data on placebo response in depression, were conducted at multiple sites and the data were accumulated over the past three decades.

Following the establishment of the anchor we conducted a literature search identifying depression clinical trials conducted over the past thirty-five years. We specifically evaluated data from depression trials that were designed to assess the role of antidepressants, psychotherapies, active intervention, and control treatments including placebo.

Our hypothesis was that the differences between the various depression treatments and controls would be relatively small. We additionally hypothesized that any differences in efficacy among these treatments would be further reduced if we applied stringent criteria for the 'blinded' status of the trial. This hypothesis is based on earlier reviews [8,14–16] as well as our own reviews of antidepressant and placebo data from pivotal antidepressant clinical trials [2,5].

In order to verify our hypothesis, we focused on evaluating the reduction of depressive symptoms experienced during depression trials by the patients assigned to the various active depression treatments and treatment controls. We controlled for rater bias by comparing the reduction of symptoms from depression trials with raters/clinicians who knew the study design, intent and potential treatment assignments compared to depression trials that included raters/clinicians who were blinded to these factors. As part of this exploration, we compared the antidepressant-placebo differences among unpublished, industry sponsored data obtained from the US FDA with published reports that were not sponsored by industry. Also, we evaluated if there were significant differences in the magnitude of symptom reduction among various psychotherapies.

Methods

Selection of Depression Trials for Evaluation

During New Drug Approval process the US FDA reviews trial level efficacy and safety data from pivotal clinical trials conducted during development programs of putative medications. In 1997 the data used by the FDA during the risk/benefit evaluations became available to the public via the Freedom of Information Act [17]. Summary Basis of Approval (SBA) reports detail data from the medication development programs and are available directly from the FDA website at www.fda.gov. If SBA reports are not available at the FDA website, the FDA staff provides data on CDRom in response to written requests.

As first part of our selection of depression treatment trials, we accessed antidepressant trial data that were reviewed by the physicians, scientists and statisticians at the FDA and reported in SBA reports. All of the data were from pivotal, placebo controlled trials that the FDA used to approve eleven antidepressants between 1987 and 2004. The efficacy dataset from these trials consisted of sixty two antidepressant clinical trials conducted between 1979 and 2001 that included 13,802 depressed patients [18,19,20].

Aside from this FDA data, we reviewed published literature regarding the efficacy data for traditionally accepted non-medicinal depression treatments and controls. We first searched the published literature for controlled trials of cognitive, behavioral, cognitive behavioral psychotherapies and derivatives of these treatments for major depressive disorder, dysthymia or postpartum depression. Following this search, we conducted a similar search for controlled trials of alternative therapies (exercise and acupuncture) for depression.

Inclusion and Exclusion of Published Depression Trials

During the span of time when these depression trials were conducted there were three versions of the Diagnostic and Statistical Manual (DSM) of the APA. These consisted of DSM-II [21], DSM-III [22] and DSM-IV [23]. In essence there are no differences in the diagnostic criteria between DSM-III and DSM-IV for major depression. However, there were significant differences in the scope and definition of depression between DSM-II and DSM-III.

In order to decrease any heterogeneity, we specifically evaluated the data from trials (n = 19) that were conducted prior to the full establishment and incorporation of DSM-III that was introduced in 1978. We specifically evaluated if the precursors of DSM-III, notably Research Diagnostic Criteria (RDC) [24] or Feighner Criteria [25] were used during diagnosis. These criteria were in fact considerably narrower than DSM-III. Four of these 19 trials used Feighner criteria and five of the nineteen used RDC criteria. Among the rest (n = 10), we included the data, if specific clinical evaluations described the sample in sufficient detail to formulate DSM-III diagnostic criteria.

Although we did not follow a published pre-specified protocol during our systematic review, the trial inclusion/exclusion criteria, search stategy and primary outcome variable were defined *a-priori* (the Prisma 2009 Checklist is Figure S1). We targeted manuscripts describing depression trials of traditionally accepted and established psychotherapies or alternative therapies for Major Depressive Disorder including the depression disorder subtypes dysthymia and postpartum depression. The published trials were representative of clinically depressed ambulatory adults between the ages of 18 and 65 years of age.

We included trials that reported acute depression treatment outcomes using the Hamilton Rating Scale for Depression (HRSD), Beck Depression Inventory (BDI), or Montgomery-Asberg Depression Rating Scale (MADRS). Trials that reported an outcome in figure format were included if we were able to estimate mean total baseline and end of acute treatment outcomes from the figure.

Exclusion criteria were as follows: 1) Trials that primarily enrolled patients that were under the age of 18 or over the age of 65, 2) Trials that targeted depressed patients with major medical or psychiatric co-morbidities (e.g., human immunodeficiency virus, cancer, cardiovascular disease, patients in recovery from stroke, patients with co-morbid substance abuse), 3) Trials that did not evaluate and report treatment outcome within one week of patient of completion of treatment, 4) Trials targeting treatment resistant or hospitalized depressed patients, 5) Trials with incarcerated depressed patients, 6) Trials that were not published in the English language. Trials that were not reported in peer-reviewed journals (for example, dissertations) were also excluded.

Trials that did not report the mean baseline symptom evaluation and treatment outcome using the HRSD, MADRS or BDI were excluded. We also excluded trials that did not include an active treatment arm with a traditionally accepted psychotherapy. For example, we excluded trials that targeted experimental therapies such as bibliotherapy (telephone therapy) or computer implemented therapy without including an active treatment arm.

Identification of Depression Trials in the Published Literature

Our primary strategy during the search for published depression treatment trials was to use a "snowball search" of the numerous published meta-analyses and reviews of psychotherapy and alternative treatments for depression.

Our literature search was conducted from September to December 2010, and targeted trials that were published between 1975 and 2009. We began by reviewing several meta-analyses designed to evaluate efficacy outcomes between psychotherapy and other treatments and controls for depression including other psychotherapies, alternative therapies, combination therapies, antidepressants, and placebos or active intervention controls [8,16,,26,27,28,29]. During this search we identified a database of 243 psychotherapy trials compiled by Dr. Pim Cuijpers and his depression research group at www.evidencebasedpsychotherapies.org [30]. Throughout this process we retrieved title and abstract of all psychotherapy for depression trials that were used for the meta-analyses and reviews as well as those from the website by Cuijpers et al.

We then conducted a similar search targeting published controlled trials of alternative therapies for depression. We conducted this second "snowball search" by accessing Cochrane Reviews website and obtaining recently completed reviews of trials of exercise and acupuncture for treatment of major depressive disorder, dysthymia or postpartum depression [11,12]. We retrieved title and abstract for each article that was included in the Cochrane Group evaluation of efficacy of exercise or acupuncture for depression.

After the "snowball search" of previously conducted reviews of published psychotherapy, exercise and acupuncture trials we conducted an additional online search for recently completed trials that may have been overlooked. We accessed Pubmed, Psychinfo and the Cochrane Register of Controlled Trials. We conducted identical searches in each database entering in turn the keywords acupuncture, exercise, and relaxation for trials of alternative therapies. For the psychotherapy trials we entered in turn the keywords psychotherapy, cognitive, behavioral, cognitive-behavioral, rational-emotive, and interpersonal. The terms "depression and placebo" or "depression and controlled" were used interchangeably in combination with the specific therapy names within each search engine.

For this search, we did not search for or include industry sponsored antidepressant trials that used a placebo control with an antidepressant, or that compared multiple antidepressants with no other established depression treatments, to avoid duplication of the FDA data. We only included antidepressant data from published trials of psychotherapy or alternative therapies for depression trials identified during the literature search outlined above. The antidepressant data from the published sources were independent from the pivotal registration trials that were reviewed by the FDA.

Organization of Data

The "snowball search" strategy produced 310 abstracts of depression treatment trials following our searches of previously published reviews, analyses and the website by Cuijpers et al. We reviewed the title and abstract of each article retrieved. Articles were retrieved and fully reviewed if they were available as English publications and did not specifically target depressed patients with physical or psychiatric co-morbidities such as Human Immunodeficiency Virus, cancer, cardiovascular disease, Bipolar Disorder, or Psychotic Spectrum Disorders. The PRISMA flow chart depicting process of exclusion for the published depression treatment trials is shown as Figure 1.

We included 106 trials from the search of previously published reviews and meta-analyses of published depression treatment trials. We identified an additional 9 trials with the online literature search. The list of references for the 115 depression treatment trials included in our study is shown as Appendix S1.

There were 328 treatment arms that enrolled 10,310 depressed patients in the 115 published depression treatment trials. Based on description by study authors, we identified four active treatments and four treatment controls. As shown in Table 1, the active depression treatments consisted of 218 trial arms enrolling 7,683 patients. Treatment controls consisted of 110 arms enrolling 2,627 patients.

The active treatments and controls, as described by the authors, are shown as Appendix S2. The active treatments were: 1) antidepressants in combination with psychotherapies or alternative treatments, 2) antidepressants with minimal clinical management, 3) psychotherapies alone that are considered to be accepted depression treatments (cognitive-behavioral, cognitive and behavioral therapies and author described derivatives), and 4) a group of treatments traditionally accepted as alternative therapies for depression. The specific names of active treatments are shown as Appendix S2 Parts1–4.

The control treatments were: 1) placebo pills, 2) procedures designated by trial authors as active intervention controls (e.g., sham acupuncture, therapies not specific to depression, partial presentations of full therapy regimens), 3) treatment-as-usual, which consisted of care by the primary care physicians or referrals to general practitioners and which may have included prescriptions for antidepressants, and 4) waiting-list controls. The specific names of the treatment controls are shown as Appendix S2 Parts 5–8.

Designation of Blinded Status

As has been shown by several groups of researchers, the outcomes of depression trials are significantly influenced by design factors that shape the expectations of clinicians and depressed patients [31–33]. Other investigators [8,14] have attempted to quantify such a possibility by evaluating the evaluator. Specifically, these earlier investigators evaluated outcome of depression trials based on the level of control that was built into trial design by blinding the symptom evaluator.

To evaluate any impact of blinding on trial outcome we used the following procedures to quantify trials as blinded or un-blinded. First, we categorized as un-blinded data from all of the depression trials that used patient ratings (BDI scale scores) as the primary dependent measure. We based this decision on the findings of Prioleau et al. that the largest treatment effects of psychotherapy relative to placebo came from studies that used undisguised self-report [14].

Second, for all trials that reported mean change in HRSD or MADRS scores we categorically evaluated the clinician/raters at the end of treatment evaluation as blinded or un-blinded following the methods outlined by Cuijpers et al. [8]. We categorized as blinded the trials that specifically described assessors at the end of treatment as independent from and blinded to the condition to which depressed patients were assigned. The trials with HRSD and MADRS that did not specify an independent symptom assessor were categorized un-blinded.

The depression trials that assigned patients to pill placebo were all categorized as blinded. Each of these trials specified that symptom assessor at end of treatment was blinded to patient assignment to antidepressant or placebo. Based on this type of demarcation, we subdivided the 115 depression treatment trials into two groups; termed group 1 with un-blinded raters ($k = 59$) and group 2 with blinded raters ($k = 56$).

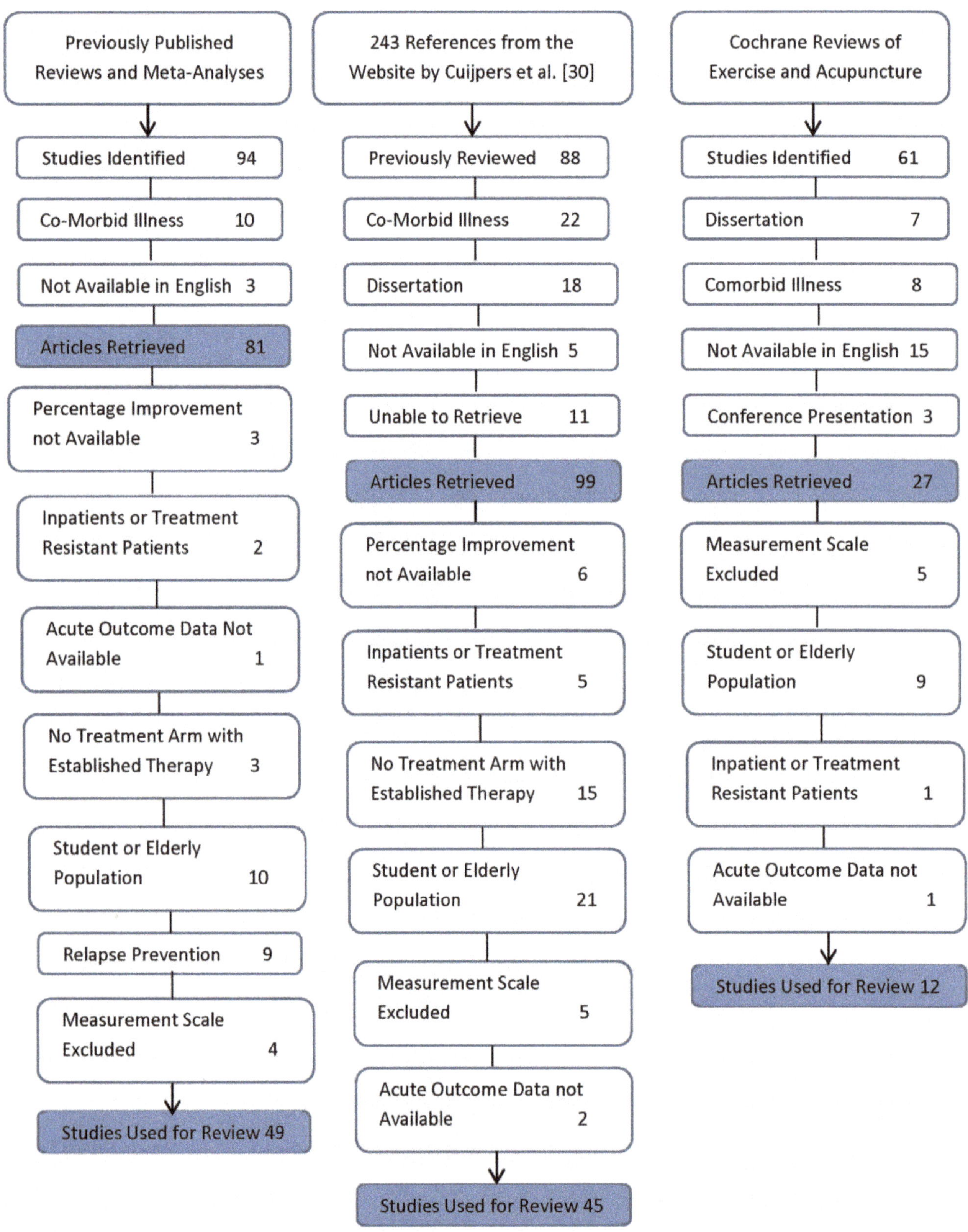

Figure 1. Process of Exclusion of Trials Identified During Search of Depression Treatment Reviews and Analyses, and the Website by Cuijpers and Colleagues.

Table 1. Summary Data from Depression Treatment Trials Based on Type of Treatment and Source of Data.

Treatment Type and Source	Number of Treatment Arms	Number of Patients
FDA Summary Basis of Approval Reports		
Investigative Agents	80	7,014
Active Comparators	31	2,220
Placebo Controls	57	4,568
Column Totals	168	13,802
Published Depression Treatment Trials		
Active Treatments		
Combination Therapy + Antidepressants	32	1,249
Antidepressants + Clinical Management	40	1,958
Accepted Psychotherapies for Depression	128	4,034
Alternative Therapies for Depression	18	442
Column Totals	218	7,683
Treatment Controls		
Pill Placebo Controls	16	412
Intervention Controls	48	1,095
Treatment as Usual Controls	12	530
Waiting-list Controls	34	590
Column Totals	110	2,627

Specific names of treatment arms for accepted depression treatments and treatment controls are shown as Appendix B.

Analysis of Data

Our analysis of data was designed to evaluate the relative efficacy of the active depression treatments and controls and to evaluate the impact that blinding the trial has on treatment outcomes. We chose the mean percentage symptom reduction as our primary outcome measure. Our selection of this outcome was based on the data available as several of the published depression trials included multiple treatment arms with a single control arm violating assumptions necessary to calculate an independent effect size. There were also trials that simply did not report data from which an effect size could be calculated.

In the event that a trial reported more than one outcome measure (for example, some trials reported BDI and HRSD outcome), we selected for evaluation the clinician administered measure. Where available we recorded the Intent-to-Treat outcome, although in some cases there were not ongoing assessments throughout the trial in which case the Completer Only results were included for analysis.

The mean weighted percentage symptom reduction as a function of blinding, therapy type, and data source for each treatment and control is displayed in Figure 2. As a preliminary analysis, we compared the antidepressant and placebo data from published non-industry depression trials to the placebo controlled antidepressant registration trials from the FDA dataset. We conducted a 2 factor univariate analysis of variance (ANOVA). We entered as binomial independent variables the data source (1 = published data, 2 = FDA data) and the comparison of antidepressant (coded 1) versus placebo (coded 2) with percentage symptom reduction being the primary outcome measure.

This was followed by a 2×8 ANOVA of the published depression trials to evaluate the role of blinding and type of treatment on outcome for the depressed patients. To conduct this ANOVA, we entered the blinding status(1 = un-blinded, 2 = blinded) and treatment type (combination = 1, antidepressant = 2, psychotherapy = 3, alternative therapy = 4, intervention control = 5, placebo control = 6, treatment as usual = 7, waiting list = 8) as independent variables and the percentage symptom reduction was the dependent variable.

Comparative efficacy between treatment outcomes was analyzed with separate one-way ANOVAs on treatment type with blinded and un-blinded studies, respectively. Tukey's Least Significant Difference post-hoc test was used to evaluate significance of any differences in percentage symptom reduction between the 4 active depression treatments and 4 treatment controls.

Lastly, we compared outcome of the psychotherapy treatment arms based on psychotherapy type. We conducted 2×5 ANOVA to evaluate impact of blinded status or psychotherapy type on outcome for the psychotherapy trial arms. We coded psychotherapy trial arms specifying use of Cognitive Behavioral Therapy (CBT) with 1, Cognitive Therapy with 2, and Behavioral Therapy with 3 and Interpersonal Psychotherapy with 4. Other therapies (e.g., Rational-emotive Therapy, Self-Control Therapy, Assertiveness Training, Post-Partum Support Group) were coded 5. The percentage symptom reduction was again used as dependent outcome measure weighted by number of patients. All analyses were conducted using SPSS version 19.0 (IBM).

Results

The preliminary comparison of percentage symptom reduction with antidepressant and placebo treatment arms from published trials to antidepressant and placebo data from the FDA files revealed two significant main effects. The ANOVA indicated that antidepressants resulted in significantly greater symptom reduction than placebo, $F(\text{df}=239)=38.5, p<.001$. There was also a significant main effect of data source, $F(\text{df}=241)=33.6, p<.001$. Percentage symptom reduction was higher for published antidepressant (published data = 51%, FDA data 42 = %) and placebo

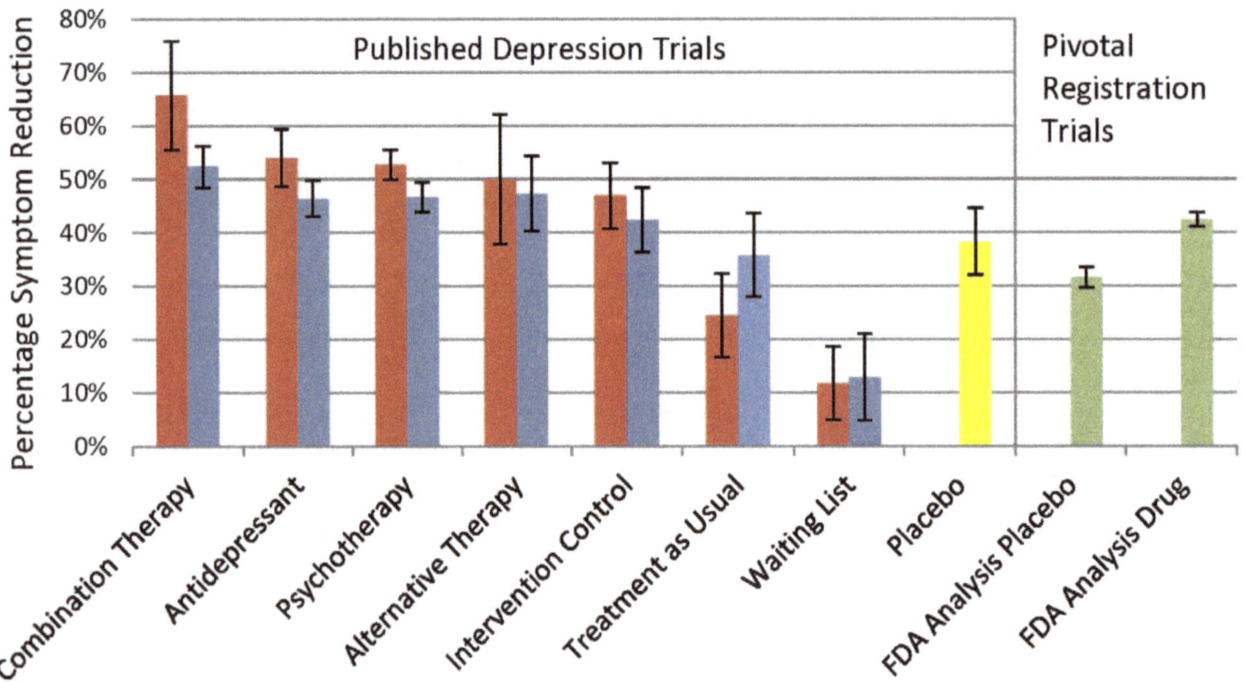

Figure 2. Mean Percentage Symptom Reduction from Un-blinded and Blinded Treatment Arms from Published Depression Trials Compared to Data from Pivotal Registration Depression Trials as Reported by the FDA. Red Bars Represent Un-Blinded Trial Arms Blue Bars Represent Blinded Trial Arms Yellow Represents Placebo Control Arms from Published Non-Registration trials Green Bars Represent Data from Pivotal Registration Trials The mean percentage symptom reduction was weighted by the number of assigned patients. Error Bars Represent 95% Confidence Intervals. Active treatment arms consist of combination antidepressant + therapy, antidepressants, psychotherapy, antidepressant therapy and alternative therapy. Control treatment arms consisted of placebo control, active intervention control, treatment-as-usual and waiting-list control. Blinded trials were operationally defined as those that utilized depression symptom raters that were blinded to treatment assignment of the patients.

(published data = 38%, FDA data = 32%) outcomes than those reported in the FDA SBA reports. The interaction between treatment type and data source was not significant, $p = 0.313$ (see Figure 2).

The 2×8 ANOVA to evaluate the role of blinding and the type of treatment on outcome in the published trials revealed a significant main effect of treatment type, $F(df = 313) = 33.7$, $p < 0.001$, and a significant interaction between treatment type and blinded status, $F(df = 313) = 2.17$, $p = 0.045$. Treatment type was a significant predictor of percentage symptom reduction in both un-blinded and blinded trials, but the magnitude and pattern of significance differed as a function of blinding.

As shown in Figure 2, the impact of blinding was most obvious in combination therapy trials with un-blinded trials resulting in 66% percentage symptom reduction versus 53% in blinded trials. The un-blinded trials also resulted in greater symptom reduction for antidepressants, psychotherapy and intervention controls. On the other hand, treatment-as-usual resulted in 24% symptom reduction for un-blinded trials with 36% symptom reduction in blinded trials.

Results from the separate one way ANOVAs to evaluate percentage symptom reduction between treatments and controls are shown as Tables 2 and 3. As shown in Table 2, in un-blinded trials combination antidepressant + therapy resulted in greater percentage symptom reduction than psychotherapy and antidepressants alone and all of the treatment controls. There were no significant differences in percentage symptom reduction between antidepressants, psychotherapy and alternative therapy. Psychotherapy and antidepressants were superior to all of the control treatments. There was no evidence of heterogeneity of outcomes across groups of un-blinded depression treatment arms based on Levene's Test of Equality of Error Variance, $F = 1.82$ (df = 150), $p = 0.099$.

As shown in Table 3, in blinded trials combination therapy was superior to psychotherapy and antidepressants alone and all of the treatment controls. There were no significant differences in percentage symptom reduction between psychotherapy, antidepressants, alternative therapies, and active intervention controls. Antidepressants, psychotherapy and active intervention controls resulted in greater percentage symptom reduction than the placebo controls, treatment-as-usual and wait-list. There was no evidence of heterogeneity of outcomes across groups of blinded depression trials based on Levene's Test of Equality of Error Variance, $F = 1.02$ (df = 163), $p = 0.420$.

There were no significant differences in percentage symptom reduction based on psychotherapy type as shown in Figure 3, $F(df = 128) = 1.42$, $p = 0.23$. There was a significant main effect of blinding, $F(df = 128) = 4.11$, $p = 0.045$.

Discussion

Much has been made of the inability of antidepressants to demonstrate clinically significant superiority to placebo in antidepressant clinical trials. The aim of this study was to compare the efficacy of combination psychotherapy + antidepressant, antidepressants, psychotherapies, alternative therapies and controls including placebo control for depression. We also evaluated the role of blinding as a factor in assessing differences between treatments.

Table 2. Percentage Symptom Reduction with Active Treatments and Controls among Depression Trials with an Un-blinded Rater.

	Combination	**Antidepressants**	**Psychotherapy**	**Alternative Therapy**	*Active Intervention Control*	*Treatment as Usual*	*Waiting List Control*
Combination (k = 8)	66%*						
Antidepressants (k = 17)	$p = 0.044$[a]	54%*					
Psychotherapy (k = 78)	$p = 0.016$[a]	NS[b]	53%*				
Alternative Therapy (k = 6)	$p = 0.049$[a]	NS[b]	NS[c]	50%*			
Active Intervention Control (k = 22)	$p = 0.001$[a]	$p = 0.057$[b]	$p = 0.055$[c]	NS	47%*		
Treatment as Usual (k = 6)	$p < 0.001$[a]	$p < 0.001$[b]	$p < 0.001$[c]	$p < 0.001$[d]	$p < 0.001$[e]	24%*	
Waiting-list Control (k = 20)	$p < 0.001$[a]	$p < 0.001$[b]	$p < 0.001$[c]	$p < 0.001$[d]	$p < 0.001$[e]	$p = 0.016$[f]	12%*

*Percentage symptom reduction values are weighted by number of patients per treatment arm for each active intervention and control for 59 un-blinded depression treatment trials with 157 treatment arms enrolling 4,083 patients.
Bolded text represents four active depression treatments. Italic text represents three treatment controls.
k = number of treatment arms for each therapy type.
Probability values show the statistical significance of comparisons between the treatment or control on the vertical access versus treatment or control on the horizontal access.
NS = Not Significant.
[a]Combination antidepressant therapy versus other treatments and controls.
[b]Antidepressant therapy versus other treatments and controls.
[c]Psychotherapy versus other treatments and controls.
[d]Alternative therapy versus treatment controls.
[e]Active intervention control versus treatment as usual and waiting-list controls.
[f]Treatment as usual versus waiting list control.
Analysis of Variance F Value (150 df) = 28.9, $p < 0.001$, statistical significance determined with Tukey's Post Hoc Test of Least Significant Difference.

Table 3. Percentage Symptom Reduction with Active Treatments and Controls among Depression Trials with a Blinded Rater.

	Combination	**Antidepressants**	**Psychotherapy**	**Alternative Therapy**	*Active Intervention Control*	*Placebo Control*	*Treatment as Usual*	*Waiting List Control*
Combination (k=24)	52%*							
Antidepressants (k=24)	$p=0.027$[a]	46%*						
Psychotherapy (k=50)	$p=0.022$[a]	NS[b]	47%*					
Alternative Therapy (k=12)	NS[a]	NS[b]	NS[c]	47%*				
Active Intervention Control (k=26)	$p=0.008$[a]	NS[b]	NS[c]	NS[d]	42%*	NS[e]		
Placebo Control (k=16)	$p<0.001$[a]	$p=0.030$[b]	$p=0.019$[c]	$p=.066$[d]	NS[e]	38%*		
Treatment as Usual (k=6)	$p<0.001$[a]	$p=0.017$[b]	$p=0.012$[c]	$p=0.035$[d]	NS[e]	NS[f]	36%*	
Waiting-list Control (k=14)	$P<0.001$[a]	$p<0.001$[b]	$p<0.001$[c]	$p<0.001$[d]	$p<0.001$[f]	$p<0.001$[e]	$p<0.001$[g]	13%*

*Percentage symptom reduction values are weighted by number of patients per treatment arm for each active intervention and control for 56 blinded depression treatment trials with 171 treatment arms enrolling 6,227 patients.
Bolded text represents four active depression treatments. Italic text represents the four treatment controls.
k = number of treatment arms for each therapy type.
Probability values show the statistical significance of comparisons between the treatment or control on the vertical access versus treatment or control on the horizontal access.
NS = Not Significant.
[a]Combination antidepressant therapy versus other treatments and controls.
[b]Antidepressant therapy versus other treatments and controls.
[c]Psychotherapy versus other treatments and controls.
[d]Alternative therapy versus treatment controls.
[e]Active intervention control versus treatment as usual and waiting-list controls.
[f]Placebo versus other treatment controls.
[g]Treatment as usual versus waiting list control.
Analysis of Variance F Value (163 df) = 11.99, $p<0.001$, statistical significance determined with Tukey's Post Hoc Test of Least Significant Difference.

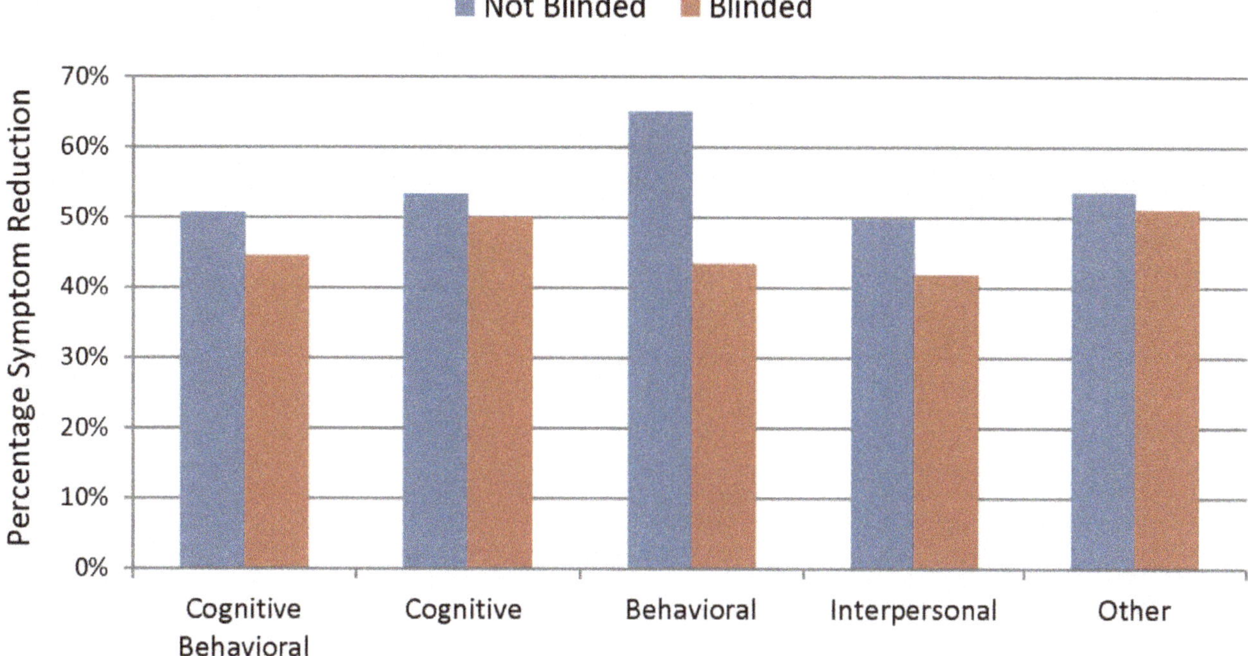

Figure 3. Mean Weighted Percentage Symptom Reduction of Psychotherapy Trial Arms from Published Depression Trials based on Type of Therapy Administered. The number of treatment arms for each therapy type was 24 for Cognitive Behavioral Therapy (16 un-blinded, 8 blinded), 39 for Cognitive Therapy (22 un-blinded, 17 blinded), 9 for Behavioral Therapy (7 un-blinded, 2 blinded), 14 for Interpersonal Therapy (7 un-blinded, 7 blinded) and 43 for therapies with other titles (26 un-blinded, 17 blinded).

Not surprisingly, blinding tended to decrease improvement in active treatment arms and increase it in control arms. This finding replicates previous analyses that have evaluated treatments by quantifying the level of blinding [8,14] suggesting that study design features do impact outcome of psychotherapy trials.

More importantly, when the raters were blinded the combined treatment of psychotherapy plus antidepressants showed only a slight advantage to antidepressants or psychotherapies alone. Although antidepressants alone and psychotherapy alone did differ significantly from placebo controls, treatment-as-usual and waiting list controls, they did not differ from alternative therapies such as exercise and acupuncture or active treatment control procedures.

It is interesting to note that although combination therapy did not statistically separate from exercise and acupuncture in the blinded trials, these alternative therapies themselves were not statistically superior to placebo ($p = 0.066$). This may be due to the small number of trials evaluating these. Aside from this fact, there is no obvious explanation for the increased variability in outcome observed in exercise and acupuncture treatment arms. Although the surface features of psychotherapy, antidepressants, exercise and acupuncture are very different, they do result in similar reduction of depressive symptoms and may have the same mechanism of action. The lack of significant differences between very diverse active treatments suggests that non-specific therapeutic factors may account for a large part of the effectiveness of these depression treatments.

Frank and Frank [34] contend that it is difficult to attribute specific outcomes to active therapies due to common therapeutic factors that patients experience during treatment. They undergo a thorough evaluation, are provided with an explanation for their distress, develop an expectation for improvement, and participate in a therapeutic ritual with an expert healer. These factors are the common threads among the conception and execution of these otherwise heterogeneous depression trials and treatments. Although such non-specific effects have been noted with comparisons of different psychotherapies for over 70 years [35,36], our study is the first to note such outcome similarities across such a diverse group of treatments and controls for depression.

One possible reason for the lack of assay sensitivity in depression trials is that common therapeutic factors are not exclusive to active depression treatments. Although the placebo pill is in essence inert and active intervention controls are devoid of the methodological rigor of active psychotherapies, the depressed patients assigned to these conditions are exposed to all other aspects of an active therapy. This reasoning might explain the finding that patients experienced similar improvement with placebo pill as compared to those assigned to treatment as usual that may have included antidepressants.

Our study has notable limitations with respect to the inferences that can be drawn from it. We know that patients that enroll in antidepressant clinical trials are not representative of depressed patients in clinical practice [37]. Depression trials of psychotherapy, exercise and acupuncture are also likely to attract a highly select group of depressed patients [38]. Thus, the generalizability of these data is limited.

Furthermore, we were not able to evaluate the roll that severity of depression may have played on treatment outcome. We do know that a higher severity of depression contributes to increased antidepressant-placebo differences in antidepressant clinical trials [33].

These data suggest that the preference of the patient, accessibility of various treatment options and riskiness of the therapy should all be factored into depression treatment decisions. It is important to note, however, that engaging in treatment is critical to improvement. These factors should be considered during cost-effectiveness analyses of potential depression treatments. For example, allowing patients to choose a preferred treatment from outset during cost-effectiveness studies may have influence on outcome and associated cost [39,40].

Our results also suggest that interpretation of clinical research evaluating relative efficacy of depression treatments using the randomized, double blind paradigm is problematic. With the exception of waiting-list control and treatment-as-usual, it is difficult to differentiate active treatments from "treatment controls" in adequately designed and highly blinded trials. This suggests alternative paradigms such as relapse prevention designs should be considered to evaluate potential treatments in the future.

In general, DSM depression is a broad and heterogeneous diagnosis, and researchers in the future might attempt to uncover specific profiles of depression which respond differentially to certain forms of treatment [41,42]. Targeting treatment effects based on age, gender, weight, pattern of symptoms and biomarkers may be worth exploring.

In conclusion, our results indicate that in acute depression trials using blinded raters the combination of psychotherapy and antidepressants may provide a slight advantage whereas antidepressants alone and psychotherapy do not significantly different from alternative therapies such as exercise and acupuncture or active intervention controls such as bibliotherapy or sham acupuncture. These data suggest that type of treatment offered is less important than getting depressed patients involved in an active therapeutic program. Thus, treatment type might best be chosen on the basis of differences in the clinical presentations, risks and patient preferences and acceptance. Future research should consider whether certain patient profiles might justify a specific treatment modality.

Supporting Information

Figure S1 Prisma 2009 Checklist.
(TIF)

Appendix S1 References and Blinded Status from 115 Depression Treatment Trials that were Included in the Analysis.
(DOCX)

Appendix S2 Active Treatment Arms (Combination Therapy + Antidepressant, Antidepressant, Psychotherapy, Alternative Therapy) and Control Treatment Arms (Placebo Control, Active Intervention Control, Treatment as Usual and Waiting-List) from 115 Published Depression Trials that Met Inclusion Criteria.
(DOCX)

Author Contributions

Conceived and designed the experiments: AK JF PL IK WAB. Performed the experiments: AK JF IK. Analyzed the data: AK JF. Contributed reagents/materials/analysis tools: AK. Wrote the paper: AK JF PL IK WAB.

References

1. Melander H, Ahlqvist-Rastad J, Meijer G, Beermann B (2003) Evidence b(i)ased medicine–selective reporting from studies sponsored by pharmaceutical industry: review of studies in new drug applications. BMJ 326(7400): 1171–1173.
2. Kirsch I, Sapirstein G (1998) Listening to prozac but hearing placebo: A meta-analysis of antidepressant medication. Prevention and Treatment 1: (Article 0002a).
3. Turner EH, Matthews AM, Linardatos E, Tell RA, Rosenthal R (2008) Selective publication of antidepressant trials and its influence on apparent efficacy. N Engl J Med 358: 252–260.
4. Fournier JC, DeRubeis RJ, Hollon SD, Dimidjian S, Amsterdam JD, et al. (2010) Antidepressant drug effects and depression severity: a patient-level meta-analysis. JAMA 303: 47–53.
5. Khan A, Leventhal RM, Khan SR, Brown WA (2002) Severity of depression and response to antidepressants and placebo: an analysis of the Food and Drug Administration database. J Clin Psychopharmacol 22: 40–45.
6. Nierenberg AA (2010) Antidepressants: can't live with them, can't live without them. CNS Spectr 15: 146–147.
7. Ullman D (2010) Homeopathy: A healthier way to treat depression. Huffington Post: Healthy Living. Available: http://www.huffingtonpost.com/dana-ullman/healthier-ways-to-treat-d_b_740720.html. Accessed 2011 May.
8. Cuijpers P, van Straten A, Bohlmeijer E, Hollon SD, Andersson G (2010) The effects of psychotherapy for adult depression are overestimated: a meta-analysis of study quality and effect size. Psychol Med 40: 211–223.
9. Belfield PW, YJ, Mulley GP (1985) Effect of aerobic exercise on depression: A controlled study. BMJ 291: 109.
10. Allen JJB, SR, Hitt SK (1998) The efficacy of acupuncture in the treatment of major depression in women. Psychol Science 9: 397–407.
11. Smith CA, Hay PPJ, MacPherson H (2010) Acupuncture for depression. Cochrane Database of Systematic Reviews Issue 1: Art. No. CD004366. doi: 10.1002/14651858.CD004046.pub3
12. Mead GE, Morley W, Campbell P, Greig CA, McMurdo M, et al. (2009) Exercise for depression. Cochrane Database of Systematic Reviews Issue 3: Art. No.: CD004366. doi: 10.1002/14651858.CD004366.pub4
13. National Collaborating Centre for Mental Health, The Royal College of Psychiatrists (2010) Depression: The NICE Guideline on the Treatment and Management of Depression in Adults. Updated edition. London: The British Psychological Society & The Royal College of Psychiatrists. 705 p.
14. Prioleau L, Murdoch M, Brody N (1983) An analysis of psychotherapy versus placebo studies. Behav Brain Sci 6: 275–310.
15. Cuijpers P, van Straten A, van Oppen P, Andersson G (2008) Are psychological and pharmacologic interventions equally effective in the treatment of adult depressive disorders? A meta-analysis of comparative studies. J Clin Psychiatry 69: 1675–1685.
16. Cuijpers P, van Straten A, Warmerdam L, Andersson G (2009) Psychotherapy versus the combination of psychotherapy and pharmacotherapy in the treatment of depression: a meta-analysis. Depress Anxiety 26: 279–288.
17. United States Department of Justice (2004) Freedom of Information Act Guide. Available: http://www.justice.gov/oip/foi-act.htm. Accessed 2012 May.
18. Khan A, Schwartz K (2007) Suicide risk and symptom reduction in patients assigned to placebo in duloxetine and escitalopram clinical trials: analysis of the FDA summary basis of approval reports. Ann Clin Psychiatry 19: 31–36.
19. Khan A, Khan SR, Leventhal RM, Brown WA (2001) Symptom reduction and suicide risk in patients treated with placebo in antidepressant clinical trials: a replication analysis of the Food and Drug Administration Database. Int J Neuropsychopharmacol 4: 113–118.
20. Khan A, Warner HA, Brown WA (2005) Symprom reduction and suicide risk in patients treated with placebo in antidepressant clinical trials: An analysis of the Food and Drug Administration database. Arch Gen Psychiatry 57: 311–317.
21. American Psychiatric Assocation (1968) Diagnostic and Statistical Manual of Mental Disorders (2nd ed.). Washington, DC.
22. American Psychiatric Association (1980) Diagnostic and Statistical Manual of Mental Disorders (3rd ed.). Washington, DC.
23. American Psychiatric Association (1994) Diagnostic and Statistical Manual of Mental Disorders (4th ed.). Washington, DC.
24. Spitzer RL, Endicott J, Robins E (1978) Research and diagnostic criteria: Rationale and reliability. Arch Gen Psychiatry 35: 773–782.
25. Feighner JP, Robins E, Guze SB, Woodruff RA, Winokur G, et al. (1972) Diagnostic criteria for use in psychiatric research. Arch Gen Psychiatry 26: 57–63.
26. Pampallona S, Bollini P, Tibaldi G, Kupelnick B, Munizza C (2004) Combined pharmacotherapy and psychological treatment for depression: a systematic review. Arch Gen Psychiatry 61: 714–9.
27. Leichsenring F (2001) Comparative effects of short-term psychodynamic psychotherapy and cognitive-behavioral therapy in depression: a meta-analytic approach. Clin Psychol Rev 21: 401–419.
28. Segal Z, Vincent P, Levitt A (2002) Efficacy of combined, sequential and crossover psychotherapy and pharmacotherapy in improving outcomes in depression. J Psychiatry Neurosci 27: 281–290.
29. Cuijpers P, van Straten A, Andersson G, van Oppen P (2008) Psychotherapy for depression in adults: a meta-analysis of comparative outcome studies. J Consult Clin Psychol 76: 909–922.
30. Cuijpers P (2008) Psychotherapy: Randomized controlled and comparative trials. Amsterdam. Available: http://www.evidencebasedpsychotherapies.org/index.php?id = 25. Accessed 2012 September.
31. Sinyor M, Levitt AJ, Cheung AH, Schaffer A, Kiss A, et al. (2010) Does inclusion of a placebo arm influence response to active antidepressant treatment in randomized controlled trials? Results from pooled and meta-analyses. J Clin Psychiatry 71: 270–279.
32. Rutherford BR, Sneed JR, Roose SP (2009) Does study design influence outcome?. The effects of placebo control and treatment duration in antidepressant trials. Psychother Psychosom 78: 172–181.

33. Khan A, Kolts RL, Thase ME, Krishnan KR, Brown W (2004) Research design features and patient characteristics associated with the outcome of antidepressant clinical trials. Am J Psychiatry 161: 2045–2049.
34. Frank JD, Frank JB (1991) Persuasion and healing: A comparative study of psychotherapy. Baltimore: The Johns Hopkins University Press.
35. Rosenzweig S (1936) Some implicit common factors in diverse methods of psychotherapy. Am J Orthopsychiat 6: 412–415.
36. Luborsky L, Rosenthal R, Diguer L, Andrusyna TP, Berman JS, et al. (2002) The dodo bird verdict is alive and well - mostly. Clin Psychol-Sci PR 9: 2–12.
37. Zimmerman M, Mattia JI, Posternak MA (2002) Are subjects in pharmacological treatment trials of depression representative of patients in routine clinical practice? Am J Psychiatry 159: 469–473.
38. Kushner SC, Quilty LC, McBride C, Bagby RM (2009) A comparison of depressed patients in randomized versus nonrandomized trials of antidepressant medications and psychotherapy. Depress Anxiety 26: 666–673.
39. Raue PJ, Schulberg HC, Heo Me, Klimstra SI, Bruce ML (2009) Patients' depression treatment preferences and initiation, adherence, and outcome: A randomized primary care study. Psychiatr Serv 60: 337–343.
40. Kwan BM, Dimidjian S, Rizvi SL (2010) Treatment preference, engagement, and clinical improvement in pharmacotherapy versus psychotherapy for depression. Behav Res Ther 48: 799–804.
41. Coryell W (2011) The search for improved antidepressant strategies: is bigger better? Am J Psychiatry 168: 664–666.
42. Lichtenberg P, Belmaker RH (2010) Subtyping major depressive disorder. Psychother Psychosom 79: 131–135.

Electro-Acupuncture Stimulation Improves Spontaneous Locomotor Hyperactivity in MPTP Intoxicated Mice

Haomin Wang[1¤a], Xibin Liang[2], Xuan Wang[3], Dingzhen Luo[3¤b], Jun Jia[3], Xiaomin Wang[3*]

1 Neuroscience Research Institute, Peking University, Key Laboratory for Neuroscience of the Ministry of Education, Beijing, PR China, **2** Department of Neurology and Neurological Sciences, Stanford University, Stanford, California, United States of America, **3** Department of Physiology, Capital Medical University, Key Laboratory for Neurodegenerative Disorders of the Ministry of Education, Beijing, PR China

Abstract

Bradykinesia is one of the major clinical symptoms of Parkinsońs disease (PD) for which treatment is sought. In most mouse models of PD, decreased locomotor activity can be reflected in an open field behavioral test. Therefore the open field test provides a useful tool to study the clinic symptoms of PD patients. Our previous work demonstrated that 100 Hz electro-acupuncture (EA) stimulation at ZUSANLI and SANYINJIAO protected the dopaminergic nigrostriatal system of C57BL/6 mice from MPTP toxicity, indicating that acupuncture might be an effective therapy for PD sufferers. In the present study, we investigated the effects of 100 Hz EA stimulation on the spontaneous locomotor activity in MPTP injured mice. Here we found that, in MPTP treated mice, the total movements significantly decreased and the movement time, velocity and distance dramatically increased, although the dopaminergic nigrostriatal system was devastated, revealed by immunohistochemistry and HPLC-ECD. After 12 sessions of 100 Hz EA stimulation, the total movements elevated and the movement time, velocity and distance decreased, in MPTP mice. 100 Hz EA increased striatal dopamine content in MPTP mice by 35.9%, but decreased its striatal dopamine turnover. We assumed that the injury of other regions in the brain, such as the A11 group in diencephalon, might be involved in the hypermotility in MPTP mice. The effects of 100 Hz EA on spontaneous locomotor activity in MPTP mice might not relate with the striatal dopamine, but with its neuroprotective and regulatory effects on motor circuits in the brain. Our study suggests that EA might be a promising treatment for neurological disorders including PD.

Editor: Huaibin Cai, National Institute of Health, United States of America

Funding: This study was supported by the National Basic Research Program of China (2011CB504100, http://www.973.gov.cn) and the National Natural Science Foundation of China (30472245, http://www.nsfc.gov.cn). The funders had no role in study design, data collection and analysis, decision to publish, or preparation of the manuscript.

Competing Interests: The authors have declared that no competing interests exist.

* E-mail: xmwang@ccmu.edu.cn

¤a Current address: Cell and Organ Transplant Institute, Fuzhou General Hospital, Xiamen University, Fuzhou, Fujian, PR China
¤b Current address: Department of Senile Neurology, Provincial Hospital Affiliated to Shandong University, Jinan, Shandong, PR China

Introduction

Parkinsońs disease (PD) is the second most frequently diagnosed neurodegenerative disease in the elderly. Its cardinal symptoms are resting tremor, rigidity, bradykinesia and postural instability, and its main pathological changes are profound loss of dopamingergic neurons in the substantia nigra pars compact (SNpc) and dopamine in the striatum. Although tremendous efforts have been made in the treatment of this disease, a long-term, effective therapy is still lacking.

Acupuncture is a branch of Traditional Chinese Medicine, which has been extensively and safely practiced in curing diseases in China for over 3,000 years. In recent decades, some studies reported that acupuncture could alleviate motor disorders, reduce the dosage of anti-Parkinsonian drugs and relieve non-motor problems of PD patients [1–4], while some other studies reported acupuncture had no effects on motor disorders of PD patients [5–7]. The controversies may be due to the difference in the treating schemes, acupuncture protocols, variable symptom profiles of patients involved and small sample sizes, etc. [5,6,8].

Compared with the clinical debates, animal experiments were in agreement with the claims that acupuncture was effective for PD by showing that acupuncture protected the dopaminergic nigro-striatal system or improved the abnormal movements in different kinds of PD animal models, i.e., the MFB-transected rat model, the 6-OHDA lesioned rat model, the MPTP lesioned mouse and rhesus monkey model [9–14].

Among all these models, the monkey MPTP model is considered the best since MPTP is known to cause Parkinsonism in humans. However, the mice MPTP model is more popularly used to value the anti-Parkinsonian therapies. Our previous studies showed that electro-acupuncture (EA) at 100 Hz could protect the dopaminergic nigrostriatal system from MPTP injury in mice via anti-oxidative effects [11]. Here, we investigated the impacts of 100 Hz EA on spontaneous locomotor activities in the same model and found that 100 Hz EA could normalize the abnormal behavior of MPTP mice.

Materials and Methods

Ethics Statement

All experimental procedures were approved by the Committee on Animal Care and Usage of Capital Medical University in which all the principles followed the Chinese Specifications for the Production, Care and Use of the Laboratory Animals. All animal experiments were performed by Haomin Wang whose permit number of the License for Performing Animal Experiments of Beijing is 12928. All efforts were made to minimize animal suffering.

Animals

Male C57BL/6J mice, weighting 22~25 g, 8 weeks old, were supplied by the Laboratory Animal Center of Peking University, and housed in a temperature-controlled room (23±1°C) under 12-h on/off light cycle with food and water *ad libitum* in the home cage. They were allowed to acclimate to the breeding environment for 7 days before experiments.

Subacute MPTP Mice Model

In the first cohort, fifty-five mice were randomly divided into a saline (NS) group (eleven mice) and a MPTP group (forty-four mice). As shown in Figure 1A, from day 1 to day 5 mice received intraperitoneal injections of MPTP (Sigma-Aldrich, St. Louis, MO, USA, 30 mg/kg, dissolved in saline) or an equivalent volume of saline once a day. Behavioral tests were performed on day 0, 6, 12, 18 and 24, and all mice in the NS group and eleven mice in the MPTP group were involved. On day 6, 12 and 18, eleven mice not participating behavioral test from MPTP group were sacrificed. On day 24, after behavioral test, the remaining mice were sacrificed.

EA Stimulation on MPTP Mice

In the second cohort, fifty-one mice were divided into four groups randomly: NS (twelve mice), saline plus EA stimulation at 100 Hz (100 Hz+NS, twelve mice), MPTP plus EA stimulation at 0 Hz (0 Hz+MPTP, thirteen mice) and MPTP plus EA stimulation at 100 Hz (100 Hz+MPTP, fourteen mice). As shown in Figure 1B, the EA stimulation was performed from day 1 to day 13 except day 7, and from day 2 to day 6, mice were received MPTP or saline (the same strategy with the first cohort of mice) half-hour after EA treatment. On day 0, 7 and 14 all mice underwent behavioral tests. EA stimulation was performed as described before [11].

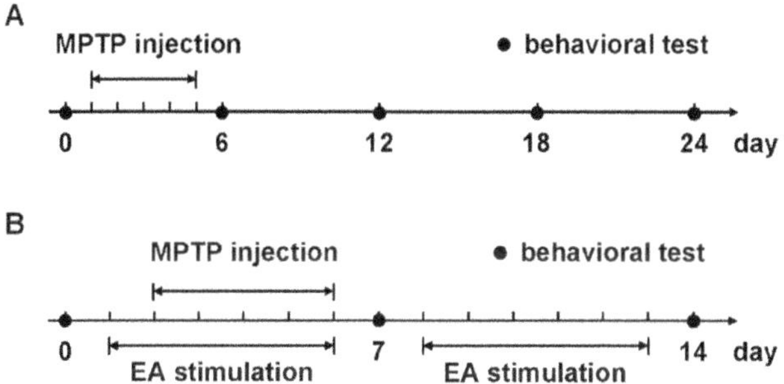

Figure 1. Experimental design of the study. (A) Subacute MPTP mice model. (B) EA stimulation on MPTP mice. Numbers represent days.

Open Field

Locomotion activity was assessed as previously described [15], using Mouse Tru Scan system (Coulbourn Instruments, USA). Briefly, each mouse was in a dark closed individual cage (25.4 x 25.4-inch-square) with a grid of infrared beams mounted horizontally every 2.5 cm, and spontaneous locomotor activity was recorded as total movements, total movement time and total movement distance across the 60 min recording period. All the assays were started at 9:00 am, and during the tests, the environment was kept quiet.

Tissue Collection and Processing

For immunohistochemistry analysis, four mice from each group on one time point were sacrificed, then the brains were removed and tissues were prepared according to the previously methods [11].

For monoamine level evaluation, seven mice from each group on one time point in the first cohort and nine to eleven mice from each group on day 14 in the second cohort were decapitated, and the bilateral striata were dissected quickly and stored at −80°C.

Immunohistochemistry and Quantification of TH-ir Neuronal Profiles

All sections spanning the SN were collected for immunohistochemistry according to the previously described method [11].

Systemic MPTP administration caused symmetrically bilateral lesions in the SNpc. Here, TH-ir neuronal profiles with distinct nuclear shapes in the left SNpc were counted in ten sections throughout the entire rostrocaudal extent of the left SNpc. All sections were coded and examined blind.

HPLC Analysis of DA and its Metabolites

Striata collected were used to detect the levels of DA and its metabolites, dihydroxyphenylacetic acid (DOPAC) and homovanillic acid (HVA), by HPLC with electrochemical detection (HPLC-ECD) according to the previously described method [11].

Statistical Analysis

Striatal monoamine levels were analyzed by one-way ANOVA followed by Least-Significant Difference (LSD) post hoc test of difference between means.

For the mouse behavior study, each animal's movement was measured at different time points, i.e. day 0, 6, 18 and 24. The day 0 mean value of each group was set as baseline. A ratio was obtained by normalizing the mean value of each time point to its own value at day 0 (the baseline). The ratios between each group were compared statistically. Statistical analyses of spontaneous locomotor activity were carried out using repeated measures ANOVA with groups as the independent variables and time as the repeated measure. When between-subjects (group) effects were significant, comparisons between the groups on each time point were performed using univariate ANOVA (in the first cohort) or univariate ANOVA with LSD post hoc test (in the second cohort).

All statistical analyses were performed by SPSS 13.0. Values are expressed as mean ± SEM. In all cases, the null hypothesis was rejected at the 0.05 level.

Results

MPTP Damages the Dopaminergic Nigrostriatal System

To this day, MPTP is mainly used to destroy the dopaminergic nigrostriatal system of animals. As shown in Figure 2, on day 6 the number of TH-ir neurons in the SNpc of the MPTP-treated mice

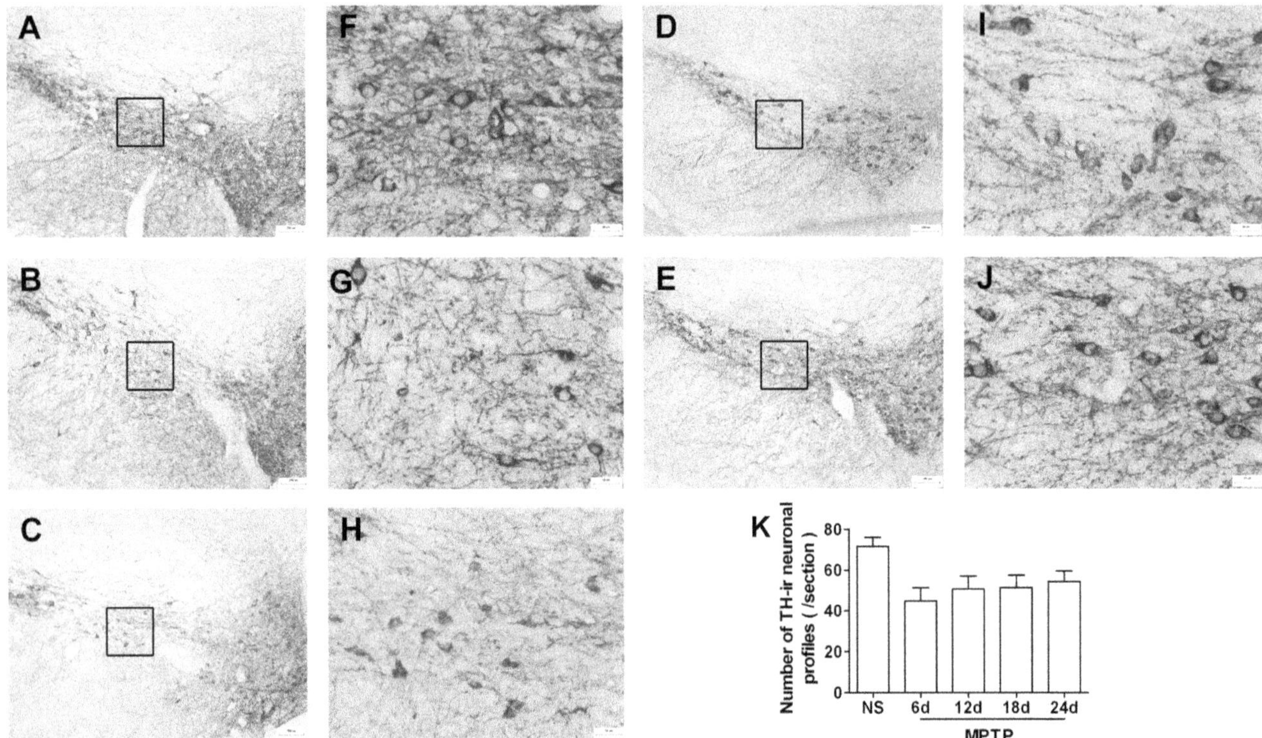

Figure 2. MPTP reduces the number of TH-ir neurons in the SNpc. (A and F) NS group. (B and G) MPTP group on day 6. (C and H) MPTP group on day 12. (D and I) MPTP group on day 18. (E and J) MPTP group on day 24. (K) Quantification of TH-ir neuronal profiles in the SNpc. Scale bar, 200 μm (A, B, C, D and E) and 50 μm (F, G, H, I and J). n = 3~4.

decreased to 62.8% of the normal amount, while from day 12 to day 24 a slight recovery occurred, keeping it at 70.8~76% of the normal level.

MPTP dramatically decreased striatal DA and its metabolites levels (DA, df = 4, F = 94.987, $p = 0.000$, Figure 3A; DOPAC, df = 4, F = 49.789, $p = 0.000$, Figure 3B; HVA, df = 4, F = 26.128, $p = 0.000$, Figure 3C), and significantly increased the DA turnover (indicated by DOPAC/DA ratio, df = 4, F = 15.214, $p = 0.000$, Figure 3D), suggesting that DA insufficiency activated the compensatory pathways. Consistent with the tendency of TH-ir neurons in the SNpc, from day 12 on, the four indices recovered significantly compared with that on day 6 (DA and DOPAC, $p < 0.01$, Figure 3, A and B; HVA and DA turnover, $p < 0.05$, Figure 3, C and D). Taking DA for example, on day 6 it dropped to 23%, yet during day 12 to day 24 it was back to 37.4~43.8%.

These data showed that in this model the dopaminergic nigrostriatal system suffered the severest injury when MPTP administration just completed (day 6), then recovered to some extent, and was in a relatively stable state from day 12 to day 24.

MPTP Increases the Spontaneous Locomotor Activity

One movement is defined as a series of successive coordinate changes without rest for at least one sample interval in the floor plane. MPTP significantly reduced the total movements in mice (df = 1, F = 5.662, $p = 0.028$, Figure 4A), suggesting either an increased movement time (hyperkinesia) or an increased rest time (hypokinesia). The total movement time in MPTP-lesioned mice markedly increased over time (df = 1, F = 8.975, $p = 0.007$, Figure 4B), indicating that the reduction of total movements in MPTP intoxicated mice was due to hyperkinesia not hypokinesia. Elevated total movement time contributed to the dramatically augmented total movement distance in MPTP mice (df = 1, F = 16.164, $p = 0.001$, Figure 4C). Movement velocity was acquired by total movement distance normalized with total movement time, and also notably raised by MPTP in mice (df = 1, F = 14.357, $p = 0.001$, Figure 4D). On day 24, the total movement time was, on average, 10% higher, movement velocity was 19% higher and total movement distance was 31% higher for MPTP mice compared with the control mice, exhibiting a phenomenon of hyperkinesia.

100 Hz EA Improves the Abnormal Behavior of MPTP Mice

In our previous study, 0 Hz EA stimulation did not show any influence on Parkinsonian mice and rats [11,16]. In this study, we used 0 Hz+MPTP group as a control because puncturing the acupoints on the legs might affect the motion of animals.

On day 14, total movements in 0 Hz+MPTP group and 100 Hz+MPTP group were still significantly lower than that in NS group ($p = 0.002$ and $p = 0.038$ respectively, Figure 5A), while total movement time in MPTP mice received 100 Hz EA administration recovered to some extent but had no statistical difference with that in the MPTP mice ($p = 0.061$, Figure 5B).

100 Hz EA had more prominent effects on movement velocity of MPTP mice, which was significantly reversed on day 14 ($p = 0.033$ *vs.* 0 Hz+MPTP group, Figure 5D). Both decreased total movement time and movement velocity accounted for the dramatically reduced total movement distance on day 14 in MPTP mice received 100 Hz EA administration ($p = 0.02$ *vs.* 0 Hz+MPTP, Figure 5C). In addition, 100 Hz EA stimulation did not influence the spontaneous locomotor activity of normal mice (Figure 5).

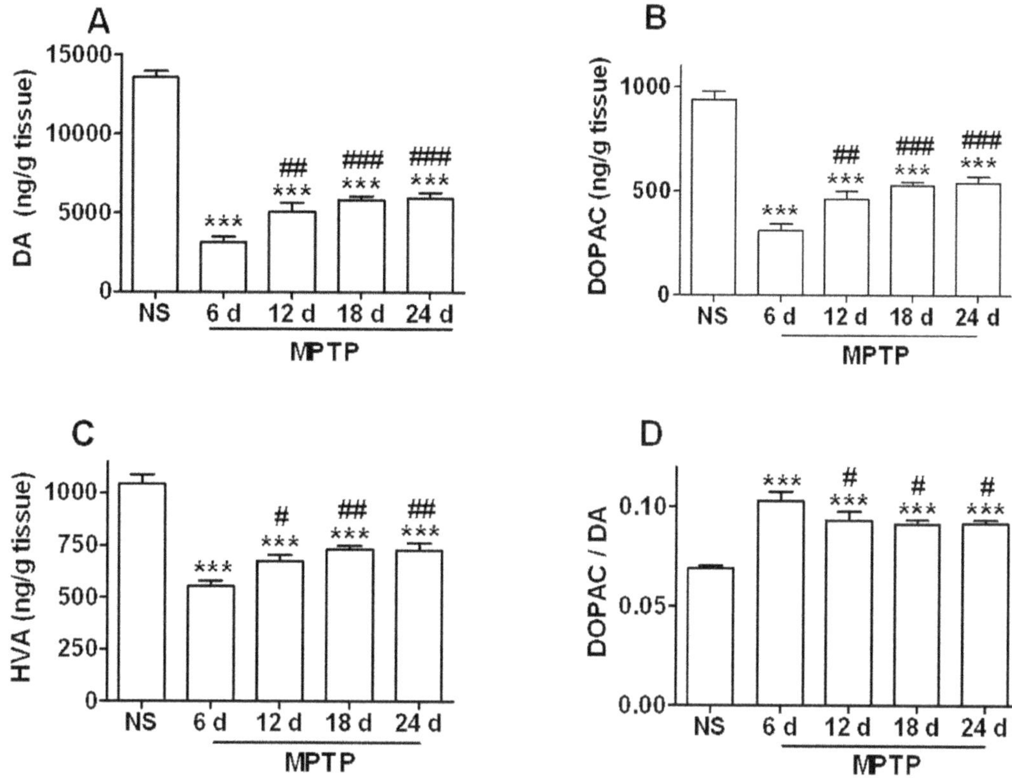

Figure 3. MPTP decreases striatal content of DA and its metabolites and increases the DA turnover. (A) DA. (B) DOPAC. (C) HVA. (D) DA turnover. *** $p<0.001$ *vs.* NS group; #$p<0.05$, ##$p<0.01$, ###$p<0.001$ *vs.* MPTP group on day 6. n = 6~7.

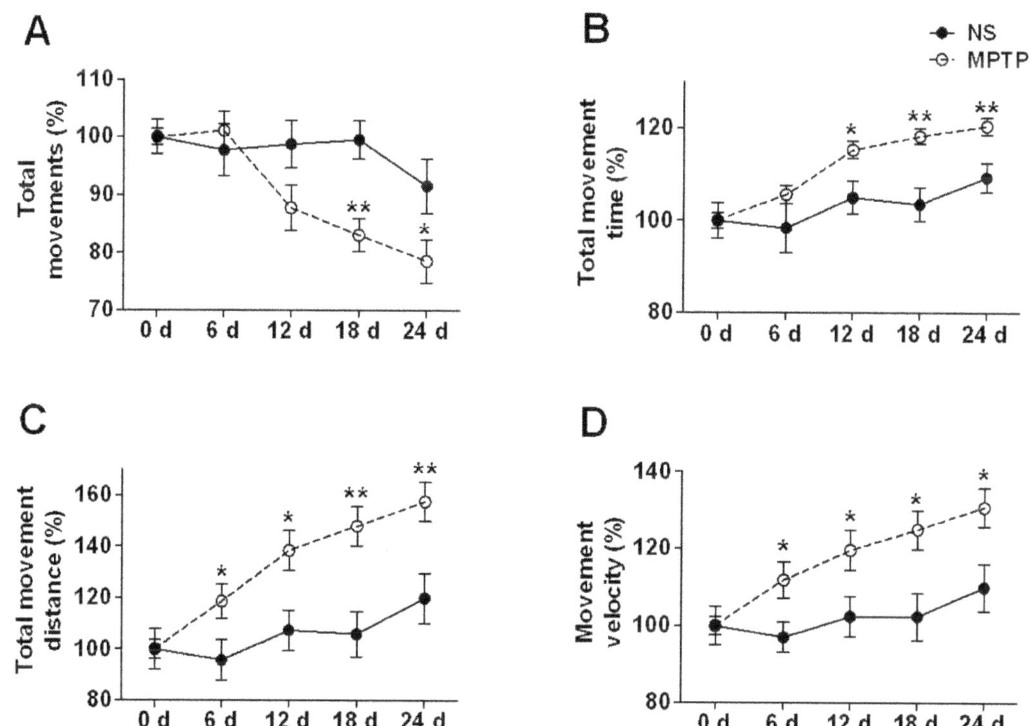

Figure 4. MPTP increases the spontaneous locomotor activity. (A) Total movements. (B) Total movement time. (C) Total movement distance. (D) Movement velocity. Filled circle with solid line represents the NS group, and hollow circle with dash line represents the MPTP group. *$p<0.05$, **$p<0.01$ *vs.* NS group on the same day. n = 10~11.

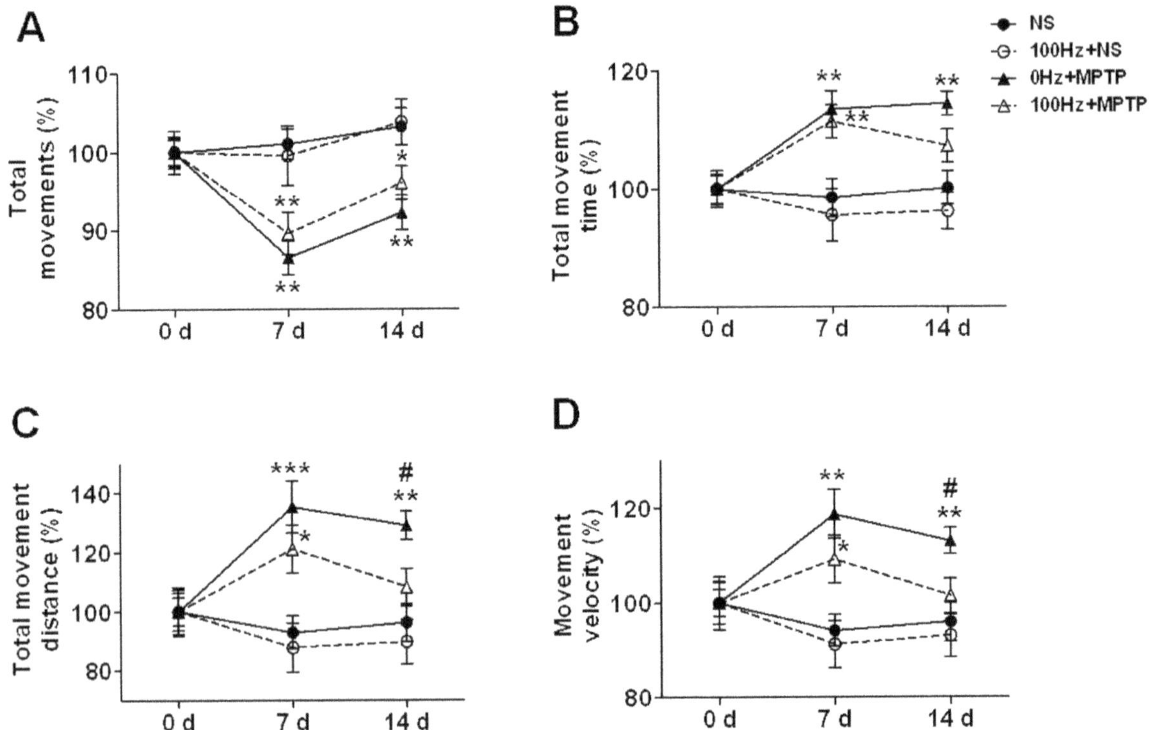

Figure 5. 100 Hz EA stimulation improves the hyperkinesia of MPTP mice. (A) Total movements. (B) Total movement time. (C) Total movement distance. (D) Movement velocity. Filled circle with solid line represents the NS group, hollow circle with dash line represents the 100 Hz+NS group, filled triangle with solid line represents the 0 Hz+MPTP group, and hollow triangle with dash line represents the 100 Hz+MPTP group. *$p<0.05$, **$p<0.01$, ***$p<0.001$ *vs.* NS group on the same day; $^{\#}p<0.05$ *vs.* 100 Hz+MPTP group on the same day. n = 12~14.

Effects of 100 Hz EA on Striatal DA and its Metabolites

On day 14, MPTP dramatically decreased the contents of DA, DOPAC and HVA but increased DA turnover in the striatum ($p=0.000$ *vs.* NS group, Figure 6). Although the DA level was 35.9% higher in the 100 Hz+MPTP group than that in the 0 Hz+MPTP group, the difference was not significant ($p=0.106$, Figure 6A). However, DOPAC and HVA levels in MPTP mice were not enhanced in such amplitude by 100 Hz EA treatment (Figure 6, B and C). Therefore, its DA turnover was significantly decreased ($p=0.000$ *vs.* 0 Hz+MPTP group, Figure 6D). In addition, 100 Hz EA stimulation did not have effects on striatal DA and its metabolites in normal mice (Figure 6).

Discussion

In this study, we observed that in a commonly used mouse PD model, although the dopaminergic nigrostriatal system was severely damaged by MPTP, the spontaneous movement time, velocity and distance increased. After stimulating acupoint ZUSANLI and SANYINJIAO with 100 Hz EA, we found that the locomotor hyperactivity in this model was normalized. 100 Hz EA increased striatal DA content in MPTP-lesioned mice, but not DOPAC and HVA content, making the DA turnover decreased. It suggested that striatal DA might not play a role in the effect of 100 Hz EA on the spontaneous locomotor activity. In addition, 100 Hz EA did not affect the striatal DA and its metabolites as well as the spontaneous locomotor activity in normal mice.

MPTP-lesioned C57BL/6 mice model is widely used to assess novel anti-Parkinsonian therapies, but conflicted results show decreased, increased and neutral phenomenon on locomotor activity, which might be due to different sources of mice or intoxication protocols [17,18].

In our study, striatal DA in MPTP mice remained 23% at its lowest level (day 6), and was about 40% when hyperkinesia became dominant (from day 12 to day 24). It is commonly assumed that a 70~90% DA deficiency is required for symptom appearance in PD [19], and a striatal DA loss greater than 80% is necessary to observe symptoms across species [17]. In our previous study on an acute MPTP C57BL/6J mice model (15 mg/kg four times at 2 h interval, i.p.), striatal DA was left 7.7%, and the spontaneous locomotor activity markedly decreased [15]. Therefore, the "suprathreshold" injury of the dopaminergic nigrostriatal sytem might contribute to the hyperkinesia.

Aside from the open field test we had also used the rotarod test, a test widely used to measure coordinated motor skills [17]. We also observed an upward tendency in MPTP mice compared with the normal control. However, no statistical difference existed between groups (n = 10 each group, data not shown).

MPTP is highly lipophilic and crosses the blood-brain barrier soon after the systemic injection. In the brain, it is transformed into the toxic form, MPP^+, in non-dopaminergic cells. MPP^+ has a high affinity for the dopamine transporters (DAT) through which it enters the DA neuron to kill the host cell. Apart from the SNpc, there distribute DA cells in other regions of the central nervous system, such as the DA A11 group in the caudal diencephalon, which projects into the spinal cord, forming the diencephalospinal pathway. Perturbation of the A11 group is thought to be involved in restless legs syndrome (RLS) [20], a common disease characterized by an intense urge to move the limbs, which can be mitigated by dopamine replacement therapy. There also exists the A11 diencephalospinal pathway in C57BL mice [21], and 6-

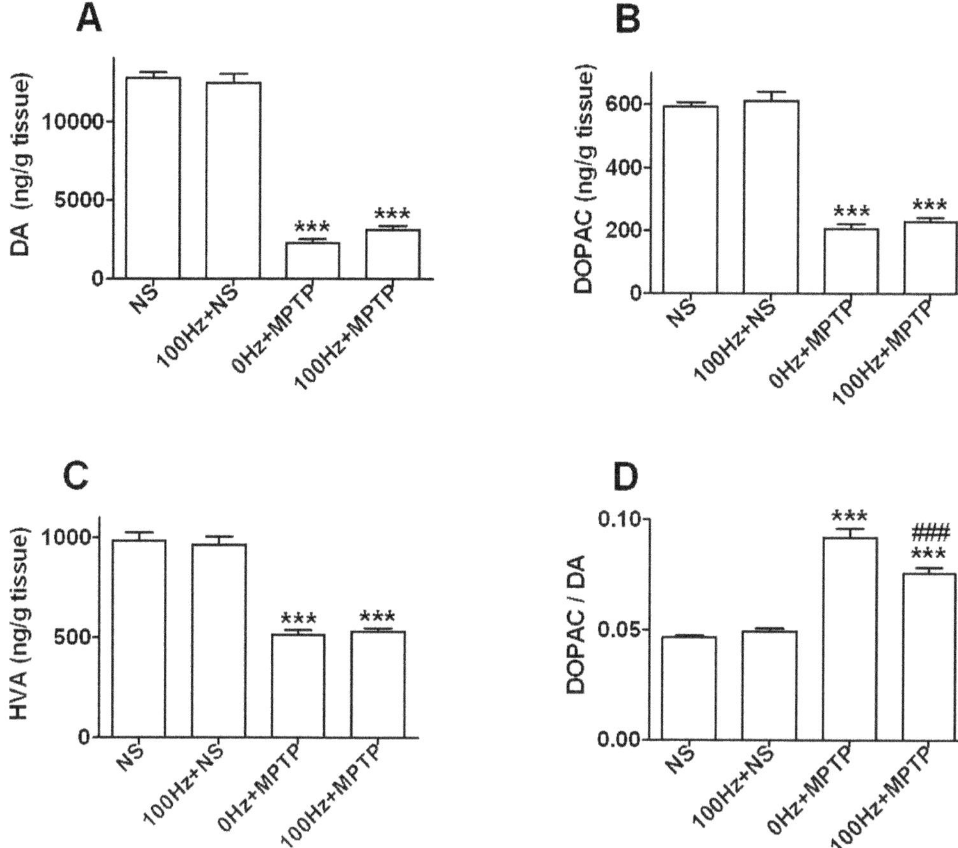

Figure 6. Impacts of 100 Hz EA stimulation on striatal DA and its metabolites. (A) DA. (B) DOPAC. (C) HVA. (D) DA turnover. ***$p<0.001$ *vs.* NS group; ###$p<0.001$ *vs.* 0 Hz+MPTP group. n = 9~11.

OHDA can lead to locomotor hyperactivity in mice by damaging the A11 group [22]. MPTP is also able to destroy the A11 group in non-human primates [23]. In our model, the A11 group might be injured and contribute to the hyperkinesia. Thus, only if it is very severely damaged (e.g. >80% loss of striatal DA), can the motor effects resulting from the devastated dopaminergic nigrostriatal system become dominant and hypokinesia emerge. In addition, our data does not suggest that this model is a potential RLS model, because contrary to it, in the SN of RLS patients there is an increased TH and no cell loss [24].

Furthermore, MPTP can destroy other monoaminergic or non-monoaminergic regions that do not express DAT [23]. Rousselet and colleagues assumed that hyperkinesia in MPTP mice might be due to the disturbance of prefrontal cortex [18]. In Rommelfanger's study, the hypokinesia did not appear in MPTP treated mice until norepinephrine loss occurred [25], however, this could not help to explain the hypermotility in MPTP mice in our study.

The mechanism of 100 Hz EA in normalizing hyperkinesia in MPTP mice is still unclear. Multiple-mechanisms might be involved in the whole process. Our previous studies showed that 100 Hz EA eased oxidative stress in this model [11], while others demonstrated that acupuncture stimulated neurotrophic factor release, and had anti-inflammatory and anti-apoptotic effects [10,12,26–28], which might also contribute to prevent neuronal damage from MPTP in this study. Our previous studies on PD rats showed that 100 Hz EA could balance neurotransimtters or neuropeptides in the motor circuits. In Jiàs study, 100 Hz EA increased GABA content and substance P content in the midbrain to improve the abnormal behavior of PD rats [16,29]. In Huòs study, it was suggested that the cortex might play the most important role in the regulation of internal balance in PD rats after 100 Hz EA treatment [9]. In addition, Huang et al. reported that acupuncture increased regional cerebral blood flow in the frontal lobe and the basal ganglia of PD patients [30].

Collectively, hyperkinesia in MPTP mice may reflect the multiple injury patterns of MPTP. Acupuncture might exert extensive neuroprotective and regulatory effects on motor circuits in PD brain.

Acknowledgments

We express sincere thanks to Miss Yilin Liang for the critical reading of the manuscript.

Author Contributions

Conceived and designed the experiments: XMW XW HMW. Performed the experiments: HMW DZL JJ. Analyzed the data: HMW XBL XW XMW. Contributed reagents/materials/analysis tools: XMW. Wrote the paper: HMW XBL. Final approval of the version to be published: XMW.

References

1. Chen L (1998) Clinical observations on forty cases of paralysis agitans treated by acupuncture. J Tradit Chin Med 18: 23–26.
2. Shulman LM, Wen X, Weiner WJ, Bateman D, Minagar A, et al. (2002) Acupuncture therapy for the symptoms of Parkinson's disease. Mov Disord 17: 799–802.
3. Ren XM (2008) Fifty cases of Parkinson's disease treated by acupuncture combined with madopar. J Tradit Chin Med 28: 255–257.
4. Zhuang X, Wang L (2000) Acupuncture treatment of Parkinson's disease–a report of 29 cases. J Tradit Chin Med 20: 265–267.
5. Lam YC, Kum WF, Durairajan SS, Lu JH, Man SC, et al. (2008) Efficacy and safety of acupuncture for idiopathic Parkinson's disease: a systematic review. J Altern Complement Med 14: 663–671.
6. Lee MS, Shin BC, Kong JC, Ernst E (2008) Effectiveness of acupuncture for Parkinson's disease: a systematic review. Mov Disord 23: 1505–1515.
7. Cristian A, Katz M, Cutrone E, Walker RH (2005) Evaluation of acupuncture in the treatment of Parkinson's disease: a double-blind pilot study. Mov Disord 20: 1185–1188.
8. Rabinstein AA, Shulman LM (2003) Acupuncture in clinical neurology. Neurologist 9: 137–148.
9. Huo LR, Liang XB, Li B, Liang JT, He Y, et al. (2012) The cortical and striatal gene expression profile of 100 Hz electroacupuncture treatment in 6-hydroxydopamine-induced Parkinson's disease model. Evid Based Complement Alternat Med 2012: 908439.
10. Liang XB, Liu XY, Li FQ, Luo Y, Lu J, et al. (2002) Long-term high-frequency electro-acupuncture stimulation prevents neuronal degeneration and up-regulates BDNF mRNA in the substantia nigra and ventral tegmental area following medial forebrain bundle axotomy. Brain Res Mol Brain Res 108: 51–59.
11. Wang H, Pan Y, Xue B, Wang X, Zhao F, et al. (2011) The antioxidative effect of electro-acupuncture in a mouse model of Parkinson's disease. PLoS One 6: e19790. doi:10.1371/journal.pone.0019790.
12. Liang XB, Luo Y, Liu XY, Lu J, Li FQ, et al. (2003) Electro-acupuncture improves behavior and upregulates GDNF mRNA in MFB transected rats. Neuroreport 14: 1177–1181.
13. Zhao F, Fan X, Grondin R, Edwards R, Forman E, et al. (2010) Improved methods for electroacupuncture and electromyographic recordings in normal and parkinsonian rhesus monkeys. J Neurosci Methods 192: 199–206.
14. Kim SN, Doo AR, Park JY, Bae H, Chae Y, et al. (2011) Acupuncture enhances the synaptic dopamine availability to improve motor function in a mouse model of Parkinson's disease. PLoS One 6: e27566. doi:10.1371/journal.-pone.0027566.
15. Luo D, Zhang Q, Wang H, Cui Y, Sun Z, et al. (2009) Fucoidan protects against dopaminergic neuron death in vivo and in vitro. Eur J Pharmacol 617: 33–40.
16. Jia J, Sun Z, Li B, Pan Y, Wang H, et al. (2009) Electro-acupuncture stimulation improves motor disorders in Parkinsonian rats. Behav Brain Res 205: 214–218.
17. Sedelis M, Schwarting RK, Huston JP (2001) Behavioral phenotyping of the MPTP mouse model of Parkinson's disease. Behav Brain Res 125: 109–125.
18. Rousselet E, Joubert C, Callebert J, Parain K, Tremblay L, et al. (2003) Behavioral changes are not directly related to striatal monoamine levels, number of nigral neurons, or dose of parkinsonian toxin MPTP in mice. Neurobiol Dis 14: 218–228.
19. Bezard E, Dovero S, Prunier C, Ravenscroft P, Chalon S, et al. (2001) Relationship between the appearance of symptoms and the level of nigrostriatal degeneration in a progressive 1-methyl-4-phenyl-1,2,3,6-tetrahydropyridine-lesioned macaque model of Parkinson's disease. J Neurosci 21: 6853–6861.
20. Paulus W, Dowling P, Rijsman R, Stiasny-Kolster K, Trenkwalder C, et al. (2007) Pathophysiological concepts of restless legs syndrome. Mov Disord 22: 1451–1456.
21. Qu S, Ondo WG, Zhang X, Xie WJ, Pan TH, et al. (2006) Projections of diencephalic dopamine neurons into the spinal cord in mice. Exp Brain Res 168: 152–156.
22. Qu S, Le W, Zhang X, Xie W, Zhang A, et al. (2007) Locomotion is increased in a11-lesioned mice with iron deprivation: a possible animal model for restless legs syndrome. J Neuropathol Exp Neurol 66: 383–388.
23. Barraud Q, Obeid I, Aubert I, Barriere G, Contamin H, et al. (2010) Neuroanatomical study of the A11 diencephalospinal pathway in the non-human primate. PLoS One 5: e13306. doi:10.1371/journal.pone.0013306.
24. Connor JR, Wang XS, Allen RP, Beard JL, Wiesinger JA, et al. (2009) Altered dopaminergic profile in the putamen and substantia nigra in restless leg syndrome. Brain 132: 2403–2412.
25. Rommelfanger KS, Edwards GL, Freeman KG, Liles LC, Miller GW, et al. (2007) Norepinephrine loss produces more profound motor deficits than MPTP treatment in mice. Proc Natl Acad Sci U S A 104: 13804–13809.
26. Liu XY, Zhou HF, Pan YL, Liang XB, Niu DB, et al. (2004) Electro-acupuncture stimulation protects dopaminergic neurons from inflammation-mediated damage in medial forebrain bundle-transected rats. Exp Neurol 189: 189–196.
27. Jeon S, Kim YJ, Kim ST, Moon W, Chae Y, et al. (2008) Proteomic analysis of the neuroprotective mechanisms of acupuncture treatment in a Parkinson's disease mouse model. Proteomics 8: 4822–4832.
28. Kang JM, Park HJ, Choi YG, Choe IH, Park JH, et al. (2007) Acupuncture inhibits microglial activation and inflammatory events in the MPTP-induced mouse model. Brain Res 1131: 211–219.
29. Jia J, Li B, Sun ZL, Yu F, Wang X, et al. (2010) Electro-acupuncture stimulation acts on the basal ganglia output pathway to ameliorate motor impairment in Parkinsonian model rats. Behav Neurosci 124: 305–310.
30. Huang Y, Jiang X, Zhuo Y, Wik G (2010) Complementary acupuncture in Parkinson's disease: a spect study. Int J Neurosci 120: 150–154.

16

Differences in Neural-Immune Gene Expression Response in Rat Spinal Dorsal Horn Correlates with Variations in Electroacupuncture Analgesia

Ke Wang[1,9], Rong Zhang[2,9], Xiaohui Xiang[2], Fei He[1], Libo Lin[1], Xingjie Ping[2], Lei Yu[3], Jisheng Han[2], Guoping Zhao[1,4]*, Qinghua Zhang[1]*, Cailian Cui[2]*

1 Shanghai-MOST Key Laboratory of Health and Disease Genomics, Chinese National Human Genome Center at Shanghai and National Engineering Research Center for Biochip at Shanghai, Shanghai, China, **2** Neuroscience Research Institute; Department of Neurobiology, Peking University Health Science Center; Key Laboratory of Neuroscience of the Ministry of Education and the Ministry of Public Health; Peking University, Beijing, China, **3** Department of Genetics and Center of Alcohol Studies, Piscataway, New Jersey, United States of America, **4** Department of Microbiology and Li Ka Shing Institute of Health Sciences, The Chinese University of Hong Kong, Prince of Wales Hospital, Shatin, New Territories, Hong Kong Special Administrative Region, China

Abstract

Background: Electroacupuncture (EA) has been widely used to alleviate diverse pains. Accumulated clinical experiences and experimental observations indicated that significant differences exist in sensitivity to EA analgesia for individuals of patients and model animals. However, the molecular mechanism accounting for this difference remains obscure.

Methodology/Principal Findings: We classified model male rats into high-responder (HR; TFL changes >150) and non-responder (NR; TFL changes ≤0) groups based on changes of their pain threshold detected by tail-flick latency (TFL) before and after 2 Hz or 100 Hz EA treatment. Gene expression analysis of spinal dorsal horn (DH) revealed divergent expression in HR and NR after 2 Hz/100 Hz EA. The expression of the neurotransmitter system related genes was significantly highly regulated in the HR animals while the proinflammation cytokines related genes were up-regulated more significantly in NR than that in HR after 2 Hz and 100 Hz EA stimulation, especially in the case of 2 Hz stimulation.

Conclusions/Significance: Our results suggested that differential regulation and coordination of neural-immune related genes might play an important role for individual variations in analgesic effects responding to EA in DH. It also provided new candidate genes related to EA responsiveness for future investigation.

Editor: Ferenc Gallyas, University of Pecs Medical School, Hungary

Funding: This work was supported by the National Basic Research Program of China (No. 973-2007CB512501), China Postdoctoral Science Foundation (No. 20100480643), and National Natural Science Foundation of China (No. 30801491). The funders had no role in study design, data collection and analysis, decision to publish, or preparation of the manuscript.

Competing Interests: The authors have declared that no competing interests exist.

* E-mail: clcui@bjmu.edu.cn (CC); qinghua_zhang@shbiochip.com (QZ); gpzhao@sibs.ac.cn (GZ)

9 These authors contributed equally to this work.

Introduction

Acupuncture has been used in China and other Asian countries for more than 2500 years and in western countries for decades [1]. Instead of traditional acupuncture manipulations, electroacupuncture (EA) has been used with electric pulses delivered to acupuncture needles to alleviate pains of diverse etiology [2,3,4]. Although EA analgesia was considered generally effective in practice, significant individual variations in analgesic effects were well documented in both animals and humans [5,6]. According to the magnitude of the analgesic response to EA, an individual can be categorized into high-responders (HR) and non-responders (NR) [6,7]. In some previous animal studies, rats showing a statistically significant increase in tail flick latency (TFL) by EA stimulation ($P<0.01$) were classified as HR, and other subjects were classified as NR [8,9,10]. In other studies, rats showing an increase more than 30% or 60% in TFL in response to EA stimulation were classified as HR, while rats showing less than a 20% or 30% increase in TFL in response to EA were classified as NR [6,11]. Because there were different criteria for definition of the HR and NR, the percentage for HR and NR in previous reports were 30.0%~61.1% and 30.0%~46.2%, respectively [6,8,9,10,11,12]. This phenomenon leaves an obstacle to clinical pain management by EA treatment, especially to the application of acupuncture compound anesthesia in clinical surgical operation.

Further research has been done to demonstrate a dynamic balance process between nociceptive and antinociceptive substances in CNS involved in acupuncture analgesia as well as individual variations in acupuncture analgesia [4]. Analgesic effect of EA has been shown to be due to the release of endogenous opioid peptides and activation of the descending inhibitory pathways in the central nervous system (CNS) [13]. The different neuropeptides are released in response to EA with different frequencies. For instance, low-frequency (2 Hz) EA accelerates the release of enkephalin, β-endorphin and endomorphin. In contrast, EA with high-frequency (100 Hz) selectively increases dynorphin release. Furthermore, many other neurotransmitters and/or receptors in CNS also play a role mediating EA analgesia [14,15]. These results of these studies suggest that the effect of EA is mediated by many substances and pathways in CNS. In addition, previous studies have demonstrated that the endogenous antiopioid peptide cholecystokinin (Cck) release and the density of the postsynaptic CCK receptors (Cck-a and -b) in the CNS are closely associated with individual sensitivity to EA [9,10,16]. Though Cck mechanisms have been well understood for individual differences in response to EA stimulation, the molecular mechanisms underlying individual differences in response to EA analgesia are largely unknown.

Gene expression in the CNS is the first measurable indicator of the interaction between genome and stimulation response [17]. Gene expression profiling of particular regions of CNS is used to decipher the molecular bases of changes in special function and behavior in response to environmental changes in modern neurobiology. Thus, we hypothesized that the differences in gene expression response may result in individual variations in EA analgesia. The spinal dorsal horn (DH) is an important direct responding region involved in EA analgesia [18,19,20], and an important relay site in the transmission of nociceptive information

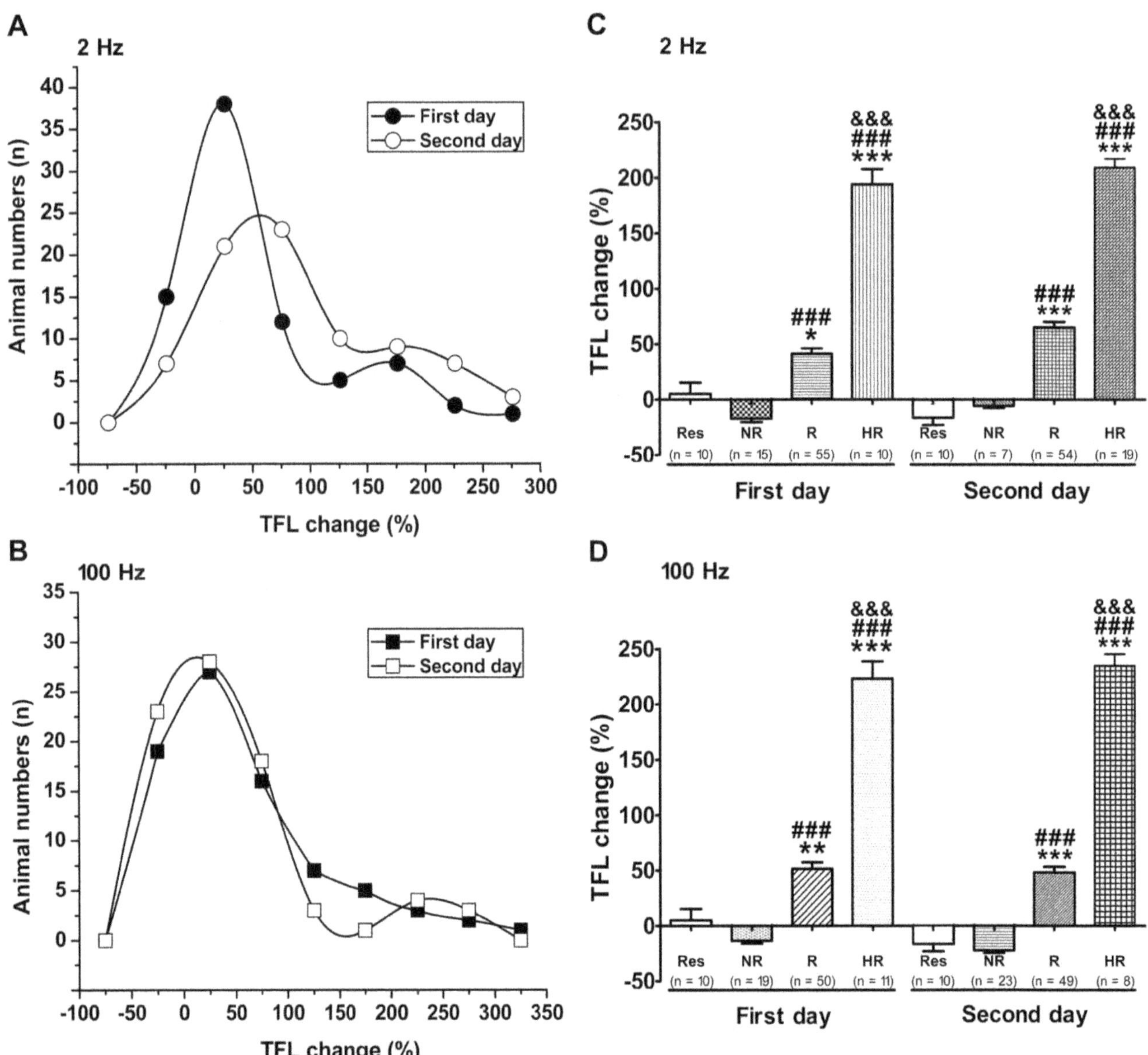

Figure 1. Analgesic effect induced by 2 Hz and 100 Hz EA in rats. The analgesic effects of EA on acute thermal pain were quantified using the TFL test, and they are expressed as percent changes from basal TFL. Either 2 Hz (A) or 100 Hz (B) EA, rats showed individual differences in sensitivity of EA analgesia for two consecutive days. A majority of rats showed sensitivity to EA analgesia (TFL change >0) and a small part appeared in contrary way (TFL change ≤0). Plan C and D showed comparison of the EA analgesic effects among the high-responder (HR), responder (R), and non-responder (NR) or restraint (Res) group in two consecutive days. Data are represented as mean ± SEM. One way ANOVA and Bonferroni's Multiple Comparison Test was used to analysis TFL change (%). *$P<0.05$, **$P<0.01$, ***$P<0.001$ vs. restraint group; $^{\#\#\#}P<0.001$, vs. compared with the corresponding NR group; $^{\&\&\&}P<0.001$, compared with the corresponding R groups.

from the periphery to the brain, and nociception modulation by descending influences from the brainstem to local mechanisms [21,22]. Aiming at elucidating the molecular basis of complex traits of behaviors in response to various kinds of stimulations, Sprage-Dawley (SD) rats were commonly used to model the human genetic complexity of individual variations in response to EA stimulation [23,24]. In the present study, in order to explore the molecular mechanisms underlying the individual variation in analgesic response to 2 Hz and 100 Hz stimulation, we studied and compared the gene expression profiles in the DH in HR versus NR rats.

Materials and Methods

Animals

All experiments were performed on male SD rats, obtained from the Experimental Animal Center, Peking University, weighing 200–220 g at the beginning of the experiment. Animals were housed in a 12 h light/dark cycle with food and water *ad libitum*. The room temperature was maintained at 22±1°C and relative humidity at 45–50%. Rats were handled daily during the first three days after arrival. All experimental procedures were approved by the Animal Care and Use Committee of Peking University Health Science Centre.

EA Stimulation

A total of 170 male rats were used in the experiment. Eighty of them were given 2 Hz EA, other 80 were given 100 Hz EA, and the rest of 10 were given restraint without EA to serve as control group to minimize the effect of restraint stress. The Zusanli (ST36) and Sanyinjiao (SP6) acupoints were chosen, which are commonly used acupoints to study acupuncture analgesic effect on diverse pain [3,25]. EA was given to the respective groups of rats once a day in two consecutive days. EA stimulations were performed as described before [26]. In brief, stainless steel needles of 0.3 mm in diameter and 3 mm in length were bilaterally inserted in the hind legs, one at the ST36 (2 mm lateral to the anterior tubercle of tibia), and the other at the SP6 (2 mm proximal to the upper border of medial melleolus, at the posterior border of the tibia). Square-wave electric output with constant current was generated by a programmed pulse generator HANS, LH 800 (manufactured at Astronautics and Aeronautics Aviation of Peking University) and1was delivered *via* the needles for a total of 30 min. The frequency of the stimulation was set at either 2 Hz or 100 Hz. The intensity of stimulation was increased stepwise from 0.5 to 1.0 and then to 1.5 mA, with each step lasting for 10 min. EA stimulation once a day in two successive days.

Nociceptive Testing

Nociceptive threshold was assessed by recording the TFL induced by radiant heat [27,28]. Focused light beam (3 mm diameter) from 12.5 W projector bulb was applied to the junction between proximal 2/3 and distal 1/3 of the tail. The projector bulb was turned off as soon as the rat flicked its tail, and a digital timer measured the TFL with the accuracy of 0.1 s. The voltage of the stimulation was adjusted to 12 V and room temperature was carefully monitored at 22±1°C to minimize the possible influence of ambient temperature on TFLs during the test [29]. We used a cut-off latency of 15 s in order to avoid possible damage to the superficial tissue of the tail. The average of three successive TFL determinations (pre-EA TFL) before EA stimulation was recorded as basal latency. The TFL, ten minutes after the ending of EA stimulation, was also assessed as EA latency. The analgesic effect of EA was represented by the average percentage change of TFL (%): [(EA latency–basal latency)/basal latency] ×100%. Results were presented as mean ± SEM and were analyzed with one-way ANOVA followed by Bonferroni's Multiple Comparison Test.

DH Tissue Harvesting

Rats were sacrificed either one hour (1 h) or 24 hours (24 h) after the last EA session on the last test day. Each rat was sacrificed by decapitation and the DH of the fifth and sixth lumbar (L5 and L6) spinal cord were quickly removed and stored immediately in cold RNAlater (Qiagen, Hilden, Germany), and then stored at −80°C till used later.

Gene Expression Profiling and cDNA Microarray Analysis

The DH tissues from HR and NR rats sacrificed at 1 hr time point were used in microarray experiment. The cDNA microarray containing 11,444 rat genes/Expressed Sequence Tags (ESTs) was used and the microarray platform was submitted to the GEO database with the accession number GPL3498 [30,31,32]. The

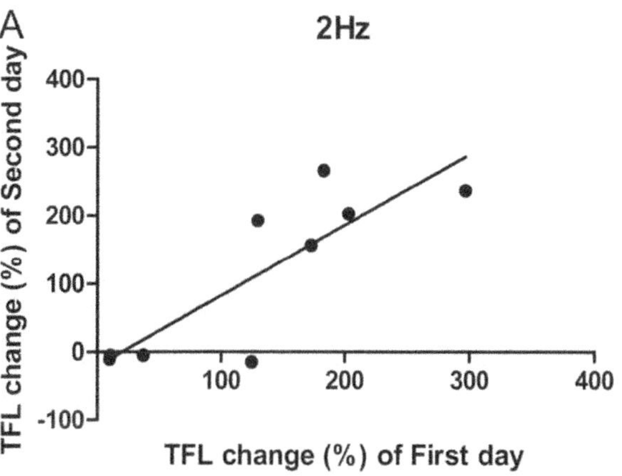

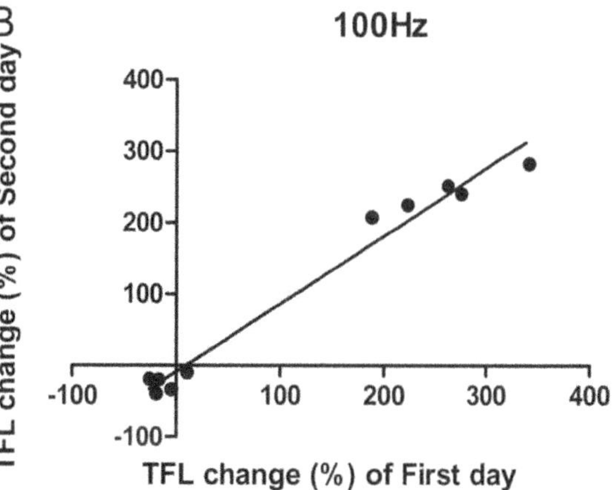

Figure 2. Scattergram of analgesic effect on two consecutive days of rats chosen in microarray experiment. In 2 Hz treated groups, the HR and NR rats have well reproducible in analgesic effect (R = 0.838, *P*<0.01 Pearson Correlation) on two consecutive days were chosen (A). Meanwhile, the rats in 100 Hz treated groups have well reproducible in analgesic effect (R = 0.988, *P*<0.001 Pearson Correlation) on two consecutive days were chosen (B).

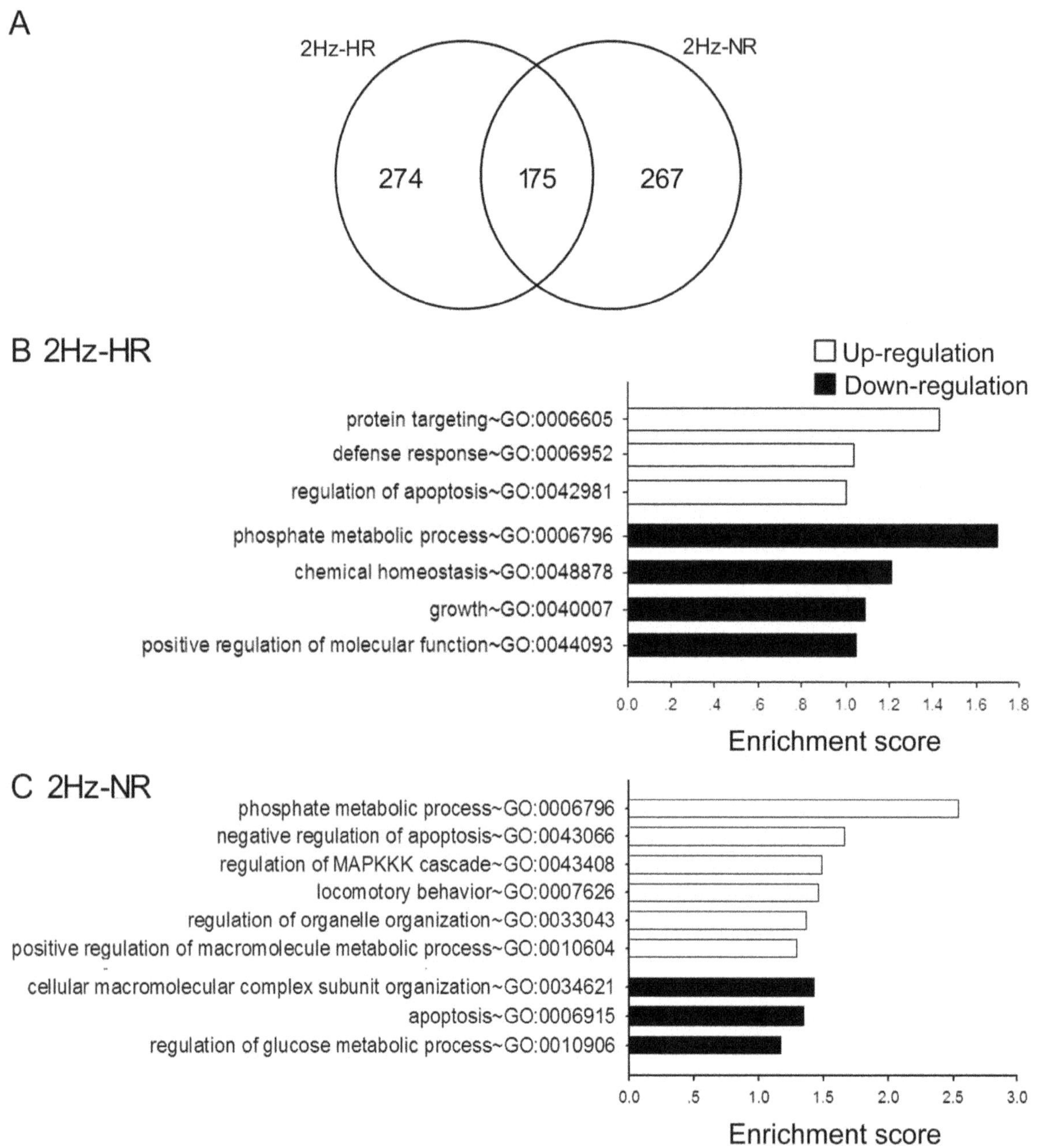

Figure 3. Overlapped and non-overlapped gene expression and enriched GO categories in 2 Hz-HR and NR rats. A: Venn diagram comparing the number of genes/ESTs identified as differentially expressed in HR and NR after 2 Hz EA stimulation at 1 hr time point. B and C: Enriched GO categories of specially regulated genes in 2 Hz-HR and 2 Hz-NR. The complete gene list of each GO category is accessible at: Table S3A.

protocol of the microarray experiments and the strategy for data extraction were described as previously [30,32]. Briefly, equal amounts of RNA samples from five restraint rat DH tissues were labeled with Cy3. The labeled RNA samples were pooled and used as reference. The RNA samples from animals following EA stimulation were individually labeled with Cy5, then Cy3-and Cy5-labeled cRNA pools were mixed to hybridize to the microarrays.

Data preprocessing was performed using Bioconductor software [33] (http://www.bioconductor.org) under the statistical programming environment R [34]. Signal intensity normalization within and between microarrays was accomplished by using intensity-dependent locally weighted scatter plot smoothing regression analysis (LOWESS). Only the genes/ESTs presenting in more than 60% samples in each group were retained for further analysis. Differentially expressed genes were then identified using the LIMMA (linear models for microarray analysis) package, and the empirical Bayes method was used to reduce the gene wise sample variances [35]. A combination of fold change $\geq$1.5 and a rigorous *P*-value $\leq$0.001 was used to identify differentially expressed genes/ESTs. The data have been submitted to GEO under accession GSE21758.

Table 1. The regulated genes of neuroactive ligand-receptor interaction and release of proinflammatory cytokines in 2 Hz-HR and 2 Hz-NR rats after 2 Hz EA stimulation.

Group	*Term*	*GenBank*	*Gene symbol*	*Log2 ratio*	*P-value*
2 Hz-HR	Neuroactive ligand-receptor interaction	NM_031349	Aplnr	0.98	0.0009316
		AF293459	Faf1	−1.06	0.000847
		L08491	Gabra2	−0.94	0.0004549
		NM_080586	Gabrg1	−1.61	5.417E-06
		NM_053296	Glrb	−1.20	0.0001422
		NM_021857	Htr1f	−1.01	2.225E-06
	Release of proinflammatory cytokines	NM_033230	Akt1	−1.22	0.0003809
		AF293459	Faf1	−1.06	0.000847
		NM_175756	Fcgr2b	1.89	1.808E-07
		NM_017090	Gucy1a3	1.82	3.023E-10
		NM_032080	Gsk3b	1.26	4.529E-06
		NM_053838	Npr2	−1.22	5.247E-05
		NM_012713	Prkcb	−1.70	2.997E-06
		NM_013012	Prkg2	−1.36	2.776E-06
		BC061979	Tsc22d3	1.17	0.0008219
2 Hz-NR	Neuroactive ligand-receptor interaction	XM_001061557	Map1b	−0.93	0.0006714
	Release of proinflammatory cytokines	NM_053619	C5ar1	1.62	0.0001809
		NM_171994	Cdc42	1.92	0.0001617
		BQ196565	Gpx2	−1.50	9.133E-05
		NM_052807	Igf1r	1.08	0.0008666
		NM_031512	Il1b	1.64	9.871E-05
		NM_012806	Mapk10	−1.92	3.064E-07
		NM_138548	Nme1	2.29	1.965E-05
		NM_175578	Rcan2	−1.27	0.0007497

Show is up-regulation (log2 ratio ≥0.585) or down-regulation (log2 ratio ≤−0.585) by ≥1.5-fold compared with control rats after EA stimulations.

Bioinformatic Analysis

Biological themes associated with differentially expressed genes were identified by the biological process of the Gene Ontology (GO) categories using the functional annotation tool of the Database for Annotation, Visualization, and Integrated Discovery (DAVID) (http://david.abcc.ncifcrf.gov/) [36], to identify important GO categories (enrichment, EASE scores ≥1.0) and to suggest their potential biological importance. The biological process of differently expressed genes was ranked by the EASE scores based on all enriched annotation terms.

To provide a functional outline for function interpretation, regulated gene pathways were explored using Kyoto Encyclopedia of Genes and Genomes (KEGG) online database (http://www.genome.jp/kegg/). The KEGG pathways of the differentially expressed genes were also matched using the DAVID Functional Annotation Tool. DAVID gives a modified Fisher Exact *P*-Value for pathway enrichment analysis.

Real-Time RT-PCR

RNA samples were from animals sacrificed at 1 hr and sacrificed at 24 hr time point after EA stimulation. Aliquots of the RNA samples were used in Real-time RT-PCR (qPCR). Two micrograms of each total RNA sample were used for cDNA synthesis using iScript™ cDNA Synthesis Kit (Bio-Rad, Hercules, CA). cDNA samples were placed on ice and stored at −20°C until further use. Prior to the analysis, 20 μl of each cDNA sample was diluted with 180 μl of MilliQ water. qPCR reactions were performed with Prism 7900 Sequence Detection System (Applied Biosystems, Foster City, CA). For each reaction, 1 μl of each diluted cDNA sample was added to a mixture containing 12.5 μl of 2× SYBR green II qRT-PCR kit (Toyobo, Osaka, Japan), 1 μl of each primer (5 μM), and 10.5 μl of MilliQ water. Cycling conditions were 10 min 95°C, followed by 40 cycles of 15 s at 95°C and 1 min at 60°C. After cycling, a melting protocol was performed with 15 s at 95°C, 1 min at 60°C, and 15 s at 95°C, to control product specificity. The fold change (FC) of target gene cDNA relative to glyceraldehyde-3-phosphate dehydrogenase (*Gapdh*) endogenous control was determined as follows: $FC = 2^{-\Delta\Delta Ct}$, where $\Delta\Delta Ct = (Ct_{Target} - Ct_{Gapdh})test - (Ct_{Target} - Ct_{Gapdh})control$. Ct values were defined as the number of the PCR cycles at which the fluorescence signals were detected. The primer sequences are listed in Table S1. Data are presented as mean ± SEM and analyzed with one-way ANOVA followed by Tukey's HSD post-hoc test.

Results

High-responders and Non-responders were Defined Based on Distinct Analgesic Effects Induced by EA at Different Frequencies

Analgesic effects induced by 2 Hz and 100 Hz EA were estimated by the TFL test in rats and the average percentage

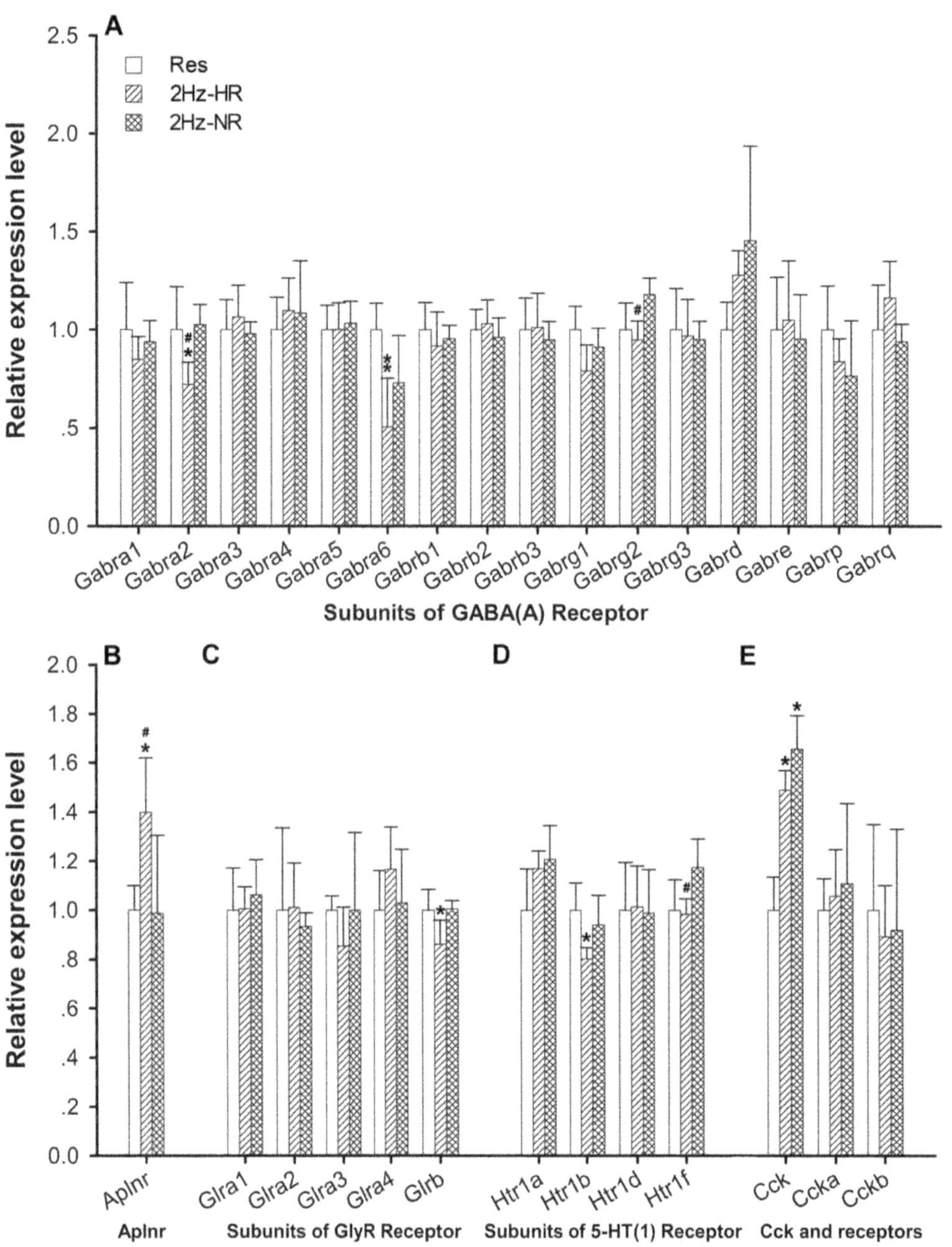

Figure 4. Expression of neurotransmitter receptors-related genes at 1 h. Data (mean ± SD) are normalized to restraint group. qPCR was conducted with triplicate experiments in each. One way ANOVA and Tukey's HSD post-hoc test was used. *P<0.05, **P<0.01 *vs.* restraint group; #P<0.05 vs. NR group.

change in TFL induced by EA stimulations once a day in two consecutive days. The distribution of sensitivity towards EA analgesia in the testing population indicated that majority of the rats (Fig. 1A. B), no matter tested in the first day or the second day, showed some sensitivity towards 2 Hz or 100 Hz EA analgesia (150≥ TFL changes >0) (responder, R). However, a small portion of them fell in either high-sensitivity (HR; TFL changes >150) or low-sensitivity (NR; TFL changes ≤0) category. There was no significant difference in the basic TFL among different treatment groups. In addition, restriction did not appear to affect their TFL (data not shown). Among the 80 rats received 2 Hz EA on the second day, 54 rats showed modest analgesic effects (mean TFL increase ratio of 65.08%) and were classified as R. Nineteen rats showed high-sensitivity with the mean TFL increased 209.15% and were classified as HR. In contrast, 7 rats were NR (mean TFL decreased 5.69%) (Fig. 1C). To the 80 rats given 100 Hz EA, 49, 8 and 23 rats fell into R (mean TFL increased 48.09%), HR (mean TFL increased 234.74%) and NR (mean TFL increased 22.04%), respectively (Fig. 1 D).

Transcriptome Modulations were Detected in the HR and NR Individuals

According to the analgesic response to EA treatment in the second day, 26 rats (19 HR *vs.* 7 NR) in 2 Hz EA and 31 rats (8

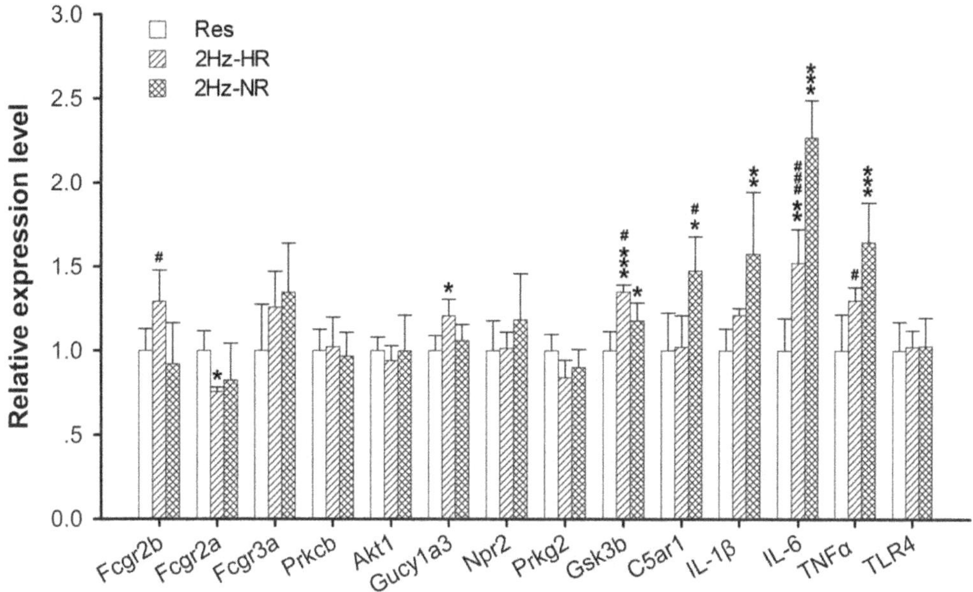

Figure 5. Expression of release of proinflammatory cytokines-related genes at 1 h. Data (mean ± SD) are normalized to restraint group. qPCR was conducted with triplicate experiments in each. One way ANOVA and Tukey's HSD post-hoc test was used. *$P<0.05$, **$P<0.01$, ***$P<0.001$ *vs.* restraint group; #$P<0.05$, ###$P<0.001$ vs. NR group.

HR *vs.* 23 NR) in 100 Hz EA were chosen for further analysis. Among these animals, individuals that presented best reproducibility in the two assessments were selected for microarray experiment based on statistical analysis of two-tailed Pearson's Correlation and paired student's *t*-test. Finally, nine rats (5 HR *vs.* 4 NR; R = 0.838, $P<0.01$; $t=0.75$, df = 8, $P=0.474$) in 2 Hz EA treatment group and 10 rats (5 HR *vs.* 5 NR; R = 0.988, $P<0.001$; $t=2.04$, df = 9, $P=0.072$) in 100 Hz EA treatment group were sacrificed at 1 hr time point after the last EA stimulation and the tissues of DH region were used to be processed for microarray experiment (Fig. 2). After filtering for high-quality array data (*See Methods*), the global transcriptional profiling of the DH region with 8442, 8382, 9498, and 9735 genes/ESTs in the 2 Hz-HR, 2 Hz-NR, 100 Hz-HR, and 100 Hz-NR groups was investigated, respectively. Using the high stringent analysis with Limma at the combination of fold change ≥1.5 and a rigorous *P*-value ≤0.001, significant differences in gene expression were observed after the EA stimulations compared with the restraint-control group. There were 449, 442, 431, 524 genes/ESTs were identified to be significantly changed level of expression in the 2 Hz-HR, 2 Hz-NR, 100 Hz-HR, and 100 Hz-NR group, respectively.

Different Gene Expression Response to 2 Hz EA between HR and NR

In the animals treated with 2 Hz EA, 175 genes/ESTs were similarly co-regulated in HR and NR. The changes in expression level were in the same direction in HR and NR (Fig. 3A, Table S2A). Besides, the expression of 274 and 267 genes/ESTs was specifically regulated in HR and NR groups, respectively (Fig. 3A; Table S2B, S2C). These differentially regulated genes were subjected to DAVID analysis to identify their potential biological themes. Genes enriched in 16 GO categories belong to the ontology of "biological process" (EASE score ≥1) (Fig. 3B, 3C; Table S3A). Among these enriched GO categories, 13 of them were mainly related with cell cycle process, which did not have direct link to the effect of EA analgesia and pain modulation [4,21,37,38]. Interestingly, the immune function related term defense response (GO:0006952) was enriched in 2 Hz-HR specific genes and the term regulation of MAPKKK cascade (GO:0043408) was enriched in 2 Hz-NR specific genes. With KEGG pathway analysis, B cell receptor signalling pathway (rno04662) was enriched in the 2 Hz-HR genes (*P*-Value ≤0.05) and three pathways (Ribosome (rno03010), Focal adhesion (rno04510) and Oocyte meiosis (rno04114)) were enriched in the 2 Hz-NR genes (Table S3B).

According to the hint that the immune function by the GO categories and KEGG pathways analysis as mentioned above and the neurochemical mechanisms implicated in pain and analgesia by literature exploration, we mapped the specially regulated genes identified in two extreme phenotype groups (HR and NR) according to these two functional characteristics. We thus identified that neuroactive ligand-receptor interaction and release of proinflammatory cytokines may play significant roles in individual variations in nociception response to 2 Hz EA (Table 1).

With respect to the neuroactive ligand-receptor interaction, *Aplnr* was up-regulated and *Gabra2*, *Gabrg1*, *Htr1f*, and *Glrb* were down-regulated in the 2 Hz-HR group. In contrast, there were no direct regulated genes related to neuroactive ligands or receptors in 2 Hz-NR group. With respect to the release of proinflammatory cytokines, mostly regulated genes implicated a trend of inhibiting the release of proinflammatory cytokines in 2 Hz-HR group, while in the 2 Hz-NR group, the regulated genes implicated a trend of inducing the release of proinflammatory cytokines.

Regulation of Neurotransmitter Receptors-related Gene Expression in 2 Hz-HR and 2 Hz-NR rats

Based on the results of the microarray analysis and suggestions regarding the neuroactive ligand–receptor interaction, qPCR was employed for detailed analysis of differential regulation of neurotransmitter receptors in 2 Hz-HR and 2 Hz-NR rats. The genes selected for this analysis included *Aplnr* and all subunits of $GABA_A$ receptor (*Gabra1–6, Gabrb1–3, Gabrg1–3, Gabrd, Gabre, Gabrp*, and *Gabrq*), glycine receptor (*Glra1–4* and *Glrb*), and 5-HT1

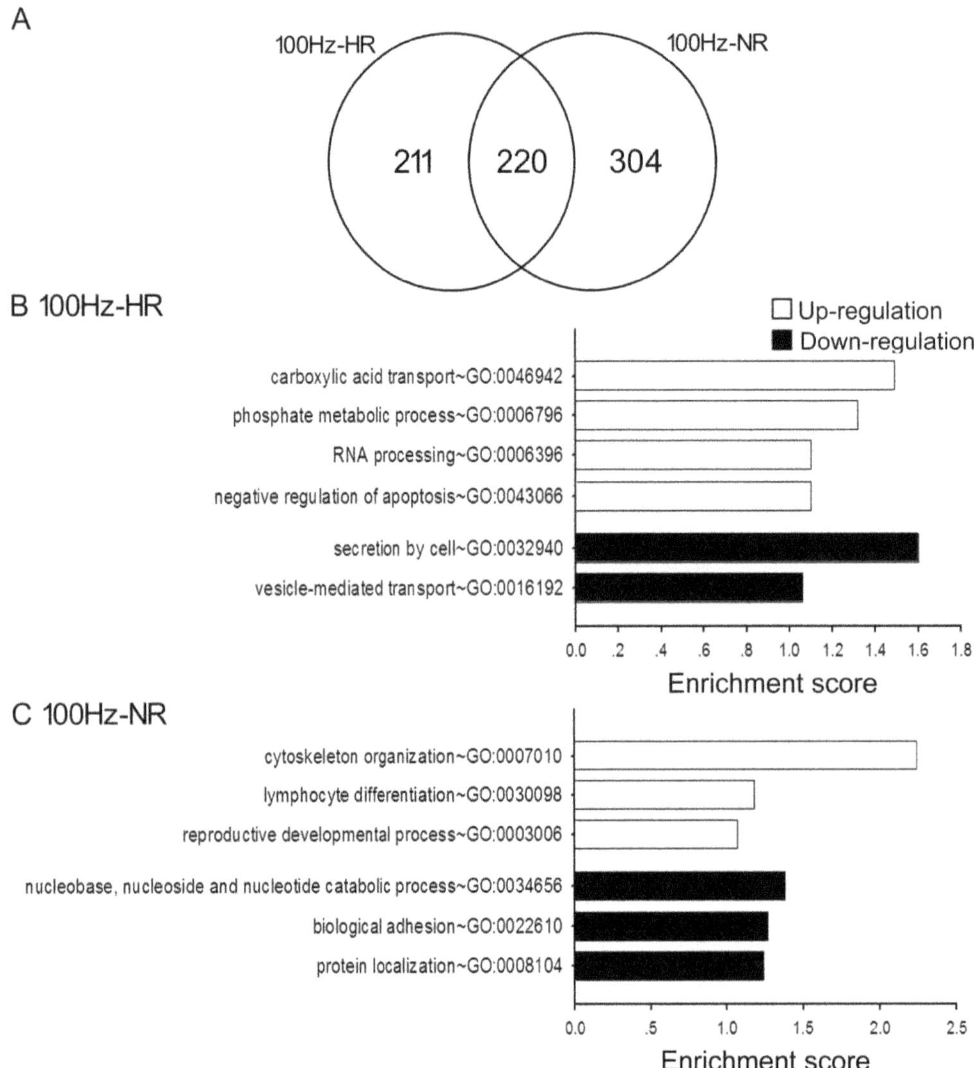

Figure 6. Overlapped and non-overlapped gene expression and enriched GO categories in 100 Hz-HR and NR rats. A: Venn diagram comparing the number of genes/ESTs identified as differentially expressed in HR and NR after 100 Hz EA stimulation at 1 hr time point. B and C: Enriched GO categories of specially regulated genes in 100 Hz-HR and 100 Hz-NR. The complete gene list of each GO category is accessible at Table S5A.

receptor (*Htr1a*, *Htr1b*, *Htr1d*, and *Htr1f*). In 2 Hz-HR group, the mRNA level of *Aplnr* was up-regulated and the mRNA levels of *Gabra2*, *Gabra6*, *Gabrg2*, *Glrb*, and *Htr1b* were down-regulated compared with the control group (Fig. 4A–4D). However, there was no significant difference in the expression of these genes in the 2 Hz-NR group comparing with that in the control group. Furthermore, the mRNA levels of *Aplnr*, *Gabra2*, *Gabrg2*, and *Htr1f* were significantly different between 2 Hz-HR and 2 Hz-NR groups (Fig. 4A–4D).

In addition, Cck is widely distributed in various brain areas and the spinal cord and exerts many physiological functions. Previous studies have clearly shown both Cck release and the density of Cck receptors are closely associated with individual sensitivity to EA [4]. NR rats had a remarkable increase in Cck release [16]. Meanwhile, the expression of *Cck-a* receptor at mRNA level was significantly higher in the rat hypothalamus of NR than HR following low-frequency EA [9]. Cck receptors (*Cck-a* and-*b*) mRNA in the hypothalamus were also increased by high-frequency EA in NR rats [10]. To assess whether the differences in expression pattern between HR and NR rats in the brain also present in DH region, the mRNA levels of *Cck*, *Cck-a* and *Cck-b* were examined using qPCR. As seen in Figure 4E, the expressions of *Cck* and its receptors (*Cck-a* and *Cck-b*) in the DH were not significantly different between HR and NR after 2 Hz EA stimulation. Compared with control group, the expression of *Cck* was significantly increased in both HR and NR in the DH after 2 Hz EA stimulation (Fig. 4E).

Regulation of Proinflammatory Cytokines-related Gene Expression in 2 Hz-HR and 2 Hz-NR Rats

The expression pattern of genes related to the release of proinflammatory cytokines was found to be different between the 2 Hz-HR and 2 Hz-NR groups. Compared with control group, the expression of *Fcgr2a* was down-regulated and the *Gucy1a3* was up-regulated in the HR group, while the expression of *C5ar1* was up-regulated in the NR group after

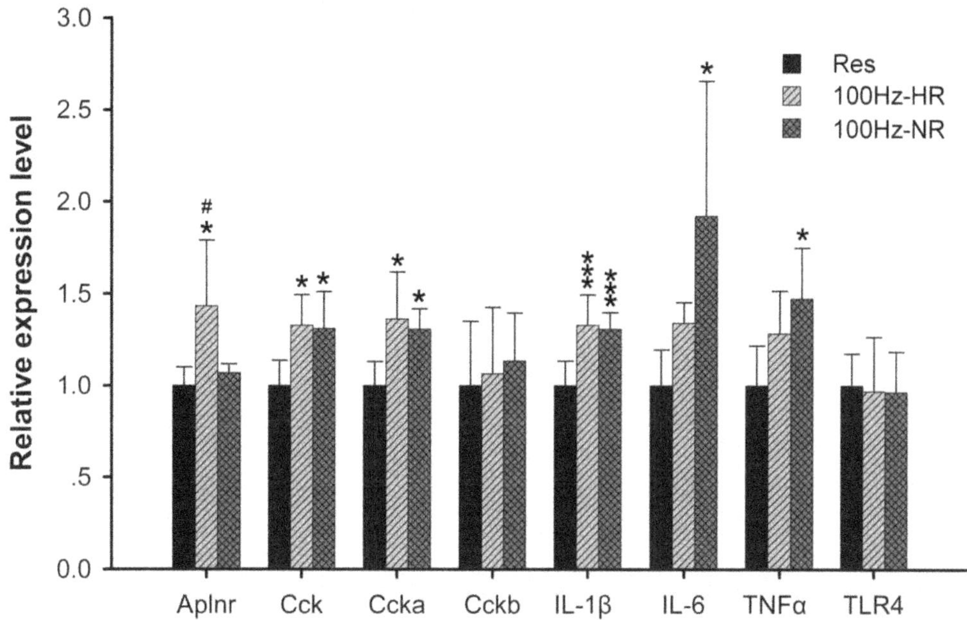

Figure 7. Gene expression detected in 100 Hz-HR and NR at 1 h by qPCR. Data (mean ± SD) are normalized to restraint group. qPCR was conducted with triplicate experiments in each. One way ANOVA and Tukey's HSD post-hoc test was used. *$P<0.05$, **$P<0.01$ *vs.* restraint group; #$P<0.05$ vs. NR group.

2 Hz EA stimulation by qPCR analysis (Fig. 5). *IL-1β*, *IL-6* and *TNFα*, three important proinflammatory cytokines, increased their expression in both HR and NR after 2 Hz EA stimulation (Fig. 5). Interestingly, the mRNA levels of *Fcgr2b* and *Gsk3b*, which could depress the proinflammatory cytokines release, were significantly increased in 2 Hz-HR group than 2 Hz-NR group (Fig. 5). Meanwhile, the expression of *C5ar1*, which could facilitate the proinflammatory cytokines release, was significantly increased in 2 Hz-NR group than 2 Hz-HR group (Fig. 5). Furthermore, higher levels of *IL-1β*, *IL-6* and *TNFα* mRNA were observed in 2 Hz-NR group compared to 2 Hz-HR group (Fig. 5). However, toll-like receptor 4 (TLR4) mRNA levels, an index of glial activation [39], had no difference between HR and NR after 2 Hz EA (Fig. 5).

Different Gene Expression Response to 100 Hz EA between HR and NR

With 100 Hz EA treatment, 211 and 304 genes/ESTs were identified to have specific regulations in HR and NR group, respectively (Fig. 6A; Table S4). Based on GO annotation, six GO categories were enriched in 100 Hz-HR specifically regulated genes and six in 100 Hz-NR specifically regulated genes (Fig. 6B, 6C; Table S5A). Importantly, GO terms of secretion by cell (GO:0032940) and vesicle-mediated transport (GO: 0016192) were enriched in the 100 Hz-HR genes, the term lymphocyte differentiation (GO:0030098) was enriched in the 100 Hz-NR group. In KEGG pathway analysis, Ribosome (rno03010) was enriched in the 100 Hz-HR group while two pathways of Ribosome (rno03010) and Fc gamma R-mediated phagocytosis (rno04666) were enriched in the 100 Hz-NR genes (Table S5B).

Unlikely multiple genes with their expression pattern significantly different between HR and NR noticed in the 2 Hz EA study, we did not see striking differences in expression pattern in genes potentially related to variations in analgesic response to 100 Hz EA. The mRNA levels of neurotransmitter receptors and proinflammatory cytokines were also detected in 100 Hz EA groups by qPCR. In neurotransmitter receptors, only the expression of *Aplnr* was significantly increased in HR rats after 100 Hz EA stimulation compared with NR group and control group (Fig. 7). The expression of *Cck* and *Cck-a* were increased in both HR and NR rats after 100 Hz EA stimulation, and there was no difference in expression pattern between HR and NR rats (Fig. 7). In respect of proinflammatory cytokines, the expression of *IL-1β* was up-regulated in both HR and NR, while *IL-6* and *TNFa* mRNA were only significantly increased in NR group after 100 Hz EA stimulation (Fig. 7). However, the mRNA level of *TLR4* was similar in HR and NR (Fig. 7).

Time Effects of EA Stimulation

In order to determine whether the gene regulation response after EA stimulation observed at 1 hr time point would sustain for a longer period of time, the gene expression activity was also examined at 24 hr time point after EA stimulation by qPCR. As shown in Figure 8, approximately 90% of the genes the expression of which has been altered at 1 hr time point returned to baseline at 24 hr time point compared the control group. However, the expression of *Cck* was still up regulated at at 24 hr time point in both HR and NR after 2 Hz and 100 Hz EA (Fig. 8). The expression of *Cck-b* gene was significant increased in 2 Hz-NR group only when compared with the control group at 24 hr time point (Fig. 8). The *Gabrg2* mRNA levels was significantly increased only in HR group following 2 Hz and 100 Hz stimulation but not in NR or control groups at 24 hr time point (Fig. 8).

Discussion

In the present study, both 2 Hz and 100 Hz EA could produce a good analgesic efficacy in most rats. On the other hand, the analgesic effects of EA on rats showed marked individual variations (Fig. 1), although there was no significant difference in

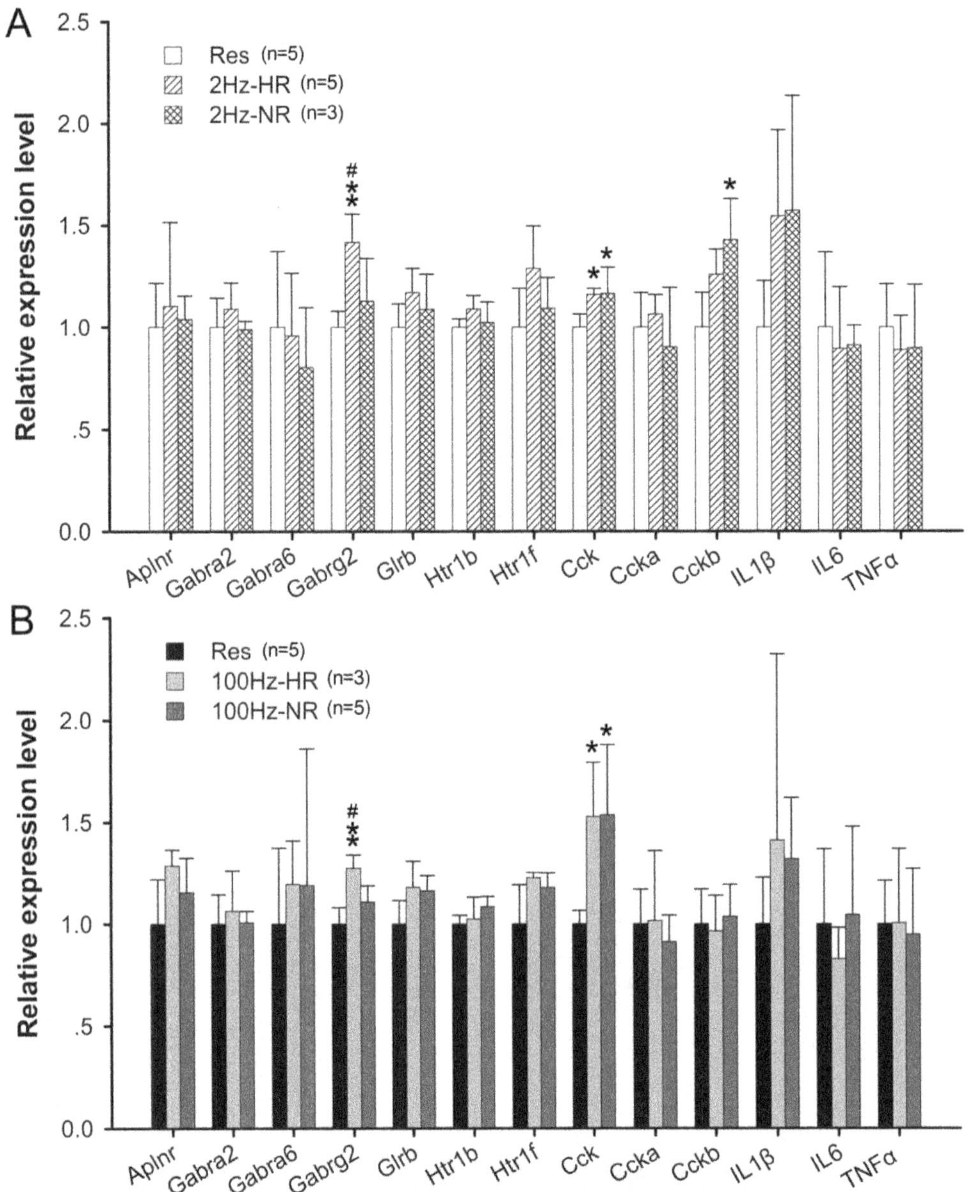

Figure 8. Gene expression at 24 hr time point after EA stimulation. Data (mean ± SD) are normalized to restraint group. qPCR was conducted with triplicate experiments in each. One way ANOVA and Tukey's HSD post-hoc test was used.

basal nociceptive threshold of HR, R, and NR rats, as measured by TFL test. It is well known that the analgesic effect of EA can be produced by transcriptional and non-transcriptional mechanisms in the nervous system. Therefore, cDNA microarray technique was used to examine the gene expression response in the DH region in order to understand the underlying mechanisms why there are individual differences in EA analgesia.

The gene expression response was profiled at 1 hr time point after EA stimulation. The time point was chosen due to the fact that the antinociceptive effects of EA were thought to be a short term response in normal animals. The gene expression profiles of DH were compared between HR and NR rats, which were classified based on their analgesic response to EA analgesia. HR and NR rats with reproducible analgesic response to EA analgesia in two consecutive days (Fig. 2), were used in the microarray experiment in order to minimize the random environmental factors. As shown in this study, HR rats and NR rats exhibited significant differences in gene expression response to 2 Hz or 100 Hz EA stimulations.

Potential Mechanisms of Individual Variations in Response to 2 Hz EA Analgesia

Compared with the gene expression profiles in response to 2 Hz EA, the genes related with neuroactive ligand-receptor interaction were more obviously regulated in the HR *vs.* NR rats and the genes related with release of proinflammatory cytokines were more dramatically up-regulated in NR (Fig. 9). For neuroactive ligand-receptor interaction, the mRNA expressions of some neurotransmitter receptors, involved in Aplnr receptor and $GABA_A$ receptor, glycine receptor, and 5-HT1 receptor, were regulated in HR rats. However, these genes were not significantly regulated in NR rats.

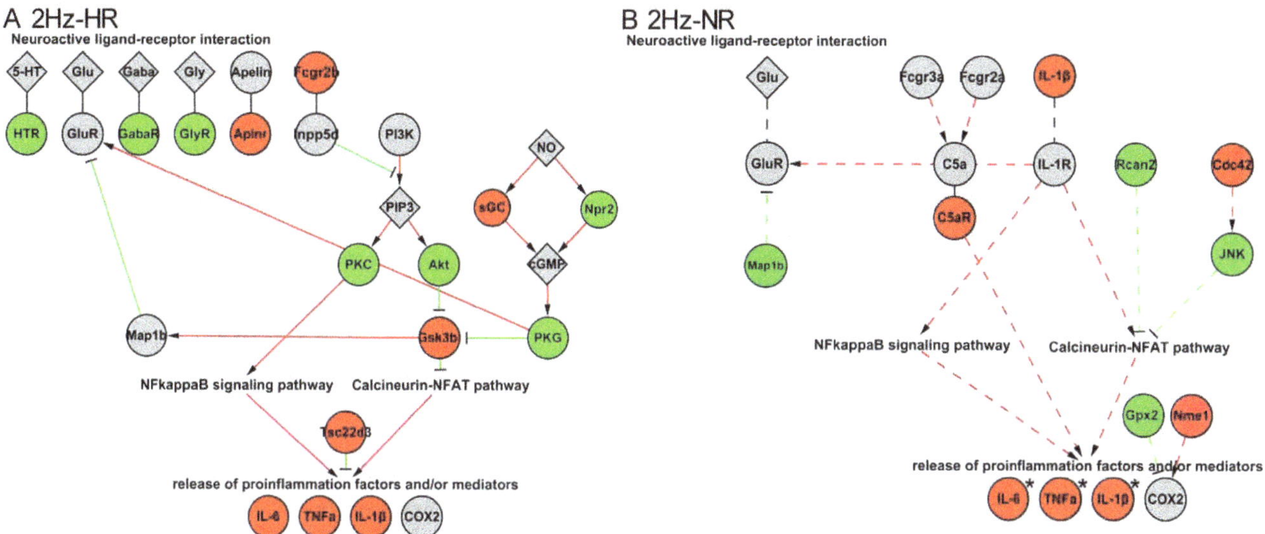

Figure 9. Ideogram illustration depicting the different regulated genes in neural-immune system in HR and NR after 2 Hz EA. Regulated gene network in the DH at 1 hr time point after 2 Hz EA of 2 Hz-HR group (A) and 2 Hz-NR group (B). The expressions of neurotransmitter receptors were regulated in HR, not in NR. Regulated genes related with the release of proinflammatory cytokines were also shown. The mRNA levels of *IL-1β*, *IL-6*, and *TNFα* were increased in both HR and NR, but higher increased in NR compared with HR. Edges (lines) connecting nodes (genes) represent regulatory interactions such as inhibits (T shape) or activates (Arrow shape). Red node indicates gene up-regulation. Conversely, blue node indicates down-regulation, grey node was non-regulation.

Consistent with the microarray analysis, qPCR further demonstrated that the expression of *Aplnr* was up-regulated and the expressions of *Gabra2*, *Gabra6*, *Gabrg2*, *Glrb*, and *Htr1b* were down-regulated in the HR rats' DH region response to 2 Hz EA (Fig. 4). Meanwhile, these genes were not significantly regulated in the NR rats' region after 2 Hz EA. Furthermore, the mRNA levels of *Aplnr*, *Gabra2*, *Gabrg2*, and *Htr1f* were significantly different between HR and NR groups (Fig. 4). Previous studies confirmed that low frequency EA was effective in treatment of neuropathic pain through mediating the neurotransmitters of GABA, 5-HT or glycine as well as their corresponding receptors [40,41]. Note worthily, the expression of *Aplnr*, a G protein-coupled receptor, was up-regulated in HR rats. The endogenous ligand for Aplnr was apelin, and the apelin-Aplnr system is widely distributed in both CNS and periphery, which inhibit the adenylate cyclase activity [42,43,44]. One study showed that intra-cerebroventricular administration of apelin could produce a dose-and time-dependent antinociceptive effect by acting on Aplnr and μ-opioid receptor [45]. Therefore, this study implicated that the apelin-Aplnr system would be a new candidate system that might participate in EA analgesia and was related with individual differences to 2 Hz EA stimulate. On the other hand, the expression of *Cck* was significantly increased after 2 Hz EA stimulation and not different between HR and NR in DH. This result that *Cck* mRNA level was increased after EA and there was no difference between HR and NR was consistent with the previous studies in DH and supraspinal regions [6,10,46], while the Cck protein level was higher in NR than HR in the midbrain periaqueductal gray and the perfusate of the rat spinal cord [6,16]. The mRNA level of the *Cck-a* receptor in DH had no significant difference in NR and HR of this study, which was inconsistent with one previous study in hypothalamus that *Cck-a* mRNA level was high expressed in NR than HR [8]. This discrepancy may be due to the differences in the examined CNS regions (DH *vs.* hypothalamus) and differences in the EA stimulation conditions used. Generally speaking, these different regulations in neurotransmitter receptors' genes in HR and NR suggested that neurotransmitter system could be mainly active in HR rats, but not in NR rats.

With respect to the release of proinflammatory cytokines, the regulated genes in HR rats mainly inhibited release of proinflammatory cytokines after EA stimulation. However, in NR rats the response genes would induce the release of proinflammatory cytokines. For example, the expression of *Fcgr2b*, *GSK3b* and *Tsc22d3* were up-regulated in HR rats, which could significantly inhibit the release of the proinflammatory cytokine [47,48,49]. The expression of *IL-1β* was up-regulated in NR rats. IL-1β is a proinflammatory cytokine, which not only induces the release of other proinflammatories but also plays a major role in nociceptive modulation in the CNS and can be nociceptive and produce hyperalgesia [50,51,52]. *IL-6* and *TNFα* mRNA expression, two other important proinflammatory cytokines, also significantly increased their expression in NR than HR after 2 Hz EA stimulation (Fig. 5). It was shown that spinal proinflammatory cytokines could be induced by multiple opioid administrate in opposing both acute and chronic opioid analgesia in normal animals [53]. This study implicated that the individuals had different reactivity in proinflammatory cytokines release, which resulted in different response with 2 Hz EA stimulation. Proinflammatory cytokines are key elements in the induction and maintenance of pain and are predominantly secreted by microglia, and some astrocytes in the CNS [51,54]. However, the expression of *TLR4*, one of glial activation marker, had no significant difference between HR and NR (Fig. 5). Therefore, it is uncertain whether the different expressions of proinflammatory cytokines between HR group and NR group were due to the different activity of glia in 2 Hz EA analgesia.

Differential Alterations of Gene Expression in HR and NR rats After 100 Hz EA Analgesia

In 100 Hz EA, HR and NR rats also exhibit differential expression response to 100 Hz analgesia in the DH. The GO enriched analysis found that category 'vesicle-mediated transport' (GO: 0016192) related to neural function was enriched with down-regulated genes in HR rats and 'lymphocyte differentiation' (GO:0030098) related to immune function was enriched with up-regulated genes in NR rats (Fig. 6). These two enriched GO categories in respective HR and NR were some similar to the findings that different regulation of neural-immune related genes in response to 2 Hz EA. Unconformity with the results of 2 Hz EA, there was no significant gene expression difference in subunits of $GABA_A$ receptor, 5-HT1 receptor or GlyR receptor between HR and NR after 100 Hz EA. However, the expression of *Aplnr* was also increased in HR rats compared with NR and the control rats, further indicating that the apelin-Aplnr system would involve in 2 Hz/100 Hz EA analgesia. In proinflammatory cytokines, although the gene expression of *IL-1β* did not differ, *IL-6* and *TNFα* were more increased in NR compared with HR response to 100 Hz EA. This result suggested that different gene expression response of spinal proinflammatory cytokines were also related with individual variations in 100 EA analgesia, which the gene of spinal proinflammatory cytokines were higher up-regulated in NR than HR.

Time Effects of EA Stimulation

Twenty-four hours after EA stimulation, major portion of the regulated genes had return to baseline compared with the control group (Fig. 8). This result suggested that the regulation of gene expression in naïve rat response to EA stimulations had time-dependent changes and the burst of gene expression changes were regulated at early stage. This time-dependent changes in gene expression response to EA stimulation were in accordance with the duration of EA analgesia effect on the physiological stat in previously studies [2,55].

It is important to uncover the mechanisms about why distinct classes of individuals differ in response to EA analgesia, which could have considerable clinical value for the practice of acupuncture and the treatment of pain. This study provides a systematic view of gene expression variations in spinal DH region with individual response to 2 Hz or 100 Hz EA analgesia. The gene expression data generated in this study can serve as a future resource to elucidate the genetic underpinnings of individual variations in response to EA analgesia. Furthermore, genes of certain neurotransmitter receptors were more prominent regulated in the HR, and proinflammatory cytokine related genes were notably up-regulated in NR compared with HR after EA stimulation. Our finding suggested that different responsiveness of neural-immune system in response to EA stimulation could have implications for elucidating the basis of individual differences in EA analgesia.

Supporting Information

Table S1 Sequences of primers for qRT-PCR.
(XLS)

Table S2 Co-regulated (A) and special-regulated genes (B, C) lists in HR and NR rats by 2 Hz EA stimulation.
(XLS)

Table S3 The genes lists of enriched GO categories (A) and KEGG pathways (B) in 2Hz-HR and 2Hz-NR rats.
(XLS)

Table S4 Co-regulated (A) and special-regulated genes (B, C) lists in HR and NR rats by 100 Hz EA stimulation.
(XLS)

Table S5 The genes lists of enriched GO categories (A) and KEGG pathways (B) in 100Hz-HR and 100Hz-NR rats.
(XLS)

Acknowledgments

Authors give their thanks to Dr. Kai Song, Dr. Jun-Song Han, and Dr. Hua-Sheng Xiao of SBC for their constructive discussions and suggestions for this work. Sincere thanks also go to Dr. Ning Guo of Shanghai University of Traditional Chinese Medicine for his help in revision of the manuscript.

Author Contributions

Conceived and designed the experiments: CC GZ QZ. Performed the experiments: KW RZ LL XX XP. Analyzed the data: KW RZ FH LY JH. Wrote the paper: KW RZ CC GZ.

References

1. (1998) NIH Consensus Conference. Acupuncture. JAMA 280: 1518–1524.
2. Ulett GA, Han S, Han JS (1998) Electroacupuncture: mechanisms and clinical application. Biol Psychiatry 44: 129–138.
3. Han JS (2011) Acupuncture analgesia: areas of consensus and controversy. Pain 152: S41–48.
4. Zhao ZQ (2008) Neural mechanism underlying acupuncture analgesia. Prog Neurobiol 85: 355–375.
5. Sun J, Qin W, Dong M, Yuan K, Liu J, et al. (2010) Evaluation of group homogeneity during acupuncture stimulation in fMRI studies. J Magn Reson Imaging 32: 298–305.
6. Tang NM, Dong HW, Wang XM, Tsui ZC, Han JS (1997) Cholecystokinin antisense RNA increases the analgesic effect induced by electroacupuncture or low dose morphine: conversion of low responder rats into high responders. Pain 71: 71–80.
7. Chae Y, Park HJ, Hahm DH, Yi SH, Lee H (2006) Individual differences of acupuncture analgesia in humans using cDNA microarray. J Physiol Sci 56: 425–431.
8. Kim SK, Moon HJ, Park JH, Lee G, Shin MK, et al. (2007) The maintenance of individual differences in the sensitivity of acute and neuropathic pain behaviors to electroacupuncture in rats. Brain Res Bull 74: 357–360.
9. Lee G, Rho S, Shin M, Hong M, Min B, et al. (2002) The association of cholecystokinin-A receptor expression with the responsiveness of electroacupuncture analgesic effects in rat. Neurosci Lett 325: 17–20.
10. Ko ES, Kim SK, Kim JT, Lee G, Han JB, et al. (2006) The difference in mRNA expressions of hypothalamic CCK and CCK-A and -B receptors between responder and non-responder rats to high frequency electroacupuncture analgesia. Peptides 27: 1841–1845.
11. Kim SK, Park JY, Koo BH, Lee JH, Kim HS, et al. (2009) Adenoviral gene transfer of acetylcholinesterase T subunit in the hypothalamus potentiates electroacupuncture analgesia in rats. Genes Brain Behav 8: 174–180.
12. Gao YZ, Guo SY, Yin QZ, Hisamitsu T, Jiang XH (2007) An individual variation study of electroacupuncture analgesia in rats using microarray. Am J Chin Med 35: 767–778.
13. Han JS (2004) Acupuncture and endorphins. Neurosci Lett 361: 258–261.
14. Wang L, Zhang Y, Dai J, Yang J, Gang S (2006) Electroacupuncture (EA) modulates the expression of NMDA receptors in primary sensory neurons in relation to hyperalgesia in rats. Brain Res 1120: 46–53.
15. Silva JR, Silva ML, Prado WA (2011) Analgesia induced by 2-or 100-Hz electroacupuncture in the rat tail-flick test depends on the activation of different descending pain inhibitory mechanisms. J Pain 12: 51–60.
16. Zhou Y, Sun YH, Shen JM, Han JS (1993) Increased release of immunoreactive CCK-8 by electroacupuncture and enhancement of electroacupuncture analgesia by CCK-B antagonist in rat spinal cord. Neuropeptides 24: 139–144.
17. Robinson GE (2004) Genomics. Beyond nature and nurture. Science 304: 397–399.
18. Lau WK, Chan WK, Zhang JL, Yung KK, Zhang HQ (2008) Electroacupuncture inhibits cyclooxygenase-2 up-regulation in rat spinal cord after spinal nerve ligation. Neuroscience 155: 463–468.
19. Koo ST, Lim KS, Chung K, Ju H, Chung JM (2008) Electroacupuncture-induced analgesia in a rat model of ankle sprain pain is mediated by spinal alpha-adrenoceptors. Pain 135: 11–19.
20. Paola FA, Arnold M (2003) Acupuncture and spinal cord medicine. J Spinal Cord Med 26: 12–20.
21. Basbaum AI, Bautista DM, Scherrer G, Julius D (2009) Cellular and molecular mechanisms of pain. Cell 139: 267–284.

22. Todd AJ (2010) Neuronal circuitry for pain processing in the dorsal horn. Nat Rev Neurosci 11: 823–836.
23. Strand AD, Aragaki AK, Baquet ZC, Hodges A, Cunningham P, et al. (2007) Conservation of regional gene expression in mouse and human brain. PLoS Genet 3: e59.
24. Wan Y, Wilson SG, Han J, Mogil JS (2001) The effect of genotype on sensitivity to electroacupuncture analgesia. Pain 91: 5–13.
25. Cidral-Filho FJ, da Silva MD, More AO, Cordova MM, Werner MF, et al. (2011) Manual acupuncture inhibits mechanical hypersensitivity induced by spinal nerve ligation in rats. Neuroscience.
26. Xing GG, Liu FY, Qu XX, Han JS, Wan Y (2007) Long-term synaptic plasticity in the spinal dorsal horn and its modulation by electroacupuncture in rats with neuropathic pain. Exp Neurol 208: 323–332.
27. d'Amore A, Chiarotti F, Renzi P (1992) High-intensity nociceptive stimuli minimize behavioral effects induced by restraining stress during the tail-flick test. J Pharmacol Toxicol Methods 27: 197–201.
28. Le Bars D, Gozariu M, Cadden SW (2001) Animal models of nociception. Pharmacol Rev 53: 597–652.
29. Tjolsen A, Hole K (1993) [Pain regulation and plasticity]. Tidsskr Nor Laegeforen 113: 2921–2924.
30. Wang K, Xiang XH, He F, Lin LB, Zhang R, et al. (2010) Transcriptome profiling analysis reveals region-distinctive changes of gene expression in the CNS in response to different moderate restraint stress. J Neurochem 113: 1436–1446.
31. Li H, Xie Z, Lin J, Song H, Wang Q, et al. (2008) Transcriptomic and metabonomic profiling of obesity-prone and obesity-resistant rats under high fat diet. J Proteome Res 7: 4775–4783.
32. Xiao HS, Huang QH, Zhang FX, Bao L, Lu YJ, et al. (2002) Identification of gene expression profile of dorsal root ganglion in the rat peripheral axotomy model of neuropathic pain. Proc Natl Acad Sci U S A 99: 8360–8365.
33. Gentleman RC, Carey VJ, Bates DM, Bolstad B, Dettling M, et al. (2004) Bioconductor: open software development for computational biology and bioinformatics. Genome Biol 5: R80.
34. Ihaka R, Gentleman R (1996) R: a language for data analysis and graphics. Journal of computational and graphical statistics 5: 299–314.
35. Smyth GK (2004) Linear models and empirical bayes methods for assessing differential expression in microarray experiments. Stat Appl Genet Mol Biol 3: Article3.
36. Huang da W, Sherman BT, Lempicki RA (2009) Systematic and integrative analysis of large gene lists using DAVID bioinformatics resources. Nat Protoc 4: 44–57.
37. Gold MS, Gebhart GF (2010) Nociceptor sensitization in pain pathogenesis. Nat Med 16: 1248–1257.
38. Kuner R (2010) Central mechanisms of pathological pain. Nat Med 16: 1258–1266.
39. Tanga FY, Nutile-McMenemy N, DeLeo JA (2005) The CNS role of Toll-like receptor 4 in innate neuroimmunity and painful neuropathy. Proc Natl Acad Sci U S A 102: 5856–5861.
40. Park JH, Han JB, Kim SK, Go DH, Sun B, et al. (2010) Spinal GABA receptors mediate the suppressive effect of electroacupuncture on cold allodynia in rats. Brain Res 1322C: 24–29.
41. Somers DL, Clemente FR (2009) Contralateral high or a combination of high- and low-frequency transcutaneous electrical nerve stimulation reduces mechanical allodynia and alters dorsal horn neurotransmitter content in neuropathic rats. J Pain 10: 221–229.
42. Lee DK, Cheng R, Nguyen T, Fan T, Kariyawasam AP, et al. (2000) Characterization of apelin, the ligand for the APJ receptor. J Neurochem 74: 34–41.
43. O'Carroll AM, Selby TL, Palkovits M, Lolait SJ (2000) Distribution of mRNA encoding B78/apj, the rat homologue of the human APJ receptor, and its endogenous ligand apelin in brain and peripheral tissues. Biochim Biophys Acta 1492: 72–80.
44. Kalea AZ, Batlle D (2010) Apelin and ACE2 in cardiovascular disease. Curr Opin Investig Drugs 11: 273–282.
45. Xu N, Wang H, Fan L, Chen Q (2009) Supraspinal administration of apelin-13 induces antinociception via the opioid receptor in mice. Peptides 30: 1153–1157.
46. Fukazawa Y, Maeda T, Kiguchi N, Tohya K, Kimura M, et al. (2007) Activation of spinal cholecystokinin and neurokinin-1 receptors is associated with the attenuation of intrathecal morphine analgesia following electroacupuncture stimulation in rats. J Pharmacol Sci 104: 159–166.
47. Kaneko Y, Nimmerjahn F, Ravetch JV (2006) Anti-inflammatory activity of immunoglobulin G resulting from Fc sialylation. Science 313: 670–673.
48. Beurel E, Michalek SM, Jope RS (2010) Innate and adaptive immune responses regulated by glycogen synthase kinase-3 (GSK3). Trends Immunol 31: 24–31.
49. Yang N, Zhang W, Shi XM (2008) Glucocorticoid-induced leucine zipper (GILZ) mediates glucocorticoid action and inhibits inflammatory cytokine-induced COX-2 expression. J Cell Biochem 103: 1760–1771.
50. Ren K, Torres R (2009) Role of interleukin-1beta during pain and inflammation. Brain Res Rev 60: 57–64.
51. Guo W, Wang H, Watanabe M, Shimizu K, Zou S, et al. (2007) Glial-cytokine-neuronal interactions underlying the mechanisms of persistent pain. J Neurosci 27: 6006–6018.
52. Weyerbacher AR, Xu Q, Tamasdan C, Shin SJ, Inturrisi CE (2010) N-Methyl-D-aspartate receptor (NMDAR) independent maintenance of inflammatory pain. Pain 148: 237–246.
53. Hutchinson MR, Coats BD, Lewis SS, Zhang Y, Sprunger DB, et al. (2008) Proinflammatory cytokines oppose opioid-induced acute and chronic analgesia. Brain Behav Immun 22: 1178–1189.
54. Uceyler N, Schafers M, Sommer C (2009) Mode of action of cytokines on nociceptive neurons. Exp Brain Res 196: 67–78.
55. Almeida RT, Duarte ID (2008) Nitric oxide/cGMP pathway mediates orofacial antinociception induced by electroacupuncture at the St36 acupoint. Brain Res 1188: 54–60.

17

CXCL10 Controls Inflammatory Pain via Opioid Peptide-Containing Macrophages in Electroacupuncture

Ying Wang[1]*, Rebekka Gehringer[1], Shaaban A. Mousa[2], Dagmar Hackel[1], Alexander Brack[1], Heike L. Rittner[1]*

1 Department of Anesthesiology, University Hospital of Würzburg, Würzburg, Germany, 2 Department of Anesthesiology and Critical Care, Charité – Universitätsmedizin Berlin, Campus Virchow-Klinikum, Berlin, Germany

Abstract

Acupuncture is widely used for pain treatment in patients with osteoarthritis or low back pain, but molecular mechanisms remain largely enigmatic. In the early phase of inflammation neutrophilic chemokines direct opioid-containing neutrophils in the inflamed tissue and stimulate opioid peptide release and antinociception. In this study the molecular pathway and neuroimmune connections in complete Freund's adjuvant (CFA)-induced hind paw inflammation and electroacupuncture for peripheral pain control were analyzed. Free moving Wistar rats with hind paw inflammation were treated twice with electroacupuncture at GB30 (Huan Tiao - gall bladder meridian) (day 0 and 1) and analyzed for mechanical and thermal nociceptive thresholds. The cytokine profiles as well as the expression of opioid peptides were quantified in the inflamed paw. Electroacupuncture elicited long-term antinociception blocked by local injection of anti-opioid peptide antibodies (beta-endorphin, met-enkephalin, dynorphin A). The treatment altered the cytokine profile towards an anti-inflammatory pattern but augmented interferon (IFN)-gamma and the chemokine CXCL10 (IP-10: interferon gamma-inducible protein) protein and mRNA expression with concomitant increased numbers of opioid peptide-containing CXCR3$^+$ macrophages. In rats with CFA hind paw inflammation without acupuncture repeated injection of CXCL10 triggered opioid-mediated antinociception and increase opioid-containing macrophages. Conversely, neutralization of CXCL10 time-dependently decreased electroacupuncture-induced antinociception and the number of infiltrating opioid peptide-expressing CXCR3$^+$ macrophages. In summary, we describe a novel function of the chemokine CXCL10 - as a regulator for an increase of opioid-containing macrophages and antinociceptive mediator in inflammatory pain and as a key chemokine regulated by electroacupuncture.

Funding: This study was supported by a grant of the German medical acupuncture association (DÄgfA), China scholarship council and University Funds from the University Hospitals of Wuerzburg. The funders had no role in study design, data collection and analysis, decision to publish, or preparation of the manuscript.

Competing Interests: The authors have declared that no competing interests exist.

* E-mail: e_wang_y@ukw.de (YW); rittner_h@ukw.de (HLR)

Introduction

Acupuncture has been shown to significantly reduce pain intensity in various pain syndromes e.g. in patients with osteoarthritis [1], low back pain [2] in most, but not all studies [3]. Indeed, due to large cohort studies in patients with low back pain and knee pain this treatment is covered by public heath insurances in some countries including Germany [4]. Despite its widespread use, the underlying mechanisms of acupuncture-induced analgesia are still only incompletely understood. Acupuncture leads to a down-regulation of pro-inflammatory cytokines such as tumor necrosis factor (TNF-alpha) and interleukin (IL)-1beta at the site of inflammation [5,6]. This anti-inflammatory as well as antinociceptive effect involved activation of the cannabinoid receptor 2 (CB2) [6]. Endogenous opioid peptides such as beta-endorphin (END) also could contribute to acupuncture-induced analgesia. They activate opioid receptors both at the level of the spinal cord [7,8] as well as on peripheral sensory neurons at the site of inflammation [9,10]. Acupuncture triggers END transcription and translational in the inflamed tissue and this was attenuated by a CB2 antagonists [11].

Opioid-mediated peripheral antinociception has been extensively studied in models of local hind paw inflammation induced by complete Freund's adjuvant (CFA) [12]. Opioid-containing leukocytes migrate into the inflamed tissue, release opioid peptides such as END, Met-enkephalin (ENK) and dynorphin A (DYN) and induce antinociception by binding to opioid receptors (μ, MOR; δ, DOR and κ, KOR) on peripheral nociceptive neurons. In the early phase of inflammation (first 24 h post induction) neutrophils are the predominant opioid-containing leukocytes whereas monocytes/macrophages are relevant at later stages ($>$ 24 h) [13,14]. Chemokines (CXCL2/3) or corticotrophin releasing hormone can trigger opioid peptide release [14–17]. These mediators are either locally injected or they were endogenously released under conditions of stress (cold water swim). The pathophysiological relevance of peripheral opioid-mediated antinociception was more recently demonstrated since bacterial products (formyl peptides) at the site of inflammation bind to formyl peptide receptors on neutrophils leading to tonic release of opioid peptides and a reduced intensity of inflammatory pain [18]. Studies on chemokines have shown that chemokine receptor CXCR2 ligands play a dual role in peripheral antinociception;

they are responsible for both the increased numbers of opioid-containing CXCR2$^+$ neutrophils to the site of inflammation and the release of opioid peptides from this leukocyte population [16]. In contrast, the role of chemokines at later stages of inflammation when monocytes and macrophages are the major opioid-containing leukocyte population is not well understood. Thus far, the chemokine receptor CCR2 that is expressed on monocytes and peripheral sensory neurons and its ligand CCL2 were shown to act as proalgesic mediators in neuropathic pain and in inflammation [4].

In our study, we explored the molecular mechanisms of peripheral opioid-mediated antinociception in late inflammation and antinociception by electroacupuncture. Specifically, we addressed i) the regulation of cytokines and chemokines by electroacupuncture, ii) the role of the chemokine CXCL10 (= IP-10, interferon gamma-inducible protein) in CFA inflammation, and iii) the function of CXCL10, opioid-containing macrophages as key regulator of electroacupuncture-induced antinociception.

Materials and Methods

Animals and model of inflammation

Animal protocols (REG 69/10) were approved by the governmental animal care committee (Regierung von Unterfranken, Würzburg, Germany) and are in accordance with the International Association for the Study of Pain [19]. Experimental procedures except electroacupuncture treatment were performed under isoflurane anesthesia. Six to ten male Wistar rats (280–350 g) per treatment group were injected intraplantarly (i.pl.) with 150 µl of CFA (Calbiochem, San Diego, CA, USA) in the right hind paw [14].

Electroacupuncture treatment

A reproducible electroacupuncture protocol in free moving rats performed right after injection of CFA and at 24 h post CFA using 3D image computer modeling was previously established [10]. Rats were randomly divided into CFA+EA (EA) and CFA control (CFA) group and were carefully habituated within the sterilized disposable paper cap three days before experiment. Before needling, the fur above GB30 was shaved on the lower back and disinfected. Briefly, disposable acupuncture needles (Ø = 0.20 mm, length = 25 mm, schwa-medico, Ehringshausen, Germany) connected to an electrical stimulator (AS Super_4_digital, schwa-medico) were slightly inserted into bilateral GB30 (Huan Tiao). GB30 is widely used to treat sciatica in patients or hind paw pain in rats located on the junction of lateral 2/3 and medial 1/3 on the line between the great trochanter and last sacral vertebrae [20]. The needle position was adjusted if sign of direct irritation of a nerve or blood vessel were noted. The intensity of electroacupuncture was delivered in a gradual and intermittent manner of 2–2.5–3 mA (frequency: 100 Hz, pulse width: 0.1 ms) for 20 min. The exact intensity for different individuals was flexibly kept between 2–3 mA. A slight muscle twitching of the entire hind limb including the paw could be observed as a sign of accurate needling on sciatic nerve underneath of GB30. Rats were kept conscious and allowed for complete free mobilization in the cage during the whole process. For sham treatment needling was performed without application [10].

Measurement of nociceptive thresholds

Thermal nociceptive thresholds (paw withdrawal latency; PWL) were obtained by the Hargreaves test (IITC Inc/Life Science, Italy) [18]. Rats were habituated in the plastic box with a glass plate underneath for 2–3 d before experiments. The heat of a radiant bulb was adjusted to obtain a paw withdrawal latency of 20 s in the non-inflamed paw. The required time (s) until paw withdrawal was taken as thermal nociceptive threshold. The cut off was set at 30 s to avoid tissue damage. The average of two measurements (with 20 s intervals) was calculated for analysis.

Mechanical nociceptive thresholds (paw pressure threshold; PPT) were evaluated with the paw pressure algesiometer (modified Randall-Selitto test; Ugo Basile, Comerio, Italy) [18]. Rats were habituated into a sterilized disposable man-made cap for several days before experiments and were gently held in the cap during the pain measurements [18]. Increasing pressure (g) was applied to the dorsal surface of paw until the rat withdrew its paw. The cut off point was set at 250 g to avoid tissue damage. Measurements were performed three times (with 10 s intervals) and averages were calculated. All the behavioral tests were performed in a blinded manner.

A value of nociceptive threshold lower than that determined in the contralateral paw usually represents hyperalgesia (= pain) and values above contralateral thresholds usually represent antinociception (= analgesia) in animals. Strictly speaking full or partial reversal of hyperalgesia can also be stated as anti-hyperalgesia.

Pharmacologic interventions

To examine the role of opioid peptides, groups of EA-treated animals were i.pl. injected with anti-opioid peptide antibodies (anti-END, anti-ENK, or anti-DYN; all rabbit anti-rat IgG antibodies, Peninsula, CA, US) at 4 d post CFA induced inflammation. In separate groups of animals, recombinant rat CXCL10 or rabbit anti-rat CXCL10 (both from Peprotech, Hamburg, Germany) was i.pl. administered daily for 5 d (day 0 to 4). Optimal doses were established in preliminary experiments or were based on previous studies [18,21]. Solvent saline or an identical dose of rabbit IgG was used as a control.

Enzyme-linked immunosorbent assay (ELISA)

Paw tissue was retrieved at 96 h post CFA injection and minced in ice cold lysis buffer (20 mM imidazole hydrochloride, pH 6.8; 100 mM potassium chloride, 1 mM magnesium chloride, 10 mM ethylene glycol tetraacetic acid, 1.0% Triton X-100, 10 mM sodium fluoride, 1 mM sodium molybdate, 1 mM ethylenediaminetetraacetic acid (Sigma-Aldrich, Munich; Merck, Darmstadt; Carl Roth GmbH, Karlsruhe, all Germany) with complete Protease Inhibitor Cocktail (Roche Diagnostics, Mannheim, Germany). The homogenate was frozen at −80°C. Before experiment, the homogenate was thawed, incubated at 4°C overnight, centrifuged at 14,000 g for 10 min and the supernatant was used for ELISA [13]. ELISA kits were used according to the manufacturer's instructions: IL-1alpha, IL-1beta and interferon (IFN)-gamma (R&D systems, London, UK); CXCL10 (Peprotech, Hamburg, Germany); TNF-alpha and IL-4 (Invitrogen, Life Technologies, Darmstadt, Germany) and IL-13 (Abcam, Cambridge, UK).

RNA extraction, cDNA transcription and real-time-polymerase chain reaction (RT-PCR)

Rat paw tissues at 72 and 96 h post CFA were homogenized with sterilized stainless steel beads (5 mm, Qiagen, Düsseldorf, Germany) by Tissuelyser (frequency: 20 Hz, Qiagen, Hilden, Germany) [22]. Total RNA was extracted by using TRIzol (Invitrogen/Life Technologies, Carlsbad, CA, USA). Purified RNA (1 µg) was reversely transcribed into cDNA using the High-Capacity cDNA Reverse Transcription Kit. cDNA was diluted 10-fold and amplified by RT-PCR with Taqman gene expression assays for rat CXCL10 (labeled with FAM, Assay ID: Rn01413889_g1) and GAPDH (glyceraldhyde-3- phosphate dehydrogenase, labeled with VIC) as a housekeeping gene (FAM and VIC are compatible fluorescein-based 5′ end reporter dye, the sequence of each primer is confidential from Applied Biosystems/ Life Technologies). Assays were performed according to the manufacturer's recommendations using 50 cycles, annealing and extension 1 min at 60°C (7300 System Sequence Detection Software v1.4.0). RT-negative control was applied by all the reagents except the enzyme mix 'ABsolute QPCR ROX Mix' (Thermo Fisher Scientific GmbH, Heiligenfeld, Germany) to access the genomic DNA contamination in reverse transcription reaction. Results were calculated using the $2^{\Delta\Delta CT}$ method for relative quantification. GAPDH was selected as a reference for quantification due to the optimal stable expression in inflamed and non-inflamed paw tissue compared to beta-actin and 18SrRNA in our preliminary experiments (data not shown).

Immunohistochemistry

Three rats/group at 96 h post CFA were deeply anesthetized with isoflurane and perfused transcardially with 0.1 M phosphate-buffered saline, pH 7.4, and with cold phosphate-buffered saline containing 4% paraformaldehyde pH 7.4 (fixative solution) [23]. The subcutaneous tissue adjacent to the skin was dissected from plantar surfaces of both hind paws, post-fixed in the fixative solution, and cryoprotected in 10% sucrose solution at 4°C overnight, embedded in tissue-Tek compound (OCT, Miles Inc., Elkhart, IN), and frozen. Seven-micrometer-thick sections were prepared on cryostat and mounted on gelatin-coated slides. For double immunostaining, the tissue sections were incubated with a) polyclonal rabbit anti-END or -ENK or -DYN (1:1000; all from Peninsula Laboratories, Merseyside, UK) in combination with monoclonal mouse anti-CD68 (ED1, 1:400; Serotec, Düsseldorf, Germany) or b) mouse anti-CXCR3 (1:500, Biosource, Inc., San Diego, USA) in combination with polyclonal rabbit anti-rat macrophage (1:200, Cedarlane Laboratories, Ontario Canada). Texas red conjugated goat anti-rabbit antibodies in combination with FITC conjugated donkey anti-mouse antibodies were used as secondary antibodies (all Vector Laboratories, Burlingame, CA). Finally, the tissues were stained with 4′,6 diamidino-2-phenylindole (DAPI) and mounted on vectashield (Vector Laboratories). To demonstrate specificity of staining, omission of the primary antibody was used. The contralateral (contra.) paws without inflammation were stained as negative control (data not shown).

A total of 3 samples from the inflamed paw tissue were imaged in each group, and counting of single- and double-labeled cells was done on confocal images randomly taken from three view fields in each section. Cell counting was performed by a blinded investigator using NIH Image J software (Bethesda, MD, USA). The percentage of double-labeled cells per single-labeled cells was used for statistical analysis.

Experimental protocols

Before experiments, all animals were randomly divided to CFA+EA, CFA+ sham and CFA control.

1. Antibodies against opioid peptides (END: 2 μg, ENK: 1.25 μg, DYN: 1 μg) were applied (i.pl.) on CFA+EA treated rats at 96 h post CFA. Mechanical and thermal nociceptive threshold changes were assessed 5 min post injection. Control animal received IgG (2 μg).

2. A cytokine array (data not shown) for detecting the relative signals of 29 cytokines/chemokines was performed with paw tissue from CFA or CFA+EA treated rats. ELISA further quantified the protein levels of selected promisingly expressed cytokines/ chemokines from cytokine array. CXCL10 was chosen as the targeted chemokine and applied for all subsequent studies due to the most significant upregulation by CFA+EA treatment as well as our former investigations on antinociceptive property of other CXC-chemokines [16].

3. Nociceptive thresholds were daily determined from CFA rats treated with CXCL10 (i.pl., 0.2 ng) or CFA+EA rats treated with the CXCL10 blocking antibody (i.pl., 2 μg) daily from 0–4 d. (a) In selected experiments rats were injected with anti opioid peptide antibodies on day 4 and nociceptive thresholds measured thereafter. (b) Double immunohistochemistry staining on paw tissue sections was conducted for macrophages with either CXCR3 (receptor of CXCL10) or END/ENK/DYN on day 4 after treatment.

Statistical analysis

All data were presented as mean ± SEM. Data of nociceptive thresholds were given as raw values. Multiple measurements at one time point between two or more than two groups were analyzed by t-test or one way analysis of variance (ANOVA), respectively, e.g. t-test was used for analysis of two groups with one variable factor (e.g. cytokine ELISA from CFA and CFA+EA groups), and one way ANOVA was applied for comparison of multiple groups at one time point (opioid peptide staining from CFA, CFA+EA, CFA+ sham groups). Multiple measurements at different time points between two or more than two groups were analyzed by two way repeated measurement (RM) ANOVA (e.g. all behavioral experiments). Holm-Sidak method was used for one way ANOVA and Student-Newman-Keuls Method was used for two way RM ANOVA. $^*P<0.05$ or $^{**}P<0.01$ was regarded as statistically significant.

Results

Antinociception by electroacupuncture is linked to peripheral opioid peptides

In a previous study, at 96 h CFA, electroacupuncture at GB30 caused antinociception in CFA inflammation which was fully blocked by peripheral injection (i.pl.) of the opioid receptor antagonist naloxone at the site of inflammation [10]. Sham-EA treatment (needling without application of current) did not elicit a comparable antinociceptive effect in both mechanical and thermal nociceptive threshold tests (**Fig. 1A, E**). Local injection of antibodies against the opioid peptides END or ENK significantly inhibited electroacupuncture-mediated mechanical and thermal antinociception at 5 min post injection compared to isotype control antibody (**Fig. 1B, C, F, G**, doses according to [18]). There was no significant difference between CFA baseline paw pressure threshold at 96 h and CFA+EA and anti-END or anti-DYN paw pressure thresholds. Anti-END or anti-ENK injection in CFA+EA rats thermal thresholds even more than baseline CFA levels at 96 h. Simultaneous injection of anti-END and anti-ENK antibodies did not cause an additive effect (data not shown). Antibodies against DYN (i.pl., doses according to [21]) completely blocked antinociception to mechanical (**Fig. 1H**) but not thermal stimuli (**Fig. 1D**). Nociceptive thresholds of non-inflamed paws from the same experiments in **Fig. 1** were not significantly altered as displayed in **Fig. S1**, manifesting the peripheral other than the central opioid peptide-related mechanism involved in the study. Due to the more pronounced effects of EA on mechanical nociceptive thresholds and different mechanisms of thermal and mechanical hyperalgesia we focused on these in subsequent experiments.

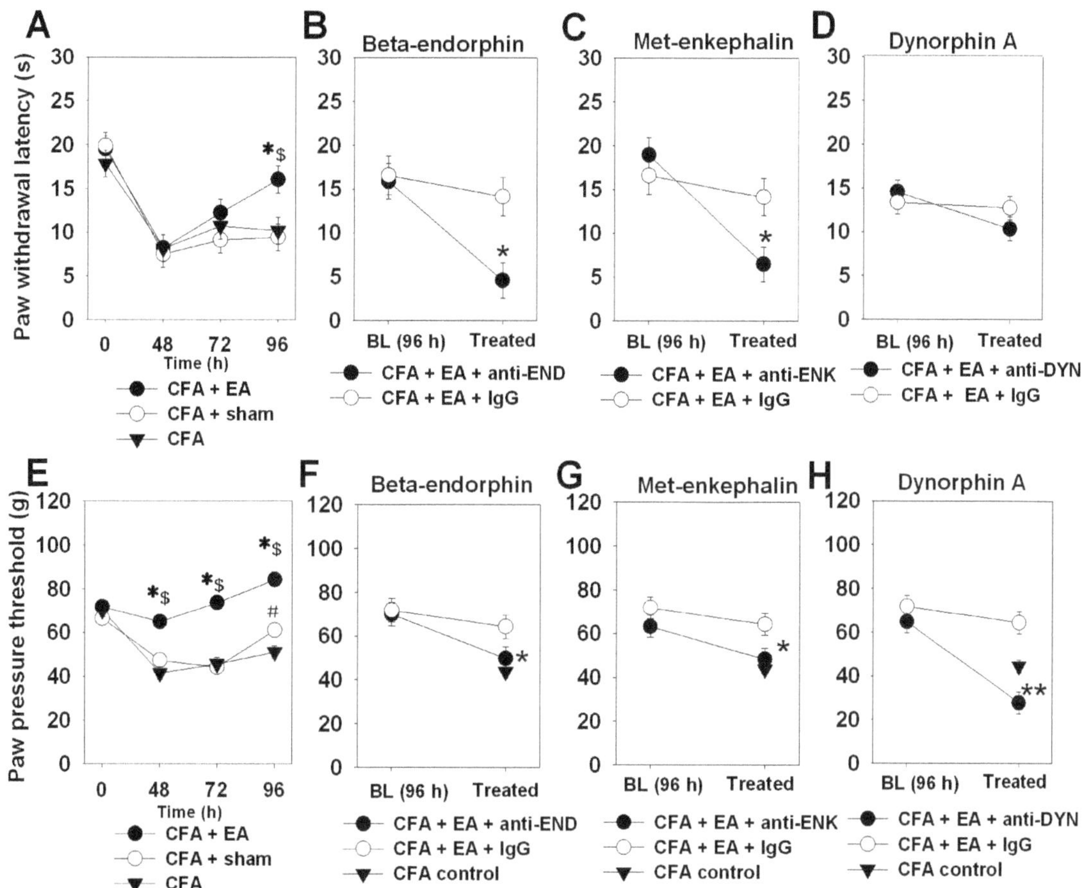

Figure 1. The antinociceptive effect of electroacupuncture (EA) via opioid peptides at the site of inflammation. Wistar rats were injected with CFA i.pl. for 48–96 h and treated with CFA and electroacupuncture (EA) at GB30 at 0 and 24 h (day 0 and 1, 100 Hz, 20 min, 2–3 mA) (CFA+EA). [**A, E**] In previous studies, sham-EA rats did not show significant difference in both mechanical and thermal nociceptive thresholds measurements at 0, 48, 72 and 96 h. Data were presented as mean ± SEM (*$p<0.05$, CFA+EA versus CFA; $^{\$}p<0.05$, CFA+EA versus CFA+ sham; $^{\#}p<0.05$, CFA+ sham versus CFA; Two-way RM ANOVA, Student-Newman-Keuls). We therefore omitted sham-EA treatment in following studies. Anti-END (2 µg [**B, F**], anti-ENK (1.25 µg [**C, G**]) or anti-DYN (1 µg [**D, H**]) was locally injected (i.pl.) at 4 d post CFA and concomitant twice EA treatment (black circles). Two control groups were added: injection with identical doses of nonspecific anti-rabbit IgG (white circle) or for comparison CFA without EA (black triangle). Paw withdrawal latency (thermal nociceptive thresholds [**A–D**]) or paw pressure thresholds (mechanical nociceptive thresholds [**E–H**]) were determined before (BL: baseline) and 5 min after injection (treated). All the data are presented as mean ± SEM (n = 6 per group, *$p<0.05$, **$p<0.01$, CFA+EA+IgG versus CFA+EA+anti-END/ENK/DYN; Two-way RM ANOVA, Student-Newman-Keuls).

Electroacupuncture regulates expression of certain cytokines in the inflamed paw

At 96 h CFA, based on a cytokine array detecting a total 29 cytokines (data not shown), we selectively quantified the protein level of several positive cytokines. Pro-inflammatory cytokines including TNF-alpha and IL-1beta (**Fig. 2A, C**) were significantly downregulated by electroacupuncture whereas IL-1alpha (**Fig. 2B**) was unaltered. The anti-inflammatory cytokine IL-4 remained unchanged whereas IL-13 was significantly upregulated (**Fig. 2D, E**). Interestingly, the only pro-inflammatory cytokine that was significantly upregulated was IFN-gamma (**Fig. 2F**).

CXCL10 expression and increased numbers of opioid-containing macrophages are associated with electroacupuncture

CXCL10 is a chemokine stimulated by IFN-gamma [24]. Since IFN-gamma was the only pro-inflammatory cytokine upregulated by electroacupuncture, we focused our subsequent experiments on CXCL10. Electroacupuncture significantly upregulated CXCL10 on both the protein (**Fig. 3A**) and mRNA level (**Fig. 3B**). No CXCL10 protein increase was seen in sham-treated animals.

Neutrophils are an important source of opioid peptides released in the early phase of CFA-inflammation (up to 24 h) whereas macrophages are considered mainly responsible for peripheral opioid peptide-mediated antinociception at later stage of inflammation (48–96 h). T cells constitute only a small subpopulation of infiltrating leukocytes (<5%) [14]. Since CXCL10 exclusively binds to the chemokine receptor CXCR3 [25], we analyzed the co-expression of CXCR3 with a rabbit anti-rat macrophage serum at the site of inflammation with or without concomitant electroacupuncture. CXCR3 was expressed on the vast majority of infiltrating macrophages (**Fig. 3C**). Furthermore, the percentage of $CXCR3^{+}$ expressing macrophages was significantly increased by electroacupuncture (**Fig. 3D**).

CXCL10 reverses CFA-induced mechanical hyperalgesia via peripheral opioid peptides

Chemokines like CXCL1 and CXCL2/3 play a dual role in peripheral opioid peptide mediated antinociception, because

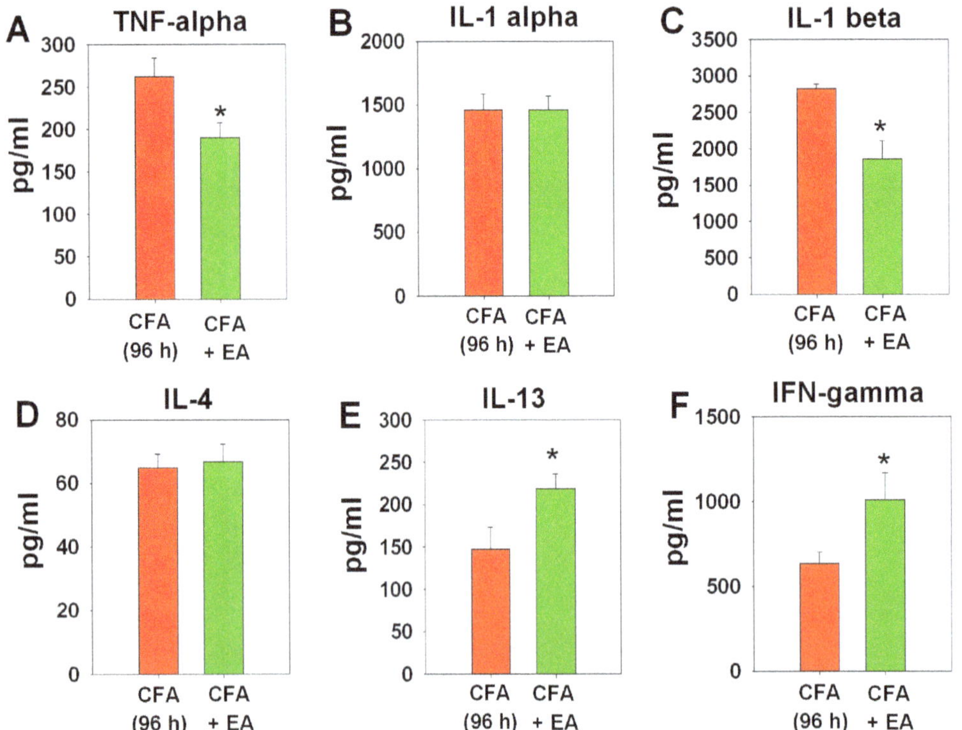

Figure 2. Differential alterations in pro- and anti-inflammatory cytokines in inflamed paw tissue by electroacupuncture (EA). Rats were injected with CFA treated with (CFA+EA) or without (CFA) EA. Based on the results from pilot experiments for immune array of 29 cytokines (data not shown), **[A–F]** *pro- and anti-inflammatory* cytokines including TNF-alpha, IL-1alpha, IL-1beta, IFN-gamma, IL-4 and IL-13 in the paws were selectively quantified by ELISA after 96 h CFA. Data are presented as mean ± SEM (n = 5–10 per group, *p<0.05, CFA+EA versus CFA; t-test).

they recruit opioid-containing neutrophils and trigger opioid peptide release via its receptor CXCR2 [16]. To address whether CXCL10 was able to attenuate inflammatory pain by CFA via increased numbers of opioid containing cells we performed multiple injection of CXCL10. Repeated daily administration of 0.2 ng CXCL10 (based on a preliminary dose-finding study, data not shown) elicited sustained mechanical antinociception at 48, 72 and 96 h (**Fig. 4A**). CXCL10-mediated antinociception was fully reversed by the concomitant i.pl. administration of CXCL10 with anti-END, anti-ENK, or anti-DYN at 96 h (**Fig. 4B**). In parallel, repeated chemokine injection was associated with a significant increase in ED1$^+$ macrophages co-expressing the opioid peptides END, ENK, and DYN in comparison to solvent control (**Fig. 4C–E**). More ED1$^+$ macrophages expressed ENK (almost 72%) compared to END (63%) and DYN (55%) (**Fig. 4F**). No change was seen in rats treated with solvent.

Electroacupuncture increases ligand availability

Next, we tested whether electroacupuncture affects the accumulation of opioid peptide. Electroacupuncture was associated with a significant increase in the number of ED1$^+$ macrophages co-expressing the three opioid peptides END, ENK and DYN (**Fig. 5A, B, C**). More ED1$^+$ macrophages expressed ENK (almost 75%) compared to END (65%) and DYN (60%) (**Fig. 5D**). No change on the co-expression of opioid peptides and ED1 was seen in sham treated rats.

Electroacupuncture-induced antinociception and increased numbers of opioid-containing macrophages is prevented by blockade of CXCL10

Since electroacupuncture-elicited antinociception correlated with the number of opioid-containing macrophages, we examined whether CXCL10 was a key regulator. Daily injections of anti-CXCL10 significantly decreased the pain threshold at 48–96 h post CFA and abolished the electroacupuncture-induced antinociception (**Fig. 6A**). Furthermore, multiple injections of the anti-CXCL10 significantly reduced the number of ED1$^+$ macrophages co-expressing the opioid peptides END, ENK, and DYN (**Fig. 6B, C, D**) stimulated by electroacupuncture. The percentage of ED1$^+$ macrophages expressed END was reduced to 53% compared to ENK (43%) and DYN (44%) (**Fig. 6E**). No change was seen in rats treated with isotype control antibody.

Discussion

Acupuncture is widely used as an alternative analgesic therapy in a broad range of pain syndromes. Despite its widespread use the role is often doubted and attributed to placebo effects. Indeed, the underlying molecular mechanisms of pain control are not well understood. In our study electroacupuncture suppressed selected pro- and enhanced anti-inflammatory cytokines in a model of inflammatory pain in rats. In contrast to this pattern, EA increased the production of the cytokine IFN-gamma and the chemokine CXCL10 at the site of inflammation leading to an increase in opioid-containing CXCR3$^+$ macrophages. Macrophage-derived opioid peptides could activate opioid receptors on peripheral

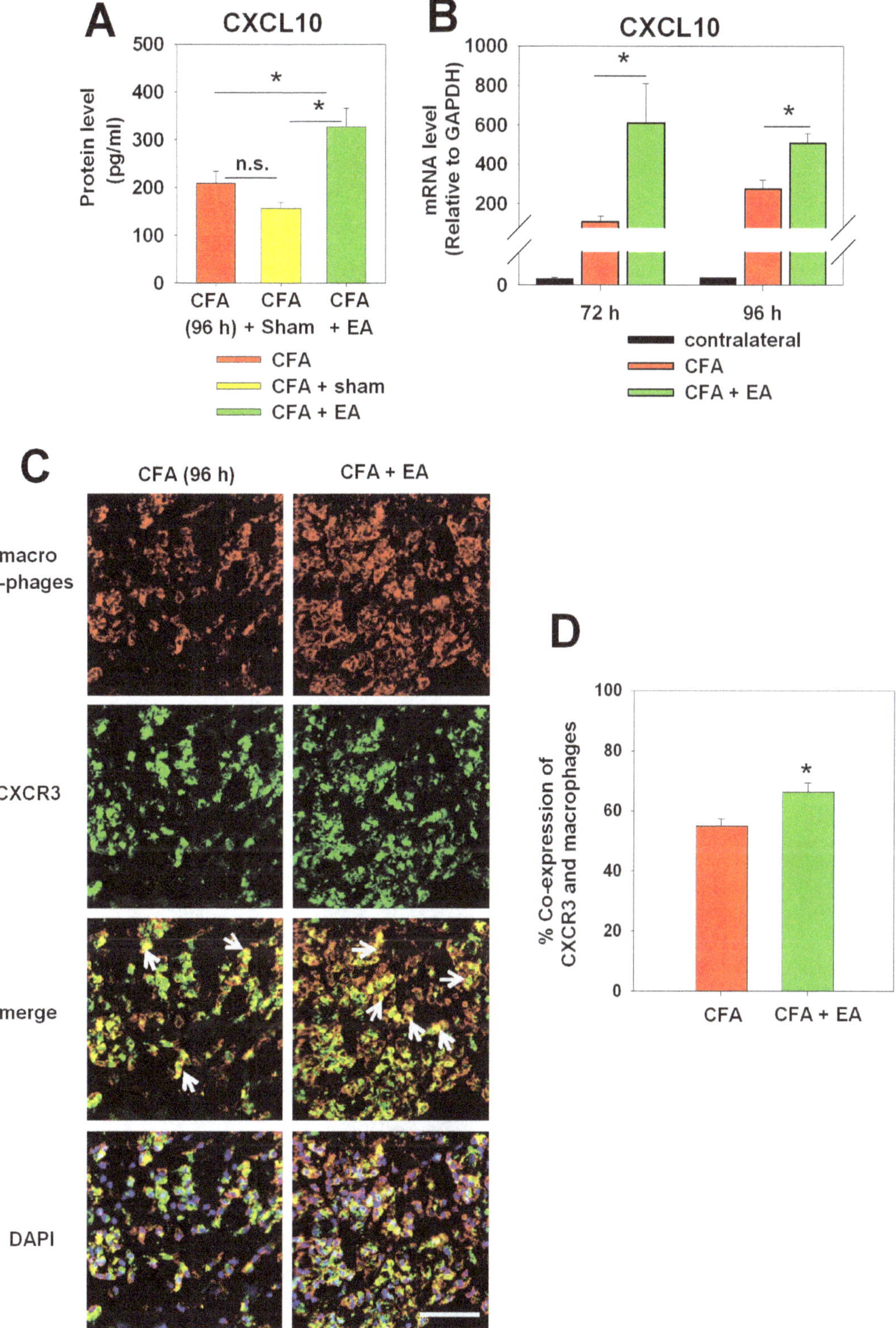

Figure 3. Upregulation of CXCL10 and an increase of CXCR3⁺macrophages in inflamed paw tissue by electroacupuncture (EA). Rats were injected with CFA and treated with (CFA+EA), (CFA+sham) or CFA only. On day 4 (96 h), CXCL10 was quantified by ELISA [**A**] and semi-quantitative RT-PCR (72 and 96 h) in subcutaneous paw tissue ([**B**] noninflamed contralateral paw (contra.) is only shown as a negative control). Data are presented as mean ± SEM (For ELISA: n = 6 per group, *$p<0.05$, one way ANOVA, Holm-Sidak method; For RT-PCR: n = 6 per group, *$p<0.05$, CFA+EA versus CFA; t-test). [**C**] Tissue sections were stained with rabbit anti-rat macrophage serum (red), mouse anti-rat CXCR3 antibody (green) and DAPI. The arrows are pointing at CXCR3 expressed macrophages. Representative sections are shown, arrows pointing on double positive cells (scale bar: 50 μm). [**D**] The percentage of macrophages and opioid positive cells was analyzed. All data are presented as mean ± SEM (n = 3 per group, *$p<0.05$, CFA+EA versus CFA; t-test).

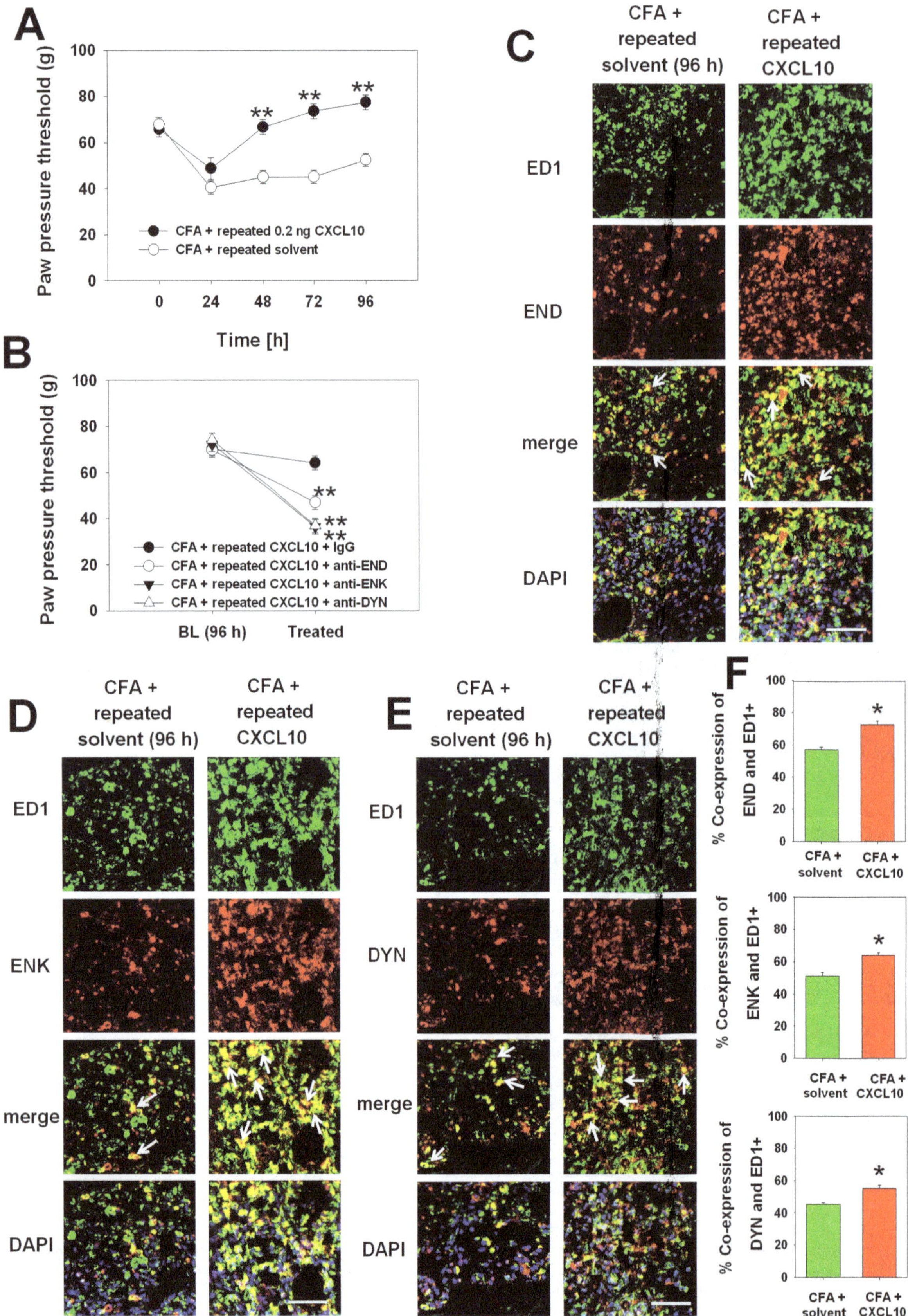

Figure 4. Opioid peptide-dependent sustained antinociception and increase opioid peptide expressed macrophages by repeated CXCL10 injection. Rats were i.pl. injected with CFA and daily with CXCL10 (0.2 ng) or solvent control. [A] Mechanical nociceptive thresholds were

determined daily before each injection. Data were presented as mean ± SEM (n = 6 per group, *p<0.05, **p<0.01, CFA+CXCL10 versus CFA+solvent; Two-way RM ANOVA, Student-Newman-Keuls). [B] Anti-END (2 µg, anti-ENK (1.25 µg) or anti-DYN (1 µg) was locally injected (i.pl.) at 4 d post CFA on rats with repeated injection of CXCL10 (0.2 ng). Identical doses of anti-rabbit IgG were used as control. Data were presented as mean ± SEM (n = 6 per group, *p<0.05, **p<0.01, CFA+CXCL10+IgG versus CFA+CXCL10+anti-END/ENK/DYN; Two-way RM ANOVA, Student-Newman-Keuls). [C] Immunohistochemical staining of paw tissue was performed at 96 h with a mouse anti-ED1 (CD68) macrophage antibody (green) and with rabbit anti-END, anti-ENK or anti-DYN antibodies (all was marked red) as well as DAPI. Representative sections are shown. Arrows pointing at double positive cells. (scale bar: 50 µm). [D] The percentage of END/ENK/DYN+ and ED1+ was quantified. All the data are presented as mean ± SEM (n = 3 per group, *p<0.05, CFA+ solvent versus CFA+CXCL10; t-test).

sensory neurons and suppressed inflammatory pain. Taken together we identified a new molecular pathway of acupuncture-induced analgesia.

Effects of electroacupuncture on the peripheral opioid system and on cytokine production

Endogenous opioid peptides inhibit pain both in the central nervous system and in the periphery. Acupuncture triggers the release of opioid peptides at the level of the spinal cord and in the brain leading to activation of MOR and sometimes other opioid receptors [7,26–29]. In the periphery, opioid peptide-induced antinociception seems to involve MOR, DOR and KOR at the site of inflammation [9,10,30]. There are some hints that acupuncture regulates the expression of the END in immune cells and in keratinocytes via activation of the cannabinoid receptor CB2 [11]. We now extended these findings by demonstrating that electroacupuncture stimulated the increased numbers of leukocytes containing the three opioid peptides END, ENK, and DYN and that all three opioid peptides mediated antinociception to thermal and mechanical stimuli (similar to stress (cold water swim)-induced antinociception [12]). In our study, DYN did not contribute to thermal antinociception induced by acupuncture. Anti-END and anti-ENK treatment even lowered thermal nociceptive thresholds more than CFA baseline at 96 h possibly due to endogenous tonic release of opioid peptides in thermal hyperalgesia [18]. In accordance with our study here, other groups also observed that electroacupuncture better controls mechanical than thermal hyperalgesia in inflammatory pain [31], probably due to different mechanisms and receptors controlling thermal and mechanical pain.

In addition to the upregulation of opioid peptides, acupuncture was previously claimed to suppress the production of the pro-inflammatory cytokines TNF-alpha, IL-1beta and IL-6 in inflammatory pain [6,11]. Studies in other models (asthma, trauma) demonstrated that T_h1 cytokines such as IL-2 and IFN-gamma were increased whereas T_h2 cytokines such as IL-4, IL-10 and IL-13 were suppressed [32–34]. In our model of inflammatory pain, electroacupuncture significantly attenuated IL-1beta and TNF-alpha as well as selectively upregulated the T_h1 cell type cytokine IFN-gamma. In contrast to the findings in models of asthma and trauma, the T_h2 cytokine IL-4 was unchanged and IL-13 was upregulated indicating the activation of both T_h1 and T_h2 cell signaling by electroacupuncture. Therefore, differential effects of EA on cytokines are observed in different models. Despite the suppression of pro-inflammatory cytokines we and others [6] found that the number of infiltrating opioid peptide-containing leukocytes (i.e. macrophages) was significantly increased by electroacupuncture. In line with our previous studies [13,14] T cells were almost absent at the site of CFA-induced inflammation (data not shown). In summary, our study in part supports the previously described anti-inflammatory effects of electroacupuncture, but some pro-inflammatory cytokines like IFN-gamma and CXCL10 seem to be upregulated in inflammatory pain.

Chemokines in inflammation and nociception

In our model of inflammatory pain, the expression of the chemokine CXCL10 and, in parallel, the numbers of macrophages expressing the corresponding chemokine receptor CXCR3 were significantly upregulated by electroacupuncture. Few studies examined the role of electroacupuncture on chemokine expression. It was reported electroacupuncture augmented the production of the chemokine CXCL12 (stromal cell-derived factor-1alpha) in cerebral ischemic injury [35] whereas the production of CCL2 (monocyte chemotactic protein-1) was downregulated in adipose tissue without any accompanying inflammation [36]. While these studies focused on acupuncture, the role of chemokines in hyperalgesia and antinociception has been studied on more general level. The monocytic chemokine CCL2 and its corresponding receptor CCR2 were shown to be proalgesic mediators in neuropathic and other pain models [37]. Interestingly, chemokine receptors (including CCR2 and CXCR4) could interact with receptors involved in antinociception (MOR) or inflammation (adenosine A2A receptor). Activation of one receptor leads to the trans-deactivation of the other. Crosstalk between chemokines and neuronal receptors bridges immune and nervous systems [38]. Studies examining the chemokine-mediated selective recruitment of isolated leukocyte subpopulations to non-inflamed skin demonstrated that the monocytic chemokine CCL2 and the neutrophilic chemokine CXCL1 or CXCL2/3 induced recruitment of the respective leukocyte population, but while nociceptive thresholds were unchanged by CXCL2/3 [39], CCL2 elicited hyperalgesia [23,40]. The role of CXCL10 in pain is not very well examined. Toll like receptor ligands can induce expression and production of pro-inflammatory chemokines and cytokines including CXCL10 or e.g. IL-1alpha, IL-1beta, and PGE_2 in dorsal root ganglia neurons, which in part have previously been shown to increase pain [41]. In summary, the role of cytokines and chemokines in the generation of hyperalgesia or antinociception depends on the model and the state of inflammation.

The broad spectrum of CXCL10-mediated actions in inflammation

Electroacupuncture augmented the CXCL10 expression both on the transcriptional and translational level and increased the number of opioid containing $CXCR3^+$ macrophages as well as long-lasting antinociception. Repeated injections of CXCL10 reversed hyperalgesia in CFA rats. Similarly, repeated anti-CXCL10 in EA-treated animals lessened the antinociceptive effect of EA. CXCL10 is upregulated by IFN-gamma, which was also increased after treatment with electroacupuncture. CXCL10 is a chemoattractant for activated T cells, monocytes/macrophages, dendritic cells and microglia [24]. In addition to recruiting inflammatory cells, CXCL10 induced astroglial proliferation and is directly neurotoxic e.g. in the HIV-1 neuropathogenesis [42]. Interestingly, the CXCL10/CXCR3 interaction played an important role in tuberculosis. Both tuberculosis and CFA-induced hind paw inflammation are caused by different strains of mycobacteria. CXCL10 production was upregulated in macro-

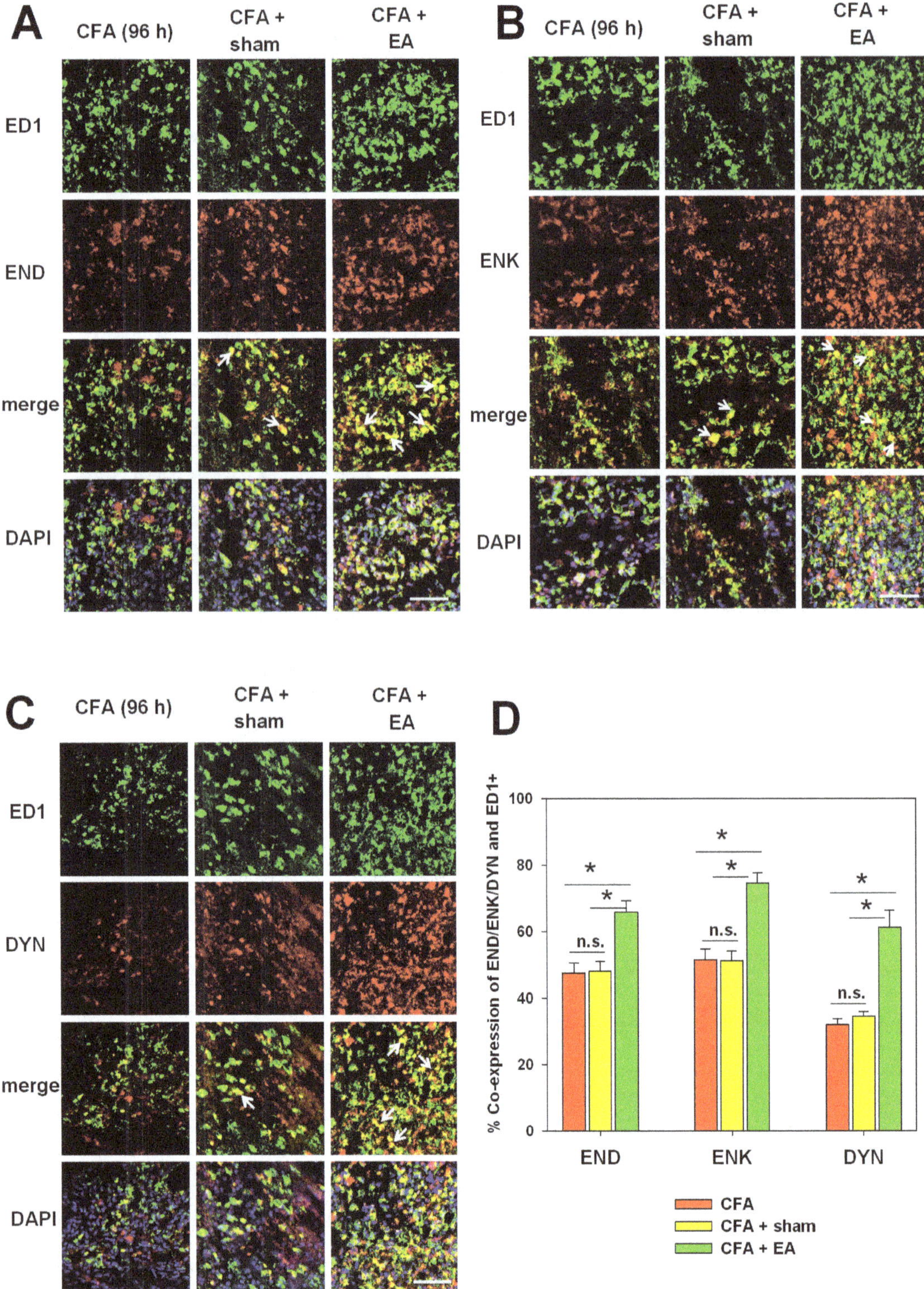

Figure 5. EA enhanced the recruitment of opioid-containing macrophages. Rats were injected with CFA with (CFA+EA), (CFA + sham) or without (CFA) EA treatment for 4 days. Immunohistochemical staining was performed for mouse anti-CD68 macrophages (green) and rabbit [**A**] anti-END, [**B**] anti-ENK or [**C**] anti-DYN antibodies respectively (red). DAPI (blue) was used to recognize cell nuclei (Representative sections are shown by arrows, scale bars: 50 μm). [**D**] The percentage of ED1 and opioid positive cells was quantified. All the data are presented as mean ± SEM (n = 3 per group, *p<0.05, one way ANOVA, Holm-Sidak method).

phages (and to a lesser degree in dendritic cells) by mycobacterium tuberculosis *in vitro* and *in vivo* [43]. This is a hallmark of active – but not latent – infection [44] similar to our study of CFA inflammation with heat killed and dried mycobacteria in oily solution as a nonspecific active inflammation. Furthermore, CXCL10 regulates the recruitment of $CXCR3^+$ macrophages to

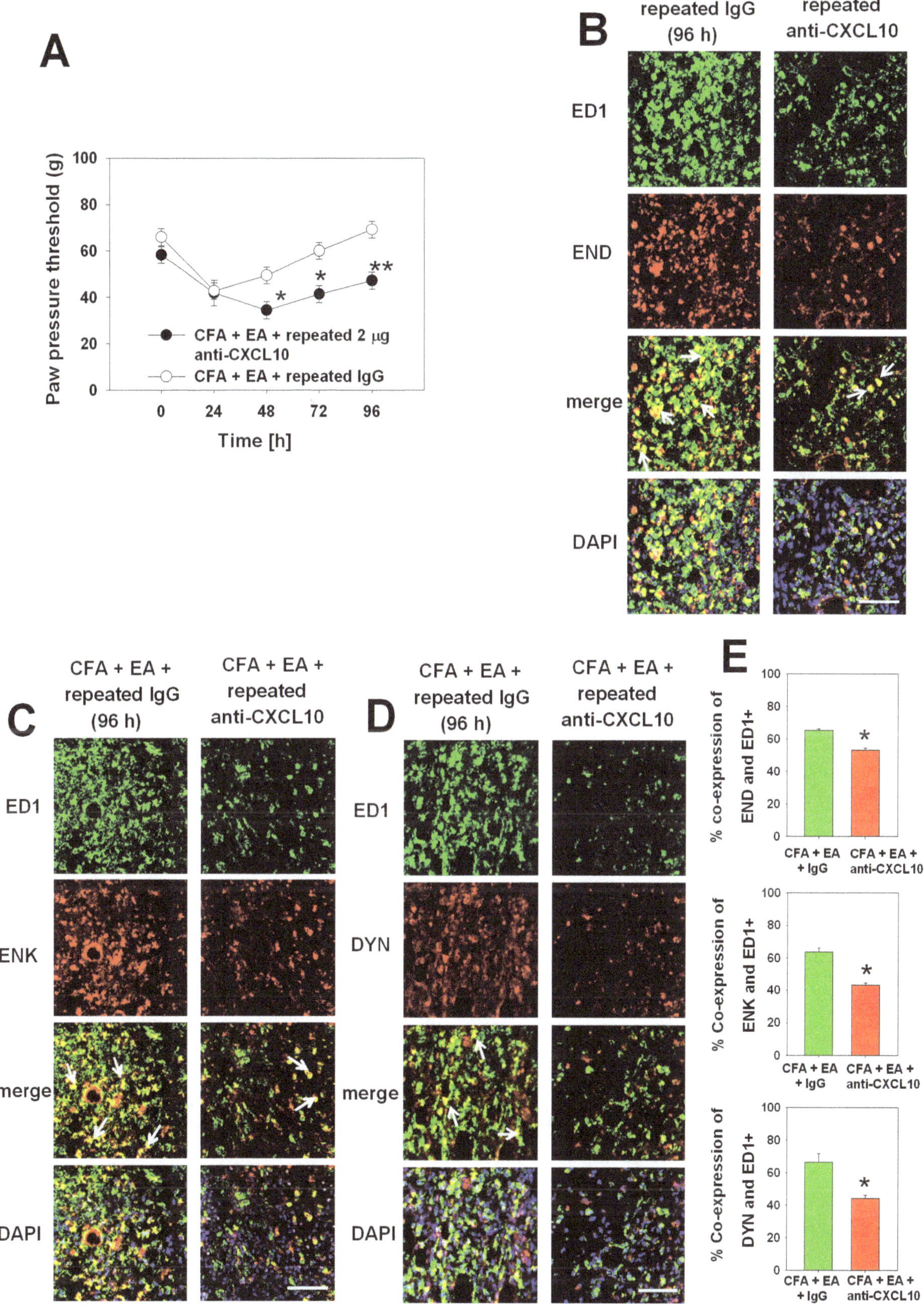

Figure 6. Neutralization of CXCL10 fully reversed electroacupuncture (EA)-induced antinociception and increase of opioid-containing monocytes/macrophages. [A] Rats with CFA inflammation and EA treatment were daily i.pl. injected with an antibody against

CXCL10. Controls were injected with anti-rabbit IgG antibody. Mechanical nociceptive thresholds were determined before (BL) and after injections. Data are presented as mean ± SEM (n = 6 per group, *p<0.05, **p<0.01, CFA+EA+IgG versus CFA+EA+anti-CXCL10; Two-way RM ANOVA, Student-Newman-Keuls). [B–D] Immunohistochemical staining was performed for mouse anti-ED1 monocytes/macrophages (green) and rabbit anti-END, anti-ENK or anti-DYN antibodies respectively (red). DAPI (blue) was used to recognize cell nuclei. Representative sections are shown, arrows pointing at double positive cells (scale bar: 50 μm). [E] Quantification for immunohistochemical staining showed the percentage of double positive ED1 and END/ENK/DYN cells. All the data are presented as mean ± SEM (n = 3 per group, *p<0.05, CFA+EA+IgG versus CFA+EA+anti-CXCL10; t-test).

the vessel wall [45]. In contrast in our CFA model, macrophages were the predominant leukocyte population, T cells were virtually absent (<5%) and NK cells have thus far not been studied [13,14]. Thus, CXCL10 seemed to preferentially interact with opioid-containing CXCR3$^+$ macrophages.

The novel role of CXCL10 – a key regulator of antinociception in acupuncture

Repeated daily injection of CXCL10 conferred sustained antinociception and lead to a parallel increase in the number of opioid peptide-expressing macrophages. Our data favor the hypothesis that electroacupuncture influenced the transcription and translation of CXCL10. How could this be mediated? One obvious candidate would be adenosine since manual acupuncture triggers its release and antinociception is mediated by adenosine A1 receptors [46]. However, adenosine receptor activation decreased, rather than increased CXCL10 production in macrophages [47]. Alternatively, cannabinoid receptors could be involved since they contributed to acupuncture-induced antinociception [5,6]. However, they also suppressed inflammation and downregulated chemokines at least in keratinocytes [48]. Although the immune regulation of peripheral acupuncture-induced antinociception appears well understood, the molecular link between the peripheral nervous system (presumably activated by acupuncture) and the immune regulation remains enigmatic to be solved.

Availability of opioid receptors and ligands for pain control

Previously, expansion of opioid-containing neutrophils by hematopoietic factors [22] or enhanced recruitment by local injection of neutrophilic chemokines [49] did not enhance peripheral opioid-mediated antinociception in early stages of inflammation since opioid receptor expression was limiting antinociception. In addition electroacupuncture did not further alter the expression of opioid receptors in the inflamed paw (data not shown). In contrast to the findings of expansion or recruitment of opioid-containing neutrophils, enhanced recruitment of opioid-containing macrophages induced antinociception in later stages of inflammation probably because the opioid receptors are already upregulated after 4 d of inflammation and not fully occupied by the available ligands. Importantly, neutralization by an anti-CXCL10 antibody time-dependently inhibited electroacupuncture-elicited antinociception by daily injection. It also largely suppressed the increased numbers of opioid-containing macrophages. In summary, intensity of antinociception is regulated differently during inflammation. Antinociception is limited by opioid receptor availability in early and ligand availability (i.e. opioid peptides) in late inflammation. Accordingly, increased numbers of opioid-containing leukocytes enhance antinociception in late but not in early inflammation.

Taken together, our data suggest that electroacupuncture enhances CXCL10 production at the site of inflammation and stimulates peripheral opioid peptide-mediated antinociception. Furthermore CXCL10 itself appears to trigger an increased number of opioid-containing monocytes/macrophages at the site of inflammation without acupuncture. Our data suggest that CXCL10 appears to be a key antinociceptive mediator also in electroacupuncture-mediated analgesia.

Supporting Information

Figure S1 [A–H] Nociceptive thresholds of non-inflamed paws in Fig. S1 were measured as contralateral controls. No statistical difference was observed between each group at given time points. All the data are presented as mean ± SEM (n = 6 per group, two way RM ANOVA).
(TIF)

Acknowledgments

The author would like to thank for the professional technical assistance of Anja Neuhoff as well as the invaluable advice of Dr. Winfried Neuhaus for experimental design.

Author Contributions

Conceived and designed the experiments: YW DH AB HLR. Performed the experiments: YW RG SAM. Analyzed the data: YW RG. Contributed reagents/materials/analysis tools: YW RG SAM. Wrote the paper: YW AB HLR.

References

1. Mavrommatis CI, Argyra E, Vadalouka A, Vasilakos DG (2012) Acupuncture as an adjunctive therapy to pharmacological treatment in patients with chronic pain due to osteoarthritis of the knee: a 3-armed, randomized, placebo-controlled trial. Pain 153: 1720–1726.
2. Manheimer E, White A, Berman B, Forys K, Ernst E (2005) Meta-analysis: Acupuncture for low back pain. Ann Intern Med 142: 651–663.
3. Vas J, Aranda JM, Modesto M, Benitez-Parejo N, Herrera A, et al. (2012) Acupuncture in patients with acute low back pain: A multicentre randomised controlled clinical trial. Pain 153: 1883–1889.
4. White FA, Sun J, Waters SM, Ma C, Ren D, et al. (2005) Excitatory monocyte chemoattractant protein-1 signaling is up-regulated in sensory neurons after chronic compression of the dorsal root ganglion. PNAS 102: 14092–14097.
5. Gondim DV, Costa JL, Rocha SS, Brito GAD, Ribeiro RD, et al. (2012) Antinociceptive and anti-inflammatory effects of electroacupuncture on experimental arthritis of the rat temporomandibular joint. Can J Phys Pharmacol 90: 395–405.
6. Su TF, Zhao YQ, Zhang LH, Peng M, Wu CH, et al. (2012) Electroacupuncture reduces the expression of proinflammatory cytokines in inflamed skin tissues through activation of cannabinoid CB2 receptors. Eur J Pain 16: 624–635.
7. Zhang RX, Lao LX, Wang LB, Liu B, Wang XY, et al. (2004) Involvement of opioid receptors in electroacupuncture-produced anti-hyperalgesia in rats with peripheral inflammation. Brain Res 1020: 12–17.
8. Zhang RX, Wang LB, Liu B, Qiao JT, Ren K, et al. (2005) Mu opioid receptor-containing neurons mediate electroacupuncture-produced anti-hyperalgesia in rats with hind paw inflammation. Brain Res 1048: 235–240.
9. Taguchi R, Taguchi T, Kitakoji H (2010) Involvement of peripheral opioid receptors in electroacupuncture analgesia for carrageenan-induced hyperalgesia. Brain Res 1355: 97–103.
10. Wang Y, Hackel D, Peng F, Rittner HL (2013) Long-term antinociception by electroacupuncture is mediated via peripheral opioid receptors in free-moving rats with inflammatory hyperalgesia. Eur J Pain 17:1447–57.
11. Su TF, Zhang LH, Peng M, Wu CH, Pan W, et al. (2011) Cannabinoid CB2 receptors contribute to upregulation of beta-endorphin in inflamed skin tissues by electroacupuncture. Mol Pain 7: 98–128.
12. Machelska H, Heppenstall PA, Stein C (2003) Breaking the pain barrier. Nat Med 9: 1353–1354.

13. Brack A, Rittner HL, Machelska H, Leder K, Mousa SA, et al. (2004) Control of inflammatory pain by chemokine-mediated recruitment of opioid-containing polymorphonuclear cells. Pain 112: 229–238.
14. Rittner HL, Brack A, Machelska H, Mousa SA, Bauer M, et al. (2001) Opioid peptide-expressing leukocytes: identification, recruitment, and simultaneously increasing inhibition of inflammatory pain. Anesthesiology 95: 500–508.
15. Czlonkowski A, Stein C, Herz A (1993) Peripheral mechanisms of opioid antinociception in inflammation: involvement of cytokines. European Journal of Pharmacology 242: 229–235.
16. Rittner HL, Labuz D, Schaefer M, Mousa SA, Schulz S, et al. (2006) Pain control by CXCR2 ligands through Ca2(+)-regulated release of opioid peptides from polymorphonuclear cells. FASEB J 20: 2627.
17. Schafer M, Carter L, Stein C (1994) Interleukin 1 beta and corticotropin-releasing factor inhibit pain by releasing opioids from immune cells in inflamed tissue. PNAS 91: 4219–4223.
18. Rittner HL, Hackel D, Voigt P, Mousa S, Stolz A, et al. (2009) Mycobacteria attenuate nociceptive responses by formyl peptide receptor triggered opioid peptide release from neutrophils. Plos Pathogens 5: e1000362.
19. Zimmermann M (1983) Ethical guidelines for investigations of experimental pain in conscious animals. Pain 16: 109–110.
20. Lao L, Zhang RX, Zhang G, Wang X, Berman BM, et al. (2004) A parametric study of electroacupuncture on persistent hyperalgesia and Fos protein expression in rats. Brain Res 1020: 18–29.
21. Schreiter A, Gore C, Labuz D, Fournie-Zaluski MC, Roques BP, et al. (2012) Pain inhibition by blocking leukocytic and neuronal opioid peptidases in peripheral inflamed tissue. FASEB J 26: 5161–5171.
22. Brack A, L Rittner H, Machelska H, Beschmann K, Sitte N, et al. (2004) Mobilization of opioid-containing polymorphonuclear cells by hematopoietic growth factors and influence on inflammatory pain. Anesthesiology 100: 149–157.
23. Pflücke D, Hackel D, Mousa SA, Partheil A, Neumann A, et al. (2013) The molecular link between C-C-chemokine ligand 2-induced leukocyte recruitment and hyperalgesia. J Pain 15: 1–14.
24. Taub DD, Lloyd AR, Conlon K, Wang JM, Ortaldo JR, et al. (1993) Recombinant human interferon-inducible protein 10 is a chemoattractant for human monocytes and T lymphocytes and promotes T cell adhesion to endothelial cells. J Exp Med 177: 1809–1814.
25. Booth V, Keizer DW, Kamphuis MB, Clark-Lewis I, Sykes BD (2002) The CXCR3 binding chemokine IP-10/CXCL10: structure and receptor interactions. Biochemistry 41: 10418–10425.
26. Han JS (2004) Acupuncture and endorphins. Neuroscience Letters 361: 258–261.
27. Clement-Jones V, McLoughlin L, Tomlin S, Besser GM, Rees LH, et al. (1980) Increased beta-endorphin but not met-enkephalin levels in human cerebrospinal fluid after acupuncture for recurrent pain. Lancet 2: 946–949.
28. Chung SH, Dickenson A (1980) Pain, enkephalin and acupuncture. Nature 283: 243–244.
29. Zhang Y, Li AH, Lao LX, Xin JJ, Ren K, et al. (2011) Rostral ventromedial medulla mu, but not kappa, opioid receptors are involved in electroacupuncture anti-hyperalgesia in an inflammatory pain rat model. Brain Res 1395: 38–45.
30. Zhang GG, Yu C, Lee W, Lao L, Ren K, et al. (2005) Involvement of peripheral opioid mechanisms in electroacupuncture analgesia. Explore (NY) 1: 365–371.
31. Huang C, Hu ZP, Long H, Shi YS, Han JS, et al. (2004) Attenuation of mechanical but not thermal hyperalgesia by electroacupuncture with the involvement of opioids in rat model of chronic inflammatory pain. Brain Res Bull 63: 99–103.
32. Wang K, Wu HX, Wang GN, Li MM, Zhang ZD, et al. (2009) The Effects of Electroacupuncture on Th1/Th2 Cytokine mRNA Expression and Mitogen-Activated Protein Kinase Signaling Pathways in the Splenic T Cells of Traumatized Rats. Anesth Analg 109: 1666–1673.
33. Carneiro ER, Xavier RAN, De Castro MAP, Do Nascimento CMO, Silveira VLF (2010) Electroacupuncture promotes a decrease in inflammatory response associated with Th1/Th2 cytokines, nitric oxide and leukotriene B4 modulation in experimental asthma. Cytokine 50: 335–340.
34. Park MB, Ko E, Ahn C, Choi H, Rho S, et al. (2004) Suppression of IgE production and modulation of Th1/Th2 cell response by electroacupuncture in DNP-KLH immunized mice. J Neuroimmunol 151: 40–44.
35. Kim JH, Choi KH, Jang YJ, Kim HN, Bae SS, et al. (2013) Electroacupuncture preconditioning reduces cerebral ischemic injury via BDNF and SDF-1 alpha in mice. BMC Complement Altern Med 13: doi: 10.1186/1472-6882-13-22.
36. Yu M, Xiao XQ, Tang CL, Liu ZL, Hou YX, et al. (2011) [Effect of different intensities of electroacupuncture on expression of monocyte chemoattractant protein-1 and TNF-alpha in adipose tissue in obesity rats]. Zhen Ci Yan Jiu 36: 79–84.
37. Miller RE, Tran PB, Das R, Ghoreishi-Haack N, Ren D, et al. (2012) CCR2 chemokine receptor signaling mediates pain in experimental osteoarthritis. PNAS 109: 20602–20607.
38. Zhang N, Oppenheim JJ (2005) Crosstalk between chemokines and neuronal receptors bridges immune and nervous systems. J Leukoc Biol 78: 1210–1214.
39. Rittner HL, Mousa SA, Labuz D, Beschmann K, Schäfer M, et al. (2006) Selective local PMN recruitment by CXCL1 or CXCL2/3 injection does not cause inflammatory pain. J Leukoc Biol 79: 1022–1032.
40. Hackel D, Pflücke D, Neumann A, Viebahn J, Mousa S, et al. (2013) The connection of monocytes and reactive oxygen species in pain. PLoS One 8: e63564.
41. Qi J, Buzas K, Fan H, Cohen JI, Wang K, et al. (2011) Painful pathways induced by TLR stimulation of dorsal root ganglion neurons. J Immunol 186: 6417–6426.
42. Yao H, Bethel-Brown C, Li CZ, Buch SJ (2010) HIV neuropathogenesis: a tight rope walk of innate immunity. J Neuroimmune Pharm 5: 489–495.
43. Jang S, Uzelac A, Salgame P (2008) Distinct chemokine and cytokine gene expression pattern of murine dendritic cells and macrophages in response to Mycobacterium tuberculosis infection. J Leukoc Biol 84: 1264–1270.
44. Lu C, Wu J, Wang H, Wang S, Diao N, et al. (2011) Novel biomarkers distinguishing active tuberculosis from latent infection identified by gene expression profile of peripheral blood mononuclear cells. PLoS One 6: e24290.
45. Zhou J, Tang PC, Qin L, Gayed PM, Li W, et al. (2010) CXCR3-dependent accumulation and activation of perivascular macrophages is necessary for homeostatic arterial remodeling to hemodynamic stresses. J Exp Med 207: 1951–1966.
46. Goldman N, Chen M, Fujita T, Xu Q, Peng W, et al. (2010) Adenosine A1 receptors mediate local anti-nociceptive effects of acupuncture. Nat Neurosci 13: 883–888.
47. Panther E, Corinti S, Idzko M, Herouy Y, Napp M, et al. (2003) Adenosine affects expression of membrane molecules, cytokine and chemokine release, and the T-cell stimulatory capacity of human dendritic cells. Blood 101: 3985–3990.
48. Gaffal E, Cron M, Glodde N, Bald T, Kuner R, et al. (2013) Cannabinoid 1 receptors in keratinocytes modulate proinflammatory chemokine secretion and attenuate contact allergic inflammation. J Immunol 190: 4929–4936.
49. Brack A, Rittner H, Machelska H, Shaqura M, Mousa SA, et al. (2004) Endogenous peripheral antinociception in early inflammation is not limited by the number of opioid-containing leukocytes but by opioid receptor expression. Pain 108: 67–75.

18

Laser Acupuncture Therapy in Patients with Treatment-Resistant Temporomandibular Disorders

Wen-Long Hu[1,2,3*§], Chih-Hao Chang[3,4§], Yu-Chiang Hung[1,5], Ying-Jung Tseng[1], I-Ling Hung[1], Sheng-Feng Hsu[6,7]

1 Department of Chinese Medicine, Kaohsiung Chang Gung Memorial Hospital and Chang Gung University College of Medicine, Kaohsiung, Taiwan, **2** Kaohsiung Medical University College of Medicine, Kaohsiung, Taiwan, **3** Fooyin University College of Nursing, Kaohsiung, Taiwan, **4** Division of Chinese Medicine, Kaohsiung Municipal Chinese Medical Hospital, Kaohsiung, Taiwan, **5** School of Chinese Medicine for Post Baccalaureate, I-Shou University, Kaohsiung, Taiwan, **6** Graduate Institute of Acupuncture Science, China Medical University, Taichung, Taiwan, **7** Department of Chinese Medicine, China Medical University Hospital, Taipei Branch, Taipei, Taiwan

Abstract

Objective: To investigate the clinical effects of laser acupuncture therapy for temporomandibular disorders (TMD) after ineffective previous treatments.

Methods: A retrospective observational study was conducted in 29 treatment-resistant TMD patients (25 women, 4 men; age range, 17–67 years). Subjects were treated 3 times per week for 4 weeks with the Handylaser Trion (GaAlAs laser diode, 810 nm, 150 mW, pulsed waves), which delivered 0.375 J of energy (5 s) to ST7, ST6, and LI4 and 3 J (40 s) to each Ashi point, 7.5–26.25 J/cm^2 in total. The visual analog scale (VAS) and maximal mouth opening (MMO) were evaluated before and after treatment.

Results: VAS analysis showed that the patients were free of pain at rest (endpoint) after 5.90±6.08 sessions of laser acupuncture for acute TMD and after 16.21±17.98 sessions for chronic TMD. The VAS score on palpation of the temporomandibular joint reduced to 0.30±0.67 for patients with acute TMD ($p=0.005$) and to 0.47±0.84 for those with chronic TMD ($p<0.001$). The MMO significantly increased in patients with acute TMD (7.80±5.43 mm, $p=0.008$) and in patients with chronic TMD (15.58±7.87 mm, $p<0.001$).

Conclusions: Our study shows that laser acupuncture therapy improves the symptoms of treatment-resistant TMD. Further studies with a more appropriate design, involving long-term follow-up examinations in a larger patient sample, are needed to evaluate its efficacy.

Editor: Jan P. A. Baak, Stavanger University Hospital, Norway

Funding: These authors have no support or funding to report.

Competing Interests: The authors have declared that no competing interests exist.

* Email: oolonghu@gmail.com

§ These authors contributed equally to this work.

Introduction

Temporomandibular disorder (TMD) is a collective term traditionally used to describe multiple disorders, including intracapsular disorders, true abnormalities of the temporomandibular joint (TMJ), and muscular disorders or myofascial pain dysfunction (MPD) syndrome [1]. TMD is a major cause of nondental pain in the orofacial region. In the adult non-patient population, approximately 33% reported at least one TMD symptom, and clinical findings revealed at least one TMD sign in 40%–75% of the population [2]. It can be a very painful condition, leading to significant deterioration in the patient's quality of life. The primary symptoms associated with TMD include facial muscle pain, preauricular (TMJ) pain, TMJ sounds (jaw clicking, popping, catching, and locking), limited mouth opening, and increased pain associated with chewing. The secondary symptoms are earache, headache, and neck ache [3]. Bruxism, teeth clenching, and chronic gum chewing are important factors influencing the production of pain in the masseter and temporalis muscles. Arthritis and degenerative changes in the TMJ, loss of teeth, ill-fitting dentures or lack of dentures, and other dental conditions can lead to TMD or MPD, which manifest as facial and masticatory muscle pain [4].

The roles of electrophysical modalities and surgery in the management of TMD have not been fully elucidated [5]. Initial conservative therapy is based on 3 general approaches: patient education, pharmacologic therapy, and physical therapy. However, patients with chronic TMD usually need a multidisciplinary approach involving a team of therapists, including a dentist, psychologist, physical therapist, and even a chronic pain physician [3].

Among the therapeutic procedures, low-level laser therapy (LLLT) has recently been proposed to reduce pain intensity and improve maximal mouth opening (MMO) in both acute and

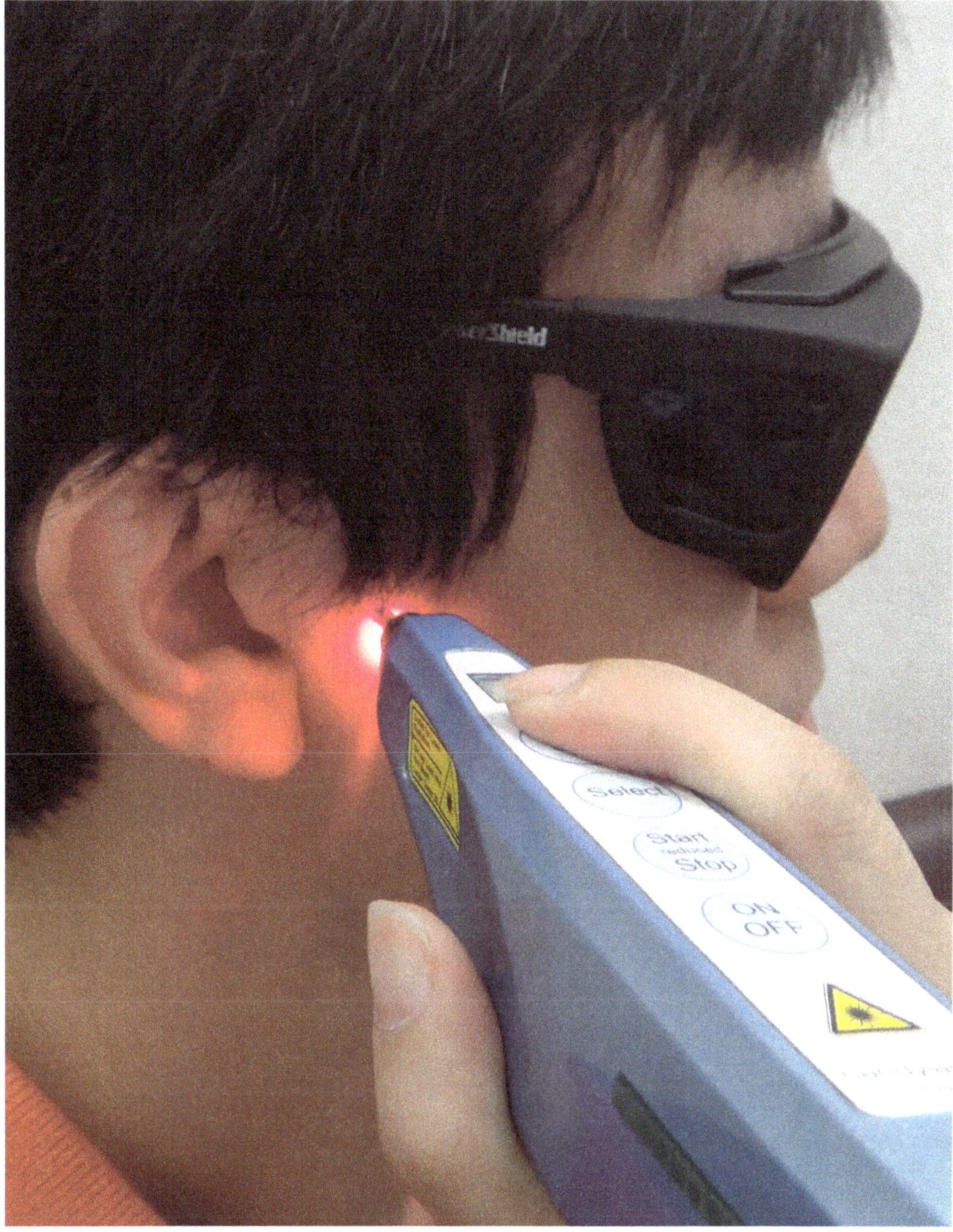

Figure 1. Laser acupuncture performed using the Handylaser Trion at ST7.

chronic TMD patients who had received no previous TMD treatment (e.g., surgical treatment, occlusal splint, or LLLT) [6]. A systematic review reported that LLLT is probably more effective for the treatment of TMJ disorders, and less effective for the treatment of masticatory muscle disorders [7]. One systematic review and meta-analysis showed that there is limited evidence for symptomatic treatment of TMD with acupuncture [8]. Another study suggested that acupuncture is a reasonable adjunctive treatment for producing a short-term analgesic effect in patients with painful TMD symptoms [9]. Furthermore, laser acupuncture therapy (LAT) has been proposed as an effective treatment modality because it alleviates the chronic pain associated with TMD without any previous treatment [10]. However, the effect of LAT on TMD symptoms in patients in whom previous treatments were unsuccessful has not been investigated. Therefore, in this study, we investigated the effect of LAT in such patients.

Materials and Methods

Patients

The study was approved by the Human Ethics Committee of our hospital (Chang Gung Medical Foundation Institutional Review Board, Permit No 102-1932B). This is a retrospective observational study in general practice. The patient's verbal

Table 1. The set parameters of the Handylaser Trion used to perform laser acupuncture in this study.

Laser medium	GaAlAs laser diode
Wavelength	810 nm
Output power - maximum	150 mW
Probe aperture	0.03 cm^2
Power density	5 W/cm^2
Time	5 s/acupuncture point; 40 s/Ashi point
Frequencies	Bahr (B1: 599.5 Hz, B2: 1199 Hz, B3: 2398 Hz, B4: 4796 Hz, B5: 9592 Hz, B6: 19184 Hz, B7: 38360 Hz) Nogier (NA′: 292 Hz, NB′: 584 Hz, NC′: 1168 Hz, ND′: 2336 Hz, NE′: 4672 Hz, NF′: 9344 Hz, NG′: 18688 Hz)
Type of application	Contact
Treatment dose	7.5–26.25 J/cm^2 in total

informed consent for treatment was recorded on the medical chart. Our ethics committee approved the verbal consent procedure. Furthermore, the individual in this manuscript (Figure 1) has given written informed consent to publish these case details. Patients who visited our outpatient acupuncture clinic between January 2009 and December 2011 were recruited for this study. In total, 25 women and 4 men (age range, 17–67 years; mean ± standard deviation, 42.48±14.77) with treatment-resistant TMD were enrolled. They were diagnosed with TMD (cardinal signs: limitation of jaw opening or function, pain with jaw opening or function, and joint sounds [11]) and treated by dentists, and referred to us because of unsuccessful previous treatments such as advice and counseling regarding their diet, cold/hot packs, administration or topical use of nonsteroidal anti-inflammatory drugs, and/or an occlusal appliance. Seven patients had bilateral TMD, and the rest had unilateral TMD. The duration of symptoms from the onset of disease ranged 1–144 months (17.45±31.64). In 10 patients, the symptoms lasted for <6 months (acute TMD), and in the remaining patients, they lasted for ≥6 months (chronic TMD) [12]. Patients were instructed not to resort to self-medication.

Laser acupuncture therapy

The patients were treated 3 times per week for 4 weeks (recommendation based on clinical experience; treatment could be extended if necessary) with the Handylaser Trion (Table 1, RJ-Laser, Germany) by an experienced physician (acupuncture specialist with total acupuncture experience of 25 years). Protective goggles were used by both the operator and the patient to inhibit visual perception during LAT. The laser was used to deliver 0.375 J of energy in pulsed waves to each of the following traditional acupoints for 5 s sequentially: ST7 (Xiaguan, B2: 1199 Hz) (Figure 1), ST6 (Jiache, B2: 1199 Hz), and LI4 (Hegu, B3: 2398 Hz). In addition, the laser was applied to the Ashi points on and near the TMJs and/or masseter muscles (2–4 points) for 40 s each, delivering 3 J of energy in pulsed wave (NC′: 1168 Hz), 7.5–26.25 J/cm^2 in total.

Outcome measures and data analysis

A 10-cm visual analog scale (0–10 points, least to greatest pain intensity, VAS) was used to measure the pain intensity at rest (spontaneous, VASS) and upon digital palpation (0.5 kg of pressure [13] applied by Dr. WLH) of the TMJ (VASP). To measure MMO, patients were asked to open their mouths as wide as possible without assistance. The interincisal distance in mm was recorded using a ruler. SPSS Statistics 17.0 (SPSS Inc., Chicago, USA) was used to analyze the data. The Wilcoxon signed-rank test was used to compare the VAS and MMO results before treatment with those obtained after LAT. All p-values were 2-tailed, and the alpha level of significance was set at 0.05.

Results

After 12.66±15.64 therapeutic sessions, the patients experienced pain relief and improvement in MMO. After 5.90±6.08 therapeutic sessions, the acute TMD patients reported that they were free of pain at rest (endpoint); in contrast, chronic TMD patients required 16.21±17.98 therapeutic sessions before they could report a similar outcome (Table 2). After 8.73±7.44 therapeutic sessions, the patients without disc displacement reported that they were free of pain at rest; in contrast, the patients with disc displacement required 15.06±18.82 therapeutic sessions before they could report a similar outcome. No negative side effects were reported during or after LAT.

Reduction in pain intensity

Before treatment, all 29 patients reported a VASS score of 6.24±1.52, and VASP score of 7.45±0.94. The mean VASS score before LAT was 5.70±1.62 for acute TMD patients and 6.53±1.43 for chronic TMD patients. The mean VASP score before LAT was 7.10±0.97 for acute TMD patients and 7.63±0.90 for chronic TMD patients.

After treatment, all 29 patients reported no pain at rest (Wilcoxon test, z = −4.828, $p<0.001$), and a VASP score of 0.41±0.78 upon palpation of the TMJ (Wilcoxon test, z = −4.753, $p<0.001$). The mean VASP score was 0.30±0.67 for acute TMD patients (Wilcoxon test, z = −2.831, $p = 0.005$) and 0.47±0.84 for chronic TMD patients (Wilcoxon test, z = −3.868, $p<0.001$; Table 3).

Improvement in maximal mouth opening

Before treatment, the MMO for all 29 patients with treatment-resistant TMD was 26.90±8.96 mm. The MMO for patients with acute TMD was 32.90±6.79 mm, whereas the MMO for patients with chronic TMD was 23.74±8.44 mm.

After treatment, the MMO for all 29 patients with treatment-resistant TMD was 39.79±2.47 mm (Wilcoxon test, z = −4.628, $p<0.001$). The MMO for patients with acute TMD was 40.70±2.67 mm (Wilcoxon test, z = −2.668, $p = 0.008$), whereas the MMO for patients with chronic TMD was 39.32±2.29 mm (Wilcoxon test, z = −3.833, $p<0.001$; Table 3).

Table 2. Patient demographics before and after LAT.

No.	Gender	Age	Site	Course (M)	VASSB	VASSA	VASPB	VASPA	MMOB	MMOA	Sessions	Disc displacement
1	M	45	R	1	4.5	0.0	6.5	0.0	40.0	41.0	1	None
2	F	26	L	1	4.0	0.0	6.0	0.0	38.0	45.0	3	R
3	F	57	R	1	4.0	0.0	6.0	0.0	32.0	42.0	14	R
4	F	48	R	1	7.0	0.0	8.0	0.0	32.0	43.0	18	None
5	F	54	L	1	7.0	0.0	8.0	0.0	33.0	42.0	6	None
6	F	58	R	1	4.5	0.0	6.5	0.0	34.0	40.0	1	R
7	F	42	L	1	8.0	0.0	8.0	2.0	39.0	39.0	10	R
8	F	39	R	2	7.0	0.0	8.0	0.0	30.0	40.0	2	None
9	M	23	B	3	4.0	0.0	6.0	0.0	35.0	40.0	1	None
10	M	58	R	4	7.0	0.0	8.0	1.0	16.0	35.0	3	None
11	M	58	L	6	9.0	0.0	9.0	0.0	16.0	38.0	72	NR
12	F	44	B	6	4.0	0.0	6.0	0.0	30.0	41.0	54	R
13	F	40	R	6	4.0	0.0	6.0	0.0	30.0	40.0	2	R
14	F	40	B	6	7.0	0.0	8.0	2.0	16.0	34.0	6	NR
15	F	26	R	6	7.0	0.0	8.0	0.0	16.0	42.0	19	NR
16	F	17	L	6	4.0	0.0	6.0	0.0	32.0	36.0	19	R
17	F	58	L	6	7.0	0.0	8.0	0.0	32.0	42.0	20	None
18	F	23	B	10	7.0	0.0	8.0	1.0	35.0	39.0	1	R
19	F	62	B	12	7.0	0.0	8.0	1.0	16.0	38.0	4	NR
20	F	39	L	12	7.0	0.0	8.0	0.0	33.0	41.0	6	None
21	F	38	R	12	7.0	0.0	8.0	3.0	16.0	40.0	13	NR
22	F	17	L	12	7.0	0.0	8.0	0.0	16.0	40.0	16	NR
23	F	21	L	12	7.0	0.0	8.0	0.0	16.0	40.0	19	NR
24	F	54	B	18	7.0	0.0	8.0	0.0	33.0	41.0	6	None
25	F	29	L	24	7.0	0.0	8.0	1.0	16.0	35.0	4	R
26	F	45	R	36	4.0	0.0	6.0	0.0	33.0	41.0	4	R
27	F	43	R	60	7.0	0.0	8.0	1.0	16.0	38.0	10	NR
28	F	61	L	96	8.0	0.0	8.0	0.0	16.0	40.0	16	None
29	F	67	B	144	7.0	0.0	8.0	0.0	33.0	41.0	17	None

LAT: laser acupuncture therapy; MMOA: Maximal mouth opening after LAT; MMOB: Maximal mouth opening before LAT; NR: without reduction; R: with reduction; VASPA: Visual analog scale upon palpation after LAT; VASPB: Visual analog scale upon palpation before LAT; VASSA: Visual analog scale, spontaneous (at rest), after LAT; VASSB: Visual analog scale, spontaneous (at rest), before LAT.

Table 3. Effect of LAT on treatment-resistant TMD.

Variable	VASS	VASP	MMO
Total, *n* = 29			
Before LAT	6.24±1.52	7.45±0.94	26.90±8.96
After LAT	0	0.41±0.78	39.79±2.47
A–B	−6.24±1.52	−7.10±1.04	12.90±7.97
Z	−4.828	−4.753	−4.628
P value	0.000	0.000	0.000
Acute TMD, *n* = 10			
Before LAT	5.70±1.62	7.10±0.97	32.90±6.79
After LAT	0	0.30±0.67	40.70±2.67
A–B	−5.70±1.62	−6.80±0.89	7.80±5.43
Z	−2.831	−2.831	−2.668
P value	0.005	0.005	0.008
Chronic TMD, *n* = 19			
Before LAT	6.53±1.43	7.63±0.90	23.74±8.44
After LAT	0	0.47±0.84	39.32±2.29
A–B	−6.53±1.43	−7.26±1.10	15.58±7.87
Z	−3.976	−3.868	−3.833
P value	0.000	0.000	0.000

Wilcoxon signed-rank test; A–B: after–before LAT; LAT: laser acupuncture therapy; MMO: Maximal mouth opening; TMD: temporomandibular disorder; VASP: Visual analog scale upon palpation; VASS: Visual analog scale, spontaneous (at rest).

Discussion

The suppression of cortical responses and brainstem reflexes is elicited by a predominantly nociceptive input in TMD patients, which suggests that chronic craniofacial pain in TMD patients may be associated with dysfunction of the trigeminal nociceptive system [14]. Increased pain intensity in patients with MPD-TMD at rest has been associated with increased gray matter in the rostral anterior cingulate cortex and posterior cingulate. In the same study, pain intensity with palpation was associated with decreased gray matter in the pons, corresponding to the trigeminal sensory nuclei. Longer pain duration was associated with greater gray matter in the posterior cingulate, hippocampus, midbrain, and cerebellum. The pattern of gray matter abnormalities found in MPD-TMD individuals suggests the involvement of trigeminal and limbic system dysregulation, as well as potential somatotopic reorganization in the putamen, thalamus, and somatosensory cortex [15].

According to the theory of traditional Chinese medicine (TCM), pain results from blood stasis due to *qi* stagnation (a pathological change in which a long-standing or severe stagnation of *qi* impedes blood flow, a condition characterized by the coexistence of *qi* stagnation and blood stasis) [16,17]. We selected the acupoints on both Yangming meridians based on the principle of "places where meridian passed, treatments thereby can be reached" [18]. According to Manfred Reininger et al., frequencies can be applied to acupuncture points to improve the meridian energy [19]. The ST7 (B2: 1199 Hz used for central tissue layer), ST6 (B2: 1199 Hz), and LI4 (B3: 2398 Hz used for surface tissue structures [20]) points are involved in freeing the meridians and collaterals, and moving *qi* to relieve pain. The combined use of these acupoints is therefore effective in activating blood and moving *qi*, anti-inflammation, and analgesia. In addition to stimulating Ashi points (NC′: 1168 Hz used for circulation, energy transfer, and locomotor disorders [20]) on and near the TMJ and/or masseter muscle, the flow of *qi* and blood in the body is realigned to restore internal homeostasis and resolve the symptoms of disease.

LAT is a noninvasive technique involving the stimulation of traditional acupoints, with low-intensity, non-thermal laser irradiation. The clinical application of LAT is widespread, although its mechanism is not well understood. LLLT has biologic effects, such as increased pain tolerance, due to changes in the potency of the cellular membrane; vasodilatation; reduction of edema; increase in intracellular metabolism; and acceleration of wound healing [21]. The biomodulatory effect of LLLT improves local microcirculation and oxygen supply to hypoxic cells in the painful areas. Simultaneously, tissue asphyxia is reduced to a minimum and collected waste products are removed. The laser-induced normalization of microcirculation interrupts the vicious cycle that originates, develops, and maintains pain; in addition, it restores the normal physiological condition of the tissue [22,23]. Research has shown that LLLT can modulate inflammation by reducing the levels of biochemical markers (prostaglandin E2, messenger ribonucleic acid cyclooxygenase-2, interleukine-1β, and tumor necrotizing factor-α), neutrophil influx, oxidative stress, edema, and hemorrhage in a dose-dependent manner [24].

Analgesia induced by LLLT is mediated by peripheral opioid receptors [25]. Laser acupuncture is a modality resulting from scientific exploration of TCM [10]. Acupuncture has both local and distant analgesic effects that may be mediated by different mechanisms. Various central opioid receptors are important in mediating the analgesic effect induced by acupuncture-related techniques of different frequencies [26]. In comparison with needle-based acupuncture for achieving *qi*, LAT is not associated with somatosensation and has the advantage of being noninvasive and aseptic. Moreover, LAT is painless and safe because no heat is generated during the procedure. It is also more effective and requires less time than needle-based acupuncture [19,27].

Although Melis et al. hypothesized that when structural or functional problems are present (for example, a displaced disc), the effects of the laser beam cannot sufficiently alleviate the symptoms until the main cause is addressed [7]. Our patients with disc displacement reported that they were free of pain at rest after 15.06±18.82 therapeutic sessions. LAT might act on the synovia and stimulate cellular energy processes [28]. The results of our study are similar to those of Ferreira et al.'s study [10], in which equivalent methodology was used. Furthermore, no side effects or complications resulting from LAT were observed in our study.

TMDs occur disproportionately in women of childbearing age in a female to male ratio of between 4:1 and 6:1; the prevalence decreases significantly in men and women above 55 years of age [11]. We also noted this disproportion in our treatment-resistant TMD patients. In this study, although most patients reported a drastic reduction in pain intensity after LAT, 2 patients with acute TMD reported a VASP score of 1–2 after treatment, and 6 patients with chronic TMD reported a VASP score of 1–3. With regard to the etiological multifactorial aspects of TMD, LR3 (Taichong) might be used in combination with LI4 to alleviate conditions of stress, depression, and anxiety, as well as pain, by promoting the free flow of energy and emotions [10]. Tunér and Hode [29] reported that there is a methodological association with local laser action in clinical practice and in some studies involving LAT. It is known that the laser in the irradiated region is also capable of promoting punctiform analgesia, particularly when the equipment is specifically adjusted [30]. Future studies are needed to verify the effect of the local laser beyond the acupoints, the selection of the acupoints; treatment intervals; therapeutic sessions; and optimal laser parameters, including wavelength, dose, and intensity, necessary to maximize the physiological benefit and cost effectiveness of LAT for treatment-resistant TMD.

Conclusions

We found that TMD symptoms improved with LAT. Given the relative scarcity of research on this topic, long-term follow-up of these cases and further studies with a larger patient sample and an appropriate design are needed to elucidate the efficacy of LAT in treatment-resistant TMD patients.

Author Contributions

Conceived and designed the experiments: WLH CHC. Performed the experiments: WLH YJT ILH. Analyzed the data: WLH CHC YCH. Contributed reagents/materials/analysis tools: WLH CHC YCH. Wrote the paper: WLH CHC. Critically review and revise the manuscript: SFH.

References

1. Rotter BE (2010) Temporomandibular Joint Disorders. In: Flint WP, Haughe BH, Lund VJ, et al., editors. Cummings Otolaryngology: Head & Neck Surgery, 5th ed., Missouri: Mosby. pp. 1279–1286.
2. De Leeuw R (2008) The American Academy of Orofacial Pain. Orofacial pain. Guidelines for assessment, diagnosis, and management, 4th ed., Chicago: Quintessence. pp.129–204.
3. Okeson JP (2012) Temporomandibular Disorders in Chapter 5 - Diseases of the Head and Neck. In: Bope ET, Kellerman RD, editors. Conn's Current Therapy 2013, 1st ed., Pennsylvania: Saunders. pp. 320–323.
4. Garza I, Swanson JW, Cheshire WP Jr, Boes CJ, Capobianco DJ, et al. (2012) Headache and Other Craniofacial Pain. In: Daroff RB, Fenichel GM, Jankovic J, Mazziotta JC, editors. Bradley's Neurology in Clinical Practice, 6th ed., Pennsylvania: Saunders. pp. 1714.
5. Emshoff R, Bösch R, Pümpel E, Schöning H, Strobl H (2008) Low-level laser therapy for treatment of temporomandibular joint pain: a double-blind and placebo-controlled trial. Oral Surg Oral Med Oral Pathol Oral Radiol Endod 105: 452–6.
6. Salmos-Brito JA, De Menezes RF, Teixeira CE, Gonzaga RK, Rodrigues BH, et al. (2013) Evaluation of low-level laser therapy in patients with acute and chronic temporomandibular disorders. Lasers Med Sci 28: 57–64.
7. Melis M, Di Giosia M, Zawawi KH (2012) Low level laser therapy for the treatment of temporomandibular disorders: a systematic review of the literature. Cranio 30: 304–12.
8. Junga A, Shin BC, Lee MS, Sim H, Ernst E (2011) Acupuncture for treating temporomandibular joint disorders: A systematic review and meta-analysis of randomized, sham-controlled trials. J Dent 39: 341–50.
9. La Touche R, Goddard G, De-la-Hoz JL, Wang K, Paris-Alemany A, et al. (2010) Acupuncture in the treatment of pain in temporomandibular disorders: a systematic review and meta-analysis of randomized controlled trials. Clin J Pain 26: 541–50.
10. Ferreira LA, De Oliveira RG, Guimarães JP, Carvalho AC, De Paula MV (2013) Laser acupuncture in patients with temporomandibular dysfunction: a randomized controlled trial. Lasers Med Sci 28: 1549–58.
11. Dym H, Israel H (2012) Diagnosis and Treatment of Temporomandibular Disorders. Dent Clin N Am 56: 149–61.
12. Merskey H, Bogduk N (1994) Classification of Chronic Pain, Second Edition, IASP Task Force on Taxonomy, Seattle: IASP Press.
13. Ohrbach R, Gonzalez Y, List T, Michelotti A, Schiffman E (2013) Diagnostic Criteria for Temporomandibular Disorders (DC/TMD) Clinical Examination Protocol. Form Version: May 12, 2013, http://www.rdc-tmdinternational.org/Portals/18/protocol_DC-TMD/DC-TMD_examform_international_2013-05-12.pdf. Accessed 2014 Jun 10.
14. Romaniello A, Cruccu G, Frisardi G, Svensson P (2003) Assessment of nociceptive trigeminal pathways by laser-evoked potentials and laser silent periods in patients with painful temporomandibular disorders. Pain 103: 31–9.
15. Younger JW, Shen YF, Goddard G, Mackey SC (2010) Chronic myofascial temporomandibular pain is associated with neural abnormalities in the trigeminal and limbic systems. Pain 149: 222–8.
16. Shi DB (2002) The encyclopedia of traditional Chinese medicine [e-book in Chinese]. Version 1.0 for PC. Taipei: Yuan-Liou.
17. World Health Organization Regional Office for the Western Pacific (WPRO) (2007) WHO International Standard Terminologies on Traditional Medicine in the Western Pacific Region. Manila: WPRO. pp. 56.
18. Hu WL, Hung YC, Chang CH (2011) Acupuncture for Disorders of Consciousness - A Case Series and Review. In: Saad M. Acupuncture - Clinical Practice, Particular Techniques and Special Issues, Rijeka: InTech. pp. 3–28.
19. Hu WL, Hung YC, Hung IL (2013) Explore Laser Acupuncture's Role. In: Chen LL, Cheng TO, editors. Acupuncture in Modern Medicine, Rijeka: InTech. pp. 205–20.
20. REIMERS & JANSSEN GmbH (2008) RJ- LASER-THERAPY, pp. 26 & 32. http://s3.amazonaws.com/zanran_storage/www.rj-laser.com/ContentPages/44313265.pdf. Accessed 2014 June 10.
21. Wilder-Smith P (1988) The soft laser: therapeutic tool or popular placebo? Oral Surg Oral Med Oral Pathol 66: 654–8.
22. Simunovic Z (1996) Low level laser therapy with trigger points technique: a clinical study on 243 patients. J Clin Laser Med Surg 14: 163–7.
23. Sandoval MC, Mattiello-Rosa SM, Soares EG, Parizotto NA (2009) Effects of laser on the synovial fluid in the inflammatory process of the knee joint of the rabbit. Photomed Laser Surg 27: 63–9.
24. Bjordal JM, Johnson MI, Iversen V, Aimbire F, Lopes-Martins RA (2006) Photoradiation in acute pain: a systematic review of possible mechanisms of action and clinical effects in randomized placebo-controlled trials. Photomed Laser Surg 24: 158–68.
25. Peres e Serra A, Ashmawi HA (2010) Influence of naloxone and methysergide on the analgesic effects of low-level laser in an experimental pain model. Rev Bras Anestesiol 60: 302–10.
26. Han JS (2011) Acupuncture analgesia: areas of consensus and controversy. Pain 152: S41–8.
27. Hu WL, Chang CH, Hung YC (2010) Clinical Observations on Laser Acupuncture in Simple Obesity Therapy. Am J Chin Med 38: 861–7.
28. Marini I, Gatto MR, Bonetti GA (2010) Effects of superpulsed low-level laser therapy on temporomandibular joint pain. Clin J Pain 26: 611–6.
29. Tunér J, Hode L (2010) The difficult dose and intensity. In: Tunér J, Hode L (eds) The new laser therapy handbook. Grängsberg: Prima Books, 505–26.
30. Shen X, Zhao L, Ding G, Tan M, Gao J, Wang L, et al. (2009) Effect of combined laser acupuncture on knee osteoarthritis: a pilot study. Lasers Med Sci 24: 129–36.

Prolonged Repeated Acupuncture Stimulation Induces Habituation Effects in Pain-Related Brain Areas: An fMRI Study

Chuanfu Li[1], Jun Yang[2]*, Kyungmo Park[3], Hongli Wu[4], Sheng Hu[5], Wei Zhang[1], Junjie Bu[6], Chunsheng Xu[1], Bensheng Qiu[5], Xiaochu Zhang[6]*

1 Laboratory of Digital Medical Imaging, Medical Imaging Center, First Affiliated Hospital, Anhui University of Chinese Medicine, Hefei, Anhui, China, **2** Department of Acupuncture and Moxibustion, First Affiliated Hospital of Anhui University of Chinese Medicine, Hefei, Anhui, China, **3** Department of Biomedical Engineering, Kyung Hee University, Yongin, Republic of Korea, **4** College of Medical Information engineering, Anhui University of Chinese Medicine, Hefei, Anhui, China, **5** School of Information Science and Technology, University of Science and Technology of China, Hefei, Anhui, China, **6** CAS Key Laboratory of Brain Function & Disease and School of Life Sciences, University of Science and Technology of China, Hefei, Anhui, China

Abstract

Most previous studies of brain responses to acupuncture were designed to investigate the acupuncture instant effect while the cumulative effect that should be more important in clinical practice has seldom been discussed. In this study, the neural basis of the acupuncture cumulative effect was analyzed. For this experiment, forty healthy volunteers were recruited, in which more than 40 minutes of repeated acupuncture stimulation was implemented at acupoint *Zhusanli* (ST36). Three runs of acupuncture fMRI datasets were acquired, with each run consisting of two blocks of acupuncture stimulation. Besides general linear model (GLM) analysis, the cumulative effects of acupuncture were analyzed with analysis of covariance (ANCOVA) to find the association between the brain response and the cumulative duration of acupuncture stimulation in each stimulation block. The experimental results showed that the brain response in the initial stage was the strongest although the brain response to acupuncture was time-variant. In particular, the brain areas that were activated in the first block and the brain areas that demonstrated cumulative effects in the course of repeated acupuncture stimulation overlapped in the pain-related areas, including the bilateral middle cingulate cortex, the bilateral paracentral lobule, the SII, and the right thalamus. Furthermore, the cumulative effects demonstrated bimodal characteristics, i.e. the brain response was positive at the beginning, and became negative at the end. It was suggested that the cumulative effect of repeated acupuncture stimulation was consistent with the characteristic of habituation effects. This finding may explain the neurophysiologic mechanism underlying acupuncture analgesia.

Editor: Jie Tian, Institute of Automation, Chinese Academy of Sciences, China

Funding: This study was supported by grants from Anhui Provincial Natural Science Foundation under Grant No. 1208085MH147 (http://220.178.98.52/zrkxjj/), Major Scientific Projects of Anhui Provincial Education Commission under Grant No. KJ2011ZD05 (http://www.ahsr.edu.cn/srmis/), the National Natural Science Foundation of China under Grant No. 81202768, 31171083, 31230032 (http://www.nsfc.gov.cn/Portal0/default152.htm), and the National Key Basic Research and Development Program (973) under Grant No. 2010CB530500 (http://www.973.gov.cn/Default_3.aspx). The funders had no role in study design, data collection and analysis, decision to publish, or preparation of the manuscript.

Competing Interests: The authors have declared that no competing interests exist.

* E-mail: yangzyun@aliyun.com (JY); zxcustc@ustc.edu.cn (XZ)

Introduction

Acupuncture, an ancient healing technique that originated in China, is used by millions of patients in many countries [1]. Continuous use of acupuncture in East Asia and more recently throughout the world has led to the assumption that acupuncture is a relatively effective and safe procedure. However, with the call for evidence based medicine, acupuncture has been tested at the forges of modern medicine [2]. Understanding the physiologic basis of acupuncture is critical to producing reliable results. Proposing and testing ideas about the underlying mechanisms of acupuncture could eventually lead to a real understanding about how acupuncture does work [3]. However, for the present it remains to be seen whether we are dealing with a specific physiological response of the brain to acupuncture, or with non-specific reactions to an undifferentiated stimulus [1]. In recent 20 years, fMRI studies have been extensively conducted to investigate the neurophysiologic mechanism of acupuncture. Although it is generally agreed that the brain and nervous system play a leading role in processing acupuncture stimuli [4,5], the specific mechanism underlying the therapeutic effects of acupuncture is still under debate. Some researchers [5–10] proposed that the deactivation of the limbic-paralimbic-neocortical system was crucial to producing acupuncture's therapeutic effects while some others [11] argued that these deactivations did not occur reliably and suggested that brain responses to acupuncture were activation-dominated.

To investigate reasons for the varying results of the previous studies, some influencing factors, including expectation [12], acupuncture sensation [13,14], methodology [15,16], pathological status [17], and time-variant characteristics [18,19], were studied. Among them, acupuncture time-variant characteristics should be one of the most important factors based on the following facts. First, the stimulation duration and paradigm in different studies varied; some studies had only one run of acupuncture stimulation for several minutes [20–28] while other studies had several runs of stimulation lasting nearly half an hour or longer [6,8,9,29–31]. The varied duration and paradigm might lead to the different findings of these acupuncture fMRI studies. Secondly, it is generally accepted in clinical practice that the acupuncture treatment ought to be longer than a few minutes in length and repeated [4,18,19,32,33]. The cumulative effects of prolonged, repeated acupuncture stimulations in the brain may differ from the instant effects of acupuncture stimulation, and the time-variant characteristics of acupuncture stimulation, which was engaged in differential temporal neural responses in a wide range of brain networks [34], might be the fundamental reason of cumulative effects.

Because of these reasons, prolonged acupuncture stimulation was suggested [4,19,32] in order to investigate the cumulative effects of typical clinical application of acupuncture. However, some of questions still remained. What the acupuncture cumulative effect could be? Is it the brain activations or deactivations of some specific brain areas or some natural neurophysiologic process? For the present it remains to be seen whether we are dealing with a specific physiological response of the brain to acupuncture, or with non-specific reactions to an undifferentiated stimulus [1]. Generally speaking, acupuncture is a kind of stimulus [4]. A wide range of experiments on organisms ranging from amoebas to humans demonstrated a natural response of habituation to a variety of external repeated stimulus [35], including the acupuncture stimulation. In 1966, a landmark paper published by Thompson and Spencer [36] clarified the definition of habituation by presenting nine characteristics of habituation. Recently, a group of researchers who study habituation redefined these characteristics based on the 40 years of research adding a new characteristic termed as long-term habituation to the original list of the nine characteristics [37]. Considering the ten characteristics of habituation, we believe that the mechanism of acupuncture analgesia, the most widely accepted and proven application of acupuncture [38], could be reasonably explained through the characteristics of habituation, especially the characteristic of generalization to other stimuli (characteristic #7) and the characteristic of long-term habituation (characteristic #10). Therefore, we hypothesized that the prolonged repeated acupuncture stimulation could produce the habituation effect in the brain response that might be useful for the clinical application of acupuncture.

To validate this hypothesis, we designed an experiment with prolonged, repeated acupuncture stimulations in which three runs of acupuncture fMRI with identical paradigms were performed. Among them, six blocks of acupuncture stimulations were applied with different acupuncture cumulative durations. With the datasets acquired from the three runs of acupuncture stimulation, the cumulative effect of acupuncture stimulation was investigated.

Materials and Methods

1. Subjects

Forty healthy volunteers, 20 males and 20 females ranging in age from 21 to 32 years old, were recruited for this experiment. This study was approved by the Institutional Review Board of the First Affiliated Hospital of Anhui University of Chinese Medicine, and written informed consent was obtained from each participant prior to the experiment. All volunteers were right-handed college students with no history of mental, psychiatric or neurological disorders, drug abuse, or abnormality in brain. Any volunteer who had acupuncture experience in the past three months was excluded.

2. Experiment Procedures

Before the experiment, the subjects were asked not to fall into sleep in the process of experiment, and then they were asked to relax and their ears were plugged with cotton balls to reduce audio stimulations. During the entire scanning process, the subjects were also asked to close their eyes and avoid any psychological activities. At the end of the experiment, the subjects were asked whether or not they had fallen asleep, and then answered questionnaires about the sensations experienced on the stimulated acupoints on the both sides. Sensations including soreness, numbness, fullness, aching, spreading and heaviness were scored in four grades (0 = no sensation felt, 1 = mild, 2 = moderate, and 3 = severe).

All of the fMRI experiments were completed on a 1.5T whole-body MRI scanner (Symphony; Siemens Medical System, Erlangen, Germany) with a standard head coil. The MR imaging sequences included: (1) T2-weighted MRI to exclude any obvious diseases in the brain; (2) first run of fMRI/EPI-BOLD parallel to the AC-PC line with 36 slices that covered the whole brain with TR/TE/FA 4000 ms/30 ms/90°, FOV 192 mm×192 mm, and matrix 64×64, at 150 time points; (3) T1-weighted 2D anatomical MRI with the same slices of the fMRI with TR/TE 500/12 ms, FOV 230 mm×230 mm, slice thickness/interval 3.0 mm/ 0.75 mm, and matrix 192×144; (4) the second run of fMRI with the same parameters of the first run of fMRI; (5) T1-weighted 3D anatomical sagittal images with a total of 176 slices that covered the whole brain using a spoiled gradient echo sequence with TR/TE/FA 2100 mm/3.93 mm/13°, FOV 250 mm×250 mm, slice thickness/spacing 1.0 mm/0.5 mm and matrix 256×256, followed by the third run of fMRI with the same parameters of the first run of fMRI (see **Figure 1A**).

3. Experimental Paradigm and Data Acquisition

Three runs (six blocks) of acupuncture fMRI were performed, with each block lasting 2 minutes. Following the fMRI, two series of 2D and 3D anatomical MRI, which lasted for about 5 minutes and 9 minutes respectively, were interposed into the three runs of acupuncture fMRI (see **Figure 1A**). The acupuncture stimulation lasted more than 40 minutes from the time of the needle-in to the time of needle-out.

4. Acupuncture Manipulation

Before the first run of fMRI, the sterile and disposable acupuncture needles with size of 25 mm×0.30 mm (Suzhou Medical Appliance Factory, China) were inserted into the bilateral acupoints of *Zhusanli* (ST36) at a depth of 15–20 mm. Once the *De-Qi* sensation was elicited, the handles of the needles were connected to an electro-acupuncture machine (Shanghai Huayi Medical Equipment Co., China) at frequency of 2 Hz and intensity of 2 mA. After finishing the third run of fMRI, the needles were disconnected from the electro-acupuncture machine and pulled out from the acupoints. All the operations of acupuncture were performed by a professional acupuncturist.

5. Data Analysis

In order to remove the possible influence of head movement, the data with head movement greater than 1 mm or 1° were excluded. As a result, six cases were excluded in this study. The remaining fMRI data involving 34 subjects (18 females and 16 males, age 25.0±2.3 years old, ranging from 22 to 32 years old)

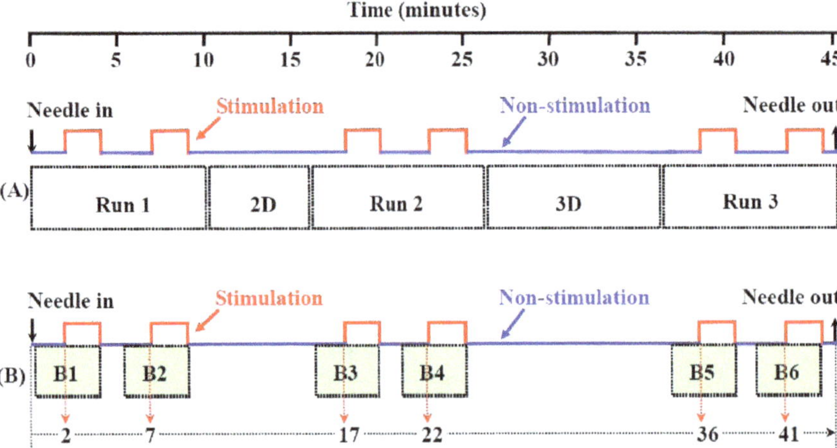

Figure 1. Diagrams of paradigm design and data selection. A: Diagram of paradigm design and data acquisition. From the time of needle-in to the time of needle-out, five series of MRI data were acquired, which were the first run of fMRI (Run 1), 2D anatomical images (2D), the second run of fMRI (Run 2), 3D anatomical images (3D) and the third run of fMRI (Run 3), respectively. Each run of fMRI data acquisition consisted of ten minutes of scan with two blocks of two minutes acupuncture stimulation, and the durations of non-stimulation state were 2 minutes, 3 minutes and 1 minute before, between and after the two blocks of stimulation, respectively. B: Diagram of data selection for each block analysis and definition of covariable of duration. Six blocks of data for block response analysis were B1, B2, B3, B4, B5, and B6, respectively. Each block consisted of two minutes data during stimulation and two minutes data before stimulation (non-stimulation). The covariable of cumulative acupuncture durations, i.e. the time delay from the time of acupuncture needle-in to the beginning of each block of stimulation, were 2, 7, 17, 22, 36 and 41 minutes respectively.

was analyzed using the general linear model (GLM). To be comparable with other previous acupuncture fMRI studies, individual data in each of the three runs were first analyzed with GLM, in which the four time points at the beginning of each run were removed. The group analyses of the first run, the second run, the third run and the three runs in total were performed with *t*-test, respectively.

Considering the possible methodological bias with GLM analysis [18], the individual brain responses to each block were analyzed. The data for the block analysis was extracted from the three runs of fMRI data, which were composed of two minutes of stimulation and two minutes of non-stimulation represented by 30 time points for the stimulation state and non-stimulation state, respectively. After removal of 4 time points at the beginning of the non-stimulation, the data for each block analysis was composed of 26 time points of the non-stimulation state and 30 time points of the stimulation state. After that, acupuncture cumulative effects, which referred to the tendency of acupuncture summed effects that could not be demonstrated in a single block of acupuncture stimulation, were analyzed with analysis of covariance (ANCOVA) to find the correlation between the degree of brain responses and the corresponding cumulative duration of acupuncture (hereafter referred as CDA). The covariance of CDA was defined as the duration from the time of needle-in to the beginning of each of the blocks. Here, the CDAs of the six blocks were 2 minutes, 7 minutes, 17 minutes, 22 minutes, 36 minutes and 41 minutes, respectively (see **Figure 1B**).

The activated or deactivated regions in the brain represented the potentiated or attenuated cumulative effects in the course of the six blocks of repeated acupuncture stimulation. In order to find whether the cumulated areas corresponded with the results of GLM analysis in the first block of acupuncture stimulation, the overlapped brain areas were found with intersection between the activated areas in the first block and the cumulated areas in the course of repeated acupuncture stimulation. Using the overlapped areas as the regions of interest (ROIs), the average and standard error of brain response degree of each ROI in the six blocks were calculated. Then, Pearson correlation coefficients were calculated as a measure of the strength and direction of the linear relationship between the average degree of brain responses and the cumulative duration of the acupuncture stimulation.

Results

Based on self-report, no subjects fell asleep during the experiment. The degrees of *De-qi* sensations such as soreness, numbness, fullness, aching, spreading and heaviness at both sides of acupoints were recorded and presented in **Figure 2**. The brain responses to acupuncture stimulation in the first run, the second run, the third run, and the aggregated runs were quite different (**Figure S1**), and the brain responses to the six blocks of acupuncture stimulation were also extremely varied (**Figure S2**). The brain response in the first block was the strongest. Only positive responses (activations) in the first block were found above the threshold ($P>0.005$, $\alpha = 0.01$, Cluster size = 21, Monte Carlo Method) after multiple comparison correction. These activated areas in the first block included the thalamus, the second somatosensory cortex (SII), the middle cingulate gyrus, the paracentral lobule, the inferior frontal gyrus, the superior frontal gyrus, the precentral gyrus, the precuneus, the inferior parietal lobule, the superior temporal gyrus, the middle temporal gyrus, the fusiform gyrus, and the cerebellum (see **Table 1**, **Figure 3**).

With ANCOVA analysis, the brain responses in the course of repeated acupuncture stimulation showed that cumulative effects in five brain areas were all attenuated and no potentiated cumulative effects were found (**Table 2**). Four of the five attenuated areas, including the bilateral middle cingulate gyrus, the bilateral paracentral lobule, the right SII, and the right thalamus, were overlapped with 35% to 71% of the activated areas in the first block of acupuncture stimulation (**Table 3**, **Figure 3**).

The brain response in the overlapped areas demonstrated an interesting bimodal characteristic of attenuation, i.e. positive brain response appeared in the first block of stimulation, then the brain response began to decrease and it became negative in the last. The

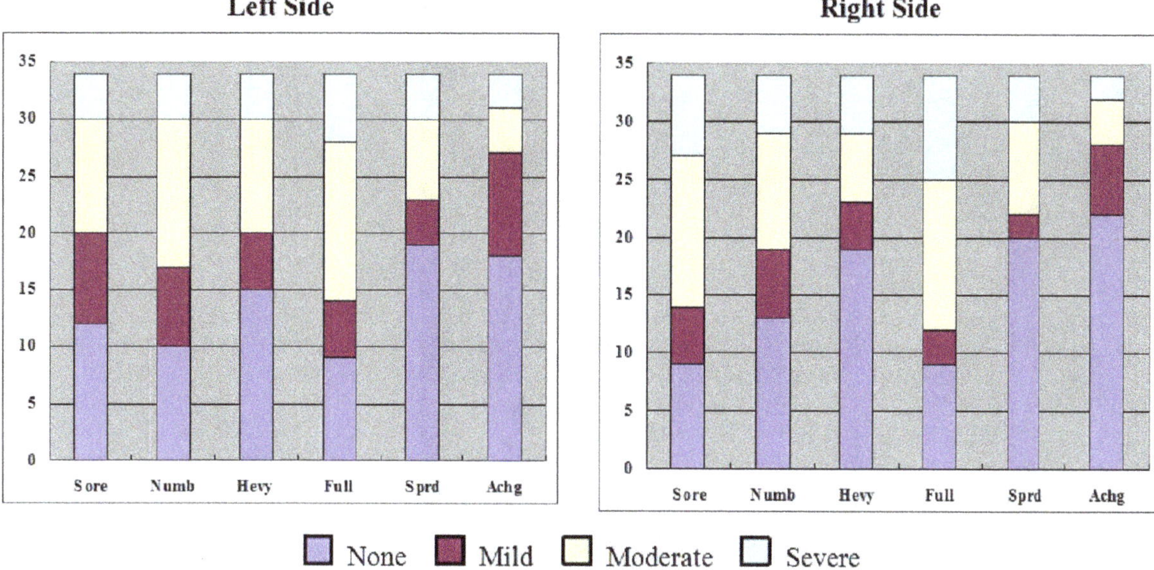

Figure 2. Demonstration of acupuncture sensation composition of different degrees in the both sides of acupoints. The acupuncture sensations were labeled on the x-axis, including soreness (Sore), numbness (Numb), heaviness (Heav), fullness (Full), spreading (Sprd) and aching (Achg). The different degrees of sensations were marked with different colors as shown in the legend. The numbers on the y-axis indicated the cases for each kind of sensation.

coefficients of correlation between the brain response and the CDA of each block ranged from 0.63 to 0.94 (**Figure 4**).

Discussion

Our results demonstrated that the brain responses to acupuncture stimulation were time-variant, in which the brain responses to

Table 1. Activated areas in the first block of acupuncture stimulation.

Regions (BA)	Side	Peak z Value	Coordinate(Talairach)			Volume
			Peak x	Peak y	Peak z	(mm³)
Fusiform Gyrus	R	3.81	−55.5	+61.5	−12.5	3753
Middle Cingulate Gyrus(24)	B	4.21	+4.5	+1.5	+41.5	3591
Middle Temporal Gyrus(37)	L	4.43	+52.5	+55.5	−6.5	3483
Superior Frontal Gyrus(9)	R	4.16	−37.5	−40.5	+32.5	3159
Paracentral Lobule (6)	B	4.69	+1.5	+19.5	+56.5	3105
Cerebellar Tonsil	L	4.17	+22.5	+43.5	−48.5	2916
Precuneus(7)	R	3.99	−1.5	+58.5	+17.5	2727
SII(40)	R	4.34	−61.5	+28.5	+17.5	2376
Cerebellum Lobule VIIb	L	4.05	+7.5	+70.5	−21.5	2241
Inferior Parietal Lobule(40)	L	4.42	+43.5	+52.5	+47.5	1782
Superior Temporal Gyrus(42)	R	3.80	−67.5	+16.5	+8.5	1242
Superior Frontal Gyrus (6)	R	3.54	−19.5	−13.5	+47.5	1107
Inferior Frontal Gyrus (45)	L	3.97	+55.5	−16.5	+5.5	1026
Superior Temporal Gyrus(22)	R	4.41	−58.5	−7.5	+2.5	972
Inferior Frontal Gyrus(45)	R	3.93	−52.5	−13.5	+2.5	864
Precentral Gyrus(4)	L	4.59	+37.5	+22.5	+59.5	864
Precuneus(7)	R	3.61	−22.5	+73.5	+53.5	837
Middle Temporal Gyrus(37)	L	4.08	+46.5	+64.5	+8.5	648
Thalamus	R	3.84	−10.5	+13.5	+14.5	621

Note: BA, Brodmann area; L, left; R, right; B: bilater; SII: secondary somatosensory cortex.

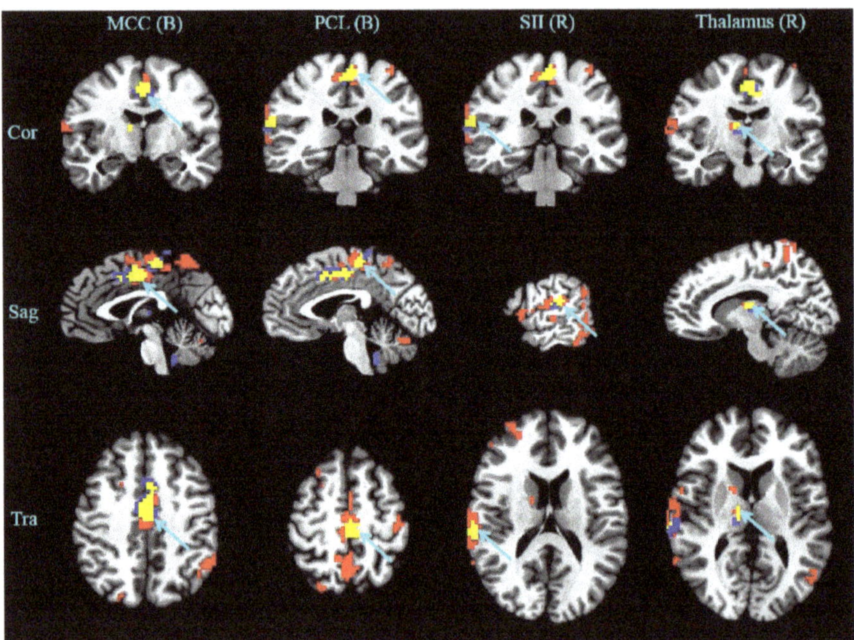

Figure 3. Demonstration of overlapped brain areas (in yellow color) between the activated areas in the first block (in red color) and the habituated areas in the course of six blocks of repeated acupuncture stimulation (in blue color). The threshold was set to $P<=0.005$, $\alpha<=0.01$ (corrected with the Monte Carlo Method). Cor: coronal; Sag: sagittal; Tra: transversal; B: bilateral; R: right; L: left. Overlapped areas included the bilateral middle cingulate cortex (MCC), the bilateral paracentral lobule (PCL), the right SII, and the right thalamus.

the initial stimulation were the strongest. This finding is consistent with the previous acupuncture fMRI studies [18,19]. The most interesting finding in this study was that the prolonged repeated acupuncture stimulation induced habituation effects in some pain-related brain areas. In these areas, acupuncture instant effects in the initial stage demonstrated as extensive brain activations and cumulative effects in the process of repeated acupuncture stimulation demonstrated as an interesting characteristic of bimodal habituation, i.e. positive brain response appeared at the beginning of acupuncture stimulation, and then it declined and became negative in the last.

1. Acupuncture Cumulative Effects and Habituation Effects

In this study, the brain responses to acupuncture stimulation demonstrated time-variant activations or/and deactivations in different runs and blocks, which was consistent with the time-variant characteristics of brain responses to acupuncture [18,19]. In order to reduce the influence of the time-variant characteristic on the results of brain responses and avoid the possible methodological problem with GLM analysis [18], we focused on the analysis of brain responses to each block of acupuncture stimulation in this study. The results demonstrated that acupuncture stimulation at the first block resulted in extensive activations in a wide range of brain areas, but no deactivation above the threshold was found. These activations in this areas, including the thalamus, the SII, the middle cingulate gyrus, the paracentral lobule, the inferior frontal gyrus, the superior frontal gyrus, the precentral gyrus, the precuneus, the inferior parietal lobule, the superior temporal gyrus, the middle temporal gyrus, the fusiform gyrus, and the cerebellum, were consistent with most of the previous acupuncture fMRI studies [39–64].

The results also demonstrated that all of the cumulative effects were attenuated and no potentiated cumulative effects were found. Interestingly, most of the cumulated brain areas (4 of 5) were overlapped with the activated areas in the first block of acupuncture stimulation, including the middle cingulate cortex,

Table 2. Cumulated areas after repeated acupuncture stimulation.

Regions (BA)	Side	Peak z Value	Coordinate(Talairach)			Volume
			Peak x	Peak y	Peak z	(mm^3)
Middle Cingulate Gyrus (24)	B	−4.93	−1.5	4.5	41.5	**3888**
Paracentral Lobule (6)	B	−3.76	−1.5	25.5	50.5	**1593**
SII (40)	R	−3.82	−61.5	25.5	17.5	**1053**
Thalamus	R	−3.79	−10.5	16.5	11.5	**729**
Cerebellar Tonsil	L	−3.80	4.5	43.5	−36.5	**702**

Note: BA, Brodmann area; L, left; R, right; B: bilater; SII: secondary somatosensory cortex.

Table 3. Overlapped areas between the activated areas in the first block and the cumulated areas and their overlapped ratio.

Overlapped areas	Overlapped volume(mm^3)	Activated volume(mm^3)	Habituated volume(mm^3)	Overlapped ratio
Bilateral Middle Cingulate Gyrus (24)	2403	3591	3888	67%
Bilateral Paracentral Lobule (6)	1134	3105	1593	71%
Right SII (40)	540	2376	1053	51%
Right Thalamus	216	621	729	35%

the paracentral lobule, the SII and the thalamus. It suggested that the cumulative effect in these brain areas might reflect some acupuncture related characteristics. In fact, there were some relevant reports about acupuncture that have found consistent results. One report [19] found linearly decreasing time-variant activation in response to both verum and sham acupuncture stimulations in sensorimotor brain regions (SII, posterior insula, premotor cortex) and bimodal time-variant characteristic, i.e. consisting of activation in early blocks, and deactivation by the end of the run, in limbic regions (amygdala, hippocampus, and substantia nigra). Another report [65] showed the similar linearly declined psychophysical response to acupuncture, i.e. the initial acupuncture sensations were the strongest, and then started to drop at 2 minutes and kept decreasing for an hour.

In particular, the results of ROI analysis demonstrated that the brain responses in the overlapped areas were bimodal, i.e. positive response in early stimulation blocks, and negative response in late stimulation blocks. It suggests that the brain response in these areas was a kind of habituation effects. Firstly, this change was consistent with the definition of habituation (characteristic #1), i.e. "given that a particular stimulus elicits a response, repeated applications of the stimulus result in decreased response and the decrease is usually a negative exponential function of the number of stimulus presentations" [35,37]. Secondly, according to the characteristic #6 of habituation [35,37], the effects of habituation training may proceed beyond the zero or asymptotic response level, which implies that the brain response could become below-zero or negative. In a word, the habituation effects demonstrated in the process of prolonged repeated acupuncture stimulation should reflect the acupuncture cumulative effects.

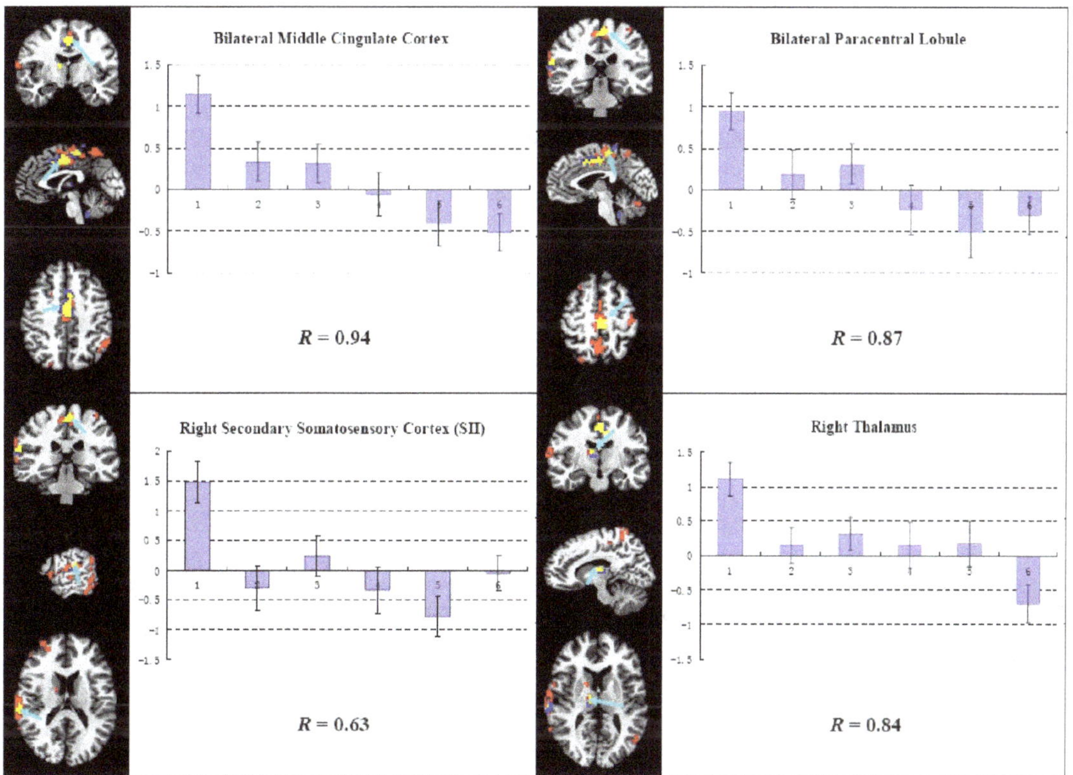

Figure 4. ROIs analysis results of the four overlapped areas between the activated areas in the first block and the habituated areas in the course of repeated acupuncture stimulation. The brain responses to acupuncture stimulation were increasingly decreased as the acupuncture cumulative duration became longer. The characteristic of habitation was bimodal, i.e. positive brain response was found in the first block of acupuncture stimulation, then it began to decrease and brain response became negative in the last (*R*: Pearson's correlation coefficient).

2. Clinical Implication of the Acupuncture Habituation Effects

Acupuncture cumulative effect was considered as an important factor closely associated with clinical efficiency [4]. Therefore, the key point is to find what the acupuncture cumulative effects reflect. Is it potentiated or attenuated? In this study, with ANCOVA analysis, we did not find any potentiated brain response in the course of repeated acupuncture stimulation, but the attenuated brain response or habituation effect was found in the middle cingulate cortex, the paracentral lobule, the second somatosensory cortex, and the thalamus. Among them, the paracentral lobule located in the upper medial part of the precentral gyrus and the postcentral gyrus (**Figure 3**) was composed of primary motor cortex (MI) and the primary somatosensory cortex (SI) according to the somatotopic map [66]. All of these interested brain areas are significantly related to the process of pain perception. In the human somatosensory system, the contralateral SI is presumed to process and encode the type and intensity of sensory inputs, whereas the bilateral SII responds bilaterally to non-painful and painful somatosensory stimuli, and is believed to perform higher order functions including sensorimotor integration, integration of information from the two body halves, attention, learning, and memory [67]. The MI as a part of motor cortical areas may be related to pain epiphenomena, such as suppression of movement or actual pain-evoked movements themselves [68]. The middle cingulate cortex played an important role in interrupting attention during pain anticipation [69]. Finally, the thalamus is a key relay station for the transmission of nociceptive information to the cerebral cortex, which may hold the key to pain consciousness and the key to understanding spontaneous and evoked pain in chronic pain conditions [70].

All of these cortical or subcortical brain structures demonstrated positive response in the initial stage of acupuncture stimulation. These findings were in accordance with their roles in pain perception because acupuncture stimulation could induce various sorts of pain sensations, such as soreness, aching, or dull pain. Interestingly, the brain responses in these areas began to decrease in the following stimulation and then became negative in the last. As far as the pain perception was concerned, stronger activations of pain-related brain areas might reflect stronger psychophysical ratings of pain [71]. In contrast, the lack of activation in these areas might correlate with weaker pain ratings, and deactivations in these areas were probably able to further reduce the pain rating and increase the pain threshold. In other words, the brain deactivations resulted from the habituation effect in pain related brain areas might play an antinociceptive role. Similar study on heat induced pain was reported by Bingel et al [72]. In their report, pain ratings induced by heat stimulus gradually decreased over time, and the related pain threshold increased over time. The analysis of fMRI data in their report found decreased activity to the thermal stimuli over time (day 1 vs. day 8) and the reduced brain response was found in the pain matrix including thalamus, putamen, insula and SII. This response pattern was consistent with our findings.

On the other hand, it is plausible that even if repeated acupuncture stimulation could result in decrease in pain ratings and increase in pain threshold, it would not necessarily be useful in clinical practice. If acupuncture is to be used as an analgesic, it should meet the following two prerequisites, i.e. the decrease in pain ratings induced by repeated acupuncture stimulation should have the possibility of extending to other sources of pain and the analgesia effects should be sustained for a certain period. In fact, these two prerequisites could be met if the acupuncture cumulative effect could be proved a kind of habituation as previously discussed. It is known that there are ten common characteristics of habituation in total [37]. The most relevant and important ones here are the characteristic #7 and the characteristic #10. The characteristic #7 states "habituation of response to a given stimulus exhibits stimulus generalization to other stimuli", which implies that the brain habituated to acupuncture stimulation would probably be the neural basis of reducing responses to other similar stimulus, such as acute or chronic pain [73,74]. Another important characteristic of habituation is characteristic #10, which states, "some stimulus repetition protocols may result in properties of the response decrement that last hours, days or weeks. This persistence of aspects of habituation is termed as long-term habituation". The characteristic of long-term habituation implies that the analgesia effect, which may result from the generalization characteristic of habituation, has the possibility of lasting for a long time. Therefore, if the acupuncture accumulative effect was of a kind of habituation and the habituation had the general effects, the mechanism of acupuncture analgesia could be easily explained with these common characteristics of the habituation.

3. Consistency and Inconsistency with Previous Relevant Studies

Compared with previous fMRI studies on acupuncture, there were some consistency and inconsistency because of the heterogeneity in previous acupuncture fMRI studies. A recent meta-analysis [71] of acupuncture fMRI studies revealed some common activation patterns in the sensorimotor cortical network and deactivation patterns in the limbic-paralimbic-neocortical network following acupuncture needle stimulation. However, another review [11] argued that the reliability of these deactivations was poor. According to the review of Sun et al, brain responses during acupuncture stimulation should be activation-dominated and the deactivations probably resulted from the average of the repeated runs [11]. Our study only found activated areas in the first block of acupuncture after the multiple comparison correction using Monte Carlo method. However, as the stimulation was repeated and the cumulative duration of stimulation increased, the brain responses of those areas, which were positively activated in the first block of acupuncture stimulation, gradually decreased and eventually reversed to deactivation. This finding supported, at least to some extent, the suggestion from Sun et al [11], i.e. the deactivation might result from repeated acupuncture stimulation. However, this standpoint did not imply that acupuncture induced deactivation, which was reported as an important characteristic by many other researchers [5–10], was not important. On the contrary, our results indicated that the deactivation was very important, because deactivations induced by prolonged repeated acupuncture stimulation might be the cumulative effect and necessary for acupuncture analgesia as discussed in previous section. Therefore, our results could integrate the previous heterogeneous results in some way, i.e., the deactivation in brain areas following acupuncture stimulation may be time related and it may play an important role in acupuncture cumulative effect but not appear at the initial stimulation stage.

4. Limitations in this Study

Although it might be a proper explanation of the mechanism of acupuncture analgesia, the most widely used and most convincingly proved application of acupuncture treatment in clinical practice [4]. However, this presumption could not be convincingly proved with the single result in this study. The first limitation was that we had not adopted sham acupuncture as a control. The main reason was that the objective of this paper was to study the characteristics of brain responses to acupuncture stimulation rather than the specificity of acupoints, i.e. the difference between the true or sham acupoint. Moreover, it was generally agreed that acupuncture, electroacupuncture and transcutaneous electrical acupoint stimulation could be regarded as a continuum of stimulation techniques [4]. As a kind of stimulation techniques, acupuncture stimuli could not be fully distinguished from sensory stimuli, especially when the uncertainty of so called 'sham acupuncture' was taken into account [75]. Most importantly, sham acupuncture may be as efficacious as true acupuncture in clinical practice [76]. The second limitation was that the subjects of this study were healthy volunteers rather than patients with chronic pain. Our previous study suggested that brain response to acupuncture of healthy may differ from that of patients [17]. Nevertheless, the ROIs in this study, which were closely related to pain and acupuncture-related brain areas, might provide some support for the presumption. The third limitation in this paper was that acupuncture stimulation was applied in multiple runs in less than an hour rather than in multiple sessions in several days or weeks, because the actual treatment program for acupuncture analgesia usually lasted for at least one or two weeks. Therefore, further longitudinal investigation should be done in the future to provide more evidence for this presumption.

The differences between our finding and another similar finding by Napadow et al [19] included the bimodal habituation which we found not only in limbic regions (middle cingulate cortex) but also in sensorimotor areas (SI, SII and MI) and subcortical areas (thalamus). This inconsistency might result from the difference between the two experimental designs. Our experimental design was a multi-run with six blocks of stimulation, in which each block lasted for two minutes and was irregularly interposed, while their design was a single run design with 31 blocks of stimulation, in which each block lasted for 30 seconds and was regularly interposed. This inconsistency might suggest that the acupuncture related bimodal habituation effect may be dependent of stimulation pattern, which might be a possible reason for heterogeneity of acupuncture effect in clinical practice. In order to conclude that habituation effects might be the mechanism of acupuncture analgesia, further investigations using patients with chronic pain need to be done in the future.

Conclusion

This study demonstrated that the cumulative effect of prolonged repeated acupuncture stimulation was a kind of habituation effects in pain-related brain areas, where the positive response appeared at the beginning of acupuncture stimulation, and then declined and became negative in the last. It suggested that these increasingly decreased changes of brain response to acupuncture stimulation over time were a kind of habituation effects, a kind of acupuncture cumulative effect. This finding might be useful to explain the neurophysiologic mechanism underlying acupuncture treatment, especially to analgesia, because all brain areas showing acupuncture cumulative effects in current study were related to pain perception. Anyway, further investigations were necessary in order to provide more evidence to support the presumption that acupuncture analgesia was due to the habituation effects of acupuncture stimulation.

Supporting Information

Figure S1 Demonstration of activation and deactivation in the first run, the second run, the third run and the three runs in total ($p=0.005$, $\alpha<=0.01$ corrected with the Monte Carlo Method). The time-variant characteristic was demonstrated because the brain responses in each run and the total run were quite different.
(TIF)

Figure S2 Demonstration of activation and deactivation in each of the six blocks ($p=0.05$, cluster size = 20, uncorrected). The time-variant characteristic was showed in the results of block analysis since the brain responses in each block were quite different. The results were not corrected with any method of multiple comparison correction because the results of some blocks failed to pass the Monte Carlo method.
(TIF)

Acknowledgments

The authors gratefully acknowledge Miss Yue Qiu and Miss Yi Wang for their contributions in making grammatical and textual recommendations, and Dr. Junping Liu, Dr. Qi Lu, Dr. Chunyun Zhang and Dr. Linying Wang for their contributions in acquisition of data.

Author Contributions

Conceived and designed the experiments: CL JY KP BQ XZ. Performed the experiments: JY HW SH WZ CX. Analyzed the data: CL HW WZ JB BQ XZ. Contributed reagents/materials/analysis tools: JY KP SH JB CX. Wrote the paper: CL.

References

1. Pandolfi M (2012) The autumn of acupuncture. Eur J Intern Med 23: 31–33.
2. MacPherson H, Hammerschlag R (2012) Acupuncture and the emerging evidence base: contrived controversy and rational debate. J Acupunct Meridian Stud 5: 141–147.
3. Moffet HH (2006) How might acupuncture work? A systematic review of physiologic rationales from clinical trials. BMC Complement Altern Med 6: 25.
4. Han JS (2011) Acupuncture analgesia: areas of consensus and controversy. Pain 152: S41–48.
5. Napadow V, Kettner N, Liu J, Li M, Kwong KK, et al. (2007) Hypothalamus and amygdala response to acupuncture stimuli in carpal tunnel syndrome. Pain 130: 254–266.
6. Fang JL, Jin Z, Wang Y, Li K, Kong J, et al. (2009) The Salient Characteristics of the Central Effects of Acupuncture Needling: Limbic-Paralimbic-Neocortical Network Modulation. Human Brain Mapping 30: 1196–1206.
7. Hui KKS, Liu J, Makris N, Gollub RL, Chen AJW, et al. (2000) Acupuncture modulates the limbic system and subcortical gray structures of the human brain: Evidence from fMRI studies in normal subjects. Human Brain Mapping 9: 13–25.
8. Hui KKS, Liu J, Marina O, Napadow V, Haselgrove C, et al. (2005) The integrated response of the human cerebro-cerebellar and limbic systems to acupuncture stimulation at ST 36 as evidenced by fMRI. Neuroimage 27: 479–496.
9. Hui KKS, Marina O, Claunch JD, Nixon EE, Fang JL, et al. (2009) Acupuncture mobilizes the brain's default mode and its anti-correlated network in healthy subjects. Brain Research 1287: 84–103.
10. Hui KKS, Marina O, Liu J, Rosen BR, Kwong KK (2010) Acupuncture, the limbic system, and the anticorrelated networks of the brain. Autonomic Neuroscience-Basic & Clinical 157: 81–90.
11. Sun J, Zhu Y, Yang Y, Jin L, von Deneen KM, et al. (2013) What Is the de-qi-Related Pattern of BOLD Responses? A Review of Acupuncture Studies in fMRI. Evid Based Complement Alternat Med 2013: 297839.
12. Kong J, Gollub RL, Rosman IS, Webb JM, Vangel MG, et al. (2006) Brain activity associated with expectancy-enhanced placebo analgesia as measured by functional magnetic resonance Imaging. Journal of Neuroscience 26: 381–388.
13. Napadow V, Dhond RP, Kim J, LaCount L, Vangel M, et al. (2009) Brain encoding of acupuncture sensation - Coupling on-line rating with fMRI. Neuroimage 47: 1055–1065.
14. Asghar AU, Green G, Lythgoe MF, Lewith G, MacPherson H (2010) Acupuncture needling sensation: The neural correlates of deqi using fMRI. Brain Research 1315: 111–118.
15. Beissner F, Henke C (2011) Methodological problems in FMRI studies on acupuncture: a critical review with special emphasis on visual and auditory cortex activations. Evid Based Complement Alternat Med 2011: 607–637.

16. Sun JB, Qin W, Jin LM, Dong MH, Yang XJ, et al. (2012) Impact of Global Normalization in fMRI Acupuncture Studies. Evidence-Based Complementary and Alternative Medicine.
17. Li C, Yang J, Sun J, Xu C, Zhu Y, et al. (2013) Brain Responses to Acupuncture Are Probably Dependent on the Brain Functional Status. Evidence-Based Complementary and Alternative Medicine 2013: 1–14.
18. Bai LJ, Qin W, Tian J, Liu P, Li LL, et al. (2009) Time-Varied Characteristics of Acupuncture Effects in fMRI Studies. Human Brain Mapping 30: 3445–3460.
19. Napadow V, Dhond R, Park K, Kim J, Makris N, et al. (2009) Time-variant fMRI activity in the brainstem and higher structures in response to acupuncture. Neuroimage 47: 289–301.
20. Dong MH, Qin W, Sun JB, Liu P, Yuan K, et al. (2012) Tempo-spatial analysis of vision-related acupoint specificity in the occipital lobe using fMRI: An ICA study. Brain Research 1436: 34–42.
21. Fang JL, Wang XL, Liu HS, Wang Y, Zhou KH, et al. (2012) The Limbic-Prefrontal Network Modulated by Electroacupuncture at CV4 and CV12. Evidence-Based Complementary and Alternative Medicine.
22. Feng YY, Bai LJ, Zhang WS, Xue T, Ren YS, et al. (2011) Investigation of Acupoint Specificity by Multivariate Granger Causality Analysis From Functional MRI Data. Journal of Magnetic Resonance Imaging 34: 31–42.
23. Li G, Jack CR, Yang ES (2006) An fMRI study of somatosensory-implicated acupuncture points in stable somatosensory stroke patients. Journal of Magnetic Resonance Imaging 24: 1018–1024.
24. Li LL, Qin W, Bai LJ, Tian J (2010) Exploring vision-related acupuncture point specificity with multivoxel pattern analysis. Magnetic Resonance Imaging 28: 380–387.
25. Liu P, Zhang Y, Zhou GY, Yuan K, Qin W, et al. (2009) Partial correlation investigation on the default mode network involved in acupuncture: An fMRI study. Neuroscience Letters 462: 183–187.
26. Liu P, Zhou GY, Yang XJ, Liu JX, Sun JB, et al. (2011) Power estimation predicts specific function action of acupuncture: an fMRI study. Magnetic Resonance Imaging 29: 1059–1064.
27. Liu P, Zhou GY, Zhang Y, Dong MH, Qin W, et al. (2010) The hybrid GLM-ICA investigation on the neural mechanism of acupoint ST36: An fMRI study. Neuroscience Letters 479: 267–271.
28. Wang ZQ, Nie BB, Li DH, Zhao ZL, Han Y, et al. (2012) Effect of Acupuncture in Mild Cognitive Impairment and Alzheimer Disease: A Functional MRI Study. Plos One 7.
29. Fang JL, Krings T, Weidemann J, Meister IG, Thron A (2004) Functional MRI in healthy subjects during acupuncture: different effects of needle rotation in real and false acupoints. Neuroradiology 46: 359–362.
30. Park SU, Shin AS, Jahng GH, Moon SK, Park JM (2009) Effects of Scalp Acupuncture Versus Upper and Lower Limb Acupuncture on Signal Activation of Blood Oxygen Level Dependent (BOLD) fMRI of the Brain and Somatosensory Cortex. Journal of Alternative and Complementary Medicine 15: 1193–1200.
31. Liu B, Chen J, Wang JH, Liu X, Duan XH, et al. (2012) Altered Small-World Efficiency of Brain Functional Networks in Acupuncture at ST36: A Functional MRI Study. Plos One 7.
32. Jiang Y, Hao Y, Zhang Y, Liu J, Wang XY, et al. (2012) Thirty minute transcutaneous electric acupoint stimulation modulates resting state brain activities: A perfusion and BOLD fMRI study. Brain Research 1457: 13–25.
33. Shi GX, Yang XM, Liu CZ, Wang LP (2012) Factors contributing to therapeutic effects evaluated in acupuncture clinical trials. Trials 13.
34. Bai LJ, Tian J, Zhong CG, Xue T, You YB, et al. (2010) Acupuncture modulates temporal neural responses in wide brain networks: evidence from fMRI study. Molecular Pain 6.
35. Thompson RF (2009) Habituation: A history. Neurobiology of Learning and Memory 92: 127–134.
36. Thompson RF, Spencer WA (1966) Habituation: A model phenomenon for the study of neuronal substrates of behavior. Psychological Review 73: 16–43.
37. Rankin CH, Abrams T, Barry RJ, Bhatnagar S, Clayton DF, et al. (2009) Habituation revisited: An updated and revised description of the behavioral characteristics of habituation. Neurobiology of Learning and Memory 92: 135–138.
38. Leung L (2012) Neurophysiological Basis of Acupuncture-induced Analgesia–An Updated Review. Journal of Acupuncture and Meridian Studies 5: 261–270.
39. Kong J, Gollub RL, Webb JM, Kong JT, Vangel MG, et al. (2007) Test-retest study of fMRI signal change evoked by electroacupuncture stimulation. Neuroimage 34: 1171–1181.
40. Liu S, Zhou WH, Ruan XZ, Li RH, Lee TT, et al. (2007) Activation of the hypothalamus characterizes the response to acupuncture stimulation in heroin addicts. Neuroscience Letters 421: 203–208.
41. Schaechter JD, Connell BD, Stason WB, Kaptchuk TJ, Krebs DE, et al. (2007) Correlated change in upper limb function and motor cortex activation after verum and sham acupuncture in patients with chronic stroke. Journal of Alternative and Complementary Medicine 13: 527–532.
42. Dougherty DD, Kong J, Webb M, Bonab AA, Fischman AJ, et al. (2008) A combined 11C diprenorphine PET study and fMRI study of acupuncture analgesia. Behavioural Brain Research 193: 63–68.
43. Ho TJ, Duann JR, Chen CM, Chen JH, Shen WC, et al. (2008) Carryover effects alter fMRI statistical analysis in an acupuncture study. American Journal of Chinese Medicine 36: 55–70.
44. Li L, Liu H, Li YZ, Xu JY, Shan BC, et al. (2008) The human brain response to acupuncture on same-meridian acupoints: Evidence from an fMRI study. Journal of Alternative and Complementary Medicine 14: 671–678.
45. Wu Y, Jin Z, Li K, Lu ZL, Wong V, et al. (2008) Effect of Acupuncture on the Brain in Children With Spastic Cerebral Palsy Using Functional Neuroitnaging (fMRI). Journal of Child Neurology 23: 1267–1274.
46. Chae Y, Lee H, Kim H, Kim CH, Chang DI, et al. (2009) Parsing Brain Activity Associated with Acupuncture Treatment in Parkinson's Diseases. Movement Disorders 24: 1794–1802.
47. Chae Y, Lee H, Kim H, Sohn H, Park JH, et al. (2009) The neural substrates of verum acupuncture compared to non-penetrating placebo needle: An fMRI study. Neuroscience Letters 450: 80–84.
48. Kong J, Kaptchuk TJ, Polich G, Kirsch I, Vangel M, et al. (2009) Expectancy and treatment interactions: A dissociation between acupuncture analgesia and expectancy evoked placebo analgesia. Neuroimage 45: 940–949.
49. Kong J, Kaptchuk TJ, Polich G, Kirsch I, Vangel M, et al. (2009) An fMRI study on the interaction and dissociation between expectation of pain relief and acupuncture treatment. Neuroimage 47: 1066–1076.
50. Na BJ, Jahng GH, Park SU, Jung WS, Moon SK, et al. (2009) An fMRI study of neuronal specificity of an acupoint: Electroacupuncture stimulation at Yanglingquan (GB34) and its sham point. Neuroscience Letters 464: 1–5.
51. Bai LJ, Yan H, Li LL, Qin W, Chen P, et al. (2010) Neural Specificity of Acupuncture Stimulation at Pericardium 6: Evidence From an FMRI Study. Journal of Magnetic Resonance Imaging 31: 71–77.
52. Cho SY, Jahng GH, Park SU, Jung WS, Moon SK, et al. (2010) fMRI Study of Effect on Brain Activity According to Stimulation Method at LI11, ST36: Painful Pressure and Acupuncture Stimulation of Same Acupoints. Journal of Alternative and Complementary Medicine 16: 489–495.
53. Quah-Smith I, Sachdev PS, Wen W, Chen XH, Williams MA (2010) The Brain Effects of Laser Acupuncture in Healthy Individuals: An fMRI Investigation. Plos One 5.
54. Sun JB, Qin W, Dong MH, Yuan K, Liu JX, et al. (2010) Evaluation of Group Homogeneity During Acupuncture Stimulation in fMRI Studies. Journal of Magnetic Resonance Imaging 32: 298–305.
55. Wu Y, Jin Z, Li K, Lu ZL, Wong V, et al. (2010) Functional Magnetic Resonance Imaging Activation of the Brain in Children: Real Acupoint Versus Sham Acupoint. Journal of Child Neurology 25: 849–855.
56. Yeo S, Choe IH, van den Noort M, Bosch P, Lim S (2010) Consecutive Acupuncture Stimulations Lead to Significantly Decreased Neural Responses. Journal of Alternative and Complementary Medicine 16: 481–487.
57. Hsieh CW, Wu JH, Hsieh CH, Wang QF, Chen JH (2011) Different Brain Network Activations Induced by Modulation and Nonmodulation Laser Acupuncture. Evidence-Based Complementary and Alternative Medicine: 1–8.
58. Liu JX, Qin W, Guo QA, Sun JB, Yuan K, et al. (2011) Divergent Neural Processes Specific to the Acute and Sustained Phases of Verum and Sham Acupuncture. Journal of Magnetic Resonance Imaging 33: 33–40.
59. Qin W, Bai LJ, Dai JP, Liu P, Dong MH, et al. (2011) The temporal-spatial encoding of acupuncture effects in the brain. Molecular Pain 7.
60. Shukla S, Torossian A, Duann JR, Leung A (2011) The analgesic effect of electroacupuncture on acute thermal pain perception-a central neural correlate study with fMRI. Molecular Pain 7.
61. Claunch JD, Chan ST, Nixon EE, Qiu WQ, Sporko T, et al. (2012) Commonality and Specificity of Acupuncture Action at Three Acupoints as Evidenced by fMRI. American Journal of Chinese Medicine 40: 695–712.
62. Liu H, Xu JY, Shan BC, Li YZ, Li L, et al. (2012) Determining the Precise Cerebral Response to Acupuncture: An Improved fMRI Study. Plos One 7.
63. Sun JB, Zhu YQ, Jin LM, Yang Y, von Deneen K, et al. (2012) Partly Separated Activations in the Spatial Distribution between de-qi and Sharp Pain during Acupuncture Stimulation: An fMRI-Based Study. Evidence-Based Complementary and Alternative Medicine.
64. Yeo S, Lim S, Choe IH, Choi YG, Chung KC, et al. (2012) Acupuncture Stimulation on GB34 Activates Neural Responses Associated with Parkinson's Disease. Cns Neuroscience & Therapeutics 18: 781–790.
65. Ho TJ, Duann JR, Shen WC, Lin JG (2007) Needling sensation: Explanation of incongruent conclusion drawn from acupuncture fMRI study. Journal of Alternative and Complementary Medicine 13: 13–14.
66. Noback CR, Strominger NL, Demarest RJ, Ruggiero DA (2005) The Human Nervous System: Structure and Function: Humana Press Inc.
67. Chen TL, Babiloni C, Ferretti A, Perrucci MG, Romani GL, et al. (2008) Human secondary somatosensory cortex is involved in the processing of somatosensory rare stimuli: an fMRI study. Neuroimage 40: 1765–1771.
68. Apkarian AV, Bushnell MC, Treede RD, Zubieta JK (2005) Human brain mechanisms of pain perception and regulation in health and disease. Eur J Pain 9: 463–484.
69. Brown CA, Jones AKP (2008) A role for midcingulate cortex in the interruptive effects of pain anticipation on attention. Clinical Neurophysiology 119: 2370–2379.
70. Yen C-T, Lu P-L (2013) Thalamus and pain. Acta Anaesthesiologica Taiwanica 51: 73–80.
71. Chae Y, Chang DS, Lee SH, Jung WM, Lee IS, et al. (2013) Inserting Needles Into the Body: A Meta-Analysis of Brain Activity Associated With Acupuncture Needle Stimulation. Journal of Pain 14: 215–222.
72. Bingel U, Schoell E, Herken W, Buchel C, May A (2007) Habituation to painful stimulation involves the antinociceptive system. Pain 131: 21–30.

73. Boensch S (2011) Stimulation-produced analgesia: TENS, acupuncture and alternative techniques. Anaesthesia & Intensive Care Medicine 12: 28–30.
74. Zheng Z, Feng SJQ, Costa Cd, Li CG, Lu D, et al. (2010) Acupuncture analgesia for temporal summation of experimental pain: A randomised controlled study. European Journal of Pain 14: 725–731.
75. Robinson NG (2009) Making Sense of the Metaphor: How Acupuncture Works Neurophysiologically. CLINICAL TECHNIQUES: 642–644.
76. Moffet HH (2009) Sham Acupuncture May Be as Efficacious as True Acupuncture: A Systematic Review of Clinical Trials. Journal of Alternative and Complementary Medicine 15: 213–216.

20

Practitioner Perspectives on Strategies to Promote Longer-Term Benefits of Acupuncture or Counselling for Depression

Hugh MacPherson[1]*, Liz Newbronner[1,2], Ruth Chamberlain[2], Stewart J. Richmond[1], Harriet Lansdown[1], Sara Perren[1], Ann Hopton[1], Karen Spilsbury[1]

1 Department of Health Sciences, University of York, York, United Kingdom, **2** Firefly Research & Evaluation, North Yorkshire, United Kingdom

Abstract

Background: Non-pharmacological interventions for depression may help patients manage their condition. Evidence from a recent large-scale trial (ACUDep) suggests that acupuncture and counselling can provide longer-term benefits for many patients with depression. This paper describes the strategies practitioners reported using to promote longer-term benefits for their patients.

Methods: A qualitative sub-study of practitioners (acupuncturists and counsellors) embedded in a randomised controlled trial. Using topic guides, data was collected from telephone interviews and a focus group, altogether involving 19 counsellors and 17 acupuncturists. Data were audio recorded, transcribed verbatim and analysed using thematic content analysis.

Results: For longer-term impact, both acupuncturists and counsellors encouraged insight into root causes of depression on an individual basis and saw small incremental changes as precursors to sustained benefit. Acupuncturists stressed the importance of addressing concurrent physical symptoms, for example helping patients relax or sleep better in order to be more receptive to change, and highlighted the importance of Chinese medicine theory-based lifestyle change for lasting benefit. Counsellors more often highlighted the importance of the therapeutic relationship, emphasising the need for careful "pacing" such that the process and tools employed were tailored and timed for each individual, depending on the "readiness" to change. Our data is limited to acupuncture practitioners using the principles of traditional Chinese medicine, and counsellors using a humanistic, non-directive and person-centred approach.

Conclusions: Long-term change appears to be an important focus within the practices of both acupuncturists and counsellors. To achieve this, practitioners stressed the need for an individualised approach with a focus on root causes.

Editor: Fan Qu, Women's Hospital, School of Medicine, Zhejiang University, China

Funding: This research is supported by the National Institute for Health Research (NIHR) under Programme Grants for Applied Research (Grant No. RP-PG-0707-10186). The views expressed in this presentation are those of the author(s) and not necessarily those of the NHS, the NIHR or the Department of Health. The funders had no role in study design, data collection and analysis, decision to publish, or preparation of the manuscript.

Competing Interests: Liz Newbronner and Ruth Chamberlain worked for Firefly Research & Evaluation and were commissioned by the Department of Health Sciences, University of York, to conduct the interviews and work with the authors to analyse the data and prepare this manuscript.

* Email: hugh.macpherson@york.ac.uk

Background

Depression is a common illness in primary care. Some of the optimism regarding the potential of selective serotonin re-uptake inhibitors (SSRIs) as a treatment for depression has faded in the light of concerns about effectiveness and safety. [1] A recent meta-analysis has concluded that antidepressants have only a modest advantage over placebo, with the magnitude of benefit increasing with severity of depression. [2] There is an ongoing interest, especially among patients, in the potential of non-pharmacological treatments for depression, with the hope that they might avoid some of the concerns about antidepressants regarding safety and dependency. [3] Furthermore, for many patients, depression is a chronic and recurring illness, and non-pharmacological treatments that seek to improve longer-term outcomes are potentially of interest.

Evidence from a recent large-scale trial (ACUDep) [4] has suggested that acupuncture and counselling can provide longer-term benefits for many patients with on-going depression in primary care. The ACUDep trial recruited 755 patients with depression via 27 participating primary care practices; 302 were randomised to up to 12 acupuncture sessions; 302 to up to 12 counselling sessions; and 151 to usual care alone. The counselling was delivered within a recognised, manualised competency framework developed by Roth et al. at the University College of London's Centre for Outcomes Research and Effectiveness. [5] The acupuncture diagnosis and treatment, including selection of points, was based on the principles of traditional Chinese medicine, the details of which are reported elsewhere. [6]

Both acupuncture and counselling were found to be effective in reducing the symptoms of depression when compared to usual care, and these differences were significant at the 3 and 6 month time points, as well as when averaged over the 12 month period. [4][7] The trial focused on the effectiveness and cost effectiveness of the interventions. However, we were keen to understand the experiences of those providing treatments (acupuncture or counselling) within the trial, and in particular the aspects of these interventions that practitioners perceived to be associated with their longer-term benefit. In doing so, these insights will help understanding of the interventions and help inform both clinical practice and any future research design.

Underreported within randomised controlled trials are qualitative analyses of strategies employed by acupuncturists and counsellors within treatment for depression that are intended to promote longer-term change. In one qualitative study, interviews with patients receiving counselling in routine practice were used to identify the key characteristics of the intervention that were experienced as beneficial in the longer term. [8] In the authors' interpretation, a key component was the client's active engagement during and between counselling sessions. In turn this enabled a change to take place in the way they conducted their lives and relationships. We are unaware of any published qualitative studies of the processes of care associated with long-term change in the case of acupuncture for depression.

This qualitative study, embedded within a clinical trial, was designed to explore the perceptions and experiences of counsellors and acupuncturists who provided the treatment interventions within the trial. The aim was to understand better the key aspects of their work and their perceptions of the 'active ingredients' of counselling or acupuncture that were intended to promote longer-term benefits for the patients and may help in our understanding of the trial results. The study also provided an opportunity to identify important issues relating to professional practice and future policy, which are not reported here, including support needs and working arrangements; the acceptability and feasibility of different treatment options; the implications for the provision of acupuncture or humanistic counselling for treating depression within primary care settings; and related commissioning issues.

Methods

Recruitment of participants

To provide treatments for trial participants, 41 counsellors and 23 acupuncturists were recruited from across the regions of Yorkshire and the North East of England. Altogether these practitioners treated 497 (out of 604) patients participating in the intervention arms of the ACUDep trial. After the end of the trial's treatment phase, acupuncturists and counsellors who had consulted with at least two patients in the trial were invited to take part in the qualitative sub-study. They were sent an information sheet and consent form and asked to indicate whether they would prefer to be involved in a one-to-one telephone interview or a focus group. The aim was to recruit up to 30 counsellors and acupuncturists (approximately 15 in each group). Ethical approval was obtained from the York NHS Research Ethics Committee (REC ref: 09/H1311/75), which included approval for procedures that required written consent from all participants.

Interview and focus group data collection

The topic guides for the interviews and focus group were developed by the ACUDep research team to address the main research question of practitioner strategies intended to promote longer-term benefits for patients – a key finding of the trial results. The initial ideas were developed into topic guides for the interviews, one for each of the practitioner groups, and one for the focus group discussion which comprised both acupuncturists and counsellors. Along with questions, the topic guides also included prompts.These were then refined further at face-to-face meetings, such that the guides covered the practitioner's professional background and experience of working with depression, their approach to treating depression, their perceptions of working within the trial, and their thoughts on the implications for policy and professional practice. These issues were considered important for interpretation of the qualitative data.

All participants provided written consent. Those who agreed to take part in a telephone interview were contacted (either by telephone or email) to arrange a convenient time for the one-to-one interview. Arrangements were confirmed by email and the topic guide to be used in the interview was attached. Only small numbers of practitioners expressed a preference for a focus group discussion and so only one group discussion was held. Many issues covered in the group discussion were similar to those expressed in the individual interviews. However, the group discussion provided an opportunity for therapists to explore together any differences and similarities in their perceptions and experiences. This added to the richness of the data. The interviews and focus group were conducted by two experienced health services researchers from the research team who were not involved in the conduct of the trial itself (LN and RC). The interviews commonly lasted around 45 minutes (range 40 to 90) and the focus group 90 minutes. They were all audio-recorded (with participants' permission) and transcribed verbatim.

Data analysis

The transcripts were analysed thematically. [9] The main areas of inquiry covered in the topic guides were used for a framework approach to thematic content analysis, which involved analysing the data across the two groups of practitioners contributing to the study. [10] The framework was created in an Excel spreadsheet and coded and populated with data from the transcripts by the two researchers who had conducted the interviews (LN and RC). An inductive process was used to identify themes, drawing on shared experiences or points of difference identified from the data. As this study was intended to broaden our understanding of practice in relation to the treatment of patients with depression, the analysis also sought to draw out findings which might inform the practice of acupuncturists and counsellors.

Results

Practitioner characteristics

Forty-one therapists consented to be involved in the study but five therapists later withdrew or didn't respond when the fieldwork was being set up. The sub-study included individual telephone interviews with15 counsellors and13 acupuncturists (n = 28) and one focus group with 4 counsellors and 4 acupuncturists (n = 8) (Table 1). The sample for the qualitative sub-study included over half (56%) of the total number of therapists involved in the main trial.

The 17 participating acupuncturists were registered members of the British Acupuncture Council with at least three years' post-qualification experience and practising with the theoretical

Table 1. Breakdown of study participants.

	Number involved in main trial	Number involved in one-to-one interviews	Number involved in the focus group	Total number participating
Counsellors	41	15	4	19
Acupuncturists	23	13	4	17
Total	64	28	8	36

approach of traditional Chinese medicine. [6] The acupuncturists were predominantly male (39% were female), with an average duration of practice of 12 years. In the trial they treated on average 9 patients, who attended on average for 10 sessions. The 19 counsellors were members of the British Association for Counselling and Psychotherapy, who were accredited or were eligible for accreditation having completed 400 supervised hours post-qualification, and provided clients a humanistic style of counselling based on competences developed for Skills for Health. [11] They were predominantly female practitioners (79%), with an average duration of practice of 7 years. In the trial they treated on average 7 patients, who attended on average for 9 sessions.

Trial patient characteristics

Practitioners were treating patients in the trial who had ongoing depression for at least 3 months and a score of 20 or more on the Beck Depression Inventory (BDI-II), with 38% having depression categorised as "moderate" and 62% "severe". [4] The mean age was 44 years and 73% were female. They were (on average) 25 years old when they experienced their first episode of depression. In terms of prescribed medication, 69% were on anti-depressants and 48% were on analgesics.

Overview of the findings from thematic analysis

A cluster of eight themes emerged from the framework analysis. Almost all of the acupuncturists and counsellors stressed the importance they attached to promoting longer-term benefits. To achieve this, practitioners commonly reported on the need to focus on the root causes, to address treatment for each individual patient, and to value small incremental changes from one session to the next as precursors to sustained benefit over the longer term. Acupuncturists more commonly reported on the need to address concurrent physical symptoms, for example helping patients relax or sleep better in order to be more receptive to change. Most also highlighted the importance of Chinese medicine theory-based lifestyle change as an approach to promoting more lasting benefit. Counsellors more often highlighted the importance of the therapeutic relationship, emphasising the need for careful "pacing" such that the process and tools employed were tailored and timed for each individual, depending on the "readiness" to change. These findings are presented in more detail below.

Importance of a long-term focus

Long-term change appears to be an important focus within the practices of both acupuncturists and counsellors. Almost all of the practitioners mentioned the long-term perspective as inherent to the way they worked.

> *with something like depression, longer term for me, longer term approach is very fundamental.*(acupuncturist1)

For acupuncturists, this perspective was drawn from the theoretical approach of traditional Chinese medicine, in which long-term change needed to be facilitated by lifestyle changes related to acupuncture theory. For counsellors it was drawn from the humanistic approach, which many contrasted with what was perceived as the "quick fix" of cognitive behavioural therapy (CBT).

> *I would like to think that the whole approach is based on longer term change, in terms of the client learning ways of coping. Not just with the present crisis, whatever it might be, but hopefully that they would take something from it that they could apply in the future.*(counsellor1)

When comparing acupuncturists and counsellors, the reported long-term focus involved some differences in approach, as described above, as well as some similarities, especially with regard to encouraging insight into root causes on an individual basis and seeking small incremental changes as important precursors of overall benefit.

Identifying root causes

The commitment to identifying and addressing the root causes of depression within the treatment process was a commonly expressed factor among both acupuncturists and counsellors. Acupuncturists commonly used the theoretical concept of "root" (ben) and "branch" (biao).

> *Within Chinese Medicine we talk about treating the root and the branch. And there is merit in treating both.*(acupuncturist2)
> *Looking for underlying causes. Obviously there's some symptomatic stuff, but always looking at the root causes and using that as where I would start to work out my treatment principles.*(acupuncturist3)

The counsellors were more interested in "going deeper" and "further back (in time)" with their clients as a way of getting to the root causes.

> *From my experience generally, you've got to get to the root causes of depression, so it's much deeper than a CBT approach, so I think if people don't do that when clients present depression, then perhaps they are failing the clients at some level.*(counsellor2)
> *I suppose for me the long term change generally stems from a clear understanding of just what's been at the root of it all.*(counsellor3)

The implications of this approach, as reported by several practitioners, are that unless the underlying causes are addressed, then it is likely that there will not be the sustained long-term change that is desired.

Individualisation

When practised within the theoretical framework of traditional Chinese medicine, acupuncture treatment has been customised to the individual, such that treatment varies not only between patients but also, for the same patient, it varies over time. Likewise for the counsellors in the trial, all of whom were committed to working within the humanistic tradition, a person-centred approach was provided.

Everybody's different, so whenever a patient comes in, obviously, you take their full medical history. And quite often there will be other key characteristics, so not everybody gets the same points diagnosis, because of the different underlying features of their condition.(acupuncturist4)

That the reason for depression for individuals and how it's processed is unique and therefore the process focuses on how the client experiences it. I also think it's useful to bear in mind the possible causes and theories to be shared with the client.(counsellor4)

Valuing incremental change

Practitioners reported a certain amount of caution about expecting sudden or cathartic changes in their patients. More common was a sense that positive benefit required a series of small incremental changes that when combined with self-help approaches would hopefully build a more sustained improvement.

Well long term change can even come about from even small changes, really. If somebody can just sleep all night, it's surprising.(acupuncturist5)

I think to try almost to help people take responsibility and realise that there maybe is something that they can do. I think sometimes people get trapped in feeling depressed and feeling unable to do anything. So almost helping empower them to find changes that they can start to make, to make those improvements for themselves, which over time build up and help them move forward.(counsellor5)

Addressing concurrent physical symptoms

Acupuncturists generally stressed the importance of addressing concurrent physical symptoms, for example helping patients relax or sleep better in order to be more receptive to change.

What I find really interesting about working on the trial is that a lot of time people came with depression but in reality there was a host of other signs and symptoms that they were not happy in their life. Just kind of bowel, musculoskeletal, anything. So when they got a sense that I was treating them as a whole person, rather than just treating the depression....... When I'd sorted out their back, their stomach, ulcers, bad knees, you know, suddenly their depression got better. To me, that's how Traditional Chinese Medicine should be – it works with everything. Rather than, you know, like depression as a standalone thing.(acupuncturist2)

By contrast, the counsellors were less focused on the physical symptoms, and worked more on the assumption that by treating the underlying causes of depression there should be a knock-on effect in terms of reducing physical symptoms.

I'm not particularly interested in just treating symptoms, but what I'm usually interested in and what people are usually asking for is that they want to understand why they're feeling the way that they are. If you can deal with that issue, then it should help them to rid themselves of the symptoms really.(counsellor6)

Lifestyle changes

Almost all of the acupuncturists highlighted the importance of giving advice about lifestyle change that was relevant to the Chinese medicine perspective.

Yeah, it's overall sort of aimed at the long-term and I think people, you know, if they get further along with the acupuncture, they realise that it's all to do with lifestyle change as well and that those things are going to be the ones that bring them lasting benefit. Because often people start to feel better after a few treatments and then when they build in the lifestyle thing, when they actually start to think, oh, this acupuncture seems to be working for me, maybe I'll follow some of the advice as well. (acupuncturist6)

Those acupuncturists who reported on the role of lifestyle change tended to stress the importance of tailoring the advice to the patient, both in terms of content related to acupuncture theory (e.g. diet, relaxation, exercise, etc) as well as likely acceptability.

The counsellors worked within a trial protocol that had a strong emphasis on working within the humanistic tradition, which included being non-directive. [11] The protocol therefore limited the extent that they could offer lifestyle advice within the trial. Some counsellors, who typically worked more eclectically elsewhere, said they might normally include lifestyle advice, especially when working with people with addictions.

Therapeutic relationship

Counsellors consistently stressed the importance of the therapeutic relationship.

I tend to think that lasting change requires a greater degree of insight [than CBT]. But I think the change often comes – I suppose this is what puts me very squarely in the humanistic camp, the existential camp, I think it's often the relationship itself – it's actually having a new experience of a relationship for some people can be transformative.(counsellor3)

But the essence of my approach is the relationship and building good levels of rapport and trust and helping the client to feel okay with you. So it's an okay space at the start and if that forms well, that's a springboard, hopefully, for sort of therapeutic practice and change for people.(counsellor2)

However for some acupuncturists, this was also reported as a component of the treatment process that helped engender longer-term gains.

And it's kind of like a trust relationship – if they believe in the acupuncture, they believe in what you're telling them. And that kind of gives them the impetus to carry on in the longer term.(acupuncturist6)

Careful "pacing" based on "readiness to change"

Many of the counsellors emphasised the need for careful "pacing" such that the process and tools employed were tailored and timed for each individual, depending on the "readiness" to change.

And what I'm very aware of in counselling is that people will come to therapy at different stages of readiness to change. And it's very difficult to measure how useful it's been. So for example, with one client I can think of in the trial, I think he would have – I think it was probably a first experience for him, from being listened to and from being taken seriously and I think that was huge. He was very stuck. In terms of how much that was going to affect outcomes, in terms of was he going to make the necessary changes, he might have been able to begin to identify, or briefly identify, what it was in his life that was making him depressed – in terms of outcomes he wasn't at the stage where he was going to make any massive changes. But I think just having that experience, that first experience. That kind of thing is so hard to measure, isn't it?(counsellor6)

I tend to go with the speed of the client. However, if I can – my personal approach would be to help them in as short a sessions as possible to get them to feel better. However, I'm very careful to work with their speed. So am I short or long term.(counsellor7)

A number of acupuncturists identified issues related to timing, expressing the point that as patients improve, ideally appointments should be spread out towards the end of the course of treatment and beyond, as a way of sustaining benefit over the longer term.

In summary, the themes capture both similarities and differences in approaches between acupuncture and counselling, with most practitioners of both interventions having a shared sense of the prerequisites for sustained long-term benefit. The impression formed from the interviews is that the various approaches do not operate in isolation. Although the emphasis may vary, the themes appear to be integrated into a coherent combination that uniquely informs the practice of each practitioner.

Generalisability issues

With regard to the extent that these findings are transferable to other settings, the majority of counsellors said that the severity of the depression amongst trial patients was not markedly dissimilar to the people they routinely saw. By contrast, the acupuncturists were generally less used to dealing with patients with moderate to severe depression, and many said that they less commonly saw patients who consulted primarily because of a diagnosis of depression. Several of the therapists reported that the trial patients had a different attitude towards treatment compared to their private patients, particularly a more limited knowledge of the therapeutic intervention and a lower level of motivation to help themselves. Therapists also noted that there were a greater proportion of patients in lower income brackets, with more long-standing depression, or with unmanaged drug/alcohol addictions.

Discussion

Principal findings

Both acupuncturists and counsellors generally delivered treatments with an eye to encouraging longer-term change with the intention that, ideally, any putative benefit would be sustained well beyond the 12 sessions that were provided within the trial. While both types of practitioners reported on the need to address the root causes, the approach differed. For the acupuncturists there was a focus drawn from Chinese medicine theory on treating the root cause (the *ben*) as well as the manifesting symptoms (the *biao*) with the precise details of the intervention customised to their patients at an individual level. Meanwhile the approach of the counsellors was to get below the surface of the clients' problems and to "go deeper" and "further back (in time)" as a way of getting a handle on the root cause and, as with the acupuncturists, this required an individualised approach.

There were further differences in approach to facilitating more sustained benefits. Acupuncturists were more focussed on physical symptoms, on whether these could be resolved by acupuncture in order to speed up the improvements in the symptoms of depression, and on providing lifestyle advice linked to the Chinese medicine diagnosis. Meanwhile counsellors were more explicit on the importance of a strong therapeutic relationship accompanied by a careful consideration of what might be a manageable pace of change.

Strengths and limitations

The sub-study is nested within the largest trial to date of acupuncture or counselling for depression, and provides unique access to clusters of practitioners who have reported here on the treatments that they provided. The patient group is clearly defined, all with "moderate" to "severe" depression as categorised by the Beck Depression Inventory (BDI-II). The methods used, involving interviews, verbatim transcripts, and thematic analysis, are consistent with many of the markers of quality in qualitative research. [12] We have helped establish the credibility and dependability of the results through involving an independent research team (LN and RC) to help conduct the study, by arranging meetings of stakeholders to review the research questions and the methods used, and by discussing the emerging themes and refining these through debate to agreement. A substantive report emerged from this process, from which a component is reported here. With regard to the transferability of the results, we have provided details of the practitioners as well as the patients who were the focus of our sub-study, such that readers can draw conclusions regarding relevance for other areas. In terms of limitations, our data is limited to patients receiving acupuncture as practised by those using the theories of traditional Chinese medicine and to clients receiving counselling as provided in the humanistic and non-directive and person-centred style.

Relationship to the wider literature

There is limited evidence in the literature for longer-term benefits associated with acupuncture for depression. [13] In a systematic review of RCTs, counselling for depression has been reported to be no better than GP care in the long term [14], though in a review of pre-post comparisons of client outcomes, benefits have been reported to last a year or more. [15] The trial, within which this sub-study was nested, provided some further evidence on longer-term effects beyond the period of treatment. [4] Within the wider literature there is a dearth of evidence on the acupuncture treatment factors that might be associated with longer-term change in the symptoms of depression. The findings from a small study involving interviews with six practitioners in a trial of acupuncture for back pain found that these acupuncturists had a goal of a positive long-term outcome, and developed a therapeutic partnership to support the active engagement of patients in their own recovery. [16] Consistent with many of the findings we report here, the authors reported that the key elements were: establishing rapport, using an interactive diagnostic process, matching treatment to the patient, and using explanatory models from Chinese medicine to aid a shared understanding and motivate lifestyle changes to reinforce the potential recovery.

In the counselling literature, a qualitative study reported on the long-term effects of counselling, with data drawn from 15 clients who had received counselling from between one and three years previously. [8] The authors' interpretation of the client interview data led them to describe a model of the change process and mechanisms that were perceived as essential to produce lasting benefit. They identified as key elements of the counselling process the active engagement of the client during and between sessions, and the acquisition of a "box of skills" to be built on further after the counselling was finished. Unlike in the current study, in which all clients of counsellors received humanistic counselling, the authors did not identify the counselling approach provided. Another difference between this study and ours, is that all patients in our study had been diagnosed with depression.

Implications for clinical practice and research

One implication for clinical practice is that, while both acupuncture and counselling for depression appear to be associated with longer-term benefits, the interventions seem to work in different ways. Further research is needed from the perspective of patients and clients on their experiences of treatment from these two modalities. To assist referral, a clearer understanding is needed of which type of person with depression would benefit from acupuncture and which from counselling. While taking into account patient preference, such a typology would provide referring clinicians with valuable guidance on suitability for referral.

Another question is in regard to the nature of depression, and the extent to which physical symptoms are also present. Evidence suggests that 69% of people experiencing depression in primary care initially present with physical symptoms [17] and 50% of people with depression are also in pain. [18] Our study has found that acupuncturists are interested in the physical symptoms that may accompany depression, and will routinely address these symptoms as part of the treatment.

One can speculate that this focus on physical symptoms may in part explain why the acupuncturists in this trial, who reported being less experienced in treating moderate to severe depression, nevertheless delivered just as good outcomes as the counsellors, who encountered this level of depression more commonly in routine practice. Further research is needed into the patient perspective on the treatment of depression with co-morbidities, and specifically the value they place on the comorbid symptoms being addressed concurrently.

Our research raises some important questions about the clinical practice of acupuncturists and counsellors when treating a population with depression when combined with unmanaged drug and alcohol addictions. Further research might be useful to explore appropriate strategies, which might be about ensuring the availability of options, including the involvement of other agencies, and practical support.

Conclusions

Long-term change appears to be an important focus within the practices of both acupuncturists and counsellors. Practitioners of both interventions generally stressed that, for longer-term benefit, there needs to be an individualised approach with a focus on root causes. Acupuncturists more often emphasised the importance of addressing concurrent physical symptoms and highlighted the importance of relevant lifestyle change. Counsellors commonly stressed the importance of the therapeutic relationship and emphasised the need for appropriate "pacing" such that the timing of the counselling process is geared to the "readiness" to change.

Supporting Information

Text S1 Consolidated criteria for reporting qualitative studies (COREQ): 32-item checklist.
(DOCX)

Acknowledgments

We acknowledge with appreciation the contributions of the practitioners who were interviewed or who attended the focus group, Janet Eldred for providing support for the management of both the trial and the sub-study, and Anne Burton for undertaking the transcriptions. This research is supported by the National Institute for Health Research (NIHR) under Programme Grants for Applied Research (Grant No. RP-PG-0707-10186). The views expressed in this presentation are those of the author(s) and not necessarily those of the NHS, the NIHR or the Department of Health. The funders had no role in study design, data collection and analysis, decision to publish, or preparation of the manuscript.

Author Contributions

Conceived and designed the experiments: HM LN RC SR HL SP AH KS. Performed the experiments: LN RC. Analyzed the data: HM LN RC. Contributed reagents/materials/analysis tools: HM LN RC KS. Contributed to the writing of the manuscript: HM LN RC. Revision of the manuscript: HM LN RC SR HL SP AH KS.

References

1. Parker G (2009) Antidepressants on trial: how valid is the evidence? Br J Psychiatry: 1–3.
2. Kirsch I, Deacon BJ, Huedo-Medina TB, Scoboria A, Moore TJ, et al. (2008) Initial severity and antidepressant benefits: a meta-analysis of data submitted to the Food and Drug Administration. PLoS Med 5: e45.
3. Mind (2002) My Choice: A Survey. Available: http://www.mind.org.uk/News+policy+and+campaigns/Press+archive/Mind+launches+campaign+for+more+choice+of+mental+health+services+at+GP+level.htm. Accessed 13 January 2008.
4. MacPherson H, Richmond S, Bland M, Brealey S, Gabe R, et al. (2013) Acupuncture and Counselling for Depression in Primary Care: A Randomised Controlled Trial. PLoS Medicine 10: e1001518. doi:10.1371/journal.pmed.1001518.
5. Centre for Outcomes Research & Effectiveness (CORE) (n.d.) Humanistic Psychological Therapies Competences Framework. Available: http://www.ucl.ac.uk/clinical-psychology/CORE/humanistic_framework.htm#. Accessed 30 September 2013.
6. MacPherson H, Elliot B, Hopton A, Lansdown H, Richmond S (2013) Acupuncture for Depression: Patterns of Diagnosis and Treatment within a Randomised Controlled Trial. Evid Based Complement Alternat Med 2013: 286048. doi:10.1155/2013/286048.
7. MacPherson H, Richmond S, Bland J, Lansdown H, Hopton A, et al. (2012) Acupuncture, Counselling, and Usual care for Depression (ACUDep): study protocol for a randomized controlled trial. Trials 13: 209.
8. Perren S, Godfrey M, Rowland N (2009) The long-term effects of counselling: The process and mechanisms that contribute to ongoing change from a user perspective. Counselling and Psychotherapy Research 9: 241–249. doi:10.1080/14733140903150745.
9. Braun V, Clarke V (2006) Using thematic analysis in psychology. Qualitative Research in Psychology 3: 77–101.

10. Ritchie J, Lewis J (2003) Qualitative Research Practice: A Guide for Social Science Students and Researchers. London:Sage.
11. Roth A, Hill A, Pilling S (2009) The competences required to deliver effective Humanistic Psychological Therapies. London, UK: University College London.
12. Hannes K (2011) Chapter 4: Critical appraisal of qualitative research. Supplementary Guidance for Inclusion of Qualitative Research in Cochrane Systematic Reviews of Interventions. Cochrane Collaboration Qualitative Methods Group. Available: http://cqrmg.cochrane.org/supplemental-handbook-guidance. Accessed 31 March 2014.
13. Smith CA, Hay PP, MacPherson H (2010) Acupuncture for depression. Cochrane Database Syst Rev: CD004046.
14. Bower P, Knowles S, Coventry PA, Rowland N (2011) Counselling for mental health and psychosocial problems in primary care. Cochrane Database Syst Rev: CD001025.
15. Research on humanistic-experiential psychotherapies (2013) Bergin and Garfield's handbook of psychotherapy and behavior change. Hoboken, NJ: John Wiley & Sons. pp. 495–538.
16. MacPherson H, Thorpe L, Thomas KJ (2006) Beyond needling - therapeutic processes in acupuncture care: a qualitative study nested within a low-back pain trial. J Altern Complement Med 12: 873–880.
17. Simon GE, VonKorff M, Piccinelli M, Fullerton C, Ormel J (1999) An international study of the relation between somatic symptoms and depression. N Engl J Med 341: 1329–1335. doi:10.1056/NEJM199910283411801.
18. Katona C, Peveler R, Dowrick C, Wessely S, Feinmann C, et al. (2005) Pain symptoms in depression: definition and clinical significance. ClinMed 5(4): 390–395.

21

Decreased Peripheral and Central Responses to Acupuncture Stimulation following Modification of Body Ownership

Younbyoung Chae[1,2]*, In-Seon Lee[2], Won-Mo Jung[1], Dong-Seon Chang[3], Vitaly Napadow[4,5], Hyejung Lee[2], Hi-Joon Park[2], Christian Wallraven[1]*

1 Department of Brain and Cognitive Engineering, Korea University, Seoul, Korea, **2** Acupuncture and Meridian Science Research Center, College of Korean Medicine, Kyung Hee University, Seoul, Korea, **3** Department of Human Perception, Cognition and Action, Max Planck Institute for Biological Cybernetics, Tübingen, Germany, **4** Martinos Center for Biomedical Imaging, Massachusetts General Hospital, Harvard Medical School, Charlestown, Massachusetts, United States of America, **5** Department of Biomedical Engineering, Kyunghee University, Yongin, Korea

Abstract

Acupuncture stimulation increases local blood flow around the site of stimulation and induces signal changes in brain regions related to the body matrix. The rubber hand illusion (RHI) is an experimental paradigm that manipulates important aspects of bodily self-awareness. The present study aimed to investigate how modifications of body ownership using the RHI affect local blood flow and cerebral responses during acupuncture needle stimulation. During the RHI, acupuncture needle stimulation was applied to the real left hand while measuring blood microcirculation with a LASER Doppler imager (Experiment 1, $N=28$) and concurrent brain signal changes using functional magnetic resonance imaging (fMRI; Experiment 2, $N=17$). When the body ownership of participants was altered by the RHI, acupuncture stimulation resulted in a significantly lower increase in local blood flow (Experiment 1), and significantly less brain activation was detected in the right insula (Experiment 2). This study found changes in both local blood flow and brain responses during acupuncture needle stimulation following modification of body ownership. These findings suggest that physiological responses during acupuncture stimulation can be influenced by the modification of body ownership.

Editor: Marcello Costantini, University G. d'Annunzio, Italy

Funding: This research was supported by the Basic Science Research Program through the National Research Foundation of Korea (NRF) funded by the Ministry of Education, Science and Technology (No. 2011-0009913 & 2014K2A3A1000166). VN was supported by the following NIH grants from the USA: NCCAM: P01-AT006663, R01-AT005280, R01-AT007550; NIAMS: R01-AR064367. The funders had no role in study design, data collection and analysis, decision to publish, or preparation of the manuscript.

Competing Interests: The authors have declared that no competing interests exist.

* Email: ybchae@khu.ac.kr (YC); wallraven@korea.ac.kr (CW)

Introduction

The importance of an accurate representation of the body by the brain has been documented in many different studies involving both healthy participants and clinical patients [1,2]. Body ownership specifically, which refers to the sense that a part of one's body belongs to oneself, has been studied as a fundamental aspect of bodily self-consciousness [3,4]. Moreover, body ownership and aspects of bodily self-awareness influence clinical outcomes because they can modulate the regulation of one's physical self [5,6,7].

The rubber hand illusion (RHI) is an experimental paradigm that manipulates body ownership of the hand and is widely used to investigate the processes that underlie various aspects of bodily self-awareness [6,8]. When participants watch a rubber hand being stroked by a paintbrush in synchrony with strokes applied to their own corresponding hand, they typically experience a change in body ownership such that the rubber hand "feels like one's own hand" [9]. This illusory feeling of body ownership is thought to be associated with the multimodal integration of visual, tactile, and proprioceptive information in the brain [10]. When participants take ownership of the artificial counterpart, the real hand exhibits a decrease in skin temperature, slower processing of tactile information, and enhanced histamine reactivity, which suggests that a cortical body matrix integrates the perceptual and homeostatic regulation of the body [2,6,11]. The experience of the RHI is associated with in a distributed network in the brain [7]. The ventral premotor cortex has been suggested as a key brain structure for the multisensory representation of one's own body during the RHI [12]. When the rubber hand is fully incorporated into the body, artificial limbs were able to evoke a similar level of activity in the insula and the anterior cingulate cortex, indicating that the bodily ownership of the rubber hand is associated with changes in the interoceptive system [13]. The experience of body ownership of the rubber hand as measured by the effect of multisensory integration and recalibration of hand position was positively correlated with activity in the right posterior insula [14].

Acupuncture, an ancient East Asian therapeutic technique, uses needles to stimulate a particular part of the body for the purpose of inducing beneficial effects during clinical treatment [15]. Acupuncture stimulation affects microcirculatory blood flow near the inserted needle as well as regional blood flow in various organs [16,17]. Neuroimaging studies investigating acupuncture have observed overlapping brain responses in a number of cortical and subcortical brain regions. For example, activation has been observed in cortical sensorimotor and salient networks such as the insula, thalamus, anterior cingulate cortex, as well as primary and secondary somatosensory cortices, whereas deactivation has been identified in the limbic-paralimbic neocortical network in areas such as the medial prefrontal cortex, caudate, amygdala, posterior cingulate cortex, and parahippocampus [18,19]. Accordingly, recent reviews of functional magnetic resonance imaging (fMRI) studies revealed common brain activations in the sensorimotor cortical network and common deactivations in the limbic-paralimbic-neocortical network following acupuncture needle stimulation [20,21]. A number of convergent results and promising new data provide some pointers for understanding the neural mechanisms of acupuncture therapy in the context of the modern medical mainstream [20,21]. Despite recent progress, however, some questions still remain controversial and a) Are specific traditional acupuncture points related to their specifically claimed functions? (Question of Point-specificity) [19,22,23], b) How is the acupuncture-specific sensation, called *DeQi* sensation, located functionally in the brain? [24,25,26], c) Are pain-related areas desensitized in the brain during or after acupuncture treatment, explaining the phenomenon of acupuncture analgesia? [27,28,29,30], d) Can the specific (physiological) effects be distinguished with non-specific (psychological or placebo) effects of acupuncture? [15,31,32,33]. e) What is the role of the interceptive attention system, such as somato-spatial attention, body awareness, and anticipation of stimulation in the physiological responses to acupuncture? [34,35] The answers to these questions have been somewhat contradictory, and left mostly controversial.

From the perspective of cognitive neuroscience, acupuncture is not only seen as a 'simple needling' but also as a complex treatment comprised of multimodal sensory stimulation that interacts with various factors, including bodily self-awareness [36,37]. The role of psychosocial and contextual factors, including body image and body schema, are thought to exert an important influence on the clinical effects of acupuncture [38]. Neuroimaging studies have suggested that the insula, which is known to modulate the interoceptive system, plays an important role in the effects of acupuncture [35,39]. The insula was activated to a greater extent during real acupuncture than during the placebo intervention in patients with osteoarthritis [39]. Considering a salient component of acupuncture analgesia, focused attention and accentuated bodily awareness on the specific body part with acupuncture-induced sensation could contribute to the top-down modulation of nociceptive afference and the central pain matrix [35]. Conversely, we can assume that acupuncture might not properly exert its influence under reduced bodily awareness. Thus, it is conceived that components of this bodily self-awareness can be involved in the modulation of physiological responses to acupuncture stimulation. In the current study, we hypothesized that modification of body ownership can reduce the neurophysiological responses to acupuncture stimulation, especially through the disruption of the interoceptive system in the brain.

The present study aimed to investigate whether modifications of body ownership would result in measurable physiological changes in response to acupuncture stimulation using LASER Doppler and fMRI, respectively.

Methods and Materials

Procedures for measuring changes in local blood flow (Experiment 1)

Participants. Advertisements were used to recruit a total of 28 right-handed participants (age: 22.8±0.5 years; 15 males and 13 females) for this study from the general population of students, staff, and visitors to Kyung Hee University in Seoul, Republic of Korea. Participants with no history of neurological, psychiatric, or visual disorders were included in this study. Handedness was self-reported by the participants in a screening questionnaire prior to the experiment, and participants were prohibited from drinking alcohol or caffeine or taking any drugs or medications on the day of the experiment. Each participant received a detailed explanation of the study, and written informed consent was obtained prior to participation. All experiments in this study were conducted in accordance with the guidelines issued by the human subjects committee and approved by the Institutional Review Board of Korea University in Seoul, Republic of Korea.

Experimental design. The setup followed standard procedure and was designed and executed almost identically to a previous study [9], placing a rubber hand in front of each participant while their left hand was hidden from sight. The experiments followed a within-subjects cross-over design in which the independent variable was a synchronous versus an asynchronous brush touch on the hand to measure illusory body ownership. In both the synchronous and asynchronous sessions, participants received 180 seconds of acupuncture needle stimulation on the hidden (real) left hand immediately after the RHI (Fig. 1A). The order was randomized such that participants were randomly assigned to one of two groups (i.e., they received either the synchronous or the asynchronous session first). The interval between the two sessions was approximately 2 days.

Tactile stimulation for the induction of the rubber hand illusion. Participants were told to fixate on the rubber hand (Korean Prosthetic Limbs Research Institute; Seoul, Korea), to not look elsewhere, and to not move any of their fingers during the experiment. Two small paintbrushes were used to stroke both the rubber hand and the participant's hidden real left hand (strokes were approximately 2 cm in length) at a frequency of 1 Hz for 180 sec. This was done synchronously under one condition (synchronous condition) and asynchronously under the other condition (asynchronous condition).

Acupuncture stimulation. First, participants were informed that physiological data, including LASER Doppler measurements, would be recorded while they received acupuncture stimulation. Then, each participant was led to the experimental room and seated with their left and right arms on a table in the same manner as in a standard RHI experiment [9]. At the beginning of the session, an acupuncture needle was inserted at acupoint LI4 on the dorsum of the left hand radial to the midpoint of the second metacarpal bone. The needles were 0.20 mm in diameter and 40 mm long (Seirin Acupuncture, Inc.; Kasei, Japan). Participants were instructed to look at the rubber hand during the acupuncture stimulation.

After the tactile stimulation on the rubber hand and the real hand, standard acupuncture needle stimulation (the same as in clinical acupuncture treatments) was applied by a licensed and experienced Doctor of Korean Medicine, which consisted of rotating the needle at a frequency of 1 Hz for the duration of 10 seconds every 1 minute. Therefore, the total duration of acupuncture insertion was 3 minutes, including a total of 30 seconds (3×10 seconds) of acupuncture needle manipulation.

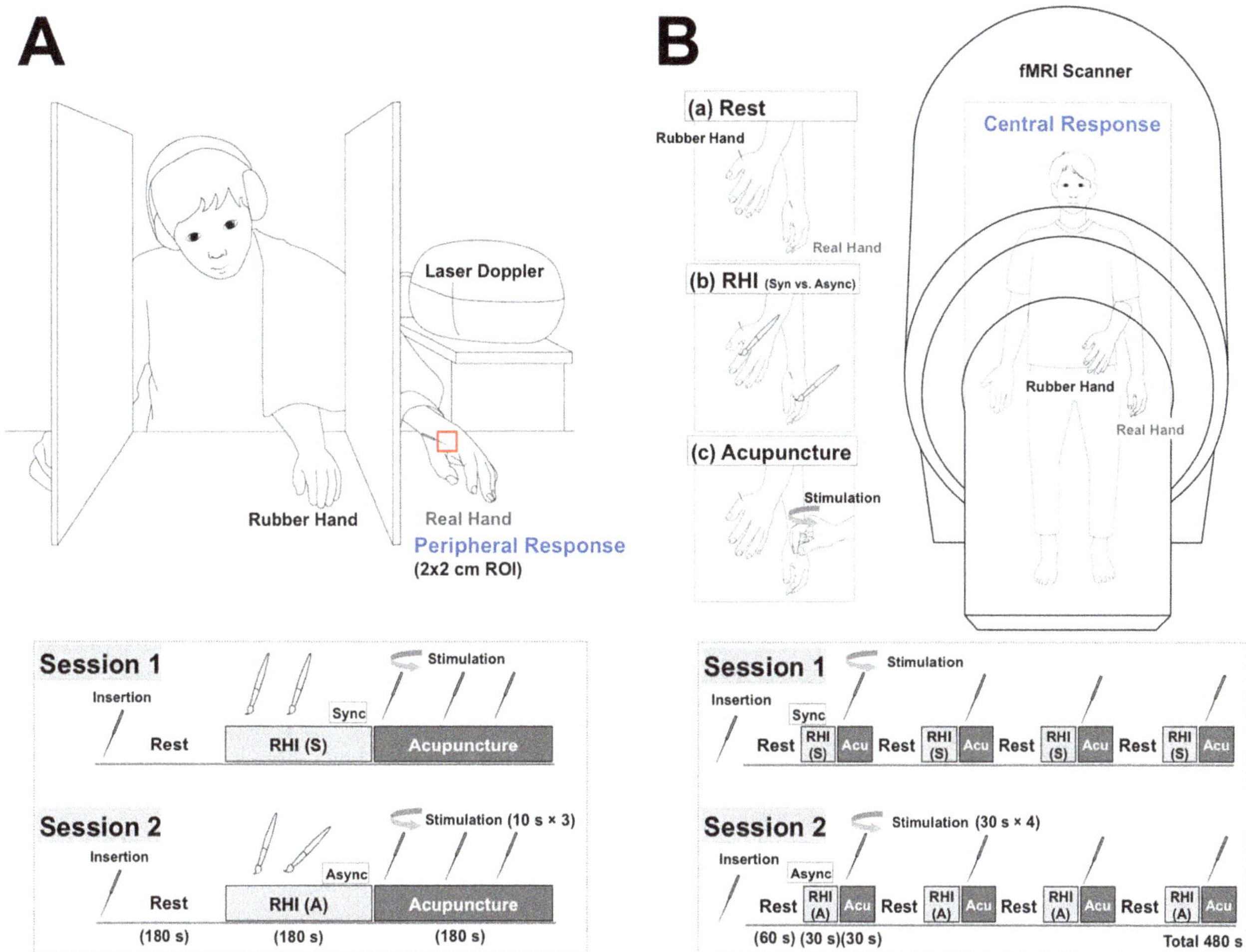

Figure 1. Experimental procedures. A: Procedures for peripheral responses (Experiment 1). Two small paintbrushes stroked the rubber hand (strokes were approximately 2 cm in length) and the hidden real left hand of the participant at a frequency of 1 Hz for 180 seconds as synchronously as possible under one condition (synchronous condition: S) and asynchronously under the other condition (asynchronous condition: A); RHI: Rubber hand illusion induction. Participants received acupuncture needle stimulation at a frequency of 1 Hz for 10 seconds every 1 minute during the 3-minute acupuncture stimulation period on the hidden (real) left hand immediately after commencing the RHI under the synchronous or asynchronous condition (Acu: Acupuncture stimulation). B: Procedures for brain responses (Experiment 2). There were two randomized sessions: a synchronous condition (S) and an asynchronous condition (A). The acupuncture needle was stimulated at the LI4 acupoint in the left hand out of sight of the participant according to the beats of a 1-Hz metronome transmitted via earphones (Acu: Acupuncture stimulation). One session included a four-block tactile-stimulation condition (30 seconds) for the RHI and a four-block acupuncture stimulation (30 seconds); these were performed successively. Tactile stimulation was synchronously or asynchronously applied with short strokes from two brushes (approximately 2 cm in length) at a frequency of 1 Hz during the tactile-stimulation block; RHI: Rubber hand illusion induction.

To confirm that the synchronous and the asynchronous sessions did not differ in terms of manual acupuncture stimulation, Acusensor2 force sensors (Stromatec Inc, Burlington, VT, USA) were attached to the needle handle to measure the degree of stimulation (rotation frequency) and the biomechanical force (torque amplitude: rotation force) [40]. The rotation frequency and torque amplitude were calculated over a period of 10 seconds based on raw data. During needle rotation, the rotation frequency was calculated using fast Fourier analyses of the raw data by Data Viewer software (Stromatec Inc.), and the torque amplitude of peaks was calculated manually as the mean value.

LASER Doppler measurement. Measurements of skin blood perfusion around the site of acupuncture stimulation (acupoint LI4) were performed using a LASER Doppler perfusion imager (LDPR; PeriScan PIM III system; Perimed AB, Sweden). Before the tactile stimulation for the induction of the RHI, the real hand (left hand) of participants was immobilized with a cylindrical object to ensure positioning, and measurements were carried out every 5 seconds for a total duration of 180 seconds. The temperature in the laboratory room was kept consistent and controlled (24–26°C) throughout the experiment. The LASER Doppler scanning was conducted on the participants' real hand out of sight without any sound and did not produce any sensation. Peripheral blood flow (PBF; symbolized as $R_{i,\ [i=1,\ 2,\ 3,\ \ldots,\ 36]}$) was defined as the mean blood flux in each scan (5 seconds) around the LI4 acupoint (2×2 cm), and the change in PBF was calculated using the following formula: $(R_i\text{-}R_1)/R_1$. For assessing the responses during and after acupuncture stimulation, each 5 sec was subtracted from a 10 s baseline prior to the initial acupuncture stimulation (onset) and averaged across the 180 s of each session, resulting in change in scores that reflected increases from the baseline.

Rubber hand illusion and self-reported DeQi sensation rating. Right after the completion of tactile stimulation on the rubber hand and real hand (synchronous and asynchronous), participants reported their perception of the RHI by answering the most relevant question (Q3) on the RHI Perception Scale: "I felt as if the rubber hand were my hand" [9]. Acupuncture is generally accompanied by the perception of a complex set of sensations, called "*DeQi*" including aching, dull, heavy, numb, radiating, spreading and tingling [41]. It is considered to be associated with acupuncture treatment outcomes [42]. After each acupuncture stimulation session, participants evaluated their acupuncture-induced *DeQi* sensation, including heaviness, soreness, and numbness, using a 100-mm visual analogue scale [43].

Data analysis. All values are expressed as means ± standard errors. RHI ratings, subjective pain ratings, and PBF changes under the synchronous brush-stroking (induction of illusory body ownership) and the asynchronous brush-stroking (control) sessions were compared using paired *t*-tests. The level of significance was set at 0.05 for all analyses. Statistical analyses were performed using the Statistical Package for Social Sciences for Windows 20.0 (SPSS Inc.; Chicago, IL, USA).

Procedures for measuring brain responses with fMRI (Experiment 2)

Participants. A total of 17 right-handed participants (age: 23.0±0.8 years; 10 males and 7 females) were recruited by advertisement from the general population of students, staff, and visitors to Kyung Hee University in Seoul, Republic of Korea for participation in this study. Participants with no history of neurological, psychiatric, or visual disorders were included in this study. Handedness was self-reported by the participants in a screening questionnaire prior to the experiment, and participants were prohibited from drinking alcohol or caffeine or taking any drugs or medications on the day of the experiment. Each participant received a detailed explanation of the study and written informed consent was obtained prior to participation. All experiments in this study were conducted in accordance with the guidelines issued by the human subjects committee and approved by the Institutional Review Board of Korea University in Seoul, Republic of Korea.

Experimental design. During the brain scans, participants lay in a supine position on the MRI table, and their left hand was comfortably placed on the MRI table while the rubber hand was placed 15 cm above their left hand so that their real hand was hidden under the rubber hand. The rubber hand was orientated in an anatomically plausible position, pointing slightly right toward the midline of the body (20°–30°). The right hand was also comfortably placed on the MRI table. A mirror attached to the head coil enabled participants to look at the rubber hand; the position of the rubber hand and/or the head-coil mirror was adjusted to ensure a clear view of the rubber hand. Before the start of scanning, the acupuncture needle was inserted at the LI4 acupoint (on the dorsum of radial to the midpoint of the second metacarpal bone) both in the left rubber hand and left real hand out of sight of the participant. Prior to scanning, we ensured that none of the participants was able to see their own hand. The two sessions (synchronous and asynchronous conditions) were conducted in a random order. Each session included four blocks of tactile stimulation (30 seconds) to invoke the RHI and four subsequent blocks of acupuncture stimulation (30 seconds) immediately after. A total of 240 volumes were acquired during each session for 480 seconds (Fig. 1B).

Induction of the rubber hand illusion and acupuncture stimulation. The participants were told to look at the rubber hand (Korean Prosthetic Limbs Research Institute), to not look elsewhere, and to not move any of their fingers during the experiment. Two small paintbrushes (approximately 2 cm in length) were used to stroke the rubber hand and the hidden real left hand of the participant at a frequency of 1 Hz for 180 seconds. This was done synchronously under one condition (synchronous condition) and asynchronously under the other condition (asynchronous condition).

Acupuncture stimulation was always applied at acupoint LI4 on the left hand by a licensed and experienced Doctor of Korean Medicine using non-magnetic titanium sterile acupuncture needles that were 40 mm long and 0.20 mm in diameter (DongBang Acupuncture Inc.; Boryeoung, Republic of Korea). All stimulations were administered according to the beat of a 1-Hz metronome transmitted via earphones. Following each trial, subjects were asked about their experience of the illusion via headphones in the scanner.

fMRI data acquisition. The fMRI scans were acquired with a MAGNETOM Trio 3 T scanner (Siemens, Erlangen, Germany) using echo planar imaging (EPI) with a 64×64 matrix (TE = 30 ms, TR = 2000 ms) across 37 slices with a thickness of 4 mm. To minimize movement artifacts, the head of each participant was fixed using a head holder. All scans were acquired by a well-trained professional operator. Each scan session contained 210 volumes of the whole brain in a 37 axial slice acquisition (TR = 2000 ms, TE = 30 ms, flip angle = 90°, field of view = 240×240 mm^2 , voxel size = 3.8×3.8×4.0 mm^3). As an anatomical reference, a 3-dimensional T1-weighted magnetization-prepared rapid gradient echo (MPRAGE) image data set was acquired using the following parameters: TR = 2000 ms, TE = 2.37 ms, flip angle = 9°, field of view = 240×240 mm^2 , voxel size = 0.9×0.9×1.0 mm^3 , 192 slices.

fMRI data analysis. Analysis of the fMRI data was performed using Statistical Parametric Mapping software (SPM8; Wellcome Institute of Imaging Neuroscience; London, UK) implemented in Matlab 7.1 (Mathworks Inc.; Natick, MA). The data were realigned and co-registered on a mean image, normalized to a template, and smoothed with an 8-mm full-width-at-half-maximum (FWHM) Gaussian kernel. The model was estimated by applying individual movement regressors.

The first four volumes of each session were discarded to allow for T1 equilibration. All the remaining functional images were corrected for slice acquisition timing and head motion. For each participant, the functional images were realigned to the first task-relevant image to correct for head motion and were co-registered to the structural T_1-weighted anatomical images. To decrease spatial noise, the images were spatially normalized using the Montreal Neurological Institute (MNI) template, resampled with an isotropic 2 mm×2 mm×2 mm voxel size, and smoothed with an 8-mm FWHM isotropic Gaussian kernel.

Each acupuncture stimulation was modeled as a boxcar function convolved with a canonical hemodynamic response function that began at the onset of each stimulation. Contrast maps were generated for brain reactivity to acupuncture stimulation, and the individual contrast images in each session were then included in a second-level random-effects analysis. Brain responses to acupuncture stimulation were recorded under both synchronous and asynchronous conditions. For statistical inference, a threshold of $P<0.05$ was used following a correction for multiple comparisons (family-wise error corrections, FWE). To plot the regions of brain activation associated with acupuncture stimulation, the neuronal activity in specific brain areas was correlated over time by extracting the averaged percent signal change in regions of interests (ROIs) separately in the common brain areas (i.e. insula and secondary somatosensory cortex (SII)). The anatomical ROIs for insula and SII were obtained using the Wake-Forest University PickAtlas tool box version 2.4 (WFU PickAtlas; [44]. Signal changes were extracted using the MarsBaR ROI toolbox for SPM8 (http://marsbar.sourceforge.net/).

A multiple regression analysis was conducted to evaluate the association of the contrast images to acupuncture stimulation between asynchronous and synchronous session with individual ratings as two separate covariate vectors (1) the differences of RHI score (synchronous – asynchronous session) and (2) the differences of *DeQi* score (asynchronous – synchronous session). For the regression analysis, activation was considered significant at $p < 0.001$ (uncorrected) with a minimum cluster extent threshold of 10 contiguous voxels.

Rubber hand illusion and self-reported DeQi sensation ratings. After finishing each session (synchronous and asynchronous), participants reported their perception of the RHI by answering question 3 on the RHI Perception Scale: "I felt as if the rubber hand were my hand" [9]. The participants also filled out the acupuncture-induced *DeQi* sensation questionnaire using a seven-point Likert scale ranging from "strongly disagree" (−3) to "strongly agree" (+3).

Data analysis. All values are expressed as means ± standard errors. RHI ratings, subjective *DeQi* ratings, and BOLD signal changes were compared between the synchronous and asynchronous sessions using paired *t*-tests. The level of significance was set at 0.05 for all analyses. Statistical analyses were performed using the Statistical Package for Social Sciences for Windows 20.0 (SPSS Inc.).

Results

Experiment 1

Changes in local blood flow following acupuncture stimulation during the RHI. Local blood flow measurements are presented as the mean PBF change over time. A significant difference was observed in the increase in local blood-flow change following acupuncture stimulation when the asynchronous and synchronous brush-stroking sessions were compared (18.6±3.3 vs. 9.3±2.8%, $t = 2.544$, $P<0.05$; Fig. 2). No significant differences were observed between the asynchronous and synchronous brush-stroke sessions in rotation frequency (degree of stimulation) or torque amplitude (biomechanical force) (frequency: 1.3±0.1 vs. 1.3±0.1 Hz, $t = -0.414$, $P>0.684$; torque: 15.4±5.0 vs. 13.8±4.2 μNm, $t = -0.295$ $P>0.771$, respectively).

Perception of the rubber hand illusion and self-reported DeQi sensation rating. We found a significant difference between the asynchronous and synchronous brush-stroke sessions in the self-reported perception of the RHI (−1.0±0.3 vs. 1.5±0.2, $t = 8.520$, $P<0.001$). No significant differences were observed in self-reported *DeQi* sensations when the asynchronous and synchronous brush-stroking sessions were compared (heaviness: 3.6±0.6 vs. 3.1±0.5, $t = 0.769$ $P>0.449$; soreness: 3.4±0.5 vs. 3.7±0.6, $t = 0.403$ $P>0.690$; numbness: 3.8±0.6 vs. 3.6±0.6, $t = 0.256$ $P>0.800$).

Experiment 2

Brain responses to acupuncture stimulation during the rubber hand illusion. Brain activations following acupuncture stimulation were observed in the contralateral secondary somatosensory cortex (SII) and insula under both the asynchronous (right SII: 44, −26, 26; $t = 11.52$; $Z = 5.9$; right insula: 44, 2, 8; $t = 9.78$; $Z = 5.5$) and synchronous (right SII: 50, −20, 20; $t = 9.33$; $Z = 5.39$; right insula: 56, 20, 0; $t = 8.9$; $Z = 5.27$) sessions (Table 1). All peaks are $p<0.05$, corrected, and all coordinates are in MNI space (Fig. 3A).

Comparison of asynchronous and synchronous sessions revealed that the brain responses following acupuncture stimulation were significantly altered in the insula during the RHI. Differences in signal change (less brain activation during the synchronous sessions) were significant in the right insula (0.32±0.04 vs. 0.23±0.05%, $t = 2.517$, $P<0.05$) but not in SII (0.34±0.05 versus 0.29±0.05%, $t = 1.413$, $P>0.177$; Fig. 3B).

Perception of the rubber hand illusion and self-reported DeQi sensation rating. In Experiment 2, a significant difference between the asynchronous and synchronous brush-stroking sessions was observed in the self-reported perception of the RHI (−0.6±0.4 vs. 0.9±0.3, $t = 4.622$, $P<0.001$). No significant differences were observed in self-reported *DeQi* sensation when comparing the asynchronous and synchronous brush-stroke sessions (1.6±0.4 vs. 2.2±0.2, $t = 1.830$, $P>0.086$).

Individual differences in rubber hand illusion score and *DeQi* score co-varied with brain activations to acupuncture stimulation during rubber hand illusion. We determined whether individual differences in RHI score (synchronous vs. asynchronous session) co-varied with functional brain activity responses to acupuncture stimulation (asynchronous vs. synchronous session). Higher RHI scores demonstrated significant co-variation with activities in the right ventral premotor cortex ($x = 52$, $y = 16$, $z = 26$, $Z = 3.34$, $r = 0.571$, $p<0.05$, Fig. 4A).

We also determined whether individual differences in *DeQi* score (asynchronous vs. synchronous session) co-varied with functional brain activity responses to acupuncture stimulation (asynchronous vs. synchronous session). Higher *DeQi* scores demonstrated significant co-variation with activities in the right posterior insula ($x = 46$, $y = -8$, $z = -10$, $Z = 4.38$, $r = 0.752$, $p< 0.001$, Fig. 4B).

Discussion

The current study demonstrated that a disrupted sense of body ownership induces significant changes in both local PBF and brain BOLD responses during acupuncture needle stimulation. Experiment 1 used LASER Doppler technology and found that the degree of increased blood flow around the site of acupuncture manipulation was significantly decreased when disembodiment (disrupted sense of body ownership) was induced in the same hand receiving the acupuncture stimulation. Experiment 2 used fMRI and found that brain activations following acupuncture stimulation were significantly reduced in the right insula when disembodiment was induced in the hand receiving the acupuncture stimulation. These findings suggest that body ownership is a crucial factor that influences physiological responses during acupuncture stimulation.

In Experiment 1, when body ownership and bodily self-awareness were preserved in a normal way (asynchronous session), an increase in PBF was observed during acupuncture stimulation (Fig. 2). These findings are consistent with previous studies that reported enhanced microcirculatory blood flow near the acupoints following acupuncture stimulation [16,17]. In contrast, when body ownership was disrupted (synchronous sessions), a significant decrease in peripheral microcirculation was observed around acupoint LI4 relative to asynchronous session. These findings indicate that the peripheral physiological responses following acupuncture stimulation are influenced by modifications of body ownership, at least around the site of acupuncture stimulation (left hand). To assure that the differences in PBF following acupuncture stimulation were not derived from discrepancies in acupuncture

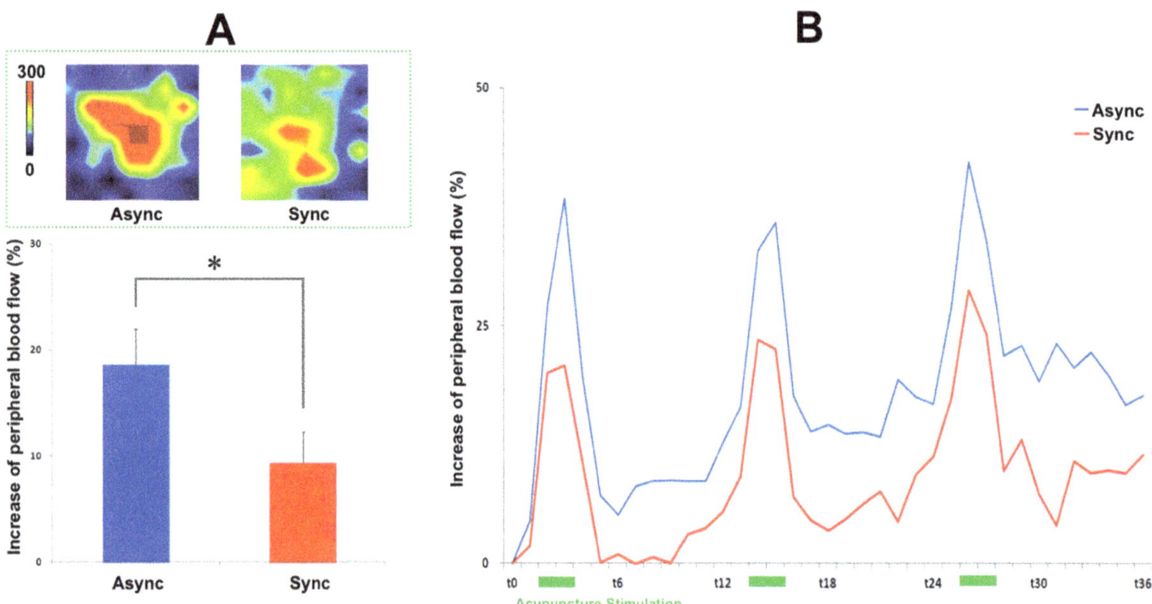

Figure 2. Peripheral responses to acupuncture stimulation during the RHI. A representative example of the peripheral responses to acupuncture stimulation around the LI4 acupoint (2×2 cm) is shown in upper column A. The increase in peripheral responses to acupuncture stimulation was significantly different between the synchronous and asynchronous brush-stroke sessions, as seen in lower column A (18.6±3.3 vs. 9.3±2.8%, $t=2.544$, $P<0.05$). Peripheral responses to acupuncture stimulation are presented as the mean peripheral blood-flow change over time. Values are means ± standard errors.

manipulations, the degree of and the biomechanical force behind the acupuncture manipulation were controlled for with force sensors. In our experiment, an experimenter conducted acupuncture manipulation immediately after he stroke both the rubber hand and the hidden real hand. In order to minimize a possible confounding factor in which a non-blinded acupuncturist could be biased to conduct acupuncture differently between the synchronous and the asynchronous sessions, we tried to make the acupuncturists conduct the manipulation using similar rotation frequencies, torques, and amplitudes during the acupuncture manipulation. The sensor measurements confirmed that there was no significant difference of the degree of stimulation (rotation frequency) and the biomechanical force (torque amplitude: rotation force) between the two sessions. Although unlikely given the professional training of the acupuncturist, we cannot exclude other possible bias to the outcome, such as tone of voice.

In Experiment 2, brain activations in the right insula and SII were observed in all sessions in which acupuncture stimulation was applied, whereas significant differences in BOLD signal change were observed only in the right insula when comparing synchronous and asynchronous brush-stroke sessions (Fig. 3). The common brain activations in the insula and SII in the both asynchronous and synchronous session were generally consistent with previous studies, which found that acupuncture stimulation leads to enhanced sensorimotor cortical network [20]. The observation of less activity in the right insula following acupuncture stimulation during the induction of the RHI (synchronous sessions) is noteworthy. The insula is known to generally modulate awareness of pain, temperature, sensual touch, and other bodily feelings using cutaneous mechanoreceptive stimuli [45]. It has often been suggested that the insular cortex is a unique neural substrate that instantiates subjective feelings from the body and feelings of emotion in the immediate present, which is highlighted by the central role of this area in "interoception" and "awareness of bodily signals" [46].

Table 1. Activated brain regions to acupuncture stimulation in asynchronous session and synchronous session (n = 17).

Activated regions	**MNI Coordinates**			**Peak *t***	***p* value (FWE corrected)**	**Cluster size**
	X	**Y**				
Async						
(R) Insula	44	2	8	9.78	<0.05	106
(R) SII	44	−26	26	11.52	<0.05	200
Sync						
(R) Insula	56	20	0	8.9	<0.05	36
(R) SII	50	−20	20	9.33	<0.05	59

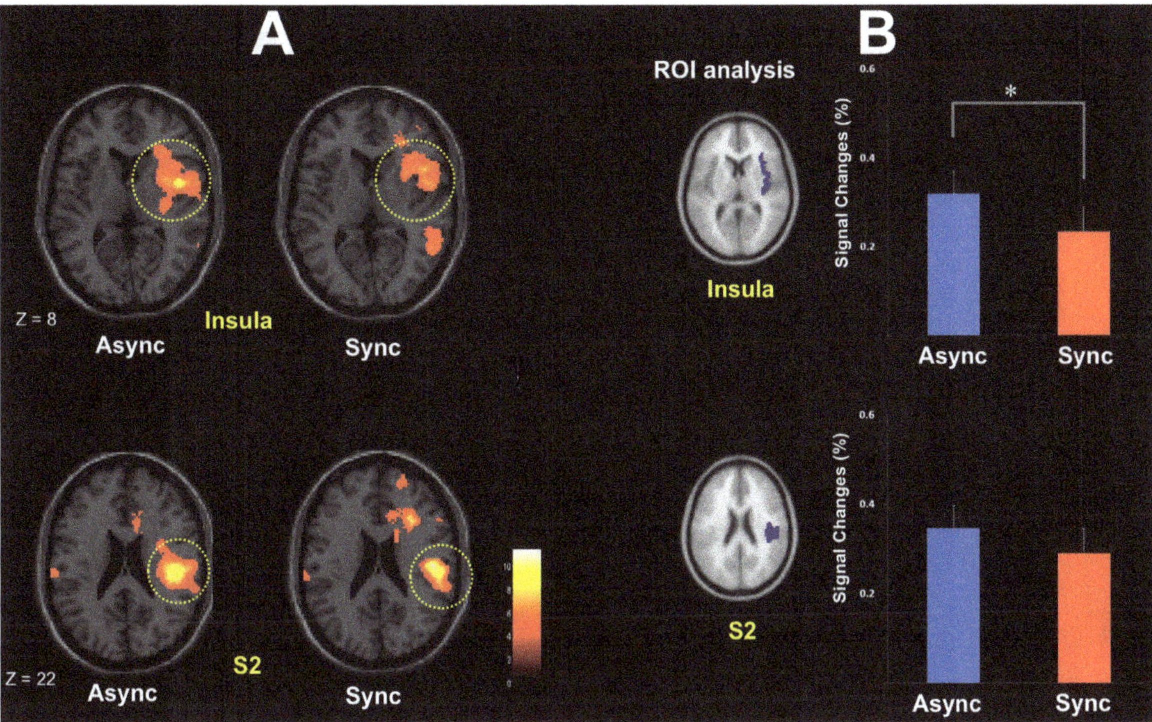

Figure 3. Brain activations in response to acupuncture stimulation. A: Brain activations in response to acupuncture stimulations were observed in the contralateral secondary somatosensory cortex (SII) and insula under both the asynchronous (right SII: 44, −26, 26; $t = 11.52$; $Z = 5.9$; right insula: 44, 2, 8; $t = 9.78$; $Z = 5.5$) and synchronous (right SII: 50, −20, 20; $t = 9.33$; $Z = 5.39$; right insula: 56, 20, 0; $t = 8.9$; $Z = 5.27$) conditions. All two peaks were $p<0.05$, corrected, and all coordinates are in MNI space. B: To plot the regions of brain activation involved in acupuncture stimulation, the averaged percent signal change in anatomical regions of interests (ROIs), including the right insula and SII, were extracted. When the acupuncture stimulation occurred, BOLD responses in the right insula (0.32±0.04 vs. 0.23±0.05%, $t = 2.517$, $P<0.05$; A) but not the SII (0.34±0.05 vs. 0.29±0.05%, $t = 1.413$, $P>0.177$; B) differed significantly under the asynchronous and synchronous sessions.

With the multiple regression analyses, we demonstrated differences in neural substrates for subjective ratings from the RHI and the *DeQi* sensation. Firstly, the RHI scores significantly correlated with the brain activations to acupuncture stimulation (asynchronous vs. synchronous session) in the ventral premotor cortex (Fig. 4A). Ventral premotor cortex has been shown to play a crucial role in multisensory integration in the context of the RHI [12,47]. Previous studies have demonstrated that neural activity in the premotor cortex was correlated with the strength of illusory perceptions during the RHI [12], and damages in fibers connecting the ventral premotor cortex with other brain regions impaired the occurrence of RHI sensations [47]. It is therefore likely that the different brain responses in premotor cortex responding to the acupuncture stimulation between asynchronous and synchronous condition were much more associated with the degrees of the RHI across the subjects. Secondly, the difference of *DeQi* sensation significantly correlated with the brain activations to acupuncture stimulation (asynchronous vs. synchronous session) in the posterior insula in the current study (Fig. 4B). The insula, as a key structure of the interoceptive system, has been studied in relation to acupuncture treatment under some conditions [35,39]. It is assumed that the differential brain responses in the posterior insula in response to acupuncture stimulation between the two sessions were reflected in the substantial variability between subjects in the change of *DeQi* sensation.

The phenomenal incorporation of the rubber hand is also reflected by brain activation in the insula, which can be explained by its association with the basic processes of self-consciousness [14]. Previous fMRI and positron emission tomography (PET) studies have observed brain activations in the insula when comparing BOLD responses during real acupuncture and sham (placebo) acupuncture stimulation. This suggests that enhanced bodily attention following acupuncture may operate as a therapeutic mechanism under some conditions [35,39]. Taken together, these findings indicate that bodily self-awareness plays a central role during acupuncture treatment and that modifications of body ownership may disturb the function of acupuncture as a somatosensory-guided mind-body therapy via modulation of the interoceptive system that is represented by the insula. Further studies using sham-acupuncture are needed to address this issue in detail.

Our results suggest important implications for acupuncture research. In East Asian cultures, acupuncture stimulation is frequently employed for various clinical treatments, and the concept of *Qi* is often used to describe a distinct kind of bodily perception that explains how people feel, control, and experience their own sense of self. Achievement of appropriate *DeQi* sensation is considered to be vital for acupuncture treatment. It is thought that such perceived needling-induced sensations not only direct patients' attention to the specific points on the body, but that they also modulate cognitive and affective aspects [20,38]. In fact, certain components ascribed to the *DeQi* sensation, or perceived *Qi* during acupuncture treatment, may share the characteristics of particular aspects of "bodily self-awareness" because feeling and the perception of oneself are crucial components of both. Recently, aspects of "bodily awareness" have been increasingly attracting the interest of researchers in many disciplines [48]. Studies in the fields of neuroscience and neurology have shown

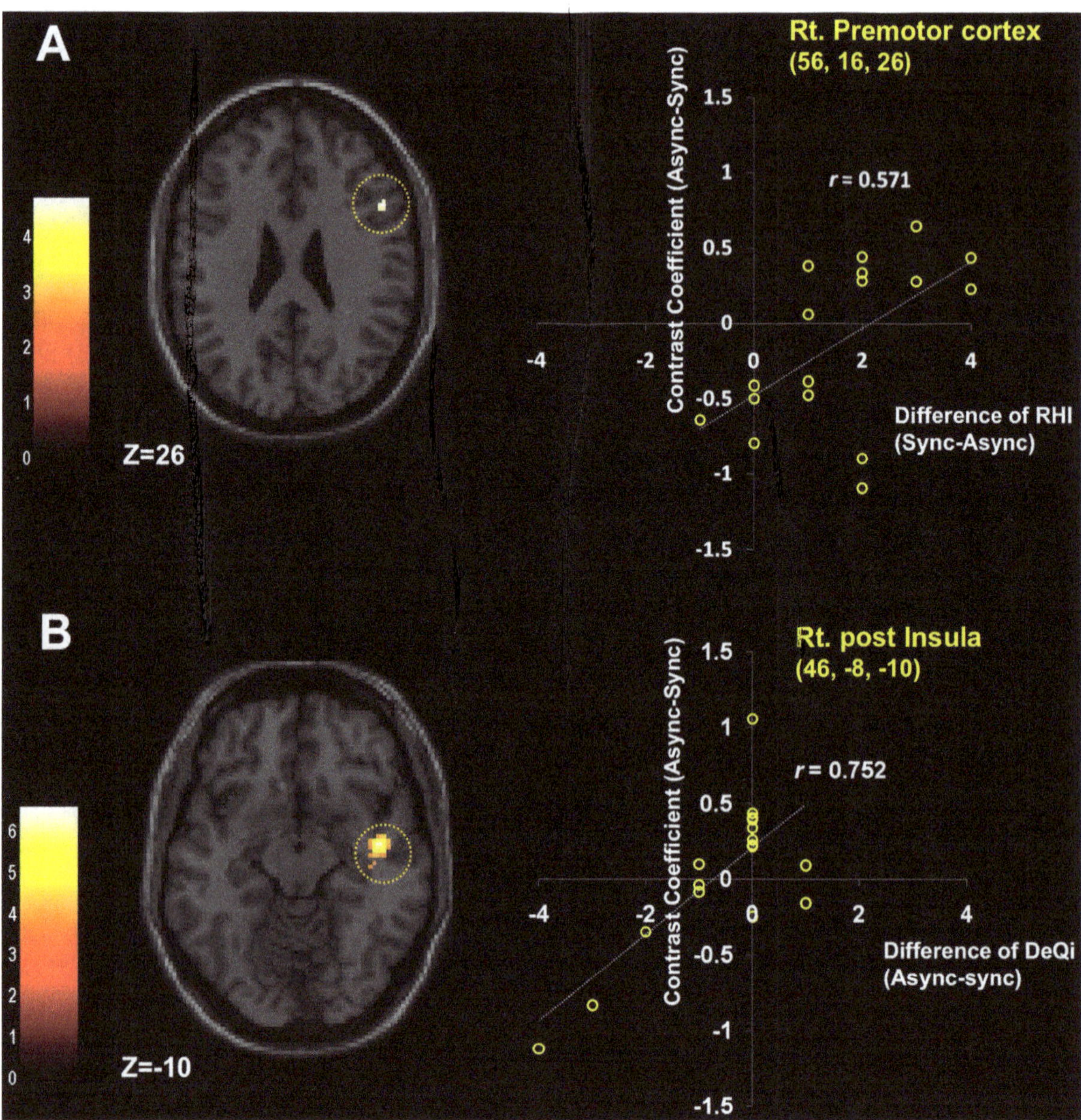

Figure 4. Individual differences in brain activations to acupuncture stimulation. A: Correlation between rubber hand illusion score and brain activations to acupuncture stimulation during reduced body ownership. Normalized SPM T-maps overlaid on the corresponding axial T1-weighted images showing statistically significant ($p<0.001$, uncorrected with 10 continuous voxels) brain activation correlations between the rubber hand illusion (synchronous vs. asynchronous session) and brain responses to acupuncture stimulation in asynchronous condition compared to synchronous condition. Brain activation was observed in the right ventral premotor cortex ($x=52$, $y=16$, $z=26$, $Z=3.34$, $r=0.571$, $p<0.05$). B: Correlation between *DeQi* score and brain activations to acupuncture stimulation during reduced body ownership. Brain activation related to *DeQi* score (asynchronous vs. synchronous session) was observed in the right posterior insula ($x=46$, $y=-8$, $z=-10$, $Z=4.38$, $r=0.752$, $p<0.001$).

that the conscious sense of one's physical self is closely linked to the physiological regulation of one's physical self [3,7]. It has also been shown that any disruption in the awareness of one's physical self can have an important impact on the physiological regulation of the self [6]. It has been suggested that a body matrix, or a multisensory representation of peri-personal space and the space directly around the body, serves to maintain the integrity of the body at both the homeostatic and psychological levels and allows for the adaptation of our body structure and orientation to changes in the environment [2]. Findings demonstrating that components of this bodily self-awareness are also involved in the modulation of the clinical effects of acupuncture may have important implications for acupuncture research. Mohan et al. have failed to demonstrate that the RHI modulate pain threshold or pain evoked by individually calibrated high and low painful stimuli delivered on the real arm [49]. Our previous study also found no significant differences in self-reported pain rating to acupuncture stimulation between the asynchronous and the synchronous session [36]. In the current study, we found no significant differences of subjective *DeQi* ratings between the two sessions. Even though there were two different characteristics of acupuncture sensations, such as the pain domain and *DeQi* domain [41], our findings are partially supporting the previous findings that there were no differences of pain ratings during the

RHI [36,49]. Although we did not find significant differences of subjective *DeQi* ratings between the two sessions, differences of brain activations to acupuncture stimulation in the posterior insula was associated with the difference of *DeQi* sensation *between the two sessions* in the current study. It is believed that the insula plays a crucial role in the enhanced body awareness on the specific body site by acupuncture evoked-*DeQi* sensation. Further studies are needed to determine whether reduced embodiment around the acupuncture points during RHI can affect the *DeQi* sensation and/or clinical outcome.

Still, our study possesses several limitations. First, as we did not implement a 2×2 (Body ownership×Intervention) factorial design using a tactile control (such as a non-penetrating placebo needle), we cannot claim that bodily self-awareness is a crucial factor influencing physiological responses that is restricted only to acupuncture stimulation. The rationale for not conducting such a control lies in the difficulty of providing non-penetrating sham acupuncture. Such needles are commonly used as a placebo control for acupuncture experiments [50]. In our previous study, we demonstrated specific patterns of brain activations related to genuine acupuncture compared to sham acupuncture, i.e. non-penetrating placebo needles [15,31]. As such a needle relies on the visual impression that a real needle is being inserted to the skin, however, researchers have claimed that its validity is limited when using such placebo acupuncture out of sight of the participant [51]. Given that participants in the present study can only see the rubber hand in front of them and are not able to see their own hand, a non-penetrating placebo needle would not work well as a placebo control stimulation. Further studies are necessary in order to explore the role of body ownership specific to acupuncture stimulation when compared to other types of tactile stimulation. Second, the acupuncture needle was inserted into only the real hand in experiment 1. In order to minimize visual differences between the rubber hand and the real hand, on the other hand, we performed experiment 2 with the acupuncture needle inserted into the real hand as well as in the rubber hand. In our previous study, the sympathetic activations to acupuncture stimulation in the real hand were markedly higher during the synchronous session compared to that of the asynchronous session only when a visual expectation of the acupuncture needle stimulation existed in the rubber hand [36]. In this case, it is assumed that the participants seemed to have already allowed the incorporation of the artificial body part into their self-representation, and can experience an additional "visual capture" of the acupuncture needling. Future research will be needed to investigate the role of the visual factor of the acupuncture needle in the rubber hand during reduced body ownership. Last but not at least, we did not include a control condition in which a rubber hand was not displayed. It is well established that some participants can still feel a sense of embodiment or ownership towards the rubber hand even without any touch. In order to minimize other confounding factor, such as touch, we were trying to compare the physiological changes of acupuncture between asynchronous and synchronous session in this study. As we did not examine the physiological responses to acupuncture in a third condition without the rubber hand, however, we cannot explicitly analyze the role of the visual factor provided by the artificial hand in our experiments.

The current study demonstrates that both local blood flow changes and brain responses following acupuncture needle stimulation are altered by modifications of body ownership. When body ownership was disrupted by the RHI during acupuncture treatment, local blood flow to the site of acupuncture stimulation was reduced and brain activations during acupuncture stimulation were significantly decreased in the insula, a key region involved in the interoceptive system. Acupuncture can be regarded as a complex treatment comprised of multimodal sensory stimulation that interacts with various factors, including bodily self-awareness [36,37]. These findings suggest that physiological responses during acupuncture stimulation can be influenced by the modification of body ownership. Further research is necessary to ascertain whether the clinical effects of acupuncture are associated with enhanced bodily self-awareness and, if so, how strongly.

Author Contributions

Conceived and designed the experiments: YC CW. Performed the experiments: YC ISL WMJ. Analyzed the data: ISL YC. Contributed reagents/materials/analysis tools: HL HJP. Contributed to the writing of the manuscript: VN DSC YC.

References

1. Lopez C, Halje P, Blanke O (2008) Body ownership and embodiment: vestibular and multisensory mechanisms. Neurophysiol Clin 38: 149–161.
2. Moseley GL, Gallace A, Spence C (2012) Bodily illusions in health and disease: physiological and clinical perspectives and the concept of a cortical body matrix'. Neurosci Biobehav Rev 36: 34–46.
3. Gallagher II (2000) Philosophical conceptions of the self: implications for cognitive science. Trends Cogn Sci 4: 14–21.
4. Newport R, Pearce R, Preston C (2010) Fake hands in action: embodiment and control of supernumerary limbs. Exp Brain Res 204: 385–395.
5. Herbert BM, Pollatos O (2012) The body in the mind: on the relationship between interoception and embodiment. Top Cogn Sci 4: 692–704.
6. Moseley GL, Olthof N, Venema A, Don S, Wijers M, et al. (2008) Psychologically induced cooling of a specific body part caused by the illusory ownership of an artificial counterpart. Proc Natl Acad Sci U S A 105: 13169–13173.
7. Tsakiris M (2010) My body in the brain: a neurocognitive model of body-ownership. Neuropsychologia 48: 703–712.
8. Folegatti A, de Vignemont F, Pavani F, Rossetti Y, Farne A (2009) Losing one's hand: visual-proprioceptive conflict affects touch perception. PLoS One 4: e6920.
9. Botvinick M, Cohen J (1998) Rubber hands feel' touch that eyes see. Nature 391: 756.
10. Makin TR, Holmes NP, Ehrsson HH (2008) On the other hand: dummy hands and peripersonal space. Behav Brain Res 191: 1–10.
11. Barnsley N, McAuley JH, Mohan R, Dey A, Thomas P, et al. (2011) The rubber hand illusion increases histamine reactivity in the real arm. Curr Biol 21: R945–946.
12. Ehrsson HH, Spence C, Passingham RE (2004) That's my hand! Activity in premotor cortex reflects feeling of ownership of a limb. Science 305: 875–877.
13. Ehrsson HH, Wiech K, Weiskopf N, Dolan RJ, Passingham RE (2007) Threatening a rubber hand that you feel is yours elicits a cortical anxiety response. Proc Natl Acad Sci U S A 104: 9828–9833.
14. Tsakiris M, Hesse MD, Boy C, Haggard P, Fink GR (2007) Neural signatures of body ownership: a sensory network for bodily self-consciousness. Cereb Cortex 17: 2235–2244.
15. Chae Y, Lee H, Kim H, Sohn H, Park JH, et al. (2009) The neural substrates of verum acupuncture compared to non-penetrating placebo needle: an fMRI study. Neurosci Lett 450: 80–84.
16. Hsiu H, Hsu WC, Hsu CL, Huang SM (2011) Assessing the effects of acupuncture by comparing needling the hegu acupoint and needling nearby nonacupoints by spectral analysis of microcirculatory laser Doppler signals. Evid Based Complement Alternat Med 2011: 435928.
17. Uchida S, Hotta H (2008) Acupuncture affects regional blood flow in various organs. Evid Based Complement Alternat Med 5: 145–151.
18. Dhond RP, Kettner N, Napadow V (2007) Neuroimaging acupuncture effects in the human brain. J Altern Complement Med 13: 603–616.
19. Fang J, Jin Z, Wang Y, Li K, Kong J, et al. (2009) The salient characteristics of the central effects of acupuncture needling: limbic-paralimbic-neocortical network modulation. Hum Brain Mapp 30: 1196–1206.
20. Chae Y, Chang DS, Lee SH, Jung WM, Lee IS, et al. (2013) Inserting needles into the body: a meta-analysis of brain activity associated with acupuncture needle stimulation. J Pain 14: 215–222.
21. Huang W, Pach D, Napadow V, Park K, Long X, et al. (2012) Characterizing acupuncture stimuli using brain imaging with FMRI–a systematic review and meta-analysis of the literature. PLoS One 7: e32960.

22. Kong J, Kaptchuk TJ, Webb JM, Kong JT, Sasaki Y, et al. (2009) Functional neuroanatomical investigation of vision-related acupuncture point specificity-a multisession fMRI study. Hum Brain Mapp 30: 38–46.
23. Liu H, Xu JY, Li L, Shan BC, Nie BB, et al. (2013) FMRI evidence of acupoints specificity in two adjacent acupoints. Evid Based Complement Alternat Med 2013: 932581.
24. Asghar AU, Green G, Lythgoe MF, Lewith G, MacPherson H (2009) Acupuncture needling sensation: the neural correlates of deqi using fMRI. Brain Res 1315: 111–118.
25. Hui KK, Marina O, Liu J, Rosen BR, Kwong KK (2010) Acupuncture, the limbic system, and the anticorrelated networks of the brain. Auton Neurosci 157: 81–90.
26. Hui KK, Nixon EE, Vangel MG, Liu J, Marina O, et al. (2007) Characterization of the "deqi" response in acupuncture. BMC Complement Altern Med 7: 33.
27. Dougherty DD, Kong J, Webb M, Bonab AA, Fischman AJ, et al. (2008) A combined [11C]diprenorphine PET study and fMRI study of acupuncture analgesia. Behav Brain Res 193: 63–68.
28. Harris RE, Zubieta JK, Scott DJ, Napadow V, Gracely RH, et al. (2009) Traditional Chinese acupuncture and placebo (sham) acupuncture are differentiated by their effects on mu-opioid receptors (MORs). Neuroimage 47: 1077–1085.
29. Napadow V, LaCount L, Park K, As-Sanie S, Clauw DJ, et al. (2010) Intrinsic brain connectivity in fibromyalgia is associated with chronic pain intensity. Arthritis Rheum 62: 2545–2555.
30. Zhang WT, Jin Z, Huang J, Zhang L, Zeng YW, et al. (2003) Modulation of cold pain in human brain by electric acupoint stimulation: evidence from fMRI. Neuroreport 14: 1591–1596.
31. Chae Y, Lee H, Kim H, Kim CH, Chang DI, et al. (2009) Parsing brain activity associated with acupuncture treatment in Parkinson's diseases. Mov Disord 24: 1794–1802.
32. Kong J, Kaptchuk TJ, Polich G, Kirsch I, Vangel M, et al. (2009) Expectancy and treatment interactions: a dissociation between acupuncture analgesia and expectancy evoked placebo analgesia. Neuroimage 45: 940–949.
33. Kong J, Kaptchuk TJ, Polich G, Kirsch I, Vangel M, et al. (2009) An fMRI study on the interaction and dissociation between expectation of pain relief and acupuncture treatment. Neuroimage 47: 1066–1076.
34. Lee J, Napadow V, Kim J, Lee S, Choi W, et al. (2014) Phantom acupuncture: dissociating somatosensory and cognitive/affective components of acupuncture stimulation with a novel form of placebo acupuncture. PLoS One 9: e104582.
35. Napadow V, Dhond RP, Kim J, LaCount L, Vangel M, et al. (2009) Brain encoding of acupuncture sensation-coupling on-line rating with fMRI. Neuroimage 47: 1055–1065.
36. Chang DS, Kim YJ, Lee SH, Lee H, Lee IS, et al. (2013) Modifying Bodily Self-Awareness during Acupuncture Needle Stimulation Using the Rubber Hand Illusion. Evid Based Complement Alternat Med 2013: 849602.
37. Langevin HM, Wayne PM, Macpherson H, Schnyer R, Milley RM, et al. (2011) Paradoxes in acupuncture research: strategies for moving forward. Evid Based Complement Alternat Med 2011: 180805.
38. Liu T (2009) Acupuncture: what underlies needle administration? Evid Based Complement Alternat Med 6: 185–193.
39. Pariente J, White P, Frackowiak RS, Lewith G (2005) Expectancy and belief modulate the neuronal substrates of pain treated by acupuncture. Neuroimage 25: 1161–1167.
40. Davis RT, Churchill DL, Badger GJ, Dunn J, Langevin HM (2012) A new method for quantifying the needling component of acupuncture treatments. Acupunct Med 30: 113–119.
41. Park H, Park J, Lee H (2002) Does Deqi (needle sensation) exist? Am J Chin Med 30: 45–50.
42. Choi YJ, Lee JE, Moon WK, Cho SH (2013) Does the effect of acupuncture depend on needling sensation and manipulation? Complement Ther Med 21: 207–214.
43. Kang OS, Chang DS, Lee MH, Lee H, Park HJ, et al. (2011) Autonomic and subjective responses to real and sham acupuncture stimulation. Auton Neurosci 159: 127–130.
44. Maldjian JA, Laurienti PJ, Kraft RA, Burdette JH (2003) An automated method for neuroanatomic and cytoarchitectonic atlas-based interrogation of fMRI data sets. Neuroimage 19: 1233–1239.
45. Craig AD (2003) Interoception: the sense of the physiological condition of the body. Curr Opin Neurobiol 13: 500–505.
46. Craig AD (2009) How do you feel–now? The anterior insula and human awareness. Nat Rev Neurosci 10: 59–70.
47. Zeller D, Gross C, Bartsch A, Johansen-Berg H, Classen J (2011) Ventral premotor cortex may be required for dynamic changes in the feeling of limb ownership: a lesion study. J Neurosci 31: 4852–4857.
48. Mehling WE, Gopisetty V, Daubenmier J, Price CJ, Hecht FM, et al. (2009) Body awareness: construct and self-report measures. PLoS One 4: e5614.
49. Mohan R, Jensen KB, Petkova VI, Dey A, Barnsley N, et al. (2012) No pain relief with the rubber hand illusion. PLoS One 7: e52400.
50. Dincer F, Linde K (2003) Sham interventions in randomized clinical trials of acupuncture-a review. Complement Ther Med 11: 235–242.
51. Tsukayama H, Yamashita H, Kimura T, Otsuki K (2006) Factors that influence the applicability of sham needle in acupuncture trials: two randomized, single-blind, crossover trials with acupuncture-experienced subjects. Clin J Pain 22: 346–349.

Effects of Acupuncture at GV20 and ST36 on the Expression of Matrix Metalloproteinase 2, Aquaporin 4, and Aquaporin 9 in Rats Subjected to Cerebral Ischemia/ Reperfusion Injury

Hong Xu[a], **Yamin Zhang**[a], **Hua Sun***, **Suhui Chen**, **Fuming Wang**

Department of Traditional Chinese Medicine, Peking Union Medical College Hospital (PUMCH), Peking Union Medical College (PUMC), Chinese Academy of Medical Sciences, Beijing, China

Abstract

Background/Purpose: Ischemic stroke is characterized by high morbidity and mortality worldwide. Matrix metalloproteinase 2 (MMP2), aquaporin (AQP) 4, and AQP9 are linked to permeabilization of the blood-brain barrier (BBB) in cerebral ischemia/reperfusion injury (CIRI). BBB disruption, tissue inflammation, and MMP/AQP upregulation jointly provoke brain edema/swelling after CIRI, while acupuncture and electroacupuncture can alleviate CIRI symptoms. This study evaluated the hypothesis that acupuncture and electroacupuncture can similarly exert neuroprotective actions in a rat model of middle cerebral artery occlusion (MCAO) by modulating MMP2/AQP4/APQ9 expression and inflammatory cell infiltration.

Methods: Eighty 8-week-old Sprague-Dawley rats were randomly divided into sham group S, MCAO model group M, acupuncture group A, electroacupuncture group EA, and edaravone group ED. The MCAO model was established by placement of a suture to block the middle carotid artery, and reperfusion was triggered by suture removal in all groups except group S. Acupuncture and electroacupuncture were administered at acupoints GV20 (governing vessel-20) and ST36 (stomach-36). Rats in groups A, EA, and ED received acupuncture, electroacupuncture, or edaravone, respectively, immediately after MCAO. Neurological function (assessed using the Modified Neurological Severity Score), infarct volume, MMP2/AQP4/AQP9 mRNA and protein expression, and inflammatory cell infiltration were all evaluated at 24 h post-reperfusion.

Results: Acupuncture and electroacupuncture significantly decreased infarct size and improved neurological function. Furthermore, target mRNA and protein levels and inflammatory cell infiltration were significantly reduced in groups A, EA, and ED vs. group M. However, MMP2/AQP levels and inflammatory cell infiltration were generally higher in groups A and EA than in group ED except MMP2 mRNA levels.

Conclusions: Acupuncture and electroacupuncture at GV20 and ST36 both exercised neuroprotective actions in a rat model of MCAO, with no clear differences between groups A and EA. Therefore, acupuncture and electroacupuncture might find utility as adjunctive and complementary treatments to supplement conventional therapy for ischemic stroke.

Editor: Thiruma V. Arumugam, National University of Singapore, Singapore

Funding: This work was supported by: 1. The National Natural Science Foundation of China (No. 81273850) http://www.nsfc.gov.cn/. 2. Peking Union Medical College Hospital (No. 2010150 http://www.pumch.cn/. The funders had no role in study design, data collection and analysis, decision to publish, or preparation of the manuscript.

Competing Interests: The authors have declared that no competing interests exist.

* E-mail: sunhuahe@vip.sina.com

[a] These authors contributed equally to this work.

Introduction

Ischemic stroke accounts for more than 80% of all stroke cases and has a high morbidity and mortality worldwide [1,2]. Reperfusion damage occurs when blood returns to the brain after a period of ischemia, continuing even after blood flow is restored [3]. Accordingly, reperfusion occupies an important position in the pathophysiology of cerebral ischemia [4], and many pathological events are associated with cerebral ischemia/reperfusion injury (CIRI). These events encompass inflammation, increased production of reactive oxygen species, blood-brain barrier (BBB) disruption, brain edema, necrosis, and apoptosis.

Inflammation in CIRI is characterized by the rapid activation of resident microglia and the infiltration of inflammatory cells, including myeloperoxidase (MPO)$^+$ neutrophils, cluster of differentiation (CD) 68$^+$ monocytes/macrophages, and leukocytes. In the early stages of ischemic stroke (hours to days), proinflammatory mediators (e.g., cytokines and matrix metalloproteinases (MMPs)) are released by resident microglia and infiltrating cells [5]. Infiltrating leukocytes release interleukin-1β, tumor necrosis factor-α, and interleukin-6, and infiltrating macrophages and neutrophils join leukocytes to induce/activate MMPs. Cerebral inflammatory responses are then amplified by the actions of cytokines and MMPs, the disruption of the BBB, and the development of brain edema [5].

The BBB crucially contributes to brain homeostasis [6] and is mostly formed by the endothelial cells of the microvasculature. The BBB facilitates selective, diffusion-mediated exchange of membrane-permeant molecules between the circulating blood and the central nervous system, and in this manner protects the brain from extraneous compounds and neurotoxic substances. Microvessel endothelial cells are connected to each other, to surrounding pericytes, and to the foot processes of astrocytes by tight junctions. These cells work together to uphold normal BBB function.

The composition and structure of the BBB includes many factors that either maintain or disturb the fluid balance in the brain during normal and pathological processes. For example, astrocytes secrete the pro-ischemic mediator, transforming growth factor-β, during pathological processes such as CIRI; transforming growth factor-β then goes on to affect the function of various cell types in the ischemic brain [7]. Ischemic stroke is similarly associated with the activation of tissue plasminogen activator, a serine protease, and the generation of thrombomodulin, an anticoagulant [8]. Furthermore, the structure and function of the vascular basement membrane/extracellular matrix [9,10], and the expression levels of aquaporin (AQP) water channels in astrocytes and endothelial cells [11], are altered during ischemic brain injury and disease. Based on these pathophysiological changes and the identified molecular targets, many directed anti-stroke therapies are now under investigation to prevent destruction of the BBB. Of the potential molecular targets, the MMPs and the AQPs form the predominant focus of our study.

MMPs belong to a family of Zn^{2+}-dependent enzymes that degrade and re-establish the extracellular matrix during normal development and growth. MMPs are also implicated in BBB permeabilization and destruction [12]. During ischemic stroke, oxygen deficiency secondary to the obstruction of blood flow precipitates the inflammatory response and the upregulation of MMPs, also termed gelatinases. MMPs/gelatinases can activate numerous proinflammatory agents, disrupt the BBB, and provoke encephaledema and cerebral hemorrhage [13]. Among the MMPs, MMP2 plays an especially important role in sustaining the water balance of the brain and is commonly present on the foot processes of astrocytes and in the extracellular matrix of vascular endothelial cells.

AQPs are mostly present on brain vessels and astrocytic endfeet around lateral ventricle and ependymal cells. AQPs (AQP4 and AQP9), like MMPs, critically participate in the destruction of the BBB after CIRI, and AQP4 deficiency reportedly attenuates acute ischemic injury by reducing brain edema in acute focal cerebral ischemia [14]. Interestingly, MMPs and AQP4 expression levels seem to be co-regulated in the modulation of water homeostasis. For example, when MMPs were upregulated during CIRI-related inflammatory processes, the concomitant overexpression of AQP4 in astrocyte endfeet "OAPs" (orthogonal arrays of particles) led to particle disruption, BBB destruction, and ensuing brain edema [15].

The function of QAP-9 is very similar to QAP-4. They are both observed in astrocytes and vascular endothelial cells after stroke, and the expression of the two proteins coincides with the accumulation of water and other small solutes [16,17]. These observations suggest that AQP-4 and AQP-9 cooperatively induce brain edema by acting as conduits to accelerate water transport between fluid compartments across the BBB and into the brain.

So far, only one drug has been approved for the treatment of ischemic stroke: the aforementioned tissue plasminogen activator, a thrombolytic agent. Unfortunately, the use of thrombolytic agents is controversial due to the increased risk of hemorrhage and neuronal death, prompting a search for safer and more efficacious ways to manage ischemic stroke. To this end, recent evidence suggests that acupuncture could be useful for the management of CIRI. Acupuncture is an alternative therapy that complements conventional medicine. Acupuncture was derived at least 2,500 years ago as an ancient Chinese treatment for illness, pain, and metabolic and pathological brain diseases. Many acupoints can be chosen for therapy, including Renzhong (governing vessel-6, GV6), Baihui (GV20), Zusanli (stomach-36, ST36), and Waiguan (triple energizer-5, TE5). Electrical stimulation in the form of electroacupuncture is usually applied to one or more acupoints for the treatment of ischemic stroke in China, enhancing the therapeutic effects of acupuncture alone. Acupuncture has recently been used to accelerate the rehabilitation of patients with brain ischemia, but its mechanism(s) of action and the added benefit of electrical stimulation for stroke remain unclear.

Our previous work indicated that electroacupuncture at GV20 and ST36 can improve neurological outcomes in CIRI model rats, and also reduce inflammation and MMP9 expression in the brain [18,19]. The current study explored the hypothesis that acupuncture alone and electroacupuncture at GV20 and ST36 can similarly confer neuroprotection in a rat model of middle cerebral artery occlusion (MCAO) via attenuation of MMP2/AQP4/AQP9 expression and inflammatory cell infiltration in the ischemic brain. As a standard treatment for CIRI, the effects of edaravone, a free radical scavenger [20], were compared with those of acupuncture and electroacupuncture.

Materials and Methods

Ethics statement

All procedures were performed in accordance with the Ethics Committees of Peking Union Medical College Hospital (PUMCH, Beijing, China) and the Chinese Academy of Medical Sciences (Beijing, China), as well as the Guide for the Care and Use of Laboratory Animals (National Institutes of Health, Bethesda, MD, USA). All efforts were made to minimize animal suffering and the number of animals employed. In addition, the Ethics Committees of PUMCH and the Chinese Academy of Medical Sciences specifically approved this study (permit No. D-002).

Rat model of CIRI

Adult male Sprague-Dawley rats (n = 80) weighing 230–250 g were housed in an environmentally controlled room at PUMCH (22±2°C with a 12 h/12 h light/dark cycle). The rats were supplied with standard rat chow and water in ad libitum. Focal cerebral ischemia was induced by MCAO, as described previously [21] with slight modifications. Briefly, MCAO was performed using an occluding suture (diameter, 0.26 mm) for 2 h, as follows. Rats were anesthetized with 10% chloral hydrate (1001g/0.3 ml) via intraperitoneal injection. The cutaneous operational area was cleaned regularly, and a 2–3 cm incision was made in the skin of the neck. The right common carotid artery, the external carotid artery, and the internal carotid artery were isolated. The external carotid artery was ligated, blood flow was blocked, and a 4–0 monofilament with a blunted tip coated with poly-L-lysine was inserted into the internal carotid artery through the external carotid artery. The suture was advanced approximately 18–20 mm beyond the carotid artery bifurcation until the origin of the middle carotid artery was blocked. After 2 h of MCAO-evoked ischemia, the suture was slowly drawn back to allow reperfusion. Rectal temperature was maintained throughout the procedure at 37±0.5°C with a temperature-regulated heating pad.

Rat groups and treatments

Rats were randomly divided into the following five groups (n = 16 rats per group): (1) sham group S, (2) MCAO model group M, (3) acupuncture group A, (4) electroacupuncture group EA, and (5) edaravone group ED. Rats in model group M received MCAO for 2 h, followed by reperfusion for 24 h. Rats in sham group S received the same surgical procedures as those in model group M, but the suture was not advanced beyond the internal carotid bifurcation. No other treatments were given in sham group S and model group M.

Animals in treatment groups A, EA, and ED received the first treatment (acupuncture, electroacupuncture, or administration of edaravone, a free radical scavenger, respectively) after MCAO for 2 h. They were then given the second acupuncture, electroacupuncture, or edaravone treatment after 22 h of reperfusion and were euthanized 2 h later, for a total reperfusion time of 24 h in all five rat groups.

The rats in group A were given acupuncture therapy for 20 min at GV20 and left ST36 with disposable, sterile acupuncture needles (diameter, 0.32 mm; length 25 mm; Tianjin Huahong Medical Company, Tianjin, China). The needle was twisted 180 degrees at a rate of 100±5 twists per min for 1 min, with the twisting procedure repeated at 10-min intervals. Rats in group EA received acupuncture therapy at GV20 and left ST36 with disposable, sterile acupuncture needles and two electrodes (Changzhou Wujin Great Wall Medical Instrument Co., Ltd., Changzou, China), with the electrode handles conjoint on GV20 and left ST36. The rats then underwent simultaneous acupuncture and continuous-wave stimulation at a frequency of 2 Hz (intensity, 1 mA) for 20 min.

Finally, the rats in the ED group received 0.35 mg/kg of edaravone (Nanjing Simcere Dongyuan Pharmaceutical Co., Ltd., Nanjing, China) by intraperitoneal injection.

Evaluation of neurological function

At 24 h post-reperfusion, neurological function was assessed in eight animals (n = 8 per group) by an observer who was blinded to the experimental conditions. The evaluation of neurological function was performed using the Modified Neurological Severity Score (mNSS) testing approach [22]. The mNSS is composed of a series of motor tests (i.e., muscle status and abnormal movements), sensory tests (i.e., visual, tactile, and proprioceptive assessment), balance tests, and reflex tests, and is graded on a composite scale of 0–18. The higher the mNSS, the more severe the injury.

Assessment of infarct volume

After assessment of neurological function, rats (n = 3 per group) were narcotized by an intraperitoneal injection of 10% chloral hydrate (100 g/0.3 ml) and sacrificed by decapitation at 24 h after reperfusion. Brains were quickly removed and chilled at −20°C for 10 min. Five consecutive 2-mm coronal sections were then prepared, beginning from the anterior pole. The sections were immediately immersed in 0.1% 2, 3, 5-triphenyltetrazolium chloride (TTC; Sigma, St. Louis, MO, USA) prepared in phosphate buffered saline for 30 min at 37°C and fixed in 4% paraformaldehyde for 1 h. The TTC-stained sections were photographed, and the infarct area was measured by an observer blinded to the experimental conditions using image analysis software (ImageJ, National Institutes of Health). To account for edema and differential shrinkage resulting from tissue processing, the infarct volume percentage was calculated as: $[(V_C-V_L)/V_C] \times 100\%$, where V_C is the volume of the control contralateral hemisphere, and V_L is the volume of the non-infarcted tissue in the lesioned ipsilateral hemisphere [23].

Hematoxylin-eosin (H&E) staining

H&E histology was conducted at 24 h after reperfusion. Rats (n = 3 per group) were narcotized by an intraperitoneal injection of 10% chloral hydrate (100 g/0.3 ml) and then perfused transcardially with saline (250 ml), followed by 4% paraformaldehyde (250 ml). Brains were removed and fixed in 4% buffered paraformaldehyde at 4°C for 72 h, and then dehydrated and embedded in paraffin blocks. Coronal sections backward from the optic chiasma were cut at a thickness of 3 μm. The sections were deparaffinized and hydrated with decreasing concentrations of alcohol, stained with H&E, and photographed under a Leica DM400 microscope (Leica, Wetzlar, Germany).

Quantitative real-time polymerase chain reaction (qPCR)

Expression levels of MMP2, AQP4, and AQP9 mRNA were determined by qPCR. Total RNA was extracted from the lesion boundary zone of the ipsilateral hemisphere (n = 3 rats per group) using an RNeasy Mini Kit (Omega Bio-Tek, Norcross, GA, USA). Extracted total RNA was then reverse transcribed to generate cDNA. The reverse transcription reaction was amplified using a Bio-Rad CFX96 Detection System (Bio-Rad, Hercules, CA, USA) with the Plexor^{TM} One-Step qRT-PCR System (Promega, Madison, WI, USA). For MMP2, AQP4, and AQP9 amplification, the following primers were used: MMP2 forward, 5′-ACGCTGATGGCGAGTACTGCA-3′, and reverse, 5′-CCATGGTAAACAAGGCTTCGTG-3′; AQP4 forward, 5′-TCCTTTGGCCCTGCAGTTATC-3′, and reverse, 5′-AGGCTTCCTTTAGGCGACGTT-3′, and AQP9 forward, 5′-GGGTCCTATGATTGGTGCTTTC-3′, and reverse, 5′-CCCAGGATACTAACCACGAAAG-3′. The fold change in relative mRNA expression was determined using the $2^{-\Delta\Delta Ct}$ method [24] and glyceraldehyde 3-phosphate dehydrogenase (GADPH) as an internal control. For GAPDH amplification, the following primers were used: GADPH forward, 5′-CACAGCAAGTTCAACGGCACAG-3′, and reverse, 5′-GACGCCAGTAGACTCCACGACA-3′.

Immunofluorescence analysis

Brain tissue sections were prepared as described above for H&E staining (n = 6 rats per group). The sections were incubated with 3% hydrogen peroxide and 5% normal goat serum at room temperature for 30 min each, followed by incubation overnight at 4°C with mouse monoclonal anti-MMP2 antibody (diluted 1:150; Novus Biologicals, Littleton, CO, USA), mouse polyclonal anti-AQP4 antibody (diluted 1:50; Santa Cruz Biotechnology, Santa Cruz, CA, USA), rabbit polyclonal anti-glial fibrillary acidic (GFAP) antibody (diluted 1:500; Dako, Glostrup, Denmark), and rabbit polyclonal anti-CD34 antibody (diluted 1:200; Abcam, Cambridge, UK). The remaining procedures conformed to standard protocols. Images were captured under a Leica Axio Observer A1 fluorescence microscope.

Immunohistochemical analysis

Brain tissue sections were prepared as described above for H&E staining (n = 6 rats per group) and incubated overnight at 4°C with rabbit polyclonal anti-NeuN antibody (diluted 1:300; Millipore, Billerica, MA, USA), mouse monoclonal anti-MMP2 antibody (diluted 1:150; Novus Biologicals), rabbit polyclonal anti-AQP4 antibody (diluted 1:150; Abcam), rabbit polyclonal anti-AQP9

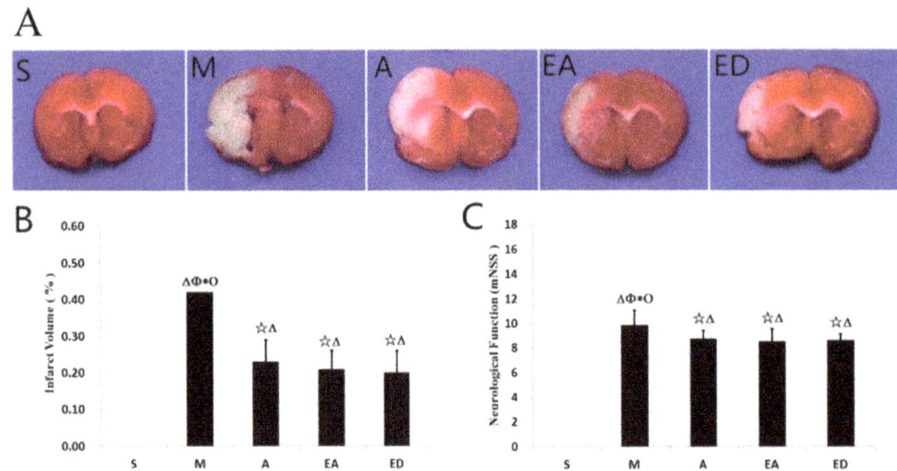

Figure 1. Evaluation of infarct volume and neurological scores in CIRI model rats. (A) TTC-stained brain sections showing the ischemic region (white) and the infarct area (red). (B) Infarct volume in the five experimental groups. (C) Neurological outcomes assessed by the mNSS. The three treatment groups (A, EA, and ED) demonstrated significant improvements in neurological function compared with MCAO model group M. Quantitative data (n = 8 animals per group) are given as the mean ± the SD. $^{\triangle}P<0.05$ vs. sham group S; $^{☆}P<0.05$ vs. MCAO model group M; $^{*}P<0.05$ vs. acupuncture group A; $^{\Phi}P<0.05$ vs. electroacupuncture group EA; $^{O}P<0.05$ vs. edaravone group ED.

antibody (diluted 1:50; Santa Cruz Biotechnology), goat polyclonal anti-MPO antibody (diluted 1:50; Santa Cruz Biotechnology), and mouse polyclonal anti-CD68 antibody (diluted 1:200; Abcam). The remaining procedures conformed to standard protocols. Brain sections were photographed under a Leica DM400 microscope and analyzed using Image J software for the semi-quantitative evaluation of the integrated optical density of MMP-2/AQP4/AQP9 labeling in the ischemic penumbra and the ischemic core zone. In addition, the numbers of MPO^{+} cells and $CD68^{+}$ cells were quantified in each 1-mm^2 area of the ischemic penumbra and the ischemic core zone.

Western blot analysis

The lesion boundary zone of the ischemic hemisphere (n = 4 rats per group) was dissected and homogenized in Radio-Immunoprecipitation Assay (RIPA) lysis buffer (Beyotime Biotechnology, Jiangsu, China), and total protein was separated by centrifugation at 13,000×g for 15 min at 4°C. Supernatants were harvested, and the protein concentration of each sample was determined using the bicinchoninic acid assay (Beyotime Biotechnology). For gel electrophoresis, samples were separated in 12% sodium dodecyl sulfate-polyacrylamide gels, and separated proteins were electrotransferred to polyvinylidene fluoride membranes (Millipore).

After transfer, the membranes were blocked for 2 h with 5% nonfat milk (BD-Becton, Dickinson and Company, San Antonio, TX, USA) and incubated overnight at 4°C with the following primary antibodies: mouse monoclonal anti-MMP2 antibody (diluted 1:500; Novus Biologicals), rabbit polyclonal anti-AQP4 antibody (diluted 1:2000; Abcam), and rabbit polyclonal anti-AQP9 antibody (diluted 1:300; Santa Cruz Biotechnology). Blots were also incubated with a primary antibody against β-actin (Santa Cruz Biotechnology), which was employed as an internal control for the normalization of protein loading. After three washes, the membranes were incubated for 2 h with species-specific horseradish peroxidase-conjugated secondary antibodies (diluted 1:5000; Jackson ImmunoResearch, Inc., West Grove, PA, USA). The immunoreactive protein bands were detected using an enhanced chemiluminescence kit (Millipore) and quantified using Labworks 4.6 image analysis software (UVP, LLC, Upland, CA, USA).

Statistical analysis

All quantitative data are expressed as the mean ± the standard deviation (SD) and were analyzed using SPSS (Statistical Package for the Social Sciences) 17.0 statistical analysis software (IBM, Chicago, IL, USA). The data were subjected to a one-way analysis of variance between different groups, followed by the least significant difference t-test. In all cases, $P<0.05$ was considered statistically significant. All final results were analyzed by observers blinded to the experimental conditions.

Results

Assessment of infarct volume in CIRI model rats

Infarct volume as a measure of stroke severity was first determined in the five rat groups (sham group S, MCAO model group M, acupuncture group A, electroacupuncture group EA, and edaravone group ED). Acupuncture and electroacupuncture both significantly decreased the volume of the MCAO-evoked infarct region (compare groups A and E with model group M), as assessed by TTC staining (Figure 1A and 1B). No significant differences in infarct volume were detected between the three treatment groups (A, EA, and ED), confirming the neuroprotective effect of acupuncture and electroacupuncture against CIRI.

Neurological outcomes

To investigate whether acupuncture or electroacupuncture can influence neurological function in CIRI model rats, neurological testing was performed using the mNSS approach at 24 h after reperfusion. Rats receiving acupuncture or electroacupuncture showed significant improvements in neurological function compared with MCAO model group M (Figure 1C). No significant differences in the mNSS were found between treatment groups A, EA, and ED.

Evaluation of cerebral histology by H&E and NeuN staining

H&E staining (Figure 2) was performed to evaluate histopathological alterations after focal ischemia, and immunohistochemical staining for NeuN, a neuronal nuclear antigen (Figure 3), was performed to evaluate neuronal loss, nuclear shrinkage, and neuronal vacuolization in CIRI model rats. Normal neurons in the contralateral hemisphere had round, lightly stained nuclei (Figure 2A), whereas dying neurons in the ipsilateral hemisphere had pyknotic nuclei (black arrows, Figure 2B and 2C) and already showed signs of vacuolization (red arrows, Figure 2B and 2C) in the core ischemic zone and the ischemic penumbra at 24 h after reperfusion. Furthermore, NeuN staining revealed a remarkable loss of neurons in MCAO model group M compared with sham group S and treatment groups A, EA, and ED, whereas the changes in the number of neurons observed between groups A, EA, and ED were not apparent (Figure 3).

Effects of acupuncture and electroacupuncture on the mRNA expression levels of MMP2, AQP4, and AQP9

The mechanistic actions of acupuncture and electroacupuncture were explored by investigating their influence on MMP2, APQ4, and AQP9 mRNA expression. The mRNA expression levels of all three target proteins were significantly increased in model group M relative to sham group S, and in model group M relative to each of the three treatment groups (Figure 4). Groups A, EA, and ED showed no significant inter-group differences between the mRNA expression levels of MMP2, but the mRNA expression levels of AQP4 and AQP9 were significantly lower in edaravone group ED than in groups A and EA.

Colocalization of MMP2 and AQP4 with GFAP and CD34 in the ischemic penumbra

To evaluate the astrocytic and vascular localization of MMP2 and AQP4 in the ischemic penumbra of CIRI model rats, immunofluorescence analysis was employed using specific primary antibodies against MMP2, AQP4, GFAP (to label astrocytes), and CD34 (to label the endothelial cell components of blood vessels). Figure 5 shows colocalization of MMP2 and GFAP (Figure 5A–5C), MMP2 and CD34 (Figure 5D–5F), AQP4 and GFAP (Figure 5G–5I), and AQP4 and CD34 (Figure 5J–5L) in MCAO model group M. These results indicate that AQP4 and MMP2 were both expressed in astrocyte endfeet and endothelial cell-derived blood vessels within the infarct area.

MMP2, AQP4, and AQP9 protein expression in the ischemic penumbra and the core zone

Next, we explored the hypothesis that acupuncture and electroacupuncture can regulate MMP2, AQP4, and AQP9 expression in the ischemic penumbra and the core zone by performing an immunohistochemical analysis of target protein expression, followed by semi-quantitative measurement of the integrated optical density of MMP2/AQP4/APQ9 labeling. Consequently, MMP2, AQP4, and AQP9 expression levels were higher in the ischemic penumbra than in the ischemic core for all five groups of rats (Figure 6A, 6B, 6D, 6E, 6G, and 6H). However, significantly lower amounts of each protein were detected in group S vs. groups M, A, EA, and ED, and in groups A, EA, and ED vs. group M. No statistically significant differences were discerned between groups A and EA (Figure 6C, 6F, and 6I).

Protein expression levels of MMP2, AQP4, and AQP9 in the lesion boundary zone of the ipsilateral hemisphere

To further investigate the influence of acupuncture and electroacupuncture on the expression patterns of MMP2, AQP4, and AQP9, Western blotting analysis was used to compare target protein levels in the lesion boundary zone in the five rat groups. The Western blotting data (Figure 7) verified the immunohistochemical findings (Figure 6), in that the protein expression levels of MMP2, AQP4, and AQP9 were all significantly higher in group M than in the other four groups ($P<0.05$). All three proteins were expressed at similar levels in groups A and EA, while the lowest protein expression levels were found in group ED (Figure 7).

Quantification of MPO^+ and $CD68^+$ cells in the ischemic penumbra and the core zone

Finally, immunohistochemical staining for MPO and CD68 was performed in the ischemic hemisphere, followed by quantification of MPO^+ and $CD8^+$ cells in the ischemic penumbra and the core (Figure 8C and 8F). Immunostaining for both antigens was more intense in the ischemic core than in the penumbra for all five rat groups (Figure 8A, 8B, 8D, and 8E). Likewise, cell counting revealed that the majority of MPO^+ and $CD68^+$ cells, indicative of neutrophils and monocytes/macrophages, respectively, were present within the ischemic core. Significantly higher numbers of MPO^+ and $CD68^+$ cells were found in both regions for group M vs. the other four groups. But no significant differences were detected between groups A and EA (Figure 8C and 8F). However, the ED group showed the lowest number of infiltrating MPO^+ and $CD68^+$ cells relative to A, EA treatment groups (Figure 8C and 8F).

Discussion

Acupuncture and electroacupuncture are both potential therapeutic strategies to repair brain injury and improve functional outcomes following acute ischemic stroke. Here, we showed that acupuncture or electroacupuncture at Baihui (GV20) and left Zusanli (ST36) significantly reduced the infiltration of inflammatory cells and the expression of the proinflammatory enzyme,

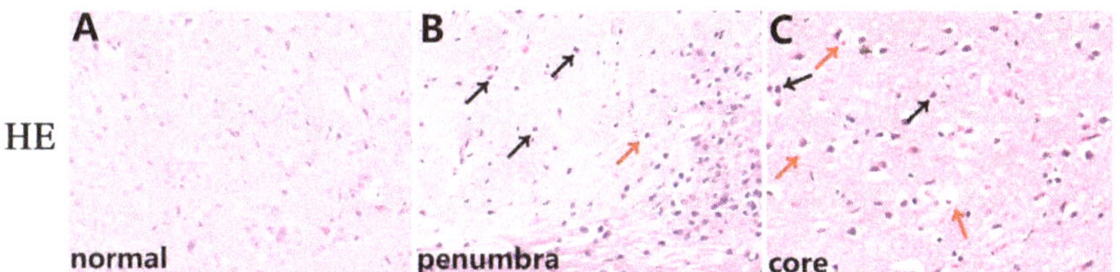

Figure 2. Evaluation of histopathological changes and neuronal damage in the ischemic penumbra and the core zone by H&E and NeuN staining. (A, B, C) H&E staining showing gross histopathological changes in normal, ischemic penumbra and the ischemic core at 24 h after reperfusion. The black arrows in (B, C) indicate significant nuclear shrinkage, and the red arrows indicate neuronal vacuolization. Scale bar = 50 μm.

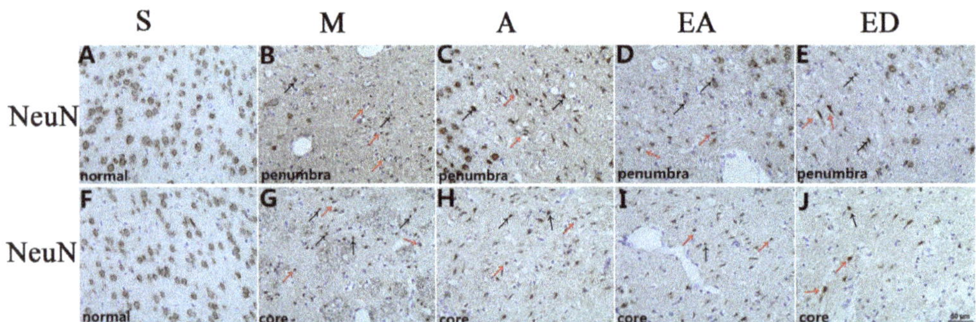

Figure 3. Evaluation of neuronal loss in the ischemic penumbra and the core zone by NeuN staining. NeuN immunohistochemical staining showing neuronal nuclei changes in the ischemic penumbra and the core zone at 24 h after reperfusion. Group M showed a marked loss of neurons compared with groups S, A, EA, and ED, whereas no apparent changes in the number of neurons was observed between groups A, EA, and ED. Note the pronounced nuclear shrinkage (black arrows) and neuronal vacuolization (red arrows) in group M. Scale bar = 50 μm.

MMP2, in CIRI model rats. Acupuncture and electroacupuncture also significantly attenuated the expression of the water channel proteins, AQP4 and AQP9, in the ischemic brain, suggesting that the protective mechanisms of these alternative treatments are partially dependent on the mitigation of inflammation-related brain edema. Consistent with the smaller observed infarct size, acupuncture and electroacupuncture both promoted significant improvements in the mNSS in CIRI model rats, indicative of enhanced neurological function.

Cerebral ischemia and edema are frequently associated with neuroinflammation, augmented production of proinflammatory mediators, and infiltration of inflammatory cells (e.g., MPO^+ neutrophils and $CD68^+$ monocyte/macrophages). The majority of the infiltrating MPO^+ and $CD68^+$ cells observed in this investigation were present within the core zone of the infarct area after CIRI, rather than in the peri-infarct penumbra. These cells were particularly prominent in model group M relative to the other four experimental groups and in A and EA groups relative to both S group. However, treatment groups A and EA showed no significant differences between the number of infiltrating MPO^+ and $CD68^+$ cells, suggesting that acupuncture and electroacupuncture are equally effective in their amelioration of certain aspects of inflammatory brain injury.

The BBB is critically involved in the maintenance of brain homeostasis. In the case of CIRI, injured brain cells (microvessel/capillary endothelial cells, pericytes, astrocytes, neurons, and others) and extracellular matter (basement membrane/extracellular matrix and tight junctions) increase the vascular permeability of the BBB and the uptake of abnormal quantities of water, thereby evoking secondary brain damage. Under normal conditions, total cessation of blood flow does not provoke dysfunction of water homeostasis, suggesting that some residual blood flow is required to develop brain edema [25]. Obviously, reperfusion worsens capillary vascular damage and augments ischemic cerebral edema. [26]. The detrimental impact of these assorted events on BBB integrity directly results in brain edema after stroke.

MMPs and other proteases are products of a molecular inflammatory cascade that damages the BBB following CIRI. BBB tight junction proteins and basal lamina proteins,which form the endothelial barrier, are vulnerable to attack by MMPs. MMP2 is especially important in astrocytes and endothelial cells, and its activation generally leads to a biphasic (transient and 24–48 h in duration) opening of the BBB [27]. For this reason, agents that protect the brain from edema by interfering with BBB are under pursuit by many researchers. Notably, our study showed that MMP2 colocalized with both GFAP in astrocytes and CD34 in endothelial cells within the ischemic penumbra, strengthening the idea that synthetic MMPs inhibitors could be used in CIRI management [28,29]. We also showed that acupuncture and electroacupuncture significantly reversed MMP2 upregulation in

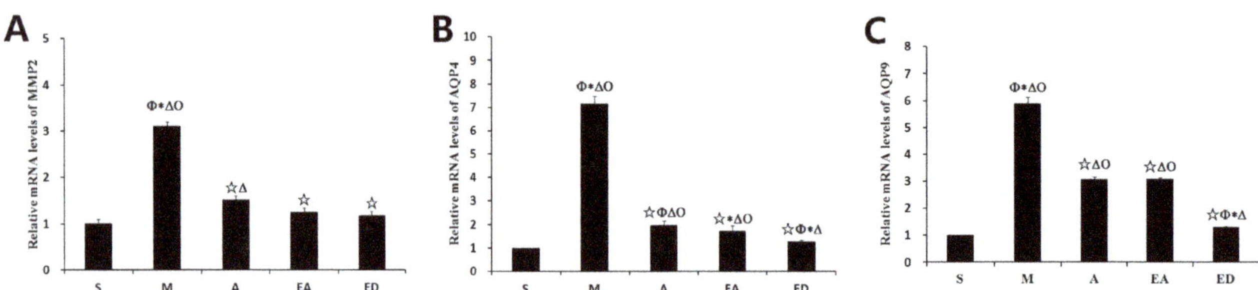

Figure 4. Effects of acupuncture and electroacupuncture on mRNA expression levels of MMP2, AQP4, and AQP9. Analysis of MMP2, APQ4, and APQ9 mRNA expression levels by qPCR. GAPDH was used as an internal control. Lower mRNA expression levels of MMP2, AQP4, and AQP9 were exhibited in group S vs. groups M, A, EA, and ED. The mRNA expression levels of all three target proteins were significantly lower in groups A and EA than in group M. Quantitative data (n = 3) are given as the mean ± the SD. $^{\triangle}P<0.05$ vs. group S; $^{☆}P<0.05$ vs. group M; $^{*}P<0.05$ vs. group A; $^{\Phi}P<0.05$ vs. group EA; $^{O}P<0.05$ vs. group ED.

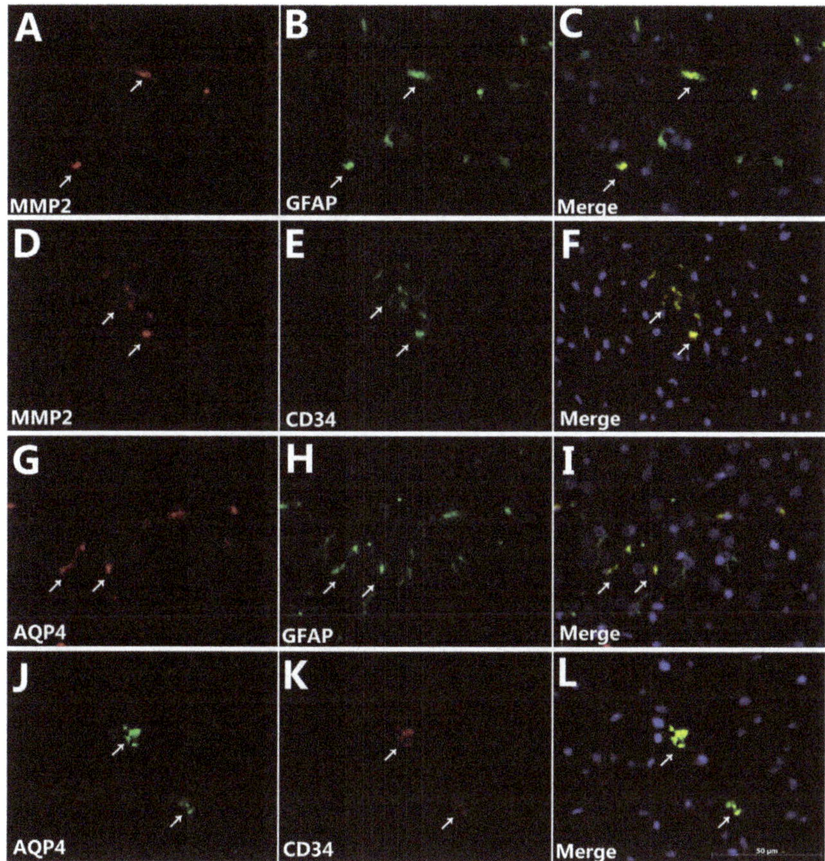

Figure 5. Colocalization of MMP2 and AQP4 with GFAP and CD34 in the ischemic penumbra. Immunofluorescence labeling for the MMP2, AQP4, GFAP, and CD34 expression levels in the ischemic hemisphere of MCAO model group M rats. MMP2 (red, A) and GFAP (green, B) staining and the MMP2/GFAP merge (C) show MMP2 expression on astrocyte endfeet; MMP2 (red, D) and CD34 (green, E) staining and the MMP2/CD34 merge (F) show MMP2 expression on endothelial cells; AQP4 (red, G) and GFAP (green, H) staining and the AQP4/GFAP merge (I) show AQP4 expression on astrocyte endfeet; and AQP4 (red, J) and CD34 (green, K) staining and the AQP4/CD34 merge (L) show AQP4 expression on endothelial cells. The yellow staining (arrows) in panels (C), (F), (I) and (L) indicates the colocalization of both antigens in the merged images. Scale bar = 50 μm.

CIRI model rats, although edaravone was more effective than either acupuncture or electroacupuncture.

AQPs, like MMP2, play essential roles in the pathogenesis of brain edema. The MCAO model, which utilizes focal brain ischemia to impart tissue damage, was previously reported to increase AQP4 expression in the infarct zone shortly after the insult [30]. On the other hand, another study suggested that AQP4 inhibition may provide a new therapeutic option for reducing brain edema [31]. Yet another study reported two peaks of brain swelling following CIRI, coinciding with two peaks of AQP4 expression in both the infarct and the peri-infarct area [32,33].

AQP9, along with AQP4, is associated with brain damage after CIRI. AQP9 is upregulated in the ischemic core and the lesion border [33], with lower expression reported in the core [34]. Our data showed elevated expression of APQ9 and AQP4 in both the ischemic penumbra and the core, but the highest expression was found in the core zone. We additionally demonstrated that acupuncture, electroacupuncture, and edaravone significantly downregulated AQP4 and AQP9 mRNA and protein levels after CIRI, again implying that AQP4 and AQP9 work together to cause brain edema.

Owing to the complex and multifaceted nature of cerebral ischemic stroke, sequential staging of therapy by a combination of different mechanistic approaches will probably prove most useful in stroke management. Nowadays, acupuncture has gained increasing popularity in modern health care, garnering new support from a myriad of scientific investigators. The popular use of acupuncture has also inspired many scientists to explore ancient traditional medical technology alongside conventional medicine. Although the precise manner in which acupuncture functions is unknown and requires further study, many researchers now claim that acupuncture and electroacupuncture are beneficial for treating ischemic stroke [35]. Indeed, the assorted effects of acupuncture and electroacupuncture on the generation and blockade of free radicals, intracellular calcium, inflammation-related cytokines, and/or vasogenic edema have all been proposed to explain their possible mechanisms of therapeutic action [36,37,38,39,40].

The list of acupoints affecting the various meridians of the body is quite long, but the Baihui (GV20), Zusanli (ST36), Neiguan (pericardium-6, PC6), Weizhong (bladder-40, BL40), Sanyinjiao (spleen-6, SP6), Chize (lung-5, LU5), Renzhong (governing vessel-6, GV6), and Waiguan (TE5) locations are the most frequently chosen acupoints. Special acupuncture manipulations are also

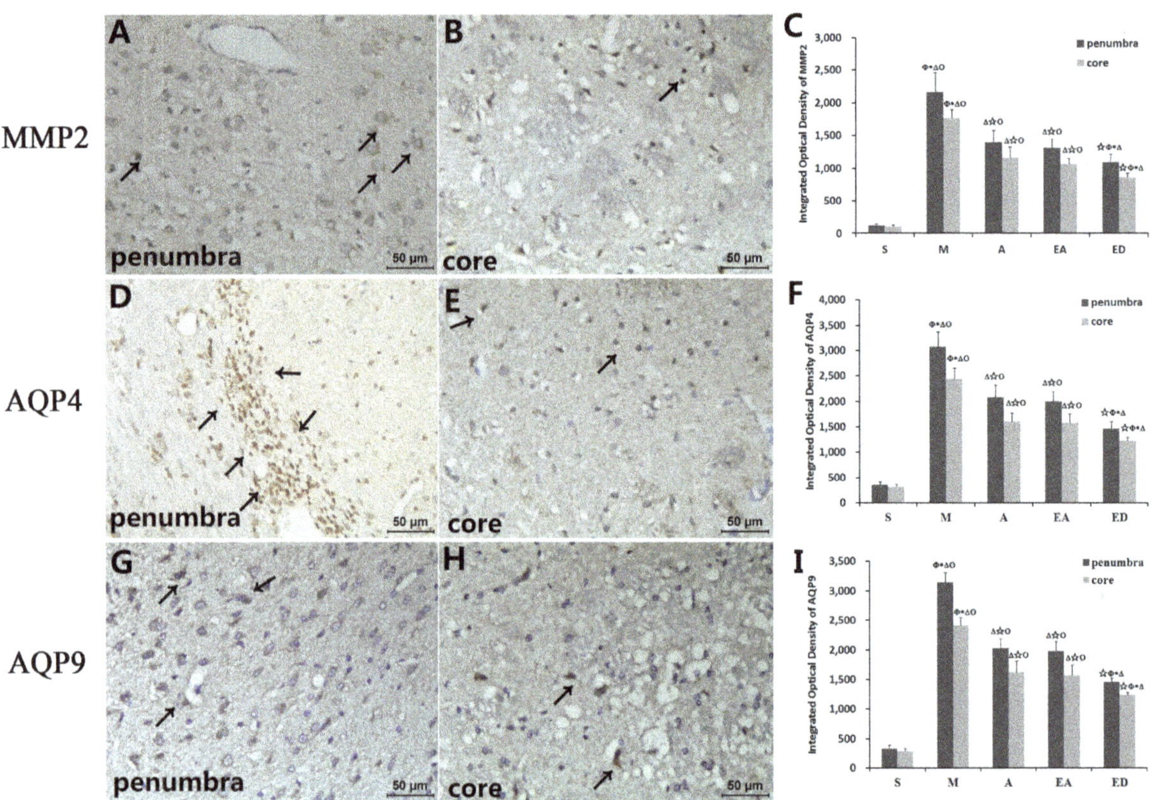

Figure 6. Protein expression of MMP2, AQP4, and AQP9 in the ischemic penumbra and the core zone. MMP2, AQP4, and AQP9 immunoreactivity (A, B, D, E, G, and H) and integrated optical density of MMP2/AQP4/AQP9 labeling (C, F, and I). Quantitative data (n = 6) are given as the mean ± the SD. △$P<0.05$ vs. group S; ☆$P<0.05$ vs. group M; *$P<0.05$ vs. group A; Φ$P<0.05$ vs. group EA; O$P<0.05$ vs. group ED. Arrows indicate the immunoreactive area for each target protein. Scale bar in (A) = 50 μm.

clinically used to improve self-care ability and quality of life in ischemic stroke patients, including scalp acupuncture and resuscitating acupuncture [41].

Traditional Chinese Medicine theory holds that GV20 belongs to the governing vessel, which in humans is located on the top of the head at the intersection of the middle sagittal line and the connection of the two ear apexes. GV20 functions to collect the yang around the body. After stimulation of GV20, the local yang is dispersed over and energizes the entire body. ST36 is located at 3 cm below Dubi (stomach-35, ST35) and one finger's breadth before the anterior crest of the tibia, and is utilized as an acupoint for treating digestive system diseases (e.g., gastroplegia, functional dyspepsia, and intestinal obstruction). ST36 is one of several acupoints of the stomach meridian, which is rich in both Qi and blood, and thus stimulation at ST36 has the capacity to modulate the function of the entire body. Once Qi and blood are enriched, the body can again be activated. Of relevance to the current study, simultaneous stimulation of GV20 and ST60 reportedly has a synergistically beneficial effect on the attenuation of brain ischemia [42].

Electroacupuncture, which can deliver continuous stimulation to acupoints, is currently under investigation for the management of ischemic stroke in experimental animals and in clinical practice [43,44]. Previous work compared the therapeutic efficacy of acupuncture at ST36 and GV20 vs. electroacupuncture at ST36 and GV20 in rats undergoing CIRI and suggested that both treatments significantly increased hippocampal cell proliferation relative to the control. However, electroacupuncture delivered potentially greater benefits than acupuncture alone in terms of neuroblast plasticity [45].

According to the results of our study, CIRI rats receiving acupuncture at GV20 and ST36 or electroacupuncture at GV20 and ST36 with continuous-wave stimulation had better neurological scores and reduced brain infarction volumes than CIRI rats receiving no post-operative treatment. However, no significant differences were found between acupuncture and electroacupuncture in MMP2/AQP9 expression or the numbers of MPO^+ and $CD68^+$ cells. In fact, the only significant difference between groups A and EA was a tempered expression of AQP4 mRNA in group EA. Thus, acupuncture and electroacupuncture may share the same mechanism of neuroprotective action, with the added stimulation of electroacupuncture conferring a slight therapeutic advantage.

Edaravone is a free radical scavenger and the first medication with demonstrated efficacy for cerebral ischemia [46]. Edaravone is commonly used in China and was therefore employed as a drug control for acupuncture and electroacupuncture in the present study. Overall, the ED group presented with the lowest number of infiltrating MPO^+ and $CD68^+$ cells, protein expression levels of MMP2, AQP4, and AQP9, and mRNA expression levels of AQP4 and AQP9 relative to the other four groups. The ED group showed improvements relative to the A and EA groups; therefore, it is possible that the acupuncture and electroacupuncture

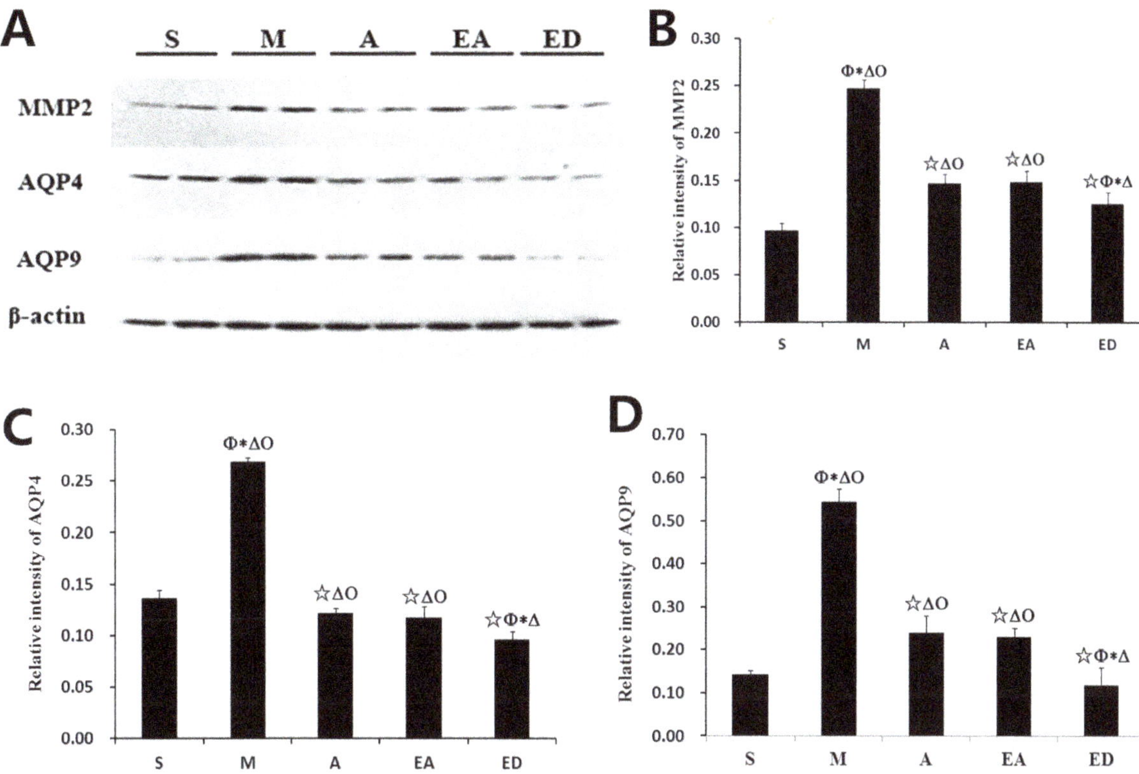

Figure 7. Western blot analysis of MMP2, AQP4, and AQP9 protein expression in the lesion boundary zone of the ipsilateral hemisphere. (A) Western blot analysis of MMP2, AQP4, and APQ9. (B–D) Relative intensity of MMP2 (B), APQ4 (C), and AQP9 (D) in each of the five rat groups. Relative intensity is defined as the intensity of the target protein normalized to that of β-actin. Quantitative data (n = 4) are given as the mean ± the SD. $^{\triangle}P<0.05$ vs. group S; $^{☆}P<0.05$ vs. group M; $^{*}P<0.05$ vs. group A; $^{\Phi}P<0.05$ vs. group EA; $^{O}P<0.05$ vs. group ED.

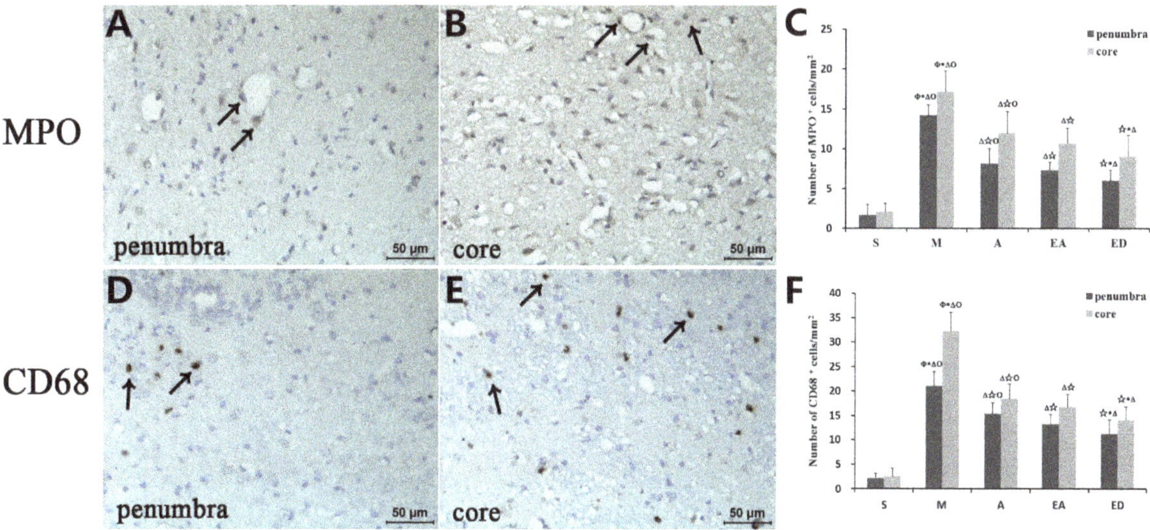

Figure 8. Quantification of MPO⁺ and CD68⁺ cells in the ischemic penumbra and the core zone. Representative photomicrographs showing immunohistochemical staining for MPO and CD68 in the ischemic penumbra (A, D) and the core zone (B, E) at 24 h after reperfusion. Brown spots indicate MPO⁺ cells, the majority of which were present within the ischemic core vs. the ischemic penumbra for all five rat groups. (B, E) The majority of CD68⁺ cells were also present in the core zone. (C, F) Bar graphs showing the quantification of MPO⁺ and CD68⁺ cells. The numbers of MPO⁺ and CD68⁺ cells were significantly higher in both the ischemic penumbra and the core zone for group M vs. the other four groups, whereas no significant differences were found between groups A and EA. Quantitative data (n = 6) are given as the mean ± the SD. $^{\triangle}P<0.05$ vs. group S; $^{☆}P<0.05$ vs. group M; $^{*}P<0.05$ vs. group A; $^{\Phi}P<0.05$ vs. group EA; $^{O}P<0.05$ vs. group ED. Arrows in (A), (B), (D), and (E) show the MPO⁺ and CD68⁺ immunoreactive cells. Scale bar = 50 μm.

techniques explored herein will require further optimization for maximum therapeutic efficacy.

In conclusion, the results of the present investigation indicate that acupuncture and electroacupuncture are effective treatments for brain tissue injury and neurological deficits following CIRI in rats. Therefore, this study adds to the growing arsenal of research supporting the view that acupuncture and electroacupuncture, which are derived from Traditional Chinese Medicine, can serve as complementary and alternative treatments to supplement the conventional management of ischemic stroke.

Author Contributions

Conceived and designed the experiments: HX HS. Performed the experiments: YMZ HX. Analyzed the data: SHC FMW. Contributed reagents/materials/analysis tools: SHC. Wrote the paper: HX YMZ.

References

1. Rosamond W, Flegal K, Furie K, Go A, Greenlund K, et al. (2008) Heart disease and stroke statistics—2008 update: a report from the American Heart Association Statistics Committee and Stroke Statistics Subcommittee. Circulation 117: e25–e146.
2. Durai PJ, Padma V, Vijaya P, Sylaja PN, Murthy JM (2007) Stroke and thrombolysis in developing countries. Int J Stroke 2: 17–26.
3. Xu D, Du W, Zhao L, Davey AK, Wang J (2008) The neuroprotective effects of isosteviol against focal cerebral ischemia injury induced by middle cerebral artery occlusion in rats. Planta Med 74: 816–821.
4. Nagahiro S, Uno M, Sato K, Goto S, Morioka M, et al. (1998) Pathophysiology and treatment of cerebral ischemia. J Med Invest 45: 57–70.
5. Amantea D, Nappi G, Bernardi G, Bagetta G, Corasaniti MT (2009) Post-ischemic brain damage: pathophysiology and role of inflammatory mediators. FEBS J 276: 13–26.
6. Krueger M, Hartig W, Reichenbach A, Bechmann I, Michalski D (2013) Blood-brain barrier breakdown after embolic stroke in rats occurs without ultrastructural evidence for disrupting tight junctions. PLoS One 8: e56419.
7. Beck K, Schachtrup C (2012) Vascular damage in the central nervous system: a multifaceted role for vascular-derived TGF-beta. Cell Tissue Res 347: 187–201.
8. Lapergue B, Dang BQ, Desilles JP, Ortiz-Munoz G, Delbosc S, et al. (2013) High-density lipoprotein-based therapy reduces the hemorrhagic complications associated with tissue plasminogen activator treatment in experimental stroke. Stroke 44: 699–707.
9. Wu Y, Wang YP, Guo P, Ye XH, Wang J, et al. (2012) A lipoxin A4 analog ameliorates blood-brain barrier dysfunction and reduces MMP-9 expression in a rat model of focal cerebral ischemia-reperfusion injury. J Mol Neurosci 46: 483–491.
10. Yang Y, Rosenberg GA (2011) MMP-mediated disruption of claudin-5 in the blood-brain barrier of rat brain after cerebral ischemia. Methods Mol Biol 762: 333–345.
11. Feng HR, Xu PC, Xu JB, Wu YP (2010) Correlation between the expression of aquaporin 4 and permeability changes of blood-brain barrier during ischemia/reperfusion in rats. Zhongguo Ying Yong Sheng Li Xue Za Zhi 26: 12–14, 18.
12. Kurzepa J, Kurzepa J, Golab P, Czerska S, Bielewicz J (2013) The significance of matrix metalloproteinase(MMP)-2 and MMP-9 in the ischemic stroke. Int J Neurosci.
13. Lee JY, Lee HE, Kang SR, Choi HY, Ryu JH, et al. (2013) Fluoxetine inhibits transient global ischemia-induced hippocampal neuronal death and memory impairment by preventing blood-brain barrier disruption. Neuropharmacology 79C: 161–171.
14. Manley GT, Fujimura M, Ma T, Noshita N, Filiz F, et al. (2000) Aquaporin-4 deletion in mice reduces brain edema after acute water intoxication and ischemic stroke. Nat Med 6: 159–163.
15. Fukuda AM, Badaut J (2012) Aquaporin 4: a player in cerebral edema and neuroinflammation. J Neuroinflammation 9: 279.
16. Badaut J, Brunet JF, Regli L (2007) Aquaporins in the brain: from aqueduct to "multi-duct". Metab Brain Dis 22: 251–263.
17. Badaut J, Petit JM, Brunet JF, Magistretti PJ, Charriaut-Marlangue C, et al. (2004) Distribution of Aquaporin 9 in the adult rat brain: preferential expression in catecholaminergic neurons and in glial cells. Neuroscience 128: 27–38.
18. Chen SH, Sun H, Xu H, Zhang YM, Gao Y, et al. (2012) Effects of acupuncture of "Baihui"(GV 20) and "Zusanli"(ST 36) on expression of cerebral IL-1beta and TNF-alpha proteins in cerebral ischemia reperfusion injury rats. Zhen Ci Yan Jiu 37: 470–475.
19. Hong X, Li-chuan H, Yan-qiu H, Su-hui C, Hua S (2010) The expression of MMP-9 and ICAM-1 in rats with cerebral ischemic/reperfusion treated by acupuncture. Basic & Clinical Medicine: 731–736.
20. Wang G, Su J, Li L, Feng J, Shi L, et al. (2013) Edaravone alleviates hypoxia-acidosis/reoxygenation-induced neuronal injury by activating ERK1/2. Neurosci Lett 543: 72–77.
21. Longa EZ, Weinstein PR, Carlson S, Cummins R (1989) Reversible middle cerebral artery occlusion without craniectomy in rats. Stroke 20: 84–91.
22. Shehadah A, Chen J, Kramer B, Zacharek A, Cui Y, et al. (2013) Efficacy of single and multiple injections of human umbilical tissue-derived cells following experimental stroke in rats. PLoS One 8: e54083.
23. Walcott BP, Kahle KT, Simard JM (2012) Novel treatment targets for cerebral edema. Neurotherapeutics 9: 65–72.
24. Livak KJ, Schmittgen TD (2001) Analysis of relative gene expression data using real-time quantitative PCR and the 2(-Delta Delta C(T)) Method. Methods 25: 402–408.
25. Candelario-Jalil E (2009) Injury and repair mechanisms in ischemic stroke: considerations for the development of novel neurotherapeutics. Curr Opin Investig Drugs 10: 644–654.
26. Walcott BP, Kahle KT, Simard JM (2012) Novel treatment targets for cerebral edema. Neurotherapeutics 9: 65–72.
27. Rosenberg GA, Yang Y (2007) Vasogenic edema due to tight junction disruption by matrix metalloproteinases in cerebral ischemia. Neurosurgical focus 22: E4.
28. Yang Y, Thompson JF, Taheri S, Salayandia VM, McAvoy TA, et al. (2013) Early inhibition of MMP activity in ischemic rat brain promotes expression of tight junction proteins and angiogenesis during recovery. J Cereb Blood Flow Metab 33: 1104–1114.
29. Lee K, Lee JS, Jang HJ, Kim SM, Chang MS, et al. (2012) Chlorogenic acid ameliorates brain damage and edema by inhibiting matrix metalloproteinase-2 and 9 in a rat model of focal cerebral ischemia. Eur J Pharmacol 689: 89–95.
30. Okuno K, Taya K, Marmarou CR, Ozisik P, Fazzina G, et al. (2008) The modulation of aquaporin-4 by using PKC-activator (phorbol myristate acetate) and V1a receptor antagonist (SR49059) following middle cerebral artery occlusion/reperfusion in the rat. Acta Neurochir Suppl 102: 431–436.
31. Manley GT, Fujimura M, Ma T, Noshita N, Filiz F, et al. (2000) Aquaporin-4 deletion in mice reduces brain edema after acute water intoxication and ischemic stroke. Nat Med 6: 159–163.
32. Zelenina M (2010) Regulation of brain aquaporins. Neurochem Int 57: 468–488.
33. Zeng X, Asmaro K, Ren C, Gao M, Peng C, et al. (2012) Acute ethanol treatment reduces blood-brain barrier dysfunction following ischemia/reperfusion injury. Brain Res 1437: 127–133.
34. Ribeiro MC, Hirt L, Bogousslavsky J, Regli L, Badaut J (2006) Time course of aquaporin expression after transient focal cerebral ischemia in mice. J Neurosci Res 83: 1231–1240.
35. Wong V, Cheuk DK, Chu V (2013) Acupuncture for hypoxic ischemic encephalopathy in neonates. Cochrane Database Syst Rev 1: D7968.
36. Xu NG, Yi W, Lai XS (2002) Effect of electro-acupuncture on calcium content in neurocytes of focal cerebral ischemia. Zhongguo Zhong Xi Yi Jie He Za Zhi 22: 295–297.
37. Chen SX, Ding MC, Dai KY (2011) Effect of electroacupuncture on nitric oxide synthase in rats with cerebral ischemia-reperfusion injury. Zhongguo Zhong Xi Yi Jie He Za Zhi 31: 784–788.
38. Lan L, Tao J, Chen A, Xie G, Huang J, et al. (2013) Electroacupuncture exerts anti-inflammatory effects in cerebral ischemia-reperfusion injured rats via suppression of the TLR4/NF-kappaB pathway. Int J Mol Med 31: 75–80.
39. Li ZB, Liu FM, Liu WJ (2013) Influence of acupuncture intervention on neurologic deficits, cerebrocortical cell apoptosis and Protein kinase A expression in rats with focal cerebral ischemia. Zhen Ci Yan Jiu 38: 106–111.
40. Inoue I, Fukunaga M, Koga K, Wang HD, Ishikawa M (2009) Scalp acupuncture effects of stroke studied with magnetic resonance imaging: different actions in the two stroke model rats. Acupunct Med 27: 155–162.
41. Shen PF, Kong L, Ni LW, Guo HL, Yang S, et al. (2012) Acupuncture intervention in ischemic stroke: a randomized controlled prospective study. Am J Chin Med 40: 685–693.
42. Tian GH, Sun K, Huang P, Zhou CM, Yao HJ, et al. (2013) Long-Term Stimulation with Electroacupuncture at DU20 and ST36 Rescues Hippocampal Neuron through Attenuating Cerebral Blood Flow in Spontaneously Hypertensive Rats. Evid Based Complement Alternat Med 2013: 482947.
43. Kim JH, Choi KH, Jang YJ, Bae SS, Shin BC, et al. (2013) Electroacupuncture acutely improves cerebral blood flow and attenuates moderate ischemic injury via an endothelial mechanism in mice. PLoS One 8: e56736.
44. Liu SY, Hsieh CL, Wei TS, Liu PT, Chang YJ, et al. (2009) Acupuncture stimulation improves balance function in stroke patients: a single-blinded controlled, randomized study. Am J Chin Med 37: 483–494.
45. Hwang IK, Chung JY, Yoo DY, Yi SS, Youn HY, et al. (2010) Comparing the effects of acupuncture and electroacupuncture at Zusanli and Baihui on cell proliferation and neuroblast differentiation in the rat hippocampus. J Vet Med Sci 72: 279–284.
46. Isahaya K, Yamada K, Yamatoku M, Sakurai K, Takaishi S, et al. (2012) Effects of edaravone, a free radical scavenger, on serum levels of inflammatory biomarkers in acute brain infarction. J Stroke Cerebrovasc Dis 21: 102–107.

23

Reporting Quality of Systematic Reviews/Meta-Analyses of Acupuncture

Yali Liu[1,2], Rui Zhang[1,3], Jiao Huang[1,3], Xu Zhao[1,4], Danlu Liu[1,2,3], Wanting Sun[1,4], Yuefen Mai[1,4], Peng Zhang[1,5], Yajun Wang[6], Hua Cao[7], Ke hu Yang[1,2,3]*

1 Evidence-Based Medicine Center, School of Basic Medical Sciences, Lanzhou University, Lanzhou, China, **2** Key Laboratory of Clinical Translational Research and Evidence-Based Medicine of Gansu Province, Lanzhou, China, **3** The First Clinical Medical College of Lanzhou University, Lanzhou, China, **4** The Second Clinical Medical College of Lanzhou University, Lanzhou, China, **5** Department of Cardiology, Qilu Hospital of Shandong University, Ji'nan, Shandong Province, China, **6** Acupuncture and Massage College, Gansu University of Traditional Chinese Medicine, Lanzhou, China, **7** Department of Neurology, Gansu Provincial Hospital of Traditional Chinese Medicine, Lanzhou, China

Abstract

Background: The QUOROM and PRISMA statements were published in 1999 and 2009, respectively, to improve the consistency of reporting systematic reviews (SRs)/meta-analyses (MAs) of clinical trials. However, not all SRs/MAs adhere completely to these important standards. In particular, it is not clear how well SRs/MAs of acupuncture studies adhere to reporting standards and which reporting criteria are generally ignored in these analyses.

Objectives: To evaluate reporting quality in SRs/MAs of acupuncture studies.

Methods: We performed a literature search for studies published prior to 2014 using the following public archives: PubMed, EMBASE, Web of Science, the Cochrane Database of Systematic Reviews (CDSR), the Chinese Biomedical Literature Database (CBM), the Traditional Chinese Medicine (TCM) database, the Chinese Journal Full-text Database (CJFD), the Chinese Scientific Journal Full-text Database (CSJD), and the Wanfang database. Data were extracted into pre-prepared Excel data-extraction forms. Reporting quality was assessed based on the PRISMA checklist (27 items).

Results: Of 476 appropriate SRs/MAs identified in our search, 203, 227, and 46 were published in Chinese journals, international journals, and the Cochrane Database, respectively. In 476 SRs/MAs, only 3 reported the information completely. By contrast, approximately 4.93% (1/203), 8.81% (2/227) and 0.00% (0/46) SRs/Mas reported less than 10 items in Chinese journals, international journals and CDSR, respectively. In general, the least frequently reported items (reported≤ 50%) in SRs/MAs were "protocol and registration", "risk of bias across studies", and "additional analyses" in both methods and results sections.

Conclusions: SRs/MAs of acupuncture studies have not comprehensively reported information recommended in the PRISMA statement. Our study underscores that, in addition to focusing on careful study design and performance, attention should be paid to comprehensive reporting standards in SRs/MAs on acupuncture studies.

Editor: Brett Thombs, McGill University, Canada

Funding: Project supported by the National Natural Science Foundation of China (Grant No. 81373882) http://www.nsfc.gov.cn/Portal0/default152.htm The funders had no role in study design, data collection and analysis, decision to publish, or preparation of the manuscript.

Competing Interests: The authors have declared that no competing interests exist.

* Email: kehuyangebm2006@126.com

Introduction

Systematic reviews (SRs) and meta-analyses (MAs) summarize large amounts of evidence and are a valuable tool for keeping clinicians up to date within their specialty [1,2]. As with all research, however, the value of SRs/MAs depends on how the analyses are performed, the actual findings, and the clarity of reporting [3]. If key information is reported poorly, the potential usefulness of the SRs/MAs is diminished.

Since 1987, numerous researchers have recognized the need to evaluate the quality of these types of reviews. For example, in 1987 Sacks and colleagues [4] evaluated reporting in SRs/MAs and found that it was inadequate. The Consolidated Standards of Reporting Trials (CONSORT) Group subsequently developed the Quality of Reporting of Meta-Analyses (QUOROM) statement to address suboptimal MA reporting. Ten years later, an updated QUOROM statement—entitled Preferred Reporting Items for Systematic Reviews and Meta-Analyses (PRISMA) statement—was developed and published [3]. The PRISMA statement consists of a checklist of 27 study reporting items such as title, abstract, methods, results, discussion, and funding sources. The checklist is intended to guide authors of SRs/MAs to improve the consistency and quality of reporting.

Acupuncture, a traditional medicine technique, has been widely used in clinical practice for thousands of years in China and many western countries. The number of published SRs/MAs of acupuncture studies has increased considerably in recent years. As the transparency and completeness of SRs/MAs in many fields is still not optimal [5–8], we examined how well SR/MA reporting standards have been followed in the field of acupuncture and compared adherence to these standards in acupuncture SRs/MAs published in three different types of journals/databases.

Methods

The protocol for this study was written in Chinese and has not been published. The study was not a classical systematic review, but we tried to report it according to PRISMA Checklist [3] (Text S1).

Inclusion/exclusion criteria

We included all SRs or MAs of acupuncture published in Chinese journals, international journals, and the Cochrane Database of Systematic Reviews (CDSR) prior to 2014. The experimental group of SRs/MAs of acupuncture studies was also compared with a control group of SRs/MAs of studies of other interventions, such as herbal medicine, massage and western medicine. Participants: human in any conditions, not animal; Intervention: acupuncture; Comparisons: sham acupuncture or other interventions, such as herbal medicine, massage, western medicine, etc; Outcomes: no limitations; Study design: SRs/MAs. We excluded SRs/MAs that focused primarily on traditional Chinese medicine (TCM) other than acupuncture (e.g., herbal medicine, massage).

Search strategy

We comprehensively and systematically searched the following literature archives for SRs/MAs published prior to 2014: CDSR, PubMed, EMBASE, Web of Science, Chinese Biomedical Literature Database (CBM), the TCM database, Chinese Journal Full-text Database (CJFD), Chinese Scientific Journal Full-text Database (CSJD), and the Wanfang database. Databases were searched three times: on March 24, 2011 for all entries submitted prior to March 2011, on June 12, 2012 for all entries submitted prior to January 2012 and on January 11, 2014 for all entries submitted prior to 2014. The search terms "acupuncture", "needling", "ear acupuncture", "electroacupuncture", "electro-acupuncture", "acupuncture points", "acupressure", "moxibustion", and "acupoint" were used with the terms "systematic review" or "meta-analysis". The search strategy is presented in Checklist S1.

Screening

The titles and abstracts of the studies were independently screened by at least two reviewers (Jiao Huang, Xu Zhao, or Rui Zhang) based on inclusion and exclusion criteria, and the full text of potentially suitable articles was retrieved for further assessment (Text S2).

Data extraction and analysis

Data were extracted independently by at least two reviewers (Rui Zhang, Jiao Huang, Xu Zhao, or Danlu Liu) in accordance with the PRISMA checklist and the assessment checklist for SRs/MAs of acupuncture studies developed for this study. Inconsistencies were subsequently resolved by discussion between the two reviewers or final decisions were made by the third principal investigator (Yali Liu). Data input utilized a standardized form and was done by trained data extractors (Wanting Sun, Pen Zhang, and Hua Cao). The form consisted of a general characteristics section (title, first author, funding source, study design, disease(s) examined, diagnostic criteria, intervention, and outcome) and a 27-item PRISMA information section (including title, abstract, introduction, method, results, discussion, and funding). Each item was assessed as "yes" if it was described in the paper or "no" if it was not (Text S3). Data were summarized with descriptive statistical analysis. For continuous data, the means ± SD was provided and one-way ANOVA was used. Data that followed a normal distribution were compared using the LSD- t test. Dichotomous data were summarized with descriptive statistical analysis (frequency, percentage). Pearson's χ^2 test and/or Fisher's exact test were used to assess differences in reporting among groups. P values less than 0.05 were considered significant. All statistical analyses were performed using Microsoft Excel (version 2007) and SPSS (version 13.0) software.

Results

Search

Our initial literature search identified 3993 potential SRs/MAs of acupuncture-related studies. After closer examination, 476 were chosen for inclusion in our analysis (Text S4). Of these, 203, 227, and 46 were published in Chinese journals, international journals, and CDSR, respectively. A flow chart of the literature search is shown in Figure 1.

General characteristics

General characteristics of the SRs/MAs analyzed are summarized in Table 1. The earliest acupuncture SRs/MAs in Chinese journals and international journals were published in 2002 and 1989, respectively. The number of acupuncture SRs/MAs in Chinese and international journals increased sharply after 2005, whereas the majority of acupuncture SRs/MAs in CDSR were published between 2008 and 2013 (Figure 2).

Acupuncture SRs/MAs in Chinese journals were conducted entirely by Chinese authors, whereas those published in international journals tended to be multinational collaborations, with Chinese first authors being most prevalent (27.31%, 62/227). Chinese authors were also most prevalent first authors in CDSR studies (34.78%, 16/46). The percentage of published acupuncture SRs/MAs in Chinese journals, international journals, and the CDSR that reported at least one funding source was 54.19% (110/203), 50.66% (115/227), and 89.13% (41/46), respectively, and the maximum number of funding sources reported was 5, 3, and 7, respectively.

The majority of SRs/MAs (95.37%, 454/476) included at least one randomized controlled trial (RCT). Nervous system diseases, musculoskeletal system diseases, and mental illness were most frequently examined (23.11, 18.91 and 13.44%, respectively). Approximately 38% (180/476) of the SRs/MAs reported western diseases or TCM syndromes in their diagnostic criteria. All acupuncture SRs/MAs examined described the interventions in detail. 39.92% (190/476) and 19.54% (93/476) SRs/MAs included adverse events and quality-of-life in the outcome which were reported as primary and/or secondary outcomes.

PRISMA information reporting

Comparison of PRISMA reporting among the three types of journals/databases (Table 2)

Among 476 SRs/MAs, only 3 reported the information completely. By contrast, approximately 4.93% (1/203), 8.81% (2/227) and 0.00% (0/46) SRs/MAs reported less than 10 items on the checklist in Chinese journals, international journals, and CDSR, respectively. In general, the least frequently reported items (reported≤50%) in SRs/MAs were item 5 ("protocol and

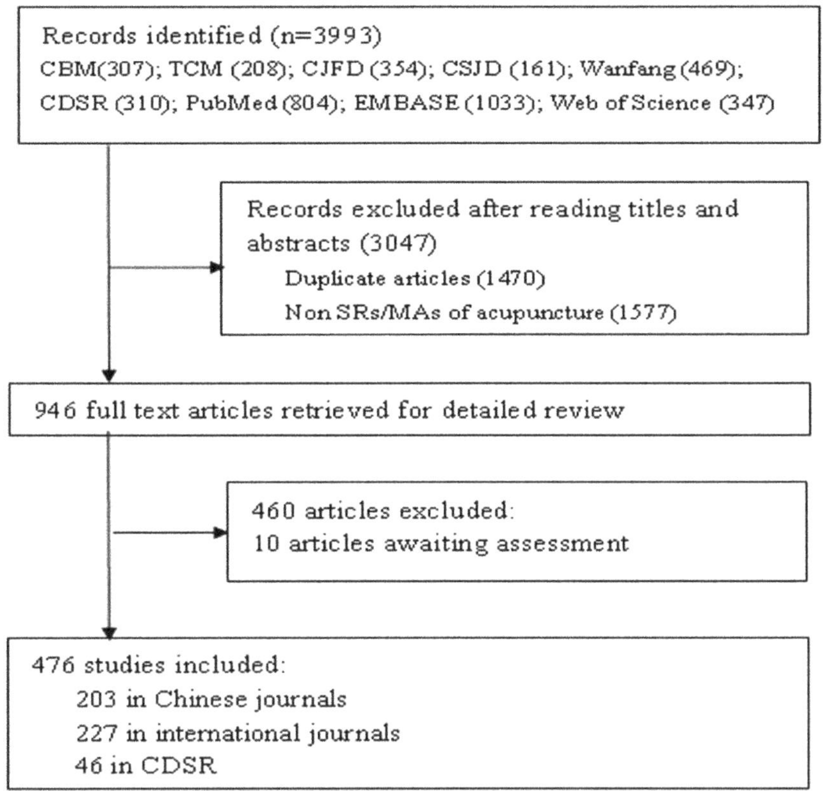

Figure 1. Flow chart of articles identified, included and excluded.

registration"), 15 and 22 ("risk of bias across studies"), and 16 and 23 ("additional analyses"). The remaining items on the checklist were adequately reported (i.e >90%), with the items listed in Table 2 being especially well reported.

Comparison of PRISMA reporting before and after release of the PRISMA statement (Table 3)

We found no statistical difference ($P>0.05$) for item 2 ("structured summary"), 5 ("protocol and registration"), 6 ("eligibility criteria"), 8 ("search"), 10 ("data collection process"), 11 ("data items"), 12 ("risk of bias in individual studies"), 16 ("additional analyses"), 17 ("study selection"), 18 ("study characteristics"), 23 ("additional analysis") and 27 ("funding") between SRs/MAs published prior to release of the PRISMA statement

Table 1. Characteristics of included studies.

Category	Characteristic	Chinese journals n = 203	International journals n = 227	CDSRs n = 46
Title	Systematic review	123 (122+1*)	167 (124+43*)	NA
	Meta analyses	66 (65+1*)	78 (35+43*)	NA
Author	The first author	203 (China)	62(China), 58(Korea), 39(England), 20(America)	16(China), 10(England), 9(Australia)
Funding source	Number of funded SRs/MAs	110 (54.19%)	110(48.46%)	40(86.96%)
Trial types	RCTs	193 (95.07%)	215(94.71%)	46 (100.0%)
Diseases	The first three	Nervous system 45 (22.17%), Musculoskeletal system 40 (19.70%), Mental illness 32 (15.76%)	Nervous system 57 (25.11%), Musculoskeletal system 42 (18.50%), Mental illness 27 (11.89%)	Musculoskeletal system 8 (17.39%), Nervous system 8 (17.39%), Mental illness 5 (10.87%)
Diagnostic criteria	Western medicine (diseases)	74(36.45%)	80(35.24%)	19(41.30%)
	Traditional medicine	44(21.67%)	6(2.64%)	0(0.00%)
Intervention		203(100.00%)	227 (100.00%)	46 (100%)
Outcome	Including adverse effect	54 (26.60%)	103 (45.37%)	33 (71.74%)
	Including quality of life	25 (12.31%)	45(19.82%)	23 (50.00%)

* Reported both "systematic review" and "meta-analysis".

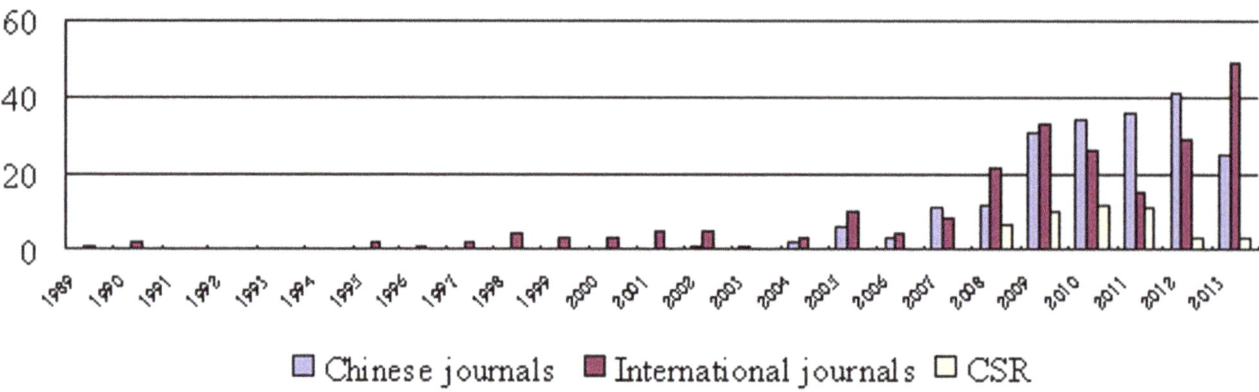

Figure 2. The number of included SRs MAs on acupuncture.

and those published after its release. Unfortunately, the rate of reporting of two items ("objective" and "information sources") had decreased in 2010–2013 compared with before 2010 ($P<0.001$).

Comparison of PRISMA reporting in Science Citation Index (SCI) and non-SCI journals (Table 3)

We found that PRISMA reporting in SRs/MAs in SCI journals was more complete overall than in non-SCI journals, especially for items 4 ("objective"), 5 ("protocol and registration"), 7 ("information sources"), 8 ("search"), 9 ("study selection"), 11 ("data items"), 23 ("additional analysis"), and 27 ("funding") ($P<0.001$).

Discussion

Over the last decade, numerous studies have assessed the quality of reporting in SRs/MAs by their compliance with assessment instruments such as the QUOROM and PRISMA statements [9–12]. These studies focused predominantly on SRs/MAs covering diagnostic research and critical care. Although some quality assessment studies have looked at acupuncture SRs/MAs [13–15], they have focused mainly on methodological diversity in database searching, risk of bias, and heterogeneity in search strategies among CDSR. Our study compared reporting quality and PRISMA compliance in acupuncture SRs/MAs between different journal types.

We found that the five PRISMA items, namely "Protocol and registration", "Risk of bias across studies" (both in the methods and results), and "Additional analyses" (both in the methods and results) in the methods and results, are not frequently reported, indicating that the overall quality of reporting in acupuncture SRs/MAs is far from adequate. Compared with SRs/MAs published in CDSR, those in Chinese and international journals were of inferior reporting quality. One possible explanation for the limited compliance may be that journals have failed to incorporate the PRISMA statement into their instructions to authors about submitting SRs/MAs [16]. We also found that SR/MA reporting was more complete in SCI journals than in non-SCI journals but that both require improvement in adherence to PRISMA standards.

Several studies have focused on the reporting quality of SRs/MAs covering the fields of TCM [17,18], physical therapy [19], orthopaedics [20], and oral implantology [21] field, which showed that the reporting quality was indeed poor. Although differences exist between these results and those we repot here, the reporting of major items in the PRISMA statement was similar to what we found in our present study. Additional, Fleming PS et al. [22] found that the quality of reporting was considerably better in reviews published in CDSR ($P<0.001$) than in non-CDSR.

Both the QUOROM and PRISMA statements encourage the use of specific terms in the titles of SRs/MAs, which help to identify these studies. Because of the special title format requirements of the CDSR, however, SRs/MAs published in this database cannot conform to the QUOROM/PRISMA recommendation.

Unequivocal descriptions of the scientific background and rationale for using acupuncture in the treatment of both western diseases and TCM syndromes provide the reader with a better understanding of the research context and rationale of SRs/MAs. In this respect, SRs/MAs in the CDSR were more explicit in their descriptions than those in international or Chinese journals.

The importance of protocol consistency and registration of SRs/MAs to the transparency of reporting is underscored by the fact that they are considered key aspects of the "reporting guidelines for systematic review protocols" in the international prospective register of systematic reviews (PROSPERO) [23,24]. We found that only SRs/MAs published in the CDSR provided protocol and registration details.

The PRISMA standards suggest that methodological details such as eligibility criteria, information sources, search strategies, study selection criteria, and data collection processes are necessary to judge the quality and accuracy of SRs/MAs. The majority of the SRs/MAs published in the CDSR adequately reported these items, whereas those published in Chinese and international journals did not. Eligibility criteria are an aspect of the PICOS criteria (participants, interventions, comparisons, outcomes, and study design) central to the PRISMA approach. We propose that it is equally important that search strategies be uniformly reported. Many international journals require information about search strategies in at least one database, and the flexibility of the CDSR layout allows reporting of search strategies for multiple databases. Chinese journals, however, rarely request search strategy information. There is also considerable need for more consistency in the databases obtain acupuncture studies. We propose that, AcuBriefs (www.acubriefs.com), AcuBase (www.acubase.fr), Acudoc2 RCT (www.acubriefs.com/), and the TCM database are the most systematic and comprehensive sources for acupuncture information. Chinese RCTs make up the highest proportion of primary studies included in acupuncture SRs/MAs. If methods for sequence generation, allocation concealment, and study blindness are not adequately described, low-quality studies [25] may mislead reviewers.

Table 2. Reporting of checklists for PRISMA statement.

Category		Item	Total n = 476	Chinese journals n = 203	International journals n = 227	CDSRs n = 46	*P* value
Title	1	Title	390(90.70%)[@]	188(92.61%)	202(88.99%)*	NA	NA
Abstract	2	Structured summary	446(93.70%)	199(98.03%)	201(88.55%)*	46(100.00%)#	0.000
Introduction	3	Rationale	380(79.83%)	152(74.88%)	182(80.18%)	46(100.00%)*#	0.001
	4	Objective	430(90.34%)	160(78.82%)	225(99.12%)*	45(97.83%)*	0.000
Methods	5	Protocol and registration	60(12.61%)	0(0.00%)	18(7.93%)	42(91.30%)*#	0.000
	6	Eligibility criteria	463(97.27%)	196(96.55%)	222(97.80%)	45(97.83%)	0.710
	7	Information sources	440(92.44%)	169(83.25%)	225(99.12%)*	46(100.00%)	0.000
	8	Search	282(59.24%)	87(42.86%)	156(68.72%)*	39(84.78%)	0.000
	9	Study selection	342(71.85%)	116(57.14%)	182(80.18%)*	44(95.65%)*	0.000
	10	Data collection process	411(86.34%)	159(78.33%)	207(91.19%)*	45(97.83%)	0.000
	11	Data items	270(56.72%)	59(29.06%)	170(74.89%)*	41(89.13%)*	0.000
	12	Risk of bias in individual studies	384(80.67%)	159(78.33%)	182(80.18%)	43(93.48%)	0.061
	13	Summary measures	387(81.30%)	182(89.66%)	164(72.25%)*	41(89.13%)	0.000
	14	Synthesis of results	402(84.45%)	191(94.09%)	167(73.57%)*	44(95.65%)#	0.000
	15	Risk of bias across studies	155(32.56%)	82(40.39%)	50(22.03%)*	23(50.00%)*#	0.000
	16	Additional analyses	191(40.13%)	77(37.93%)	76(33.48%)	38(82.61%)*#	0.000
Results	17	Study selection	430(90.34%)	188(92.61%)	197(86.78%)	45(97.83%)	0.024
	18	Study characteristics	431(90.55%)	176(86.70%)	209(92.07%)	46(100.00%)*#	0.012
	19	Risk of bias within studies	387(81.30%)	155(76.35%)	189(83.26%)	43(93.48%)*	0.016
	20	Results of individual studies	411(86.34%)	196(96.55%)	172(75.77%)*	43(93.48%)#	0.000
	21	Synthesis of results	389(81.72%)	192(94.58%)	156(68.72%)*	41(89.13%)#	0.000
	22	Risk of bias across studies	176(36.97%)	91(44.83%)	66(29.07%)*	19(41.30%)	0.003
	23	Additional analysis	165(34.66%)	49(24.14%)	75(33.04%)	41(89.13%)*#	0.000
Discussion	24	Summary of evidence	432(90.76%)	170(83.74%)	216(95.15%)*	46(100.00%)*	0.000
	25	Limitations	455(95.59%)	188(92.61%)	222(97.80%)	45(97.83%)	0.024
	26	Conclusions	464(97.48%)	193(95.07%)	226(99.56%)*	45(97.83%)	0.012
Funding	27	Funding	324(68.07%)	104(51.23%)	179(78.85%)*	41(89.13%)*	0.000

[@]n = 430;
* # : there were statistical differences compared with Chinese journals and international journals, respectively.

Table 3. The comparison for Reporting of checklists for SRs/MAs on PRISMA statement.

Category	Item		≦2009 year n = 186	>2009 year n = 290	*P* value	SCI n = 204	Non-SCI n = 272	*P* value
Title	1	Title	143(84.62%[$])	247(95.00%[#])*	0.022	145(92.36%[&])	245(90.07%)*	0.000
Abstract	2	Structured summary	171(91.94%)	275(94.83%)	0.205	188(92.16%)	258(94.85%)	0.231
Introduction	3	Rationale	113(60.75%)	268(92.41%)*	0.000	172(84.31%)	208(76.47%)*	0.035
	4	Objective	185(99.46%)	246(84.83%)*	0.000	201(98.53%)	229(84.19%)*	0.000
Methods	5	Protocol and registration	24(12.90%)	36(12.41%)	0.875	56(27.45%)	4(1.47%)*	0.000
	6	Eligibility criteria	184(98.92%)	279(96.54%)	0.076	199(97.55%)	265(97.43%)	0.933
	7	Information sources	179(96.24%)	261(90.00%)*	0.012	202(99.02%)	238(87.50%)*	0.000
	8	Search	110(59.14%)	172(59.31%)	0.971	160(78.43%)	122(44.85%)*	0.000
	9	Study selection	124(66.67%)	224(75.68%)*	0.011	173(84.80%)	169(62.13%)*	0.000
	10	Data collection process	165(88.71%)	245(84.48%)	0.193	187(91.67%)	224(82.35%)*	0.003
	11	Data items	98(52.69%)	171(58.97%)	0.178	153(75.00%)	117(43.01%)*	0.000
	12	Risk of bias in individual studies	143(76.88%)	240(82.76%)	0.115	172(84.31%)	212(77.94%)	0.081
	13	Summary measures	141(75.81%)	246(84.83%)*	0.014	160(78.43%)	227(83.46%)	0.164
	14	Synthesis of results	147(79.03%)	255(87.93%)*	0.009	162(79.41%)	240(88.24%)*	0.009
	15	Risk of bias across studies	39(20.97%)	118(40.69%)*	0.000	66(32.35%)	90(33.09%)	0.866
	16	Additional analyses	66(35.48%)	125(43.10%)	0.098	97(47.55%)	95(34.93%)*	0.005
Results	17	Study selection	162(87.10%)	268(92.41%)	0.055	183(89.71%)	247(90.81%)	0.687
	18	Study characteristics	165(88.71%)	266(91.72%)	0.273	193(94.61%)	238(87.50%)*	0.009
	19	Risk of bias within studies	140(75.27%)	247(85.17%)*	0.007	176(86.27%)	212(77.94%)*	0.020
	20	Results of individual studies	139(74.73%)	272(93.79%)*	0.000	169(82.84%)	242(88.97%)	0.054
	21	Synthesis of results	134(72.04%)	255(87.93%)*	0.000	154(75.49%)	235(86.40%)*	0.002
	22	Risk of bias across studies	49(26.34%)	129(44.48%)*	0.000	69(33.82%)	108(39.71%)	0.189
	23	Additional analysis	57(30.65%)	107(36.90%)	0.161	94(46.08%)	71(26.10%)*	0.000
Discussion	24	Summary of evidence	182(97.85%)	249(85.86%)*	0.000	193(94.61%)	239(87.87%)*	0.012
	25	Limitations	183(98.39%)	272(93.79%)*	0.017	198(97.06%)	257(94.49%)	0.176
	26	Conclusions	185(99.46%)	279(96.21%)*	0.033	202(99.02%)	262 (96.32%)	0.063
Funding	27	Funding	129(69.35%)	200(68.97%)	0.929	170(83.33%)	154(56.62%)*	0.000

[$]n = 169,
[#]n = 260,
[&]n = 157.
*: there were statistical differences compared with non-SCI journals/>2009 y and SCI journals/2009 y, respectively.

We found that there is also considerable inconsistency in reporting of study selection criteria. For example, many primary studies on acupuncture report a random allocation design but are not specific enough for the reader to determine if they are actual RCTs. We propose that these uncertainties should be clarified by contacting the primary authors to determine the appropriateness of including the studies in the SRs/MAs. Because it has been suggested that only 6.8% of acupuncture efficacy studies published in Chinese journals are based on actual RCTs [25], we strongly propose that authors of SRs/MAs verify this information prior to inclusion of studies.

Acupuncture is considered an alternative or complementary treatment to western medical interventions such as drugs and surgery, and it can be considered a separate specialty. Thus, SRs/MAs on acupuncture require not only compliance with general PRISMA reporting standards but also accurate reporting of acupuncture information. As a result, it is necessary to develop an extension of the PRISMA statement for acupuncture.

There are several limitations to our study. First, our analyses were limited to acupuncture-specific SRs/MAs and therefore may not be applicable to SRs/MAs in other fields. Second, our assessment process was not blinded, and therefore the outcomes may be influenced by publication date and other factors. Third, our assessment criteria (yes or no) did not allow partial information to be used. Fourth, our study focused primarily on acupuncture rather than other TCM. We failed to distinguish acupuncture from herbal medicine massage, or western medicine because individual SRs/MAs we included in our analysis often contained several control groups rather than one group.

In summary, SRs/MAs of acupuncture studies have not comprehensively reported the information recommended in the PRISMA statement. Our study underscores that, in addition to focusing on careful study design and performance, attention should be paid to comprehensive reporting standards when publishing SRs/MAs of acupuncture studies.

Supporting Information

Checklist S1 PRISMA Checklist.
(DOC)

Text S1 The English and Chinese databases search strategy.
(DOC)

Text S2 Inclusion Exclusion Section.
(DOC)

Text S3 Definitions of reporting items.
(DOC)

Text S4 476 SRs/MAs of acupuncture.
(DOC)

Acknowledgments

We thank Yongteng Xu, Xianxia Yan, Shengping Yang, Xin Tian, Yannan Zhou,Yiming Lu, Qingshan Guo (Lanzhou University) for previous work that contributed to the development in this study. We thank BiomEditor for providing assistance with final revision of the manuscript.

Author Contributions

Conceived and designed the experiments: YLL KHY. Performed the experiments: RZ JH XZ DLL WTS PZ HC. Analyzed the data: YFM JH. Contributed reagents/materials/analysis tools: YJW. Wrote the paper: YLL RZ.

References

1. Oxman AD, Cook DJ, Guyatt GH (1994) Users' guides to the medical literature. VI. How to use an overview. 238 Evidence-Based Medicine Working Group. JAMA 272:1367–1371.
2. Swingler GH, Volmink J, Ioannidis JP (2003) Number of published systematic 239 reviews and global burden of disease: database analysis. BMJ 327:1083–1084.
3. Moher D, Liberati A, Tetzlaff J, Altman DG, PRISMA Group (2009) Preferred reporting items for systematic reviews and meta-analyses: the PRISMA statement. BMJ 339: b2535.
4. Sacks HS, Berrier J, Reitman D, Ancona-Berk VA, Chalmers TC (1987) Meta-analysis of randomized controlled trials. New Engl J Med 316: 450–455.
5. Moher D, Tetzlaff J, Tricco AC, Sampson M, Altman DG (2007) Epidemiology and reporting characteristics of systematic reviews. PLoS Med 4:e78. [PMID: 17388659].
6. Kelly KD, Travers A, Dorgan M, Slater L, Rowe BH (2001) Evaluating the quality of systematic reviews in the emergency medicine literature. Ann Emerg Med 38:518–526.
7. Richards D (2004) The quality of systematic reviews in dentistry. Evid Based Dent 5:17.
8. Delaney A, Bagshaw SM, Ferland A, Manns B, Laupland KB, Doig CJ (2005) A systematic evaluation of the quality of meta-analyses in the critical care literature. Crit Care 9:R575–582.
9. Willis BH, Quigley M (2011) The assessment of the quality of reporting of meta-analyses in diagnostic research: a systematic review. BMC Med Res Methodol 11:163.
10. Delaney A, Bagshaw SM, Ferland A, Manns B, Laupland KB, Doig CJ (2005) A systematic evaluation of the quality of meta-analyses in the critical care literature. Crit Care 5:R575–82. [PMID: 16277721].
11. Moher D, Cook DJ, Eastwood S, Olkin I, Rennie D, et al (1999) Improving the quality of reports of meta-analyses of randomised controlled trials: the QUOROM statement. Quality of Reporting of Meta-analyses. Lancet 354: 1896–1900.
12. Delaney A, Bagshaw SM, Ferland A, Manns B, Laupland KB, et al (2005) A systematic evaluation of the quality of meta-analyses in the critical care literature. Crit Care 9: 575–582.
13. Sood A, Sood R, Bauer BA, Ebbert JO (2005) Cochrane systematic reviews in acupuncture: methodological diversity in database searching. J Altern Complement Med 11(4):719–722.
14. Liu Y, Yang S, Dai J, Xu Y, Zhang R, Jiang H, Yan X, Yang K (2011) Risk of Bias Tool in Systematic Reviews/Meta-Analyses of Acupuncture in Chinese Journals. PLoS One 6(12):e28130.
15. Lui S, Smith EJ, Terplan M (2010) Heterogeneity in search strategies among Cochrane acupuncture reviews: is there room for improvement? Acupunct Med 28(3):149–153.
16. Tao KM, Li XQ, Zhou QH, Moher D, Ling CQ, Yu WF (2011) From QUOROM to PRISMA: A Survey of High-Impact Medical Journals' Instructions to Authors and a Review of Systematic Reviews in Anesthesia. PLoS One 6(11):e27611.
17. Ma B, Guo JW, Qi GQ, , Li H, Peng J, Zhang Y, et al. (2011) Epidemiology, Quality and Reporting Characteristics of Systematic Reviews of Traditional Chinese Medicine Interventions Published in Chinese Journals. Plos One 6(5):e20185.
18. Ma B, Qi GQ, Lin XT, Wang T, Chen ZM, Yang KH (2012) Epidemiology, quality, and reporting characteristics of systematic reviews of acupuncture interventions published in Chinese journals[J]. J Altern Complement Med 18(9): 813–817.
19. Padula RS, Pires RS, Alouche SR, Chiavegato LD, Lopes AD, Costa LO (2012) Analysis of reporting of systematic reviews in physical therapy published in Portuguese. Rev Bras Fisioter 16(4):381–8.
20. Gagnier JJ, Kellam PJ (2013) Reporting and methodological quality of systematic reviews in the orthopaedic literature. J Bone Joint Surg Am 5, 95(11):e771–7.
21. Kiriakou J, Pandis N, Fleming PS, Madianos P, Polychronopoulou A (2013). Reporting quality of systematic review abstracts in leading oral implantology journals. J Dent 41(12):1181–7.
22. Fleming PS, Seehra J, Polychronopoulou A, Fedorowicz Z, Pandis N (2013) A PRISMA assessment of the reporting quality of systematic reviews in orthodontics. Angle Orthod 83(1): 158–163.
23. PROSPERO. international prospective register of systematic reviews. Available. http://www.crd.york.ac.uk/prospero/.
24. Moher D, Shamseer L, Clarke M, et al (2011) Reporting 270 Guidelines for Systematic Review Protocols. The19 Cochrane Colloquium.
25. Wu T, Li Y, Bian Z, et al (2009) Randomized trials published in some Chinese journals: how many are randomized?. Trials 10(1): 46.

24

Phantom Acupuncture: Dissociating Somatosensory and Cognitive/Affective Components of Acupuncture Stimulation with a Novel Form of Placebo Acupuncture

Jeungchan Lee[1], Vitaly Napadow[1,2], Jieun Kim[2], Seunggi Lee[3], Woojin Choi[3], Ted J. Kaptchuk[4], Kyungmo Park[1]*

1 Department of Biomedical Engineering, Kyung Hee University, Yongin, Gyeonggi, South Korea, **2** Martinos Center for Biomedical Imaging, Department of Radiology, Massachusetts General Hospital, Charlestown, Massachusetts, United States of America, **3** Department of Neuropsychiatry, College of Korean Medicine, Sangji University, Wonju, Gangwon, South Korea, **4** Program in Placebo Studies, Beth Israel Deaconess Medical Center, Harvard Medical School, Boston, Massachusetts, United States of America

Abstract

In a clinical setting, acupuncture treatment consists of multiple components including somatosensory stimulation, treatment context, and attention to needle-based procedures. In order to dissociate somatosensory versus contextual and attentional aspects of acupuncture, we devised a novel form of placebo acupuncture, a visual manipulation dubbed phantom acupuncture, which reproduces the acupuncture needling ritual without somatosensory tactile stimulation. Subjects (N = 20) received both real (REAL) and phantom (PHNT) acupuncture. Subjects were retrospectively classified into two groups based on PHNT credibility (PHNTc, who found phantom acupuncture credible; and PHNTnc, who did not). Autonomic and psychophysical responses were monitored. We found that PHNT can be delivered in a credible manner. Acupuncture needling, a complex, ritualistic somatosensory intervention, induces sympathetic activation (phasic skin conductance [SC] response), which may be specific to the somatosensory component of acupuncture. In contrast, contextual effects, such as needling credibility, are instead associated with a shift toward relative cardiovagal activation (decreased heart rate) during needling and sympathetic inhibition (decreased SC) and parasympathetic activation (decreased pupil size) following acupuncture needling. Visual stimulation characterizing the needling ritual is an important factor for phasic autonomic responses to acupuncture and may undelie the needling orienting response. Our study suggests that phantom acupuncture can be a viable sham control for acupuncture as it completely excludes the somatosensory component of real needling while maintaining the credibility of the acupuncture treatment context in many subjects.

Editor: Xi Luo, Brown University, United States of America

Funding: The authors would like to thank the Korean National Research Foundation funded by the Ministry of Science, ICT and Future Planning (NRF-2011-0028968, NRF-2009-0076345), and the Ministry of Health & Welfare and Seoul Metropolitan Government (Traditional Korean Medicine R&D Project, HI13C0700). The study was also supported by the National Center for Complementary and Alternative Medicine (NCCAM), at the United States of America National Institutes of Health (NIH) (P01-AT006663, R01-AT007550, R01-AT004714 to VN, K24-AT004095 to TJK). The content is the sole responsibility of the authors and does not necessarily represent the official views of our funding agencies. The funders had no role in study design, data collection and analysis, decision to publish, or preparation of the manuscript.

Competing Interests: The authors have declared that no competing interests exist.

* Email: saenim@khu.ac.kr

Introduction

While acupuncture has been shown to reduce pain in many previous clinical trials, statistically significant differences between real and sham acupuncture have not been consistently demonstrated [1,2,3,4]. This may be due to the fact that sham acupuncture commonly has included a somatosensory or tactile component. In fact, previous studies have not separated the complex acupuncture ritual into its constituent components, which could better determine the specific effects of this therapeutic intervention [1]. In this study, we propose an experimental design that allows for a separation of the acupuncture ritual into a somatosensory and contextual component, with autonomic outflow and psychophysical outcome metrics.

Sham acupuncture, which has been used as a control in many acupuncture studies, has been shown to produce a physiological effect [5,6], as it affects skin receptors, which are known to be even more dense than muscle and fascial somatosensory and nociceptors [7,8]. In fact, sham acupuncture can produce similar somatosensory or pain intensity even without skin penetration [9,10]. Acupuncture is a multi-dimensional intervention, and usage of sham acupuncture techniques as controls in clinical trials would be aided by a better understanding of the different components related to the therapeutic effect of acupuncture [11]. For instance, the tactile component in sham acupuncture is considered essential for credibility of the needling ritual. But this may not be the case. Because tactile stimulation produces a

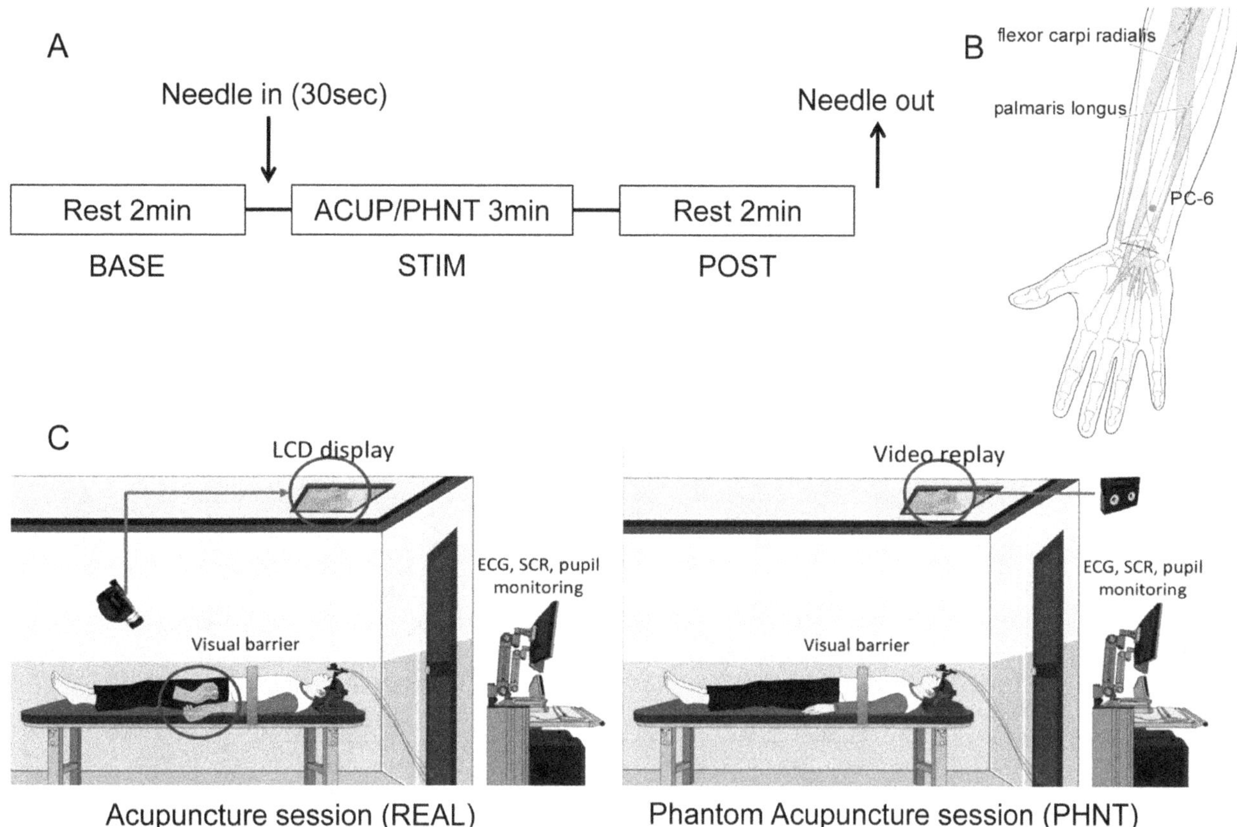

Figure 1. Experimental protocol. A. The paradigm consisted of 3-minute event-related stimulation (STIM, 3-second stimulation, ISI mean = 19.5 sec) surrounded by two 2-minute rest sessions (BASE and POST). **B.** Acupuncture stimulation location (PC6). **C.** Experimental setup for REAL and PHNT sessions. n.b. Figure in **B.** was modified from an image in 'WHO Regional Office for the Western Pacific, 2008, WHO Standard Acupuncture Point Locations in the Western Pacific Region, Manila'.

physiological response and may overlap therapeutic components of verum acupuncture, usage of sham acupuncture as a placebo control may be compromised, and there is great need for the development of a credible sham acupuncture procedure that does not include somatosensory (tactile) stimulation [12].

In this study we employed several outcome measures to assess different components of acupuncture. Physiological measures estimated autonomic nervous system (ANS) activity. ANS responses have been reported to have clinical relevance to many disease processes. For example, heart rate changes have been associated with clinical improvements for PTSD [13] and chronic pain [14], and have been linked with memory recall [15], somatosensory processing [16] and emotional memory processing [17]. Moreover, many studies have explored acupuncture's effects on ANS activity. Yao et al. showed that acupuncture induces a temporary increase in sympathetic tone, followed by a more prolonged depression [18]. Other investigators have also noted increased sympathetic tone during acupuncture stimulation [19] and increased parasympathetic tone after the stimulation [20,21]. Other studies have linked acupuncture-induced HR decrease, with immune system modulation [22]. However, Lee et al. [23] found no definitive evidence of association between heart rate variability and clinical outcomes, perhaps due to variability in stimulation methods (e.g. needling intensity, duration and frequency), experimental conditions (e.g. measurement timing), or between-subject variability. In fact, individual autonomic response is easily influenced by subtle changes of experimental setup, necessitating a well-controlled design. Our previous study measured concurrent autonomic and brain responses in a neuroimaging study [5]. We showed that, on average, acupuncture produced HR decrease and SCR increase after manual needle stimulation, though individual stimuli could produce both HR increase and decrease. These variable responses were modulated by distinct neural circuitries. In summary, acupuncture induced ANS response may vary based on needling location, needling technique, and needling dose as well as psychological factors and temporal variability.

In this study, we developed a novel form of sham acupuncture which was credible for many subjects, but did not include somatosensory stimulation. This allowed us to dissociate three different components of acupuncture. These included a tactile stimulation-specific component, an attentional shift component (due to visual/somatosensory stimulation), and a cognitive component related to a credibility of the needling procedure. Psychophysical and psychophysiological outcomes were used to dissociate these different components of acupuncture.

Materials and Methods

All research procedures were approved by the Institutional Review Board (IRB) committee of Sangji University (IRB approval number: SJ 2007-071201), and investigations were conducted in accordance with the principles of the Declaration of Helsinki. All participants in the study provided written informed consent.

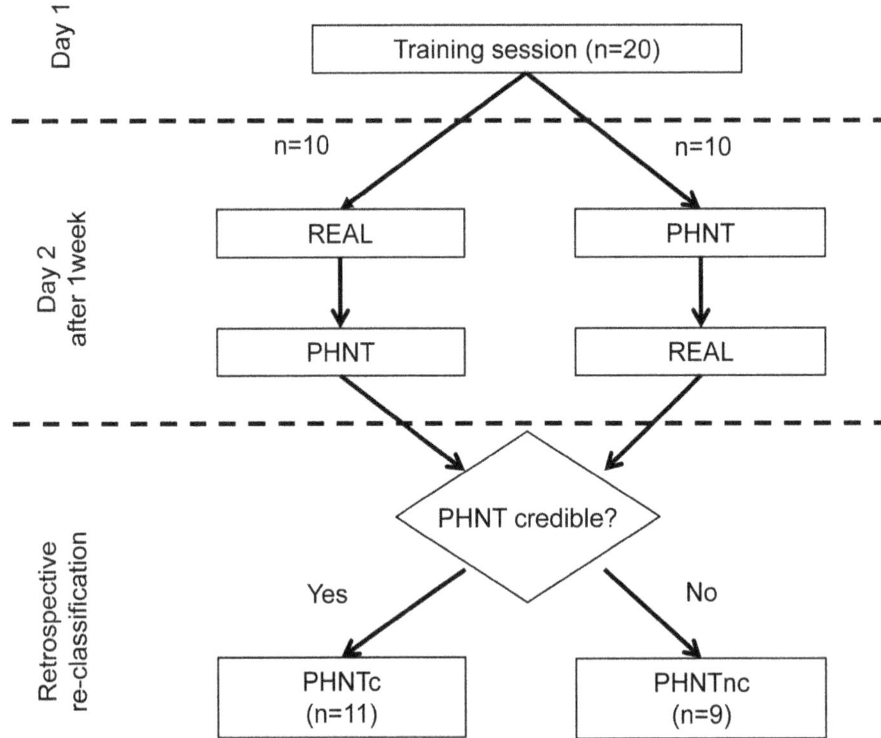

Figure 2. Study flow. Among twenty healthy subjects, ten received real acupuncture (REAL) first, while the rest received phantom acupuncture (PHNT) first, and they were re-classified into phantom credible (PHNTc) and phantom non-credible (PHNTnc) according to the needling credibility in phantom acupuncture (PHNT).

Subjects and Experimental Design

Twenty healthy, right handed female adults (21.8±2.6 years old) participated in both real acupuncture and sham control (phantom acupuncture) sessions in a crossover design. Subjects were recruited via fliers/webpage at the university and its neighborhood. Subjects were screened to exclude any autonomic dysfunction and asked not to take any pharmacological or autonomic modulating substance (e.g. caffeine) prior to testing.

A behavioral training session was completed 1 week prior to either experimental session, during which acupuncture stimulation was applied to the subjects in exactly the same way as during the real acupuncture (REAL) session to record a video clip of acupuncture needling prior to the actual acupuncture sessions. During this session, the acupuncture expectancy questionnaire was completed by study subjects to quantify individual variability in expectancy for acupuncture efficacy [24]. Subjects also completed the Edinburgh Handedness questionnaire [25]. The acupuncturist for this all subsequent sessions was an experienced practitioner (WC) with five years of clinical practice.

Real acupuncture (REAL) and phantom acupuncture (PHNT) sessions, separated by at least 40 min, were performed with pseudo-randomized order. For REAL, a 2-minute duration resting baseline (BASE) was followed by needle insertion (completed within 30 seconds, **Figure 1B**). The needle (0.3 mm*30 mm stainless steel needle, Dongbang Co., Korea) was inserted at left acupoint PC6 on the medial side of the right forearm and rotated manually at a rate of ~2 Hz. This acupoint is 2 cun (approximately 5 cm) proximal to the transverse wrist crease, between the tendons of the palmaris longus and flexor carpi radialis muscles, and is innervated by the median and antebrachial cutaneous nerves. This point is thought to be useful for cardiac conditions, as well as to control nausea and vomiting. It was chosen for this study because clinically, stimulation at this point has been used to modulate autonomic function and is known to induce robust acupuncture sensation [26].

The acupuncturist approached his hand to the acupoint and rotated the needle according to the stimulation timing that was implemented by computer (Psychtoolbox and Matlab, The MathWorks Inc., MA, USA) and relayed to the acupuncturist by auditory signals via headphones. Needle stimulation (STIM) comprised eight stimuli (3-second durations) at pseudo-randomized inter-stimulus interval ($\mu = 19.5$ second) over a duration of 3 minutes. Another 2 minute resting period (POST) followed this STIM period, where the acupuncture needle was retained in the arm (**Figure 1A**). The entire procedure (lasting ~7.5 minutes) was video-recorded and simultaneously displayed to the subject, who could not see the procedure directly due to a visual barrier.

For PHNT, the acupuncturist did not provide any tactile input to the subjects, and only approached his hand toward the acupoint. However, the video clip of prior acupuncture needling which was recorded at the previous REAL or training session was replayed to the subject, thus creating an illusion of needle insertion and stimulation (**Figure 1C**).

In order to perform the needle stimulation at the exact timing according to the experimental protocol, the acupuncturist followed auditory cues. After the stimulation timing signals were sent to the acupuncturist, the approaching time of acupuncturist's hand to the acupoint (PC6) in the video display were calculated retrospectively. The average time delay from onset of hand motion to reaching the acupoint was 0.77±0.26 second (mean±STD). Thus, actual acupuncture stimulations were applied about 0.8 second after the subject observed visual motion for the acupuncturist's hand.

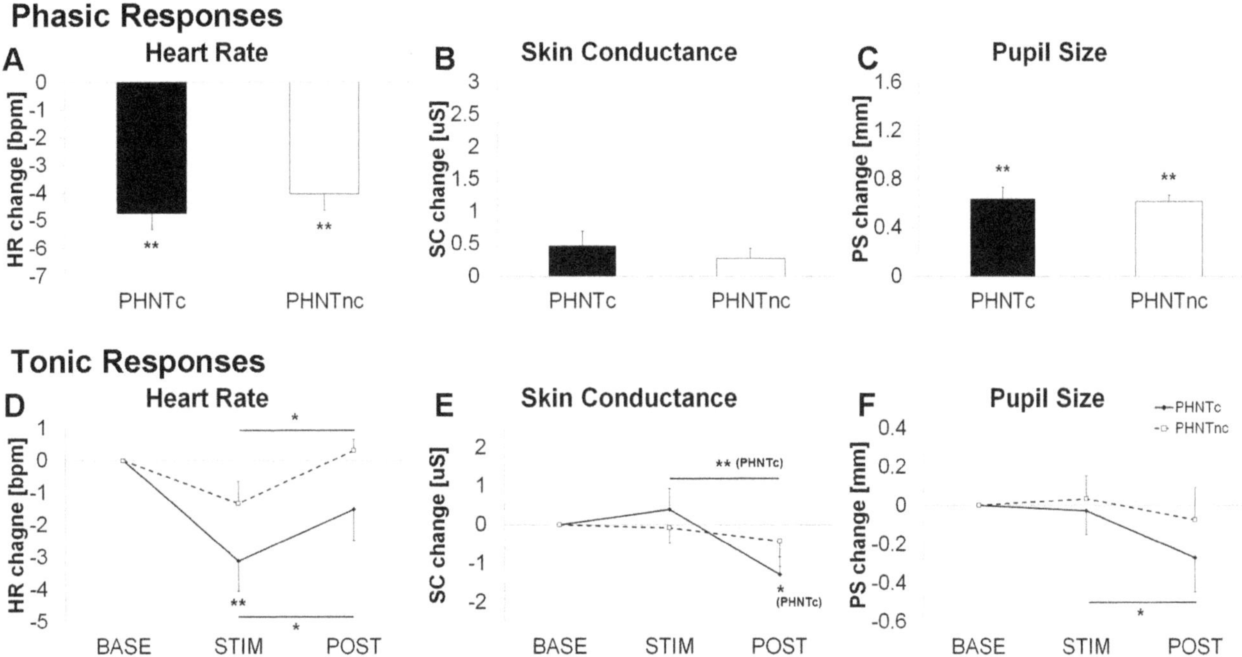

Figure 3. Influence of credibility on autonomic response modulation to phantom acupuncture. Phasic and tonic responses for heart rate (**A** and **D**), skin conductance (**B** and **E**), and pupil size (**C** and **F**) were contrasted between credible (PHNTc) and non-credible (PHNTnc) phantom acupuncture. n.b. *<0.05, **<0.01. Error bars represent standard error of the mean.

Subjects were either acupuncture-naïve (n = 2) or had only a few experiences with acupuncture treatment (n = 18, 6.0±6.7 times, mean±STD), and were informed that there would be two identical experimental acupuncture sessions. Subjects laid supine with their vision of distal body regions blocked by a barrier. They were told to look at the video display projected onto a monitor on the ceiling and were thus prevented from viewing the intervention occurring at the acupuncture point in their periphery (**Figure 1C**).

The PHNT session aimed to control for 'needling credibility,' but without somatosensory afference. In turn, the REAL session included both the 'somatosensory stimulation' as well as the needling credibility inherent to acupuncture.

Psychophysical Data Collection and Analysis

After each session, subjects were presented with a 10-point VAS and were asked to rate the intensity of different sensations they felt during the STIM period. We used an in-house Korean version of MGH Acupuncture Sensation Scale [27] comprising different "*deqi*" sensations (i.e. aching, soreness, pressure, heaviness, fullness, warmth, cool, numbness, tingling, and dull pain). In order to quantify the total intensity of acupuncture sensation experienced, we used the previously described MASS-Index [27]. This index attempts to balance breadth and depth of sensations as well as the number of different sensations chosen by the subject. The MASS index (MI) and individual sensation intensities were compared between stimulation groups using a paired *t*-test, significant at $p<0.05$.

Retrospective Re-classification According to Needling Credibility

After finishing both REAL and PHNT sessions, subjects were retrospectively separated into phantom credible (PHNTc, high needling credibility, n = 11) and phantom non-credible (PHNTnc, low needling credibility, n = 9) groups using a questionnaire and interview that evaluate the credibility of the procedure – e.g., whether or not they were able to differentiate the difference between real and phantom acupuncture, and if they believed they received real needle acupuncture in both sessions. Four subjects in the PHNTnc subgroup recognized the procedure as placebo when they noticed that the video clip of acupuncture needling was not synchronized with their hand's spontaneous movement. Five subjects in the PHNTnc subgroup had low credibility because they did not have any acupuncture sensation at the acupoint or surrounding region (**Figure 2**).

Multi-modal Physiological Data Collection and Analysis

To investigate any autonomic modulation specific to somatosensory afference or needling credibility following acupuncture, we recorded heart rate (HR), skin conductance (SC), and pupil size (PS) throughout the entire session (7.5 min). Subjects rested for at least 10 minutes prior to initiation of data collection. Electrocardiogram and electrical skin conductance were measured using commercial devices (PowerLab/800, ADinstruments, Australia) with a 1 kHz sampling rate. Pupil diameter was measured using a custom constructed pupilometry system that includes an image acquisition system (an IR camera and optical devices attached on a helmet) and analysis software enabling the estimation of precise pupil diameter for every image frame (30 frames/sec) using geometric correction, which compensate the errors induced by lens of the camera and by projection on two-dimensional image plane [28].

ANS outflow metrics (HR, SC, and PS) were computed for estimation of both a tonic response and a phasic event-related response. For the tonic response, the mean HR, SC and PS were calculated for three separate windows: BASE, STIM, and POST. For the phasic responses, the maximum change scores (typically decrease for HR, and increase for SC and PS) were calculated in a

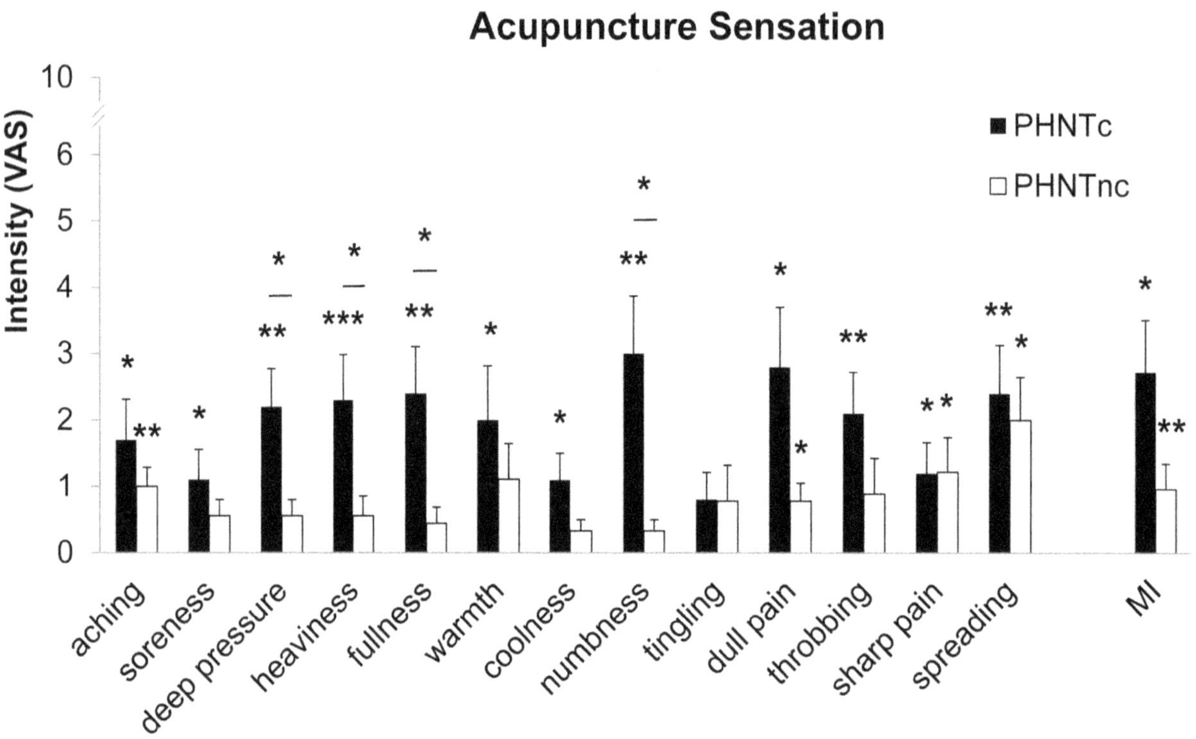

Acupuncture Sensation

Figure 4. Influence of credibility on acupuncture sensations to phantom acupuncture. PHNTc reported significantly greater sensation intensity for numbness and dull pain (i.e. *deqi* sensations). n.b. *<0.05, **<0.01, ***<0.001. Error bars represent standard error of the mean.

6 second window (0~6 seconds after each stimulation onset), which was contrast to a baseline window (preceding 5 seconds, accounting for acupuncturist hand motion as previously mentioned; i.e., −5.8 to −0.8 sec, with −0.8 to 0 second excluded due to acupuncturist's reaction time).

Results

For the 20 subjects, order of REAL or PHNT session was pseudo-randomized such that 10 received real acupuncture first, while the rest received phantom acupuncture first. There was no significant difference in age (REAL first: 21.1±2.9 years old, PHNT first: 22.5±2.3 years old; mean±STD), handedness (REAL first: 73.4±28.9%, PHNT first: 68.3±54.7%; 100%: right handed, −100%: left handed), positive expectation about acupuncture efficacy (REAL first: 2.4±0.2, PHNT first: 2.3±0.5; out of 1 to 5 range) or state/trait anxiety (STAI-state: REAL first: 27.8±7.5, PHNT first: 26.8±5.6; STAI-trait: REAL first: 33.7±5.2, PHNT first: 31.8±8.3) between the two order groups. From retrospective credibility questionnaires, we classified our subjects into PHNTc (PHNT credible; who reported high needling credibility for PHNT, n = 11) and PHNTnc (PHNT non-credible; who reported low needling credibility, n = 9).

Needling credibility effects: PHNTc vs PHNTnc

For phasic ANS responses, regardless of needling credibility, we noted decreased HR (PHNTc = −4.75±0.58 BPM, P<0.001; PHNTnc = −4.01±0.62 BPM, P<0.001, mean±SEM) and increased PS (PHNTc = 0.64±0.10 mm, P<0.001; PHNTnc = 0.62±0.05 mm, P<0.001) in response to visual stimulation. We did not note a phasic SC response. No significant differences were noted between PHNTc and PHNTnc in terms of phasic ANS response (**Figure 3A–C**).

For tonic ANS responses, we noted significant decrease in tonic HR for PHNTc (Δ = −3.12±0.94 BPM, P<0.01) but not for PHNTnc (Δ = −1.33±0.68 BPM, P = 0.09) during STIM (compared to BASE). During POST, the tonic HR rebounded back to BASE levels. For SC and PS, only PHNTc showed significant tonic decreases during POST compared to STIM (SC response: Δ = −1.27±0.45 μS, P<0.001; PS response: Δ = −0.27±0.18 mm, P<0.05) (**Figure 3D–F**).

Interestingly, following PHNTc, subjects reported many different acupuncture sensations (e.g. aching = 1.7±0.6, P<0.05; soreness = 1.1±0.5, P<0.05; deep pressure = 2.2±0.6, P<0.01; heaviness = 2.3±0.7, P<0.001; fullness = 2.4±0.7, P<0.01; warmth = 2.0±0.8, P<0.05; coolness = 1.1±0.4, P<0.05; numbness = 3.0±0.9, P<0.01; dull pain = 2.8±0.9, P<0.05; throbbing = 2.1±0.6, P<0.01; sharp pain = 1.2±0.5, P<0.05; spreading = 2.4±0.7, P<0.01). For PHNTnc, reported sensations were more mild and fewer in number (i.e. aching = 1.0±0.3, P<0.01; dull pain = 0.8±0.3, P<0.05; sharp pain = 1.2±0.5, P<0.05; and spreading = 2.0±0.6, P<0.05). Significant differences between credible versus non-credible PHNT subgroups were noted for deep pressure (PHNTc = 2.2±0.6, PHNTnc = 0.6±0.2, P<0.05), heaviness (PHNTc = 2.3±0.7, PHNTnc = 0.6±0.3, P<0.05), fullness (PHNTc = 2.4±0.7, PHNTnc = 0.4±0.2, P<0.05), and numbness (PHNTc = 3.0±0.9, PHNTnc = 0.3±0.2, P<0.05) – all classic *deqi* sensations. Trending differences were noted for dull pain (PHNTc = 2.8±0.9, PHNTnc = 0.8±0.3, P = 0.06) and MI (PHNTc = 2.7±0.8, PHNTnc = 1.0±0.4, P = 0.08) (**Figure 4**).

Acupuncture somatosensory stimulation effects: REAL vs PHNTc

Comparisons between REAL and PHNTc were based on the data collected only from subjects who regarded phantom acupuncture as real (i.e., PHNTc) and was done using paired *t*-

tests. For phasic ANS response, there was significant phasic SC increase in response to somatosensory stimulation, for REAL (1.56±0.50 μS, P<0.001) but only trending response for PHNTc (0.47±0.23 μS, P = 0.07). We also noted significant phasic HR decreases (REAL = −5.07±0.87 BPM, P<0.001; PHNTc = −4.75±1.92 BPM, P<0.001) and PS increases (REAL = 0.70± 0.10 mm, P<0.001; PHNTc = 0.64±0.10 mm, P<0.001) for both REAL and PHNTc sessions (**Figure 5A–C**).

We also noted significant tonic SC increase (STIM vs. BASE) for REAL (1.31±0.37 μS, P<0.01) but not PHNTc (0.39± 0.54 μS, P = 0.49). Additionally, significant tonic SC decreases were noted from STIM to POST for both REAL (Δ = −1.67±1.15 μS, P<0.001) and PHNTc (Δ = −1.66±0.98 μS, P< 0.001). For tonic HR response, significant decreases for STIM vs. BASE were noted for both REAL and PHNTc (PHNTc = −3.12±1.79 BPM, P<0.05; REAL = −2.24±1.35 BPM, P< 0.01). Tonic HR rebounded back to baseline levels during POST (Δ = 1.60±0.98 BPM in PHNTc, P<0.05; Δ = 1.64±1.15 in REAL, P<0.001). Significant tonic PS decreases were found for POST (vs STIM) only in PHNTc (Δ = −0.31±0.66, P<0.05), but not in REAL (Δ = −0.24±0.48, P = 0.22) (**Figure 5D–F**).

Acupuncture sensations, such as aching, soreness, deep pressure, sharp pain etc., were reported following real acupuncture stimulation (REAL). Interestingly after PHNTc, even without any direct somatosensory stimulation, similar acupuncture sensation intensities as following REAL were also reported (aching pain: PHNTc = 1.7±0.6, REAL = 3.5±0.7, P = 0.07; deep pressure pain, PHNTc = 2.2±0.6, REAL = 2.9±0.7, P = 0.23; heaviness, PHNTc = 2.3±0.7, REAL = 2.6±0.7, P = 0.56; fullness, PHNTc = 2.4±0.7, REAL = 2.9±0.7, P = 0.43; numbness, PHNTc = 3.0± 0.9, REAL = 2.3±0.7, P = 0.24; dull pain, PHNTc = 2.8±0.9, REAL = 2.5±0.6, P = 0.72). Greater sensation intensity was noted for REAL for a few other sensations, such as soreness (PHNTc = 1.1±0.5, REAL = 3.2±0.9, P<0.05), tingling pain (PHNTc = 0.8± 0.4, REAL = 3.8±0.9, P<0.01) and sharp pain (PHNTc = 1.2±0.5, REAL = 4.1±0.7, P<0.01) (**Figure 6**).

Significant correlation between acupuncture sensation and autonomic response was found in PHNTc (deep pressure vs. phasic HR decrease: r = 0.73, P<0.05; deep pressure vs. phasic PS increase: r = −0.83, P<0.05; dull pain vs. phasic PS increase: r = −0.90, P<0.05) but not in REAL.

Temporal evolution of ANS response to REAL and PHNT

During the needle insertion, before the needle manipulation (1st –8th stim.), significant HR deceleration was observed in the three groups (REAL = −8.25±3.85 BPM, P<0.0001; PHNTc = −9.67±4.02, P<0.0001; PHNTnc = −9.25±4.59, P<0.0001). The amplitude of HR decrease, in subsequent needle manipulation, was then reduced but still significant compared to the baseline (P<0.05 for all events, **Figure 7A** for individual response, **Figure 3A** for average response of eight stimuli). No significant difference was found between groups at each event.

Pupil size also showed maximum increase at needle insertion in all groups (REAL = 1.57±0.74 mm, P<0.0001; PHNTc = 1.56± 0.62 mm, P<0.0001; PHNTnc = 1.62±0.63 mm, P<0.0001), and maintained greater than the baseline (P<0.01 for all events, except the response from PHNTc at 8th stimulation; Δ = 0.48±0.79 mm, P = 0.09) (**Figure 7C** for individual response, **Figure 3C** for average response of eight stimuli). Significantly greater PS increase was observed at 8th needle manipulation in REAL than PHNTc (REAL = 0.64±0.35 mm, PHNTc = 0.36± 0.28, P<0.05) (**Figure 7C**).

Significant SC increase was also produced by needle insertion (REAL = 4.81±3.56 μS, P<0.0001; PHNTc = 4.02±4.30 μS, P< 0.05; PHNTnc = 3.01±1.78 μS, P<0.001), and the responses were reduced in subsequent manipulation but significantly

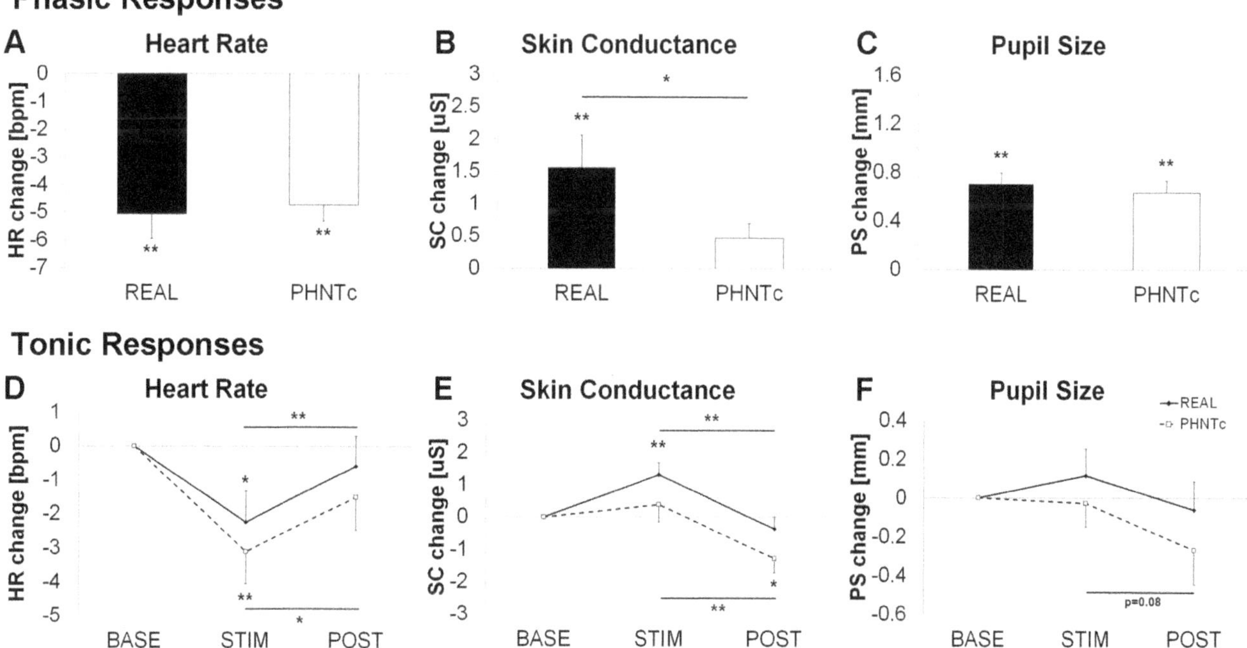

Figure 5. Influence of somatosensory needling on autonomic response modulation to real and phantom acupuncture. Phasic and tonic responses for heart rate (**A** and **D**), skin conductance (**B** and **E**), and pupil size (**C** and **F**) were contrasted between real (REAL) and credible (PHNTc) phantom acupuncture. Comparisons between REAL and PHNTc were based on the data collected only from subjects who regarded phantom acupuncture as real (i.e. PHNTc) and was done using paired *t*-tests. n.b. *<0.05, **<0.01. Error bars represent standard error of the mean.

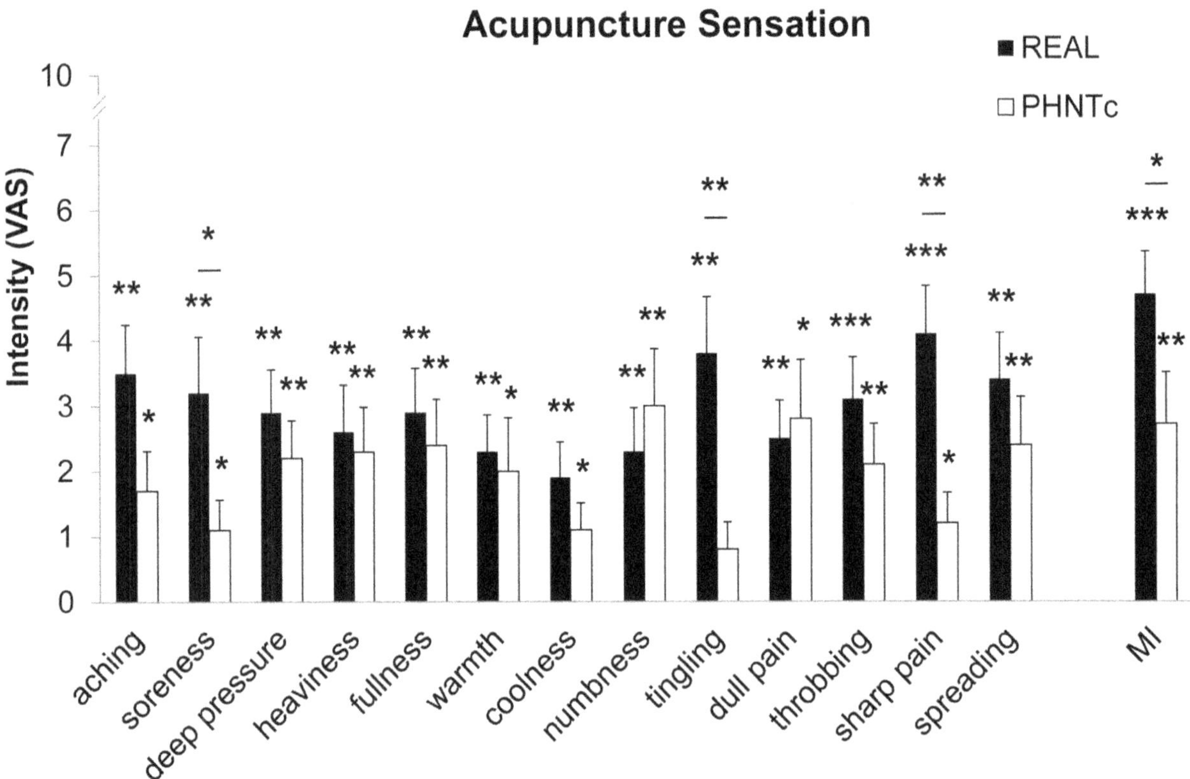

Figure 6. Influence of somatosensory needling on acupuncture sensations to real (REAL) and credible (PHNTc) phantom acupuncture. PHNTc reported similar sensation intensity as REAL for several *deqi*-related sensations (e.g., deep pressure, heaviness, fullness, numbness, dull pain). REAL produced greater sensation intensity for soreness, tingling, and sharp pain, as well as overall *deqi* sensation (i.e. MI). Comparisons between REAL and PHNTc were based on the data collected only from subjects who regarded phantom acupuncture as real (i.e. PHNTc) and was done using paired *t*-tests. n.b. *<0.05, **<0.01, ***<0.001. Error bars represent standard error of the mean.

maintained compared to the baseline in REAL ($P<0.05$ for all event) but not in PHNTc ($P>0.07$ for all events) and PHNTnc ($P>0.2$ for all events) (**Figure 7B** for individual response, **Figure 3B** for average response of eight stimuli).

Discussion

In this study, we have developed and tested a new form of placebo acupuncture, referred to as phantom acupuncture, which was characterized by an acupuncture needling intervention induced solely by visual display. We applied real (REAL) and phantom (PHNT) acupuncture and retrospectively re-classified subjects into two groups based on PHNT credibility (PHNTc, who found phantom acupuncture credible, n = 11; and PHNTnc, who did not find phantom acupuncture credible, n = 9). Physiological responses to REAL and PHNT were measured via autonomic response (heart rate, skin conductance, pupil size), while psychophysical responses were assessed by subjective ratings of needle sensation (Table 1). Real acupuncture induced greater skin conductance response, suggesting that the somatosensory component of acupuncture underlies the sympathetic outflow produced by acupuncture needle stimulation. We found that both real and phantom acupuncture (when credible) induced notable acupuncture sensation. The credibility of the ritual, a contextual component of acupuncture, was important for inducing robust *deqi* sensation, but was less important for autonomic response to purely visual phantom acupuncture, suggesting that some stimulus-associated autonomic response may be the result of subconscious processing that does not play a role in conscious cognitive re-evaluation of a ritual as credible or not.

Needling Credibility Effect: increased parasympathetic and decreased sympathetic activity

Physiological response to visual stimuli purporting to reflect needles entering the subject's skin, and being twisted, depended on whether or not the subjects believed the procedure to be credible. By contrasting PHNTc with PHNTnc, we were able to explore the acupuncture needling context independent from any somatosensory afference. Our data demonstrated that while phasic autonomic response to visual scenes of needle stimulation were not influenced by needling credibility (i.e. PHNTnc vs PHNTc), tonic autonomic responses were influenced. Specifically, compared to PHNTnc, PHNTc demonstrated HR deceleration during the stimulation period and decreased SCR/PS following stimulation (see **Figure 3**). Needling credibility may be associated with greater positive expectation of acupuncture efficacy and a generally more relaxed state, reflected in increased parasympathetic and decreased sympathetic activity, consistent with our data.

Our results showed that needling credibility influenced multi-organ autonomic response to needle-related stimuli. Previous studies have found that several brain regions implicated in placebo responses, such as pregenual anterior cingulate cortex, amygdala, and periaqueductal gray [29] are also associated with peripheral autonomic outflow and are components of a central autonomic network [30]. Other studies have noted that expectancy enhances heart rate change and sympathetic responses to deep brain

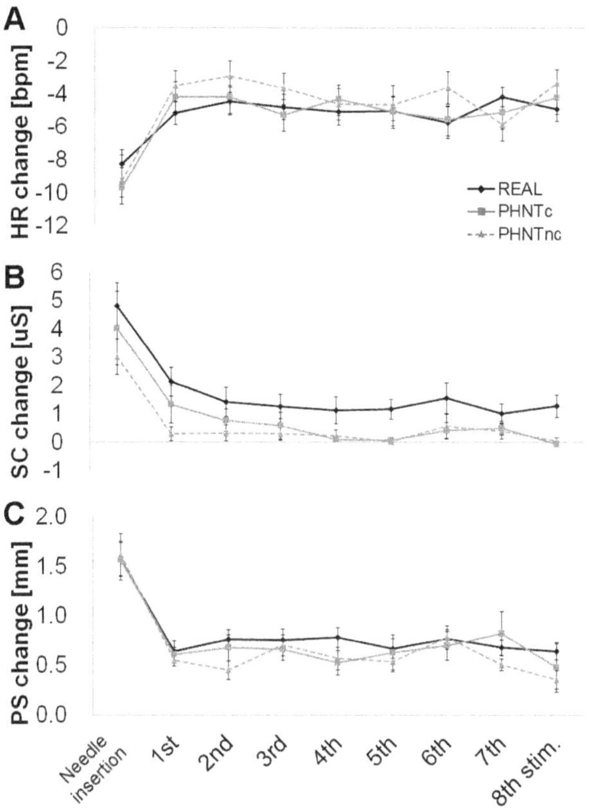

Figure 7. Temporal evolution of autonomic response to real (REAL) and phantom (credible, PHNTc; non-credible, PHNTnc) acupuncture. Needle insertion, whether real or phantom, produced significantly greater (A) HR decrease, (B) SC increase and (C) PS increase, compared to needle manipulation. ANS response to needle manipulation was relatively stable over all 8 manipulations for REAL (n = 20), PHNTc (n = 11), and PHNTnc (n = 9). SC increase was greater for REAL compared to PHNTc and especially PHNTnc, consistently over all stimuli. Error bars represent standard error of the mean.

stimulation of subthalamic limbic region in Parkinson patients [31]. In addition, placebo analgesia has been linked with reduced beta-adrenergic (not cardiovagal) heart response [32,33]. Thus, autonomic response may be an important factor in expectation and placebo-mediated outcomes. Phantom acupuncture clearly produces autonomic response and future studies should also link these multi-organ outflows with clinical outcomes in patient populations.

Interestingly, both phasic and tonic ANS response was evident for all three groups (REAL, PHNTc, PHNTnc), though more prominent in PHNT when the stimulus was judged to be credible. Visual feedback may be an important factor in augmenting a placebo intervention. Kaptchuk et al. have suggested that medical devices have an enhanced placebo effect and, specifically, that sham acupuncture is more effective than placebo pill on self-reported pain and symptom severity [34,35]. This hypothesis was recently corroborated in a systematic review of migraine prophylaxis [36]. Most prior sham acupuncture procedures include tactile (in addition to visual) stimulation, and can be characterized by adequate needling credibility. However, tactile stimulation may be an important component of a specific acupuncture effect, and some researchers have raised this point in questioning previous efficacy clinical trials which included both real and sham control acupuncture procedures [11,12]. While the visual component of acupuncture was found to also induce notable physiological response, particularly when phantom acupuncture was credible, our novel procedure was able to remove the somatosensory component and may be a viable procedure in future clinical trials aimed at dissociating the somatosensory versus visual components of acupuncture therapy.

Interestingly, the rated intensity of several acupuncture sensations (e.g. dull pain, heaviness, fullness, and numbness) associated with *deqi* sensation [27], were similar for PHNTc and REAL (see **Figure 6**). Hence, needling credibility leads to a mental rationalization of a perception anticipated by real needling (as all subjects experienced this at their initial session), even when a lack of somatosensory afference was incongruent to visual afference associated with needle insertion and stimulation. This effect may be similar to the rubber hand illusion, where body ownership is extended to an inanimate object, in this case a video recording [37]. Future studies should specifically explore if acupuncture sensation intensity can serve as a marker for needling credibility, and whether such sensations are closely linked to therapeutic efficacy in acupuncture trials. If sensation is the important variable for clinical outcomes, and if the sensation can be produced by needling credibility with no somatosensory afference, then this can be linked to the acupuncture placebo effect.

Somatosensory stimulation effect: sympathetic activation in SC response

To investigate the somatosensory stimulation effect, REAL and PHNTc were compared. Both REAL and PHNTc included a visual feedback component and were both credible acupuncture interventions, though PHNTc did not involve somatosensory afference. REAL showed significantly greater phasic and tonic SC responses, while PHNTc did not demonstrate significant SC response. This suggests that sudomotor activity is specifically driven by the tactile component of acupuncture needle stimulation. Somatosensory afference can be delivered by acupuncture

Table 1. Summarization of the physiological responses to real and phantom acupuncture stimulation.

	Parasympathetic tone	Sympathetic tone	Orienting response	Deqi sensation
REAL		↑ (SC-phasic/tonic)	↓ HR-phasic, ↑ PS-phasic	+++ (for most sensation items)
PHNTc	↑ (SC-tonic, PS-tonic)		↓ HR-phasic, ↑ PS-phasic	++ (for deep pressure, heaviness, fullness, numbness, dull pain, and spreading)
PHNTnc			↓ HR-phasic, ↑ PS-phasic	+ (for dull and sharp pain)

HR: Heart Rate, SC: Skin Conductance, PS: Pupil Szie, tonic: tonic response, phasic: phasic response, +++: around 2–4 out of 10 scale, ++: around 2–3 out of 10 scale, +: around 1 out of 10 scale.

through an ascending pathway, which carries information from spinal cord to reticular formation, PAG and thalamus, and then to ACC, SI/SII, insula and prefrontal cortex, where tactile input can have broader cognitive/affective influence [7]. In our study, SCR was mainly observed with REAL stimulation, which suggests that somatosensory afference specifically supports the previously noted sympathetic response to acupuncture [5,36] and may be similar to sympathetic modulation by other pain or pain-like stimuli [38].

Visual stimulus effects: the orienting response

As previously noted, the visual stimulus itself may induce physiological response regardless of needling credibility. In fact, PHNTc, PHNTnc, and REAL all shared the same visual stimulus and produced physiological activity consistent with an orienting response (OR). Physiologically, OR is characterized by parasympathetically driven HR deceleration, sympathetically driven SCR increase, and behavioral orienting toward novel stimuli [39]. OR is also associated with pupil dilation linked to emotional processing of stimuli [40,41]. These mixed autonomic responses likely reflect supra-spinal feedback and may be differentially associated with different aspects of cognitive and affective processing involved with attention distribution towards novel stimuli. Particularly for needle insertion, which was done before needle manipulation (see **Figure 7**), all three groups showed significant HR deceleration, SC increase, and PS dilation compared to the baseline, suggesting that the visual component of needle insertion (and perhaps needle manipulation) leads to a physiological OR. Subsequent needle manipulation events during the STIM period showed less robust ANS response compared to needle insertion, suggesting diminished salience to the subject leading to diminished physiological arousal. Importantly, lack of notable habituation across repeated needle manipulation stimuli for all three groups suggests that saliency was conserved and difference analyses using summary ANS outcome measures (pooled over all stimuli) were not confounded by preferential habituation in one or more groups.

The fact that all three groups demonstrated robust ANS response may have significant implications in terms of understanding the placebo effect. Most discussions of the placebo postulate that environmental learning cues mediated through either conscious expectations or classical conditioning are the principle psychological mechanism of placebo responses [42]. Recently there has been evidence that suggests that non-conscious and implicit framing may play a key role [43]. Our study found robust ANS outflow in response to phantom acupuncture, even when credibility was compromised. As sensation and autonomic response were likely to be classically conditioned from subjects' experience in the training session with real acupuncture, any ANS outflow following phantom acupuncture, whether credible or not, may feed back to the brain via afferent autonomic pathways and play an important role in subsequent sub-conscious placebo effects.

Psychophysical response to real and phantom acupuncture

Interestingly, while overall *deqi* sensation (i.e. MASS Index) was greater for REAL compared to PHNT, when the latter was credible, many key *deqi* sensations (e.g. dull pain, numbness, and deep pressure) were similar in intensity. This suggests that *deqi* sensations can be induced not only by somatosensory afference but also by visual suggestion of needle stimulation and needling credibility [37,44]. In fact, when PHNT was credible, greater *deqi* sensation intensity (e.g. deep pressure) was associated with greater phasic HR decrease and with smaller phasic PS increase, suggesting that credibility-mediated acupuncture sensation raised parasympathetic activity, and the increased activity may be linked with clinical outcomes in patients (i.e. placebo effect) as the parasympathetic shift or the sympathetic drop has been believed to be one of underlying mechanisms in clinical acupuncture efficacy.

Several limitations should be noted. Our study was performed in healthy subjects (i.e., young university students) and not patient populations, and sample size of this study was quite small. As acupuncture is a therapeutic intervention applied for various pathological states, these results may not extend to, for instance, chronic pain patients. Thus, further study on large sample of patients should be performed for clinical implication. Additionally, our outcomes included autonomic outflow and psychometric outcomes. More clinically-relevant outcomes such as evoked pain modulation, should also be explored. Other physiological outcomes, such as brain response measured by neuroimaging should also be investigated.

In conclusion, our study developed and tested a new form of placebo acupuncture, referred to as phantom acupuncture, which was characterized by an acupuncture needling intervention induced solely by visual display. We found that both real and phantom acupuncture (when credible) induced notable acupuncture sensation. Real acupuncture induced greater skin conductance response, suggesting that the somatosensory component of acupuncture underlies the sympathetic outflow produced by acupuncture needle stimulation. We also found that credibility of the ritual, a contextual component of acupuncture, was important for inducing robust *deqi* sensation, but was less important for autonomic response to purely visual phantom acupuncture, suggesting that some stimulus-associated autonomic response may be the result of sub-conscious processing that does not play a role in conscious cognitive re-evaluation of a ritual as credible or not.

Author Contributions

Conceived and designed the experiments: JL JK SL WC KP. Performed the experiments: JL JK SL WC KP. Analyzed the data: JL VN KP. Contributed to the writing of the manuscript: JL VN TJK KP.

References

1. Langevin HM, Wayne PM, Macpherson H, Schnyer R, Milley RM, et al. (2011) Paradoxes in acupuncture research: strategies for moving forward. Evid Based Complement Alternat Med. 2011: 180805.
2. Linde K, Streng A, Jürgens S, Hoppe A, Brinkhaus B, et al. (2005) Acupuncture for patients with migraine: a randomized controlled trial. JAMA. 293: 2118–2125.
3. Yao E, Gerritz PK, Henricson E, Abresch T, Kim J, et al. (2012) Randomized controlled trial comparing acupuncture with placebo acupuncture for the treatment of carpal tunnel syndrome. PM R. 4: 367–373.
4. Hempel S, Taylor SL, Solloway MR, Miake-Lye IM, Beroes JM, et al. (2014) Evidence Map of Acupuncture [Internet]. Washington (DC): Department of Veterans Affairs. Available: http://www.ncbi.nlm.nih.gov/books/NBK185072/.
5. Napadow V, Lee J, Kim J, Cina S, Maeda Y, et al. (2013). Brain correlates of phasic autonomic response to acupuncture stimulation: an event-related fMRI study. Hum Brain Mapp. 34: 2592–2606.
6. Madsen MV, Gøtzsche PC, Hróbjartsson A (2009) Acupuncture treatment for pain: systematic review of randomised clinical trials with acupuncture, placebo acupuncture, and no acupuncture groups. BMJ. 338: a3115. doi: 10.1136/bmj.a3115.
7. Almeida TF, Roizenblatt S, Tufik S (2004) Afferent pain pathways: a neuroanatomical review. Brain Res. 1000: 40–56.
8. McGlone F, Reilly D (2010) The cutaneous sensory system. Neurosci Biobehav Rev. 34: 148–159.

9. Streitberger K, Kleinhenz J (1998) Introducing a placebo needle into acupuncture research. Lancet. 25: 271–275.
10. Park J, White A, Lee H, Ernst E (1999) Development of a new sham needle. Acupunct Med. 17: 110–112.
11. White P, Lewith G, Hopwood V, Prescott P (2003) The placebo needle, is it a valid and convincing placebo for use in acupuncture trials? A randomised, single-blind, cross-over pilot trial. Pain. 106: 401–409.
12. Lundeberg T, Lund I, Näslund J (2012) The needling sensation: A factor contributing to the specific effects of acupuncture? Acupuncture and related Therapies. 1: 2–4.
13. Shalev AY, Sahar T, Freedman S, Peri T, Glick N, et al. (1998) A prospective study of heart rate response following trauma and the subsequent development of posttraumatic stress disorder. Arch Gen Psychiatry. 55: 553–559.
14. Sparrow K (2007) Analysis of heart rate variability in acupuncture practice: can it improve outcome? Medical Acupuncture. 19: 37–41.
15. Abercrombie HC, Chambers AS, Greischar L, Monticelli RM (2008) Orienting, emotion, and memory: phasic and tonic variation in heart rate predicts memory for emotional pictures in men. Neurobiol Learn Mem. 90: 644–650.
16. Critchley HD, Mathias CJ, Josephs O, O'Doherty J, Zanini S, et al. (2003) Human cingulate cortex and autonomic control: converging neuroimaging and clinical evidence. Brain. 126: 2139–2152.
17. Anderson AK, Yamaguchi Y, Grabski W, Lacka D (2006) Emotional memories are not all created equal: evidence for selective memory enhancement. Learn Mem. 13: 711–718.
18. Yao T, Andersson S, Thorén P (1982) Long-lasting cardiovascular depression induced by acupuncture-like stimulation of the sciatic nerve in unanaesthetized spontaneously hypertensive rats. Brain Res. 240: 77–85.
19. Knardahl S, Elam M, Olausson B, Wallin BG (1998) Sympathetic nerve activity after acupuncture in humans. Pain. 75: 19–25.
20. Cao XD, Xu SF, Lu WX (1983) Inhibition of sympathetic nervous system by acupuncture. Acupunct Electrother Res. 8: 25–35.
21. Haker E, Egekvist H, Bjerring P (2000) Effect of sensory stimulation (acupuncture) on sympathetic and parasympathetic activities in healthy subjects. J Auton Nerv Syst. 79: 52–59.
22. Mori H, Nishijo K, Kawamura H, Abo T (2002) Unique immunomodulation by electro-acupuncture in humans possibly via stimulation of the autonomic nervous system. Neurosci Lett. 320: 21–24.
23. Lee S, Lee MS, Choi JY, Lee SW, Jeong SY, et al. (2010) Acupuncture and heart rate variability: a systematic review. Auton Neurosci. 155: 5–13.
24. Dennehy EB, Webb A, Suppes T (2002) Assessment of beliefs in the effectiveness of acupuncture for treatment of psychiatric symptoms. J Altern Complement Med. 8: 421–425.
25. Oldfield RC (1971) The assessment and analysis of handedness: the Edinburgh inventory. Neuropsychologia. 9(1): 97–113.
26. Beissner F, Deichmann R, Henke C, Bär KJ (2012) Acupuncture–deep pain with an autonomic dimension? Neuroimage. 60: 653–660.
27. Kong J, Gollub R, Huang T, Polich G, Napadow V, et al. (2007) Acupuncture de qi, from qualitative history to quantitative measurement. J Altern Complement Med. 13: 1059–1070.
28. Kim J, Park K, Khang G (2004) A method for size estimation of amorphous pupil in 3-dimensional geometry. Conf Proc IEEE Eng Med Biol Soc. 2: 1451–1454.
29. Zubieta JK, Stohler CS (2009) Neurobiological mechanisms of placebo responses. Ann N Y Acad Sci. 1156: 198–210.
30. Beissner F, Meissner K, Bär KJ, Napadow V (2013) The autonomic brain: an activation likelihood estimation meta-analysis for central processing of autonomic function. J Neurosci. 33(25): 10503–10511.
31. Lanotte M, Lopiano L, Torre E, Bergamasco B, Colloca L, et al. (2005) Expectation enhances autonomic responses to stimulation of the human subthalamic limbic region. Brain Behav Immun. 19: 500–509.
32. Pollo A, Vighetti S, Rainero I, Benedetti F (2003) Placebo analgesia and the heart. Pain. 102: 125–133.
33. Meissner K (2011) The placebo effect and the autonomic nervous system: evidence for an intimate relationship. Philos Trans R Soc Lond B Biol Sci. 366(1572): 1808–1817.
34. Kaptchuk TJ, Goldman P, Stone DA, Stason WB (2000) Do medical devices have enhanced placebo effects? J Clin Epidemiol. 53: 786–792.
35. Kaptchuk TJ, Stason WB, Davis RB, Legedza AR, Schnyer RN, et al. (2006) Sham device v inert pill: randomised controlled trial of two placebo treatments. BMJ. 332: 391–397.
36. Knardahl S, Elam M, Olausson B, Wallin BG (1998) Sympathetic nerve activity after acupuncture in humans. Pain. 75(1): 19–25.
37. Botvinick M, Cohen J (1998) Rubber hands 'feel' touch that eyes see. Nature. 391: 756.
38. Piché M, Arsenault M, Rainville P (2010) Dissection of perceptual, motor and autonomic components of brain activity evoked by noxious stimulation. Pain. 149: 453–462.
39. Sokolov E, Cacioppo J (1997) Orienting and defense reflexes: Vector coding and cardiac response. In: Lang P, Simons R, Balaban M, editors. Attention and Orienting: Sensory and Motivational Processes. Mahwah, NJ: Lawrence Erlbaum Associates Publishers.
40. Bradley MM (2009) Natural selective attention: orienting and emotion. Psychophysiology. 46: 1–11.
41. Lang PJ, Bradley MM (2010) Emotion and the motivational brain. Biol Psychol. 84: 437–450.
42. Finniss DG, Kaptchuk TJ, Miller F, Benedetti F (2010) Biological, clinical, and ethical advances of placebo effects. Lancet. 375(9715): 686–695.
43. Jensen KB, Kaptchuk TJ, Kirsch I, Raicek J, Lindstrom KM, et al. (2012) Nonconscious activation of placebo and nocebo pain responses. Proc Natl Acad Sci U S A. 109(39): 15959–15964.
44. Beissner F, Marzolff I (2012) Investigation of Acupuncture Sensation Patterns under Sensory Deprivation Using a Geographic Information System. Evid Based Complement Alternat Med. 2012: 591304.

Permissions

All chapters in this book were first published in PLOS ONE, by The Public Library of Science; hereby published with permission under the Creative Commons Attribution License or equivalent. Every chapter published in this book has been scrutinized by our experts. Their significance has been extensively debated. The topics covered herein carry significant findings which will fuel the growth of the discipline. They may even be implemented as practical applications or may be referred to as a beginning point for another development.

The contributors of this book come from diverse backgrounds, making this book a truly international effort. This book will bring forth new frontiers with its revolutionizing research information and detailed analysis of the nascent developments around the world.

We would like to thank all the contributing authors for lending their expertise to make the book truly unique. They have played a crucial role in the development of this book. Without their invaluable contributions this book wouldn't have been possible. They have made vital efforts to compile up to date information on the varied aspects of this subject to make this book a valuable addition to the collection of many professionals and students.

This book was conceptualized with the vision of imparting up-to-date information and advanced data in this field. To ensure the same, a matchless editorial board was set up. Every individual on the board went through rigorous rounds of assessment to prove their worth. After which they invested a large part of their time researching and compiling the most relevant data for our readers.

The editorial board has been involved in producing this book since its inception. They have spent rigorous hours researching and exploring the diverse topics which have resulted in the successful publishing of this book. They have passed on their knowledge of decades through this book. To expedite this challenging task, the publisher supported the team at every step. A small team of assistant editors was also appointed to further simplify the editing procedure and attain best results for the readers.

Apart from the editorial board, the designing team has also invested a significant amount of their time in understanding the subject and creating the most relevant covers. They scrutinized every image to scout for the most suitable representation of the subject and create an appropriate cover for the book.

The publishing team has been an ardent support to the editorial, designing and production team. Their endless efforts to recruit the best for this project, has resulted in the accomplishment of this book. They are a veteran in the field of academics and their pool of knowledge is as vast as their experience in printing. Their expertise and guidance has proved useful at every step. Their uncompromising quality standards have made this book an exceptional effort. Their encouragement from time to time has been an inspiration for everyone.

The publisher and the editorial board hope that this book will prove to be a valuable piece of knowledge for researchers, students, practitioners and scholars across the globe.

List of Contributors

Bin Ma, Guoqing Qi, Haimin Li, Yanqin Ding andKehu Yang
Evidence-Based Medicine Center, Institute of Traditional Chinese and Western Medicine, School of Basic Medical Sciences, Lanzhou University, Lanzhou, Gansu, China

JiyePeng
The Library of Lanzhou University, Lanzhou, Gansu, China

JiwuGuo and Yulong Zhang
Evidence-Based Medicine Center, Institute of Traditional Chinese and Western Medicine, School of Basic Medical Sciences, Lanzhou University, Lanzhou, Gansu, China
Second School of Clinical Medicine of Lanzhou University, Lanzhou, Gansu, China
The Library of Lanzhou University, Lanzhou, Gansu, China

Youbo You, LijunBai, Ruwei Dai, Zhenyu Liu, Wenjuan Wei,Zhenyu Liu and Wenjuan Wei
Key Laboratory of Molecular Imaging and Functional Imaging, Institute of Automation, Chinese Academy of Sciences, Beijing, China

Hao Cheng
Department of Anesthesiology, Beijing Ditan Hospital affiliated to Capital Medical University,Beijing, China

Zhiqun Wang, Zhilian Zhao and Jie Lu
Department of Radiology, Xuanwu Hospital of Capital Medical University, Beijing, China

BinbinNie and Baoci Shan
Institute of High Energy Physics, Chinese Academy of Sciences, Beijing, China

Donghong Li and Jianyang Xu
General Hospital of Chinese People's Armed Police Forces, Beijing China

Ying Han and Haiqing Song
Department of Neurology, Xuanwu Hospital of Capital Medical University, Beijing, China

Kuncheng Li
Department of Radiology, Xuanwu Hospital of Capital Medical University, Beijing, China
Key Laboratory for Neurodegenerative Diseases, Ministry of Education, Beijing, China

Hua Liu
Institute of High Energy Physics, Chinese Academy of Sciences (CAS), Beijing, China
Graduate University of Chinese Academy of Sciences, Beijing, China
KeyLaboratory of Nuclear Analysis Techniques (LNAT), CAS, Beijing, China

Jianyang Xu
General Hospital of Armed Police Forces, Beijing, China

Yongzhong Li
Xuanwu Hospital, Capital MedicalUniversity, Beijing, China

Lin Li, JingquanXue, BinbinNie and Baoci Shan
Institute of High Energy Physics, Chinese Academy of Sciences (CAS), Beijing, China
KeyLaboratory of Nuclear Analysis Techniques (LNAT), CAS, Beijing, China

Yang Wang, Jinna Yu, Jiani Wu, Jing Wang and Zhishun Liu
Guang'anmen Hospital, China Academy of Chinese Medical Sciences, Beijing, China

Baoyan Liu
China Academy of Chinese Medical Sciences, Beijing, China

Yali Liu and Kehu Yang
Evidence-Based Medicine Center, School of Basic Medical Sciences, Lanzhou University, Lanzhou, China
Institute of Integrated Traditional Chinese and Western Medicine, Lanzhou University, Lanzhou, China

Shengping Yang, Junjie Dai, Yongteng Xu, Rui Zhang, Huaili Jiangand Xianxia Yan
Evidence-Based Medicine Center, School of Basic Medical Sciences, Lanzhou University, Lanzhou, China

The First Clinical Medical College of Lanzhou University, Lanzhou, China

Minghao Dong, Kai Yuan, Jinbo Sun, Jixin Liu, Karen M. vonDeneen and Wei Qin
School of Life Sciences and Technology, Xidian University, Xi'an, Shaanxi, China

Dahua Yu
School of Life Sciences and Technology, Xidian University, Xi'an, Shaanxi, China
Information Processing Laboratory, School of Information Engineering, Inner Mongolia University of Science and Technology, Baotou, Inner Mongolia, China

JieTian
School of Life Sciences and Technology, Xidian University, Xi'an, Shaanxi, China
Institute of Automation, Chinese Academy of Sciences, Beijing, China

JieTian
Key Laboratory of Molecular Imaging and Functional Imaging, Institute of Automation, Chinese Academy of Sciences, Beijing, China
Life Science Research Center,School of Electronic Engineering, Xidian University, Xi'an, Shaanxi, China

Ling Zhao,Fang Zeng and Fanrong Liang
The 3rd Teaching Hospital, Chengdu University of Traditional Chinese Medicine,Chengdu, Sichuan, China

Youbo You, LijunBai, Ruwei Dai, Chongguang Zhong, Hu Wang, Zhenyu Liu and Wenjuan Wei
Intelligent Medical Research Center, Institute of Automation, Chinese Academy of Sciences, Beijing, China

Ting Xue
Life Science Research Center, School of ElectronicEngineering, Xidian University, Xi'an, Shaanxi, China

JieTian
Intelligent Medical Research Center, Institute of Automation, Chinese Academy of Sciences, Beijing, China
Life Science Research Center, School of ElectronicEngineering, Xidian University, Xi'an, Shaanxi, China

Yin Jiang, Liuzhen Wu, Jisheng Han, Cailian Cui andXiaohui Xiang
Neuroscience Research Institute, Peking University, Beijing, China
Department of Neurobiology, School of Basic Medical Sciences, Peking University, Beijing, China
Key Laboratory of Neuroscience, The Ministry of Education and Ministry of Public Health, Beijing, China

LijunBai, JieTian and Zhenyu Liu
Institute of Automation, Chinese Academy of Sciences, Beijing, China

Hong Wang and Yuru Dong
Department of Magnetic Resonance, General Hospital ofArmed Police Forces, Beijing, China

Yue Dong
Department of Neurobiology, School of Basic Medical Sciences, Peking University, Beijing, China

Xinsheng Lai, Chunzhi Tang and Junjun Yang
Department of Acupuncture and Moxibustion, School of Acupuncture and Moxibustion, Guangzhou University of Chinese Medicine, Guangzhou, China

Jiayou Wang, MufengHao, Zhonghua Yang, Chunmei Ma, Jin Zhang and Zhenquan He
Departmentof Human Anatomy, School of Fundamental Medical Sciences, Guangzhou University of Chinese Medicine, Guangzhou, China

Neel R. Nabar, Helen Chew, Jun Liang and Shu-Feng Zhou
Department of Pharmaceutical Sciences,College of Pharmacy, University of South Florida, Tampa, Florida, United States of America

Kevin B. Sneed
Department of Pharmacotherapeutics and Clinical Research, College of Pharmacy, University ofSouth Florida, Tampa, Florida, United States of America

Yong Huang
Department of Acupuncture and Moxibustion, School of Chinese Medicine, Southern Medical University, Guangzhou, China

Jian Zhang
Department ofSurgery, The Third Hospital of Nanchang, Nanchang, Jiangxi, China

Sanqiang Pan and Baogui Su
Department of Human Anatomy, School of Medicine, Jinan University, Guangzhou, China

Seung-Nam Kim
Studies of Translational Acupuncture Research, Acupuncture and Meridian Science Research Center, Kyung Hee University, Seoul, Republic of Korea
Department ofOriental Medical Science, Kyung Hee University, Seoul, Republic of Korea

Ah-Reum Doo, Ji-Yeun Park, HyungjinBae, YounbyoungChae, Insop Shim,Hyangsook Lee, Woongjoon Moon, Hyejung Lee and Hi-Joon Park
Studies of Translational Acupuncture Research, Acupuncture and Meridian Science Research Center, Kyung Hee University, Seoul, Republic of Korea

Shu-Ping Fu, Su-Yun He, Bin Xu, Sheng-Feng Lu, Wei-Xing Shen, Yan Huang,Hao Hong, Qian Li, Ning Wang, Xuan-Liang Liu and Bing-Mei Zhu
Key Laboratory of Acupuncture and Medicine Research of Ministry of Education, Nanjing University of Chinese Medicine, Nanjing, Jiangsu, China

Chen-Jun Hu
School of Information Technology, Nanjing University of Chinese
Medicine, Nanjing, Jiangsu, China

Fanrong Liang
School ofAcupuncture and Tuina, Chengdu University of Traditional Chinese Medicine, Chengdu, Sichuan, China

Kun Hyung Kim
Department of Acupuncture and Moxibustion Medicine, Korean Medicine Hospital, Yangsan, South Korea

Jae Cheol Kong
Department of Rehabilitation Medicine, College of KoreanMedicine, Wonkwang University, Iksan, South Korea,

Jun-Yong Choi
Department of Korean Medical Science, School of Korean Medicine, Pusan National University, Yangsan, SouthKorea

Tae-Young Choi and Myeong Soo Lee
Medical Research Division, Korea Institute of Oriental Medicine, Daejeon, South Korea

Byung-Cheul Shin
Department of Rehabilitation Medicine, School of Korean Medicine,
Pusan National University, Yangsan, South Korea

Steve McDonald
Australasian Cochrane Centre, School of Public Health and Preventive Medicine, Monash University, Melbourne,Victoria, Australia

Arif Khan
Northwest Clinical Research Center, Bellevue, Washington, United States of America
Department of Psychiatry, Duke University Medical School, Durham, NorthCarolina, United States of America,

James Faucett
Northwest Clinical Research Center, Bellevue, Washington, United States of America

Pesach Lichtenberg
Herzog Hospital, and the School of Medicine of the Hebrew University, Department of Psychiatry, Jerusalem, Israel

Irving Kirsch
Program inPlacebo Studies, Beth Israel Deaconess Medical Center, Harvard Medical School, Boston, Massachusetts, United States of America
University of Plymouth, Plymouth,United Kingdom

Walter A. Brown
Department of Psychiatry and Human Behavior, Brown University, Providence, Rhode Island, United States of America
Department of Psychiatry,Tufts University, Boston, Massachusetts, United States of America

Haomin Wang
Neuroscience Research Institute, Peking University, Key Laboratory for Neuroscience of the Ministry of Education, Beijing, PR China

Xibin Liang
Department of Neurology andNeurological Sciences, Stanford University, Stanford, California, United States of America

Xuan Wang, Dingzhen Luo, Jun Jia and Xiaomin Wang
Department of Physiology, Capital Medical University, Key Laboratory forNeurodegenerative Disorders of the Ministry of Education, Beijing, PR China

Ke Wang, Fei He, Libo Lin and Qinghua Zhang
Shanghai-MOST Key Laboratory of Health and Disease Genomics, Chinese National Human Genome Center at Shanghai and National Engineering Research Center forBiochip at Shanghai, Shanghai, China

Rong Zhang, Xiaohui Xiang, Xingjie Ping, Jisheng Han and Cailian Cui
Neuroscience Research Institute; Department of Neurobiology, Peking University Health Science Center; Key Laboratory ofNeuroscience of the Ministry of Education and the Ministry of Public Health; Peking University, Beijing, China

Lei Yu
Department of Genetics and Center of Alcohol Studies,Piscataway, New Jersey, United States of America

Guoping Zhao
Shanghai-MOST Key Laboratory of Health and Disease Genomics, Chinese National Human Genome Center at Shanghai and National Engineering Research Center forBiochip at Shanghai, Shanghai, China
Department of Microbiology and Li KaShing Institute of Health Sciences, The Chinese University of Hong Kong, Princeof Wales Hospital, Shatin, New Territories, Hong Kong Special Administrative Region, China

Ying Wang, RebekkaGehringer, Dagmar Hackel, Alexander Brack and Heike L. Rittner
Department of Anesthesiology, University Hospital of Würzburg, Würzburg, Germany

Shaaban A. Mousa
Department of Anesthesiology and Critical Care, Charité - UniversitätsmedizinBerlin, Campus Virchow-Klinikum, Berlin, Germany

Wen-Long Hu
Department of Chinese Medicine, Kaohsiung Chang Gung Memorial Hospital and Chang Gung University College of Medicine, Kaohsiung, Taiwan
Kaohsiung MedicalUniversity College of Medicine, Kaohsiung, Taiwan, Fooyin University College of Nursing, Kaohsiung, Taiwan,

Chih-Hao Chang
Fooyin University College of Nursing, Kaohsiung, Taiwan
Division of Chinese Medicine, Kaohsiung MunicipalChinese Medical Hospital, Kaohsiung, Taiwan

Yu-Chiang Hung
Department of Chinese Medicine, Kaohsiung Chang Gung Memorial Hospital and Chang Gung University College of Medicine, Kaohsiung, Taiwan
School of Chinese Medicine for Post Baccalaureate, I-Shou University, Kaohsiung, Taiwan

Ying-Jung Tseng and I-Ling Hung
Department of Chinese Medicine, Kaohsiung Chang Gung Memorial Hospital and Chang Gung University College of Medicine, Kaohsiung, Taiwan

Sheng-Feng Hsu
Graduate Institute ofAcupuncture Science, China Medical University, Taichung, Taiwan
Department of Chinese Medicine, China Medical University Hospital, Taipei Branch, Taipei, Taiwan

Chuanfu Li, Wei Zhang and Chunsheng Xu
Laboratory of Digital Medical Imaging, Medical Imaging Center, First Affiliated Hospital, Anhui University of Chinese Medicine, Hefei, Anhui, China

Jun Yang
Department ofAcupuncture and Moxibustion, First Affiliated Hospital of Anhui University of Chinese Medicine, Hefei, Anhui, China

Kyungmo Park
Department of Biomedical Engineering, Kyung HeeUniversity, Yongin, Republic of Korea

Hongli Wu
College of Medical Information engineering, Anhui University of Chinese Medicine, Hefei, Anhui, China

Sheng Hu and BenshengQiu
School of InformationScience and Technology, University of Science and Technology of China, Hefei, Anhui, China

Junjie Bu and Xiaochu Zhang
CAS Key Laboratory of Brain Function & Disease and School of Life Sciences,University of Science and Technology of China, Hefei, Anhui, China

Hugh MacPherson, Stewart J. Richmond, Harriet Lansdown,Sara Perren, Ann Hopton and Karen Spilsbury
Department of Health Sciences, University of York, York, United Kingdom

Ruth Chamberlain
Firefly Research & Evaluation, North Yorkshire, United Kingdom

Liz Newbronner
Department of Health Sciences, University of York, York, United Kingdom
Firefly Research & Evaluation, North Yorkshire, United Kingdom

YounbyoungChae
Department of Brain and Cognitive Engineering, Korea University, Seoul, Korea
Acupuncture and Meridian Science Research Center, College of Korean Medicine,Kyung Hee University, Seoul, Korea

In-Seon Lee, Hyejung Lee and Hi-Joon Park
Acupuncture and Meridian Science Research Center, College of Korean Medicine,Kyung Hee University, Seoul, Korea

Won-Mo Jung and Christian Wallraven
Department of Brain and Cognitive Engineering, Korea University, Seoul, Korea

Dong-Seon Chang
Department of Human Perception, Cognition and Action, Max Planck Institute for Biological Cybernetics, Tübingen, Germany

VitalyNapadow
Martinos Center for Biomedical Imaging, Massachusetts General Hospital, Harvard Medical School, Charlestown, Massachusetts, United States of America
Departmentof Biomedical Engineering, Kyunghee University, Yongin, Korea

Hong Xu, Yamin Zhang, Hua Sun, Suhui Chen and Fuming Wang
Department of Traditional Chinese Medicine, Peking Union Medical College Hospital (PUMCH), Peking Union Medical College (PUMC), Chinese Academy of MedicalSciences, Beijing, China

Yali Liu
Evidence-Based Medicine Center, School of Basic Medical Sciences, Lanzhou University, Lanzhou, China
Key Laboratory of Clinical Translational Research andEvidence-Based Medicine of Gansu Province, Lanzhou, China

Rui Zhang and Jiao Huang
Evidence-Based Medicine Center, School of Basic Medical Sciences, Lanzhou University, Lanzhou, China
The First Clinical Medical College of Lanzhou University, Lanzhou, China

Xu Zhao, Wanting Sun and Yuefen Mai
Evidence-Based Medicine Center, School of Basic Medical Sciences, Lanzhou University, Lanzhou, China
The Second Clinical MedicalCollege of Lanzhou University, Lanzhou, China

Danlu Liu andKehu Yang
Evidence-Based Medicine Center, School of Basic Medical Sciences, Lanzhou University, Lanzhou, China
Key Laboratory of Clinical Translational Research andEvidence-Based Medicine of Gansu Province, Lanzhou, China

Peng Zhang
Evidence-Based Medicine Center, School of Basic Medical Sciences, Lanzhou University, Lanzhou, China
Department of Cardiology, Qilu Hospital of Shandong University, Ji'nan, Shandong Province, China

Yajun Wang
Acupuncture andMassage College, Gansu University of Traditional Chinese Medicine, Lanzhou, China

Hua Cao
Department of Neurology, Gansu Provincial Hospital of Traditional ChineseMedicine, Lanzhou, China

Jeungchan Lee and Kyungmo Park
Department of Biomedical Engineering, Kyung Hee University, Yongin, Gyeonggi, South Korea

VitalyNapadow
Department of Biomedical Engineering, Kyung Hee University, Yongin, Gyeonggi, South Korea

Jieun Kim
Martinos Center for Biomedical Imaging, Department of Radiology,
Massachusetts General Hospital, Charlestown, Massachusetts, United States of America

Seunggi Lee and Woojin Choi
Department of Neuropsychiatry, College of Korean Medicine, Sangji University,Wonju, Gangwon, South Korea

Ted J. Kaptchuk
Program in Placebo Studies, Beth Israel Deaconess Medical Center, Harvard Medical School, Boston, Massachusetts, United States of
America

Index

A
Acetylation Regulation, 100
Acupoint Specificity, 58-59, 178
Acupuncture, 2-5, 7-56, 58-60, 62-84, 86-98, 100-101, 106-109, 111-121, 123, 129-130, 132, 137-139, 141, 150-153, 156, 159, 162-204, 206-208, 210, 213-223
Acupuncture Reviews, 111-112, 114-120, 213
Acupuncture Training, 50-51
Acupuncturists, 41, 50-56, 58, 77, 180-185
Acupuncturists Forms, 50
Alzheimer Disease, 17, 19-20, 30, 77, 178
Angiogenesis, 100-101, 105-109, 206
Antidepressants, 121-123, 125-130, 180, 185
Antinociception, 151-156, 158-159, 161-163
Artificial Counterpart, 187, 195

B
Benign Prostate Hyperplasia, 38, 43
Bias Tool, 44, 46, 49, 213
Biomedical Information, 58
Blood Oxygenation-level Dependent (bold), 32
Bradykinesia, 132
Brain Neuroplasticity, 50

C
Cardioprotective Effects, 100-101, 107, 109
Central Responses, 187
Cerebral Response, 32, 178
Chinese Journal, 1-2, 6, 43-45, 49, 207-208
Cochrane Reviews, 6, 111-119, 121
Comparative Efficacy, 121, 125
Conventional Frequency Bands, 9, 15-16, 58

D
Data Extraction, 5, 45, 114, 208
Default Mode Network (dmn), 7, 69
Depression, 21, 90, 116, 121-131, 169, 180-186, 215, 223
Diagnostic Criteria, 46-47, 122, 130, 208-209
Discrepancies, 45, 68-69, 191
Diverse Pains, 139
Dopamine Availability, 91, 96-97, 138
Drug Administration, 121, 130, 185

E
Electric Pulses, 139
Electro-acupuncture Stimulation, 98, 132, 138
Electroacupuncture, 37-38, 43, 66-68, 76-77, 90, 98, 100-101, 108-109, 132, 138-139, 150-157, 159, 161-163, 177-178, 197-204, 206, 208
Electroacupuncture Analgesia, 139, 150-151, 162-163
Electrophysiological Imaging, 58, 65
Epidemiology, 1, 3, 6, 40, 43, 213
Exogenous Stimuli, 100

F
Functional Magnetic Resonance Imaging, 7, 19, 37, 57, 59, 76, 177, 187

G
Gene Expression, 89, 100, 104, 107-108, 138-142, 145-151, 206

H
Habituation Effects, 170, 174-175, 177
Hub Configurations, 7-16
Hypertension, 37, 78-79, 84, 86-90
Hypertensive Rats, 78-80, 90, 223

I
Inflamed Tissue, 152, 163
Inflammatory Pain, 152, 156, 159, 163
Internal Validity, 44, 47-48
International Prostate Symptom Score, 38-39
Interquartile Range, 2
Intrinsic Property, 50

K
Korean Databases, 111-112, 115-117, 119

L
Laser Acupuncture Therapy, 164, 166-168
Lesioned Rat Model, 132
Locomotor Hyperactivity, 132, 136-137

M
Macrophages, 152-163, 197-198, 201-202
Magnetoencephalography, 7, 17, 58-59, 66-67
Matrix Metalloproteinase, 197, 206

Mechanism of Acupuncture, 42, 68, 76, 100, 170-171, 176-177
Mild Cognitive Impairment, 19, 30-31, 178
Modalities of Acupuncture, 68-69, 71, 74-75
Motor Function, 91-92, 94-98, 138
Mouse Model, 91, 98, 138
Multifactorial Condition, 78
Multimodal Investigation, 7
Myocardial Ischemia, 100-102, 106-107, 109

N
Neuroimaging, 7, 16, 19, 57, 92, 188, 195, 215, 222-223
Neuropathological Changes, 19
Non-acupuncture Factors, 32, 36

O
Occlusal Splint, 165
Opioid Peptide Release, 152

P
Parametric Mapping, 11, 17, 19, 22, 33, 190
Parkinson's Disease, 18, 67, 91, 98-99, 138
Phantom Acupuncture, 196, 214, 216-222
Pharmacological Treatments, 180
Placebo Acupuncture, 18, 195-196, 214, 220, 222
Plastic Brain Changes, 50
Preferred Reporting Items for Systematic Reviews and Meta-analyses, 49
Professional Acupuncturists, 50-51
Prostate Gland, 38
Prostatic Hyperplasia, 38, 43
Proteomic Response, 78-79, 86-87, 89

R
Randomized Controlled Trials, 6, 44, 49, 66, 111-112, 116, 120, 130, 169, 213
Rat Spinal Dorsal Horn, 139
Real Acupuncture (ra), 32-33
Reperfusion Injury, 109, 197, 206
Risk of Bias (rob), 44

S
Scientific Representations, 58
Sensorimotor Areas, 68-69, 177
Striatal Dopamine (da), 91
Surgical Treatment, 6, 165
Sustained Effects, 58, 68-70
Systematic Reviews (srs), 1, 44, 207

T
Temporomandibular Disorders, 164, 169
Traditional Chinese Medicine, 1-2, 6-7, 10, 19, 38-40, 45, 49-50, 58, 66, 72, 100, 120, 132, 150, 168-169, 180, 182-183, 197, 204, 206-207

U
Unanesthetized Rats, 78

www.ingramcontent.com/pod-product-compliance
Lightning Source LLC
Chambersburg PA
CBHW061251190326
41458CB00011B/3645
9781632398925